Healing
with
Whole Foods

Asian Traditions and Modern Nutrition

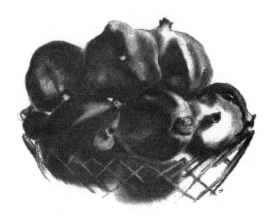

Healing
with
Whole Foods

Asian Traditions and Modern Nutrition

Revised, Updated, and Expanded Third Edition

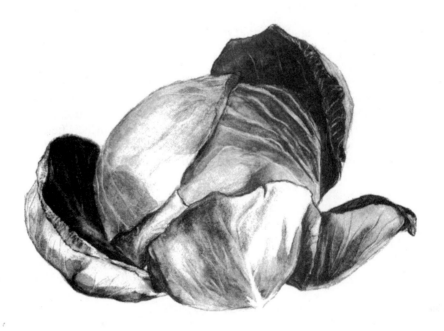

Paul Pitchford

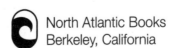

North Atlantic Books
Berkeley, California

Notice: *Healing with Wh* 3 1712 01082 4814 th information about health tailored to a varie... ...ysical patterns. However, due to differences in background and constitution, individual responses to any health plan may vary greatly. In your pursuit of well-being, especially if you are ill or embarking on a new dietary plan or treatment described in this (or any other) reference work, you may need the services of a qualified doctor, physician, or other duly licensed health provider who understands your needs and direction. The information in this book is not intended as a replacement for those services, nor is it intended as a substitute for any treatment prescribed by your physician.

Published by
North Atlantic Books
P.O. Box 12327
Berkeley, California 94712

Cover art by Divit Cardoza
Other artwork by Jennifer Harding,
Deborah Darner, Bethany Fancher,
and Ariana Strozzi Heckler

Cover and book design by Paula Morrison

Printed in the United States of America

Healing with Whole Foods: Asian Traditions and Modern Nutrition is sponsored by the Society for the Study of Native Arts and Sciences, a nonprofit educational corporation whose goals are to develop an educational and cross-cultural perspective linking various scientific, social, and artistic fields; to nurture a holistic view of arts, sciences, humanities, and healing; and to publish and distribute literature on the relationship of mind, body, and nature.

Library of Congress Cataloging-in-Publication Data

Pitchford, Paul.
    Healing with whole foods : Asian traditions and modern nutrition / by
Paul Pitchford.— 3rd ed.
        p. cm.
    Previous ed. published with subtitle: Oriental traditions and modern
    nutrition.
    Includes bibliographical references and index.
    ISBN 1-55643-471-5 (cloth)
    ISBN 1-55643-430-8 (pbk.)
    1. Diet therapy.   2. Medicine, Chinese.   3. Nutrition.   I. Title.
    RM217 .P55 2002
    613.2—dc21
                                                      2002015010

20   21   22   23   24   25 / 07   06   05   04   03   02

To you, the reader,
that you find Guidance
and choose to follow it
toward healing, awareness, and peace.

and

To your Compassionate Nature—*Gwan Shr Yin*—
that it shine forth
and inspire you to help others.

Acknowledgments

I am indebted to the many friends and associates for the faith they placed in me to do this work; and to my teachers in the healing and awareness arts, whose ancient, timeless messages inspire me continuously.

Special thanks to nutritional consultant Suzanne Shaw of the Heartwood Institute in California for her kind assistance in many areas of the project; to those who have studied with me, for their innovative spirit that enlivens the healing message of this book; to Rebecca Lee, for her vision that formed the early versions of this text, especially the recipe section; and to Mary Buckley of New Dimensions Radio for the monumental editing task she undertook with this volume.

I also thank my son Finnegan, who came, as he now says, "as a gift from God"—midway through this project: he saw when I needed to play. My deepest gratitude is for Nelle Conroy Pitchford, my mother, who passed on during her ninety-second year. Her expression of selfless service to others has been a constant example of love.

Preface

Healing with Whole Foods provides the essential information for becoming skillful in healing through diet. While recognizing the value of animal products for certain imbalances and deficiencies, it encourages the reader to move in the direction of a vegetarian diet. To do this successfully in a meat-based culture—particularly one without any obvious vegetarian traditions—requires most people to learn substantial new material on diet such as that presented in this volume, including an evaluation of one's personal condition and the various therapeutic properties of foods.

The rise in nutritional awareness occurring at a rapid pace in the West has elements of Far Eastern traditions, in which a balanced diet has been integral to health and enlightenment practices for millennia. This book is a synthesis of vital elements of Eastern and Western food practices and philosophies. Experiencing such an East/West union brings one into fresh areas of awareness and can lead to renewal in all areas of life.

Writing *Healing with Whole Foods* was a magical, wonderful, yet disciplined experience for me; I want you, the reader, to share in this kind of experience, and to find healing and harmony at a level beyond your expectations.

Paul Pitchford

How to Use this Book Efficiently

There are many possibilities. You may want to look up foods and healing methods in the index, sample the recipes, or simply read various sections that are appealing. However, one of the best ways is to gradually go through all the parts in order. This approach is ideal, since each section contains information to help clarify the material that follows it. This is particularly the case with Chapter 1, which contains Access to Healing with Whole Foods—a section that introduces important new material for the Third Edition as well as prepares one for the numerous integrative aspects of this book.

If you delve in to find information, for example, on a certain disease imbalance, fasting, or the properties of a food, it is best to first have at least a fair grasp of a few basic diagnosis and treatment terms used throughout the text, such as *exterior, heat, cold, damp, deficiency,* and so on. These terms, which have special meanings in the Chinese healing arts, are defined and developed in Part I, and summarized in the charts on pages 94–96 and 99–101. You can get a good basic sense of their meanings from these charts; nonetheless, for a more complete and useful understanding, read Part I. Part I also features a section on concepts related to immunity, among them oxygenation, yeast overgrowth, and free radicals. These concepts too are referred to regularly in later chapters. After Part I, you may appreciate reading the Summary (page 640), which provides a lively overview of the guiding principles of this book.

The information in Part III, "The Five Element and Organ Systems," gives us an awareness of our unity with nature. It brings the seasonal and environmental connections of traditional Chinese medicine into full view. Its organ systems is the crowning achievement of East Asian diagnosis. It provides penetrating images of the workings of the internal organs, their major disease syndromes, the affected emotions and body systems, and dietary and herbal remedies. This information is invaluable when deciding among healing options for long-term imbalances.

Notes on the Revisions

First revision (Second Edition): The principal traditions and teachings of this volume were not revised; however, in response to what appears to be an approaching epidemic of microbe and parasite infestations, an effective, extended anti-parasite program has been added (in the Appendix). Also in the Appendix is an article that sheds light on root canals—a serious dental problem overlooked by many health practitioners. Weston Price, a legendary force in modern nutrition, spent the better part of his life researching root canals, only to have the dental establishment turn a deaf ear on his findings.

The Index of this book has been enhanced to provide both the casual reader and researcher better access to specific information. Furthermore, a number of areas throughout the text have been updated and clarified.

A final addition is a Summary at the end of the book. It includes a new perspective on the fundamental principles of this volume through the eyes of Ayurveda, the traditional medicine of India. The Summary describes the "Sattvic" approach to diet as well as life, focusing on the awareness that enduring physical and mental health come from living in equilibrium, and from being mindful of our spiritual origins.

Second revision (Third Edition): Three major Sections, known collectively as "Access to Healing with Whole Foods," have been added to Chapter 1. This new information underscores the whole-food imperative in counteracting overweight and obesity, diabetes, heart disease, and a number of other common degenerations.

In addition, this chapter provides for the discussion of the underlying relationship between food and consciousness and offers insights to support long-term dietary improvements. To acquaint the reader with the basic dietary intentions of *Healing with Whole Foods,* a new section introduces wholesome eating patterns developed from traditional and ancient diets. In addition, this chapter presents an introductory cleansing and renewal program that prepares one for healing transformation. Moreover, various updates have occurred throughout the book to reflect recent research.

Table of Contents

Origins

Inspiration for *Healing with Whole Foods* originated from the experiences of the author and several close associates who lived and studied the major dietary and herbal traditions of the West and the East. Among our clients, a subject of intense interest was dietary healing, particularly those practices that clear and energize the body so that the spirit can flourish.

In the late twentieth century, food finally began to be recognized in the West as an important healing force. For the first time in United States history, the Surgeon General acknowledged (in 1988) the value of a good diet, while simultaneously condemning typical American eating patterns. According to his statement, fully two-thirds of all deaths are directly affected by improper diet, and poor eating habits play a *large part* in the nation's most common killers—coronary heart disease, stroke, atherosclerosis, diabetes, and some cancers.

Holistic practitioners have always seen marked improvements when individuals make appropriate dietary changes. These changes are actually a revival of ancient principles, but only in recent years has this consciousness reached mainstream America, as evidenced by the above government recognition. What is needed now are not only higher quality foods and better basic diets, but a clearer picture of which of these foods are best for overcoming personal imbalances and for maximizing vitality in each individual.

In my healing and teaching work with several thousand students and clients over the last two decades, I have gradually uncovered a more accurate way to determine which foods belong in a wholesome diet. It is based on insights generated by the interplay of East Asian traditions and modern nutrition. Frequently food therapies are used with little or no result or, worse yet, undesired results. In other cases, results are positive.

The information in this book will help ensure better results. Healing with food is not haphazard. Food acts according to its various therapeutic properties, although its properties are often less specific and its actions less drastic than those of herbs or other medicines. Food also acts as a foundation medicine. It is sometimes slower to take effect, but more profoundly affects all systems of the body. If diet is used correctly for prevention and treatment, other medicines are required less, if at all.

A major complaint of people who begin the study of diet is conflicting views in almost all sources of information. This book is written in part to resolve those conflicts by acting as a guide for individual diagnosis and the healing properties of various foods. With knowledge of how foods act in the body and the ability to self-evaluate, the reader can learn which foods and diets are best for his or her particular constitution and condition. Knowing only vitamin, mineral, and general nutrient properties is not enough.

1

East Asian medicine offers another dimension to food analysis. Thousands of years ago, master healers in China perceived a way to classify food and disease according to simple, easily observed patterns: one eats cooling foods for over-heated conditions, and warming foods are best for people who feel too cold. Detox-ifying foods are for those who carry excess toxins, building foods are good for deficient persons, and so on. This system can be highly effective even if the med-ical name of a disease is not known. For this reason we* have included the foun-dations of traditional Chinese diagnosis and treatment, so that all imbalances, regardless of their disease name, can be treated dietarily.

This does not mean, of course, that these dietary treatments are all that is ever required. Certainly, other therapies from herbology, homeopathy, healing touch, acupuncture, modern medical treatments, and all others are more effective when based on a solid dietary foundation.

Eastern traditions are fascinating to many Westerners, just as our developments in technology have been adopted so enthusiastically by the Japanese and, more recently, the Chinese and East Indians. Even this flow of cultural energy must fol-low a basic law of cosmic harmony revealed in diet and health. Most traditions in the Far East conceive this basic law as the dual principle of *yin* and *yang,* or as similar polarities when the terms *yin/yang* themselves are not used. These same princi-ples are understood by people of wisdom in the West, but expressed in different terms. The traditional *yin/yang* system we have chosen to apply throughout this book is invaluable because it precisely and simply describes the essential features of the reality of natural medicine. Western nutrition can benefit from the simplicity and subtlety of traditional Chinese medicine; Chinese medicine, in its turn, needs to awaken to the hard lessons learned in the West about denatured food.

Another purpose of this book is to integrate the most important food therapies from both the East and West. In the West we speak of proteins, carbohydrates, fats, and other components of food. These are clearly important dimensions also being studied in the Far East. However, as indicated above, various traditions in the East focus on other dimensions: the warming and cooling values of food, the abil-ity to moisten, strengthen energy, calm the mind, reduce watery or mucoid accu-mulations, and others. Knowledge of these qualities is indispensable for using food as medicine. There are still other advantages to incorporating such a system into modern nutrition: it works with subtle flows of energy, reaching diagnosti-cally far in advance to predict and prevent approaching illness; it benefits people without access to expensive diagnostic tools, since East Asian diagnosis is pow-erful in its simplicity; and it helps one select the most useful remedies from the myriad possibilities.

---

*The "we" that appears from time to time in the text represents the especially signifi-cant areas of consensus among the author, his teachers, and others who assisted with this work.

Looking at personal diagnosis and individual properties of food, one may conclude a universal diet does not exist, i.e., balance in diet is unique for each person. To find balance, it is helpful to know not only one's own needs and the properties of foods, but the correct preparation, and to exercise skill in eating by not overeating, by choosing high-quality foods, avoiding too many food combinations, and by knowing a broad range of nutritious foods including the chlorophyll-rich plants, the best sources of certain fatty acids, the least dangerous of the concentrated sweeteners, and so on. When a good attitude and sufficient exercise are combined with a balanced and disciplined diet, one finds no limit to health. This book encourages wellness and awareness beyond a neutral stage where "disease" is absent.

The best foods to use as a basis for long-term balance are not extreme; they do not overly cleanse, build, or stress one's body or mind, but form an axis around which other, more extreme parts of the diet can revolve. These are the complex carbohydrates. One finds them in traditional diets throughout the world—farmers in the Ukraine eating hand-milled bread and cabbage soup, children in southern India sitting with bowls of rice and curried lentils and vegetables. Germans are as fond of sauerkraut and rye bread as they are of liverwurst.

The complex carbohydrates are sometimes lumped together, as if they were all basically equal. Though they have properties in common, each carbohydrate has unique healing attributes. A rich variety of foods is in this group: grains, vegetables and sea vegetables, legumes (beans, peas, lentils), nuts and seeds, and the many products made from these. Fruits, which are cleansing "simple carbohydrates," play a role that depends on the person's health, constitution, the climate, and the degree of need for purification. To represent this diet, we use the term "grains and vegetables," since they are the most widely used of the carbohydrates.

In recent years, numerous studies have detailed the benefits of grains and vegetables, and of the complex carbohydrates in general. A quality of these foods, expressed by the term "fiber," has become somewhat celebrated because of its powers of disease prevention and renewal. In addition, the foods in this group offer ample protein as well as a variety of vitamins and minerals—much more nutrition than is generally acknowledged.

Recommendations in the United States for a grain-and-vegetable diet based on Asian traditions tend to be identified with macrobiotics, a distinct dietary philosophy focusing on health and longevity through lifestyle principles. One of the first macrobiotic teachers, George Ohsawa, considered anyone who was truly healthy and happy to be macrobiotic regardless of what he or she ate. This attitude corresponds with our view of emphasizing not food but the Essence within every aspect of reality, including food.

We agree with the basic macrobiotic prescriptions for unrefined regional food, a minimum of animal products, and recognizing food selection, preparation, and eating as a healing art. However, in the early days of macrobiotics, salty products and lengthy cooking methods were emphasized by some as a way of becoming more *yang*. (See *Yin and Yang and Beyond* chapter.) This did not work consistently for

Americans as it did for the rather small group of Japanese macrobiotics. Dietary incompatibility with a certain segment of the Western population —even some vegetarians—has been a result of the macrobiotic system of diagnosis and food analysis, which uses a highly generalized, unorthodox *yin/yang* system. Such a system is useful for deciding what food groups are beneficial in general, but is nearly impossible to apply to the complex health issues of individuals, or the often contradictory properties of any single food.

The system in this text is based on the standard Chinese *yin/yang* theories, medical diets, and herbal systems developed over thousands of years. Being quite precise and complete, such a system increases healing and prevention options. In recent years, growing numbers of macrobiotic adherents have come to accept more comprehensive systems such as those described in this text.

Both the traditional Chinese and East Indian Ayurvedic systems have been used with pinpoint accuracy to diagnose disease conditions and to categorize food as medicine. We have chosen to use primarily the Chinese system because its remedies and diagnostic measures are more appropriate for North American climates. Merging the Chinese healing arts with major features of modern nutrition and Ayurveda has given a flexible and uniquely workable dimension to this text. For more background information see the Chinese and Ayurvedic titles in the Appendix.

A real advantage of living in a developed and mercantile region of the earth is the widespread distribution of many products from our own as well as other cultures. Throughout the American marketplace, we find stores that carry foods such as unrefined grains, unsprayed fruit and vegetables, naturally leavened breads, whole-grain pasta, organic nuts and seeds, and quality traditional Eastern products such as miso, tempeh, tofu, amasake, and new varieties of sea vegetables. Additionally, the East Asian products are very often no longer from Asia but are manufactured by many thriving European and American businesses. For example, there are many kinds of miso soy pastes made in America, and they are usually of much higher quality than those used by the average Japanese.

Now that it has become common knowledge that complex carbohydrates should play a larger role in the modern diet, it is only natural that the West should borrow from the expertise of the the Far East. For many centuries, the Eastern diet was not meat-based, and still is not in many areas.

The fact that *traditional* Chinese healing systems and Far Eastern foods appear in this text is not a recommendation for Asian food practices in general. A great number of people in Asia do not eat particularly healthy diets. An exception are those in agrarian areas of China, Viet Nam and other areas of Southeast Asia who follow their traditional rural diets. White sugar production in China is increasing at an alarming rate, yet always falls short of demand. And Chinese people have been known to stand in long lines in urban areas to get a rare treat—refined white bread. The traditional teachings of Chinese medicine, however, were written when only organically grown whole foods were available, and very nutritious products were developed from vegetable foods. We have used and recommended many of these products, since they often make the difference between success and failure for those in transition to a vegetarian diet.

In spite of the emphasis on whole foods in this book, there are exceptions consisting primarily of a few optional nutrient supplements. Oxygen supplements in the form of ozone (O_3) and various stabilized oxygen compounds are treatment options in certain degenerations. However, such concentrated oxygen treatments are not necessary for most people.

The diet we ultimately recommend does not include animal products that require the taking of life, and except for options in the "congee" recipes, the extensive cookbook section is vegan (without any animal products whatsoever). Thus our recipes are free of two of the most prevalent allergens—dairy and eggs. There are countless recipe books based on meat, eggs, and dairy, and people in the West usually need no further encouragement to eat animal products. However, it is not our intention that such products be excluded entirely; many of their positive and negative properties are discussed in upcoming sections. We realize the value of meats in certain types of deficiencies, and we have described a way to prepare meat for medical use in cases when other measures are unsuccessful. The value of dairy is also defined, along with the types of people it may benefit. We do not expect people coming from a background of the "Standard American Diet" (SAD) to instantly give up all animal products. We encourage creative use of the recipes, and when animal food is used, it may be added as a condiment or ingredient.

Most Americans have a limited awareness of the value of grains and vegetables as the focus of a meal, and limited ideas for preparing them. When they learn the variety of simple factors involved in the preparation of vegetarian food, vital energy is added to their meals. Part of this vitality comes from correct preparation procedures that preserve and concentrate nutrients. Another important factor is the attention and respect paid to the food during its preparation; in subtle but noticeable ways a meal prepared with mindfulness will taste and look better. Our book is written in the spirit of Brother Lawrence, the legendary English friar of several centuries ago who noticeably transformed everyone who tasted his cooking. His method was to "practice the Presence" while preparing food.

In order to heighten understanding and respect for the healing essence in simple food, information about key foods appears throughout the book as well as in the recipe section. Much of the information describes how the food acts on the body, and especially whether or not it is good for certain imbalances. This information enlarges the dimension of food and complements standard nutrient measurements such as vitamin and mineral content.

A central feature of this book is that it offers remedies for overcoming various minor health problems, as well as more serious metabolic disorders such as cancer and diabetes. In these latter cases, detailed treatment plans have been laid out, generated in part from the diagnostic/treatment systems in the text. In addition, they contain new therapies that specifically address degenerative conditions.

This opening discussion has not yet touched on the basic issue of food and consciousness: Is food one kind of entity and mind another? When food is seen as an object separate from other aspects of our personality, we create imbalance regardless of the quality of the food. Preoccupation with food *per se* creates the illusion of a mind/food separation, and shows a lack of faith that we are ultimately provided for according to our needs.

This does not mean that we should not be knowledgeable about what we eat. If spiritual inclination comes first, food and other objects become its reflections. This suggests that food becomes an ultimate medicine when we recognize it as a facet of our Mind. But these philosophies must be verified by personal experience, or they remain ideas with no roots and inevitably cause confusion.

The major religions teach this level of unity between food and mind, even if the teachings have been subverted or forgotten. They also advise against extreme dietary practices. Customarily prohibited are gluttony and the overuse of intoxicants. Although there are few absolute prohibitions against meat, very often such teachings do appear in the form of suggestions and examples. Christ and Buddha were both known for their extensive fasting. Although neither explicitly forbade meat-eating, Buddha recommended that flesh animal products, pungent plants, and intoxicants not be used by those wanting to cultivate "the Way" because of their effects on consciousness. For similar reasons, the dietary restrictions that Christ regularly taught, primarily through example, were characterized by fasting and prayer.

Considering the value to modern people of these traditional dietary practices, we have included a section on fasting and purification. Throughout the text as well are recommendations regarding eating, preparing, and using food for healing, which if followed, will result in fewer mental and physical obstructions, thereby making awareness practices easier.

We find that applying spiritual awareness in daily life is of primary importance and is the one principle most often neglected in regard to food. For example, some teachings suggest that diet is the only answer. On the other hand, certain individuals refuse to have anything to do with food consciousness because they feel that spiritual teachings are superior. We recognize both aspects: the spirit teaches about correct diet, and good diet supports spiritual practice.

For ourselves and the great majority of people with whom we work, a diet based on grains and vegetables is the most beneficial. The option to choose the appropriate grains and other vegetal foods, to add animal products or raw food, and to emphasize sprouts, herbs, cereal grass, micro-algae, certain cooking methods, foods for healing specific disorders, and many other factors make such a dietary plan very adaptable and, with the right information, highly therapeutic.

Since animals are only about one percent efficient at transferring grain and other food into meat, many more people may be drawn by necessity to a grain- and vegetable-based diet as the population of the world increases. This transition is difficult for some and resisted by others. In general, it is liberating for those able to do it skillfully.

Our goal is that more people begin to follow their inner guidance, in diet and all other areas of their lives. We offer this book with encouragement for the reader to make the changes that ultimately support a life of kindness and compassion.

Access to Healing with Whole Foods

Welcome to the Third Edition of *Healing with Whole Foods*. This chapter will introduce you to the central themes of this book as well as make its information more meaningful and accessible.

Throughout this volume are a number of updates and minor revisions to the previous editions, but the main thrust of the book, which blends East Asian traditions and modern Western nutrition, has not been altered.

I have placed the majority of the new material for this edition in this chapter, which is designed to help you understand and enjoy this book. My ultimate intention is for you to gain an ever-increasing sense of vitality in your life, whether you are a newcomer to whole foods or a "seasoned" follower of this dietary lifestyle.

Specifically, this introductory chapter, which is divided into three sections, provides you with an enhanced nutritional foundation for the dietary direction of this book. Understanding nutritional science can be enlightening to everyone, while its interplay with traditional Chinese medicine can be a valuable option for modern holistic health care.

I have added more depth to subjects already covered in the book by including recent research studies. The topics of Section 1, "Whole Foods," for example, include convincing research showing the phytonutrient value of eating wholesome, unrefined foods and an East-West vision of genetic engineering.

In Section 2, "Integrative Nutrition," we will consider the vital, fundamental roles of awareness practices and activity, including exercise, as they merge with nutrition in successful, long-term dietary transformation. Starting the book in this way will heighten the likelihood of your healing success.

This chapter is also designed to address several changes of perception in the public mind about nutrition during the past decade. For instance, in Section 3, "Dietary Patterns and Directions," I provide insights into the usefulness of popular protein-centric, low carbohydrate diets. It is not difficult to construct food plans based on a few recent studies, short-term successes, and anecdotal evidence, but will these diets be sustainable? Related to this is a discussion of what we can adapt from the diets of our Paleolithic ancestors and the advantages of plant-based and rural Chinese-style diets. I also introduce our Integrative Nutrition Pyramid and a preliminary cleansing, immune-boosting program to help initiate dietary transition.

Let us now turn our attention to a subject that is oftentimes taken for granted—the nutritional value of unprocessed, unrefined foods. Important healing properties have been discovered in common whole foods in the last few years. These discoveries can elevate our appreciation of two of our most essential, widely eaten planetary foods: wheat and rice.

Section 1: Whole Foods

The Incalculable Value of Unrefined Plant Foods: Mineral Deficiencies in the Land of Excess

Ironically, in the United States, a land of plenty—indeed excess—many people are highly deficient in minerals as a result of our food production and processing methods. As such, these deficiencies can lead to degenerative diseases.

The discussion of nutrients that follows applies to whole vegetal foods in general. However, we use wheat as a starting point because this remarkable food, known in the traditional medicines of China and India to strengthen the body and nurture the mind and heart, serves as a foundation in our cultural and dietary heritage. Sadly, in the form that it is most often eaten, wheat is stripped of its essential value.

Consider this grain before it is milled into flour—"wheat berries." These whole-wheat seeds can comprise dozens of minerals and microminerals if grown in rich soil. They can also contain immuno-protective phytonutrients as well as vitamins and precious oils. In refining, as is done in the milling of wheat berries to obtain "white" flour used in common pastries, donuts, pastas, and breads, the majority of these nutrients are lost.

Every nutrient in whole wheat has an interesting and important health story. While wheat is a common allergen, virtually no one is allergic to sprouted wheat, which contains the same amount of minerals, but more vitamins, per berry. (Refer to *Sprouts,* Chapter 40.)

To get a sense of how important nutrients in wheat can be, let's look at just two minerals that are lost in the refining of whole-wheat berries and assess the impact of this loss.

Selenium: Whole wheat is one of the best food sources of selenium, especially if grown in selenium-rich soil. For 20 years, based in part on demographic studies, it has been known that cancer rates are lower in areas where selenium is abundant in the soil.[1] A 1996 study reported in the *Journal of the American Medical Association* suggests that selenium can cut certain cancer death rates by fifty percent. Other health functions of this key mineral:

- Selenium deficiency can cause hypothyroidism or low thyroid.[2] With a near epidemic of thyroid gland imbalance in the United States, especially among women, who have five times more thyroid disorders than men, it behooves everyone to make certain they are obtaining adequate selenium as well as all other minerals in their diets. It should be noted, however, that a single mineral does not work well in isolation; each mineral works best in association with all other minerals and trace minerals, the way they are found in unrefined, whole foods.

- Obesity and low thyroid are directly related. Selenium influences the transformation of thyroxin (T_4) into triiodothyronine (T_3), which makes possible the metabolism of nutrients.[3,4] Thus, if selenium is deficient, sluggish metabolism results and weight gain is more likely.

- Toxic heavy metals such as lead and mercury can be bound up with selenium, and thereby become harmless.[5]

- Viruses of many types, including HIV, are often deactivated when adequate selenium exists in the body.[6-8]

- Premature aging, heart disease, arthritis, and multiple sclerosis are frequently related to selenium deficiency.[9-12]

Magnesium: This mineral is deficient in many modern people who eat refined foods. Approximately 70% of the United States population suffers magnesium deficiency, which is considered one of the most under-diagnosed deficiencies[13,14]—yet one so easily solved. In a number of economically poor countries, people consume a great deal of magnesium in legumes (beans, soy products, peas and lentils), vegetables—especially the green variety, and most whole grains and seeds. It should be noted that animal products are not abundant in magnesium compared with plant sources.

Magnesium provides the body with a smooth, flowing nature and therefore is useful for many diseases where there are stagnancies or erratic changes. According to the Chinese healing arts, stagnation, accompanied by erratic changes in the body, emotions, or mind, represents liver/gallbladder imbalance. Thus, magnesium foods usually help nurture one's liver (and health) in numerous ways. The applications of dietary magnesium listed next nearly all parallel liver/gallbladder pathology in the view of ancient Chinese medicine.

The healing properties and uses of magnesium-rich foods include the following: They calm nerve function; harmonize various mental and emotional imbalances, including irritability, depression, bipolar disorder, sleep disorders, and PMS (premenstrual syndrome); relax functioning of the muscles, including the heart muscle; soothe erratic changes such as migraine, sudden infant death syndrome, cramps, and spasms anywhere in the body (including eclampsia); create better flows in digestion to help relieve constipation; and overcome the fast-cycling blood sugar imbalances in alcoholism and diabetes.[15-17]

Another attribute of foods concentrated in magnesium is their ability to strengthen the structural aspects of the body to counteract conditions such as chronic fatigue syndrome, fibromyalgia, arthritis, and osteoporosis.[18-24]

One way magnesium does this is by "pushing" calcium excesses in the soft tissues into the bones. Too much soft-tissue calcium is weakening and can exacerbate syndromes such as fibromyalgia that stress the muscles and nerves. Excellent research suggests that absolutely no calcium enters the bones without adequate magnesium (see *Calcium,* Chapter 15). Consequently, even though Americans ingest abundant calcium, in general they still have weaker bones than those of people in developing countries such as China, who take in adequate, but comparatively low amounts of calcium. However, the rural Chinese diet (discussed further in Section 3) is rich in magnesium.

Clearly, **bone loss or osteoporosis** is a major health issue in the West. Nonetheless, massive calcium intake without adequate dietary magnesium can lead to another sinister event: calcium tends to deposit in the soft tissues rather than entering the skeleton.[25] Thus, soft-tissue calcium excess, a problem that has been avidly researched for at least 30 years, may predispose one to virtually any degeneration,[26,27] particularly those of the kidneys, skeleton, heart, and vascular system.[28]

In some situations, the accretion of soft-tissue calcium is an early step in developing excessive intracellular calcium in the neuronal brain cells as in **Alzheimer's disease** (AD). The occurrence of increased calcium induces toxic beta-amyloid plaque to deposit, which deranges nerve cells as well as clogs the cerebral blood vessels.[29,30] Studies suggest that, in contrast, dietary magnesium helps control intracellular processes and maintains calcium in dynamic equilibrium.[31,32] Medical researcher and author Carolyn Dean, M.D., N.D., describes the cellular role of magnesium: "… recent research indicates that calcium enters the cells by way of calcium channels that are jealously guarded by magnesium. Magnesium allows a certain amount of calcium to enter a cell to create the necessary electrical transmission, and then immediately ejects the calcium once the work is done."[33]

Calcium excess can also occur in the specialized, immune-enhancing white blood cells known as lymphocytes, where it disrupts functions. This occurrence not only adds an extra pathogenic component to Alzheimer's disease,[34] but may also adversely influence overall immunity.

Another etiology in the development of AD is oxidative stress and inflammation.[35] Antioxidants show some promise in the treatment of AD if they are in the form of food.[36] For example, foods rich in vitamin E reduced the risk of developing AD, whereas vitamins E, C and beta carotene in capsules did not. It should be noted that foods with vitamin E will additionally contain a variety of antioxidants and phytonutrients that will extend oxidant protection. Potent antioxidant examples are given in the brown-rice section later.

In addition, *magnesium-rich plants*, such as vegetable greens, barley grass, chlorella, sea vegetables, aloe vera gel, whole grains, and all legumes, have varying degrees of anti-inflammatory activity. Animal studies indicate that lack of tissue magnesium contributes to both inflammation and the formation of radical oxygen species, which in turn, cause oxidative lesions.[37]

Calcium excess is related to diseases of the **heart and arteries** because it provokes coronary artery calcification, which leads to atherosclerosis—the most typical form of arterial degeneration. Another pathway to atherosclerosis involves the tearing of the inner lining of the arteries as a result of various causes, one of the more common being stress-induced quick episodes of high blood pressure. One additional cause, discussed later, is the xanthine-oxidase damage occurring from ingestion of homogenized milk. In any event, certain substances begin to repair the tear, among them collagen and platelets, as well as white blood cells, which can contain oxidized cholesterol. This oxidized form of cholesterol, which often results from poor quality fat ingestion, forms soft plaques in the arteries. Calcium is then attracted to the site, hardens the plaques, which, with further calcium accumulation, become increasingly difficult to remove.

However, by eating magnesium and other nutrient-rich whole vegetal foods, including unrefined wheat and its products, major symptoms of reduced artery volume and decreased blood flow may improve in as little as 30 days,[38] making coronary by-pass surgery and calcium channel blocker drugs unnecessary. In fact, magnesium is sometimes known as "nature's calcium channel blocker." In addition to reducing soft-tissue calcium and calcified plaque, magnesium also dilates coronary arteries and the peripheral vessels, relaxes smooth muscle (such as muscle tissue of the heart), helps prevent blood clotting, and exerts anti-arrhythmic effects, thereby improving irregular heartbeat.[39] Magnesium-rich, unrefined plant foods along with greatly limited salt intake are frequently useful for reducing high blood pressure as well.[40,41]

When we grasp such potent, scientifically demonstrated effects of just one nutrient—magnesium—and consider the hundreds of other beneficial nutrients and phytochemicals in a varied diet of unrefined plant foods, we begin to fathom that symptom relief is indeed possible in many cases of heart and artery degeneration, even within a few short weeks.

We should be aware, however, that symptoms can improve with relatively slight gains in arterial volume and other healing effects of excellent nutrition, although marked improvements in the arteries and extensive plaque reduction often involve from one to several years of appropriate diet and lifestyle change.[42] (If you take medication for your heart, the prescribing physician can ascertain dosage requirements or need for the medication—as you make dietary improvements.)

The simple art of cleansing the heart and arteries with healing diet and lifestyle is widely acknowledged among medical and research persons and has been a pervasive topic in the media. Hence, we present a useful plan along with relevant information to this effect on pages 160–169. There are also retreat and therapy centers that provide similar plant-based diets accompanied by complementary mental, emotional, and exercise programs.[43] (See note 43 on page 682 for information.)

Considering how effectively and quickly these integrative nutrition therapies can begin to cleanse the vascular system, it is surprising how few people in need even hear about them. Certainly it's a little too easy to blame the medical and drug establishments. A wiser insight may be to observe that we receive the medical treatments that match our beliefs. Thus, before some people open to nutritional cleansing and renewal therapies for the heart, there must be a fundamental shift in their beliefs, which comes about through education and increased awareness (discussed further in Section 2).

A final topic connecting low dietary magnesium with calcium-in-the-soft tissues encompasses **calcic disorders, including arthritis**. Nearly everyone has seen in themselves or others evidence of these imbalances in the form of bone spurs, calcic growths, and swollen soft cysts that appear in the joints, or perhaps has even felt sharply painful calcium crystals during a foot rub.

Magnesium-rich foods, abundantly recommended throughout this book, can reduce these and other soft-tissue calcium excesses and create better flows to clear degenerative stagnations, thereby thwarting not only calcic/arthritic disorders, but also, as we have seen, addressing a number of our most prevalent health challenges today.

By age sixty-five as much as 75% of the American population has x-ray evidence of osteoarthritis in the hand, foot, knee, or hip.[44] I estimate, based on statistics for people purchasing unrefined foods and quality animal products free of hormones or antibiotics, that more than 75% of the American population has lived almost exclusively, for the greater part of their lives, on poor-quality meats, eggs, and dairy products; oxidized, refined, and/or hydrogenated oils and fats; and completely denatured, "white" wheat-flour products. Many have eaten far too few fruits, vegetables, and legumes. In addition to excessive calcium in the soft tissue, other excesses relating to modern diet and lifestyle include residues from chemicals, heavy metals, drugs, intoxicants, and non-foods. (The reduction of these residues occurs naturally with high quality nutrition and exercise; nevertheless, the process can be expedited: see "Excesses and Toxins" section, beginning on page 111.) These folks are invariably overfed on calories but unknowingly starving for minerals (including magnesium), vitamins, essential fatty acids, enzymes, antioxidants, and especially, real food with true life force.

Such nutritional deficiencies in most people do not mean that degenerations cannot stem from causes other than diet, including predisposition due to genetic factors and constitution. Nonetheless, serious calcic disorders often require regeneration of all systems of the body (refer to the Regeneration Diets beginning on page 407 and the "Rheumatic and Arthritic Conditions" section, page 425).

Brown Rice—Rediscovered

After wheat, rice is used more extensively in human nutrition than any other grain. Brown rice, like whole wheat, contains a plethora of nutrients, including magnesium, that are all but lost during milling into white rice. An exception is that in Asian countries, refined rice is often only partly milled and therefore contains substantial nutrition compared with "white rice" in the West.

An essential topic for understanding the healing value of whole-grain brown rice is blood sugar levels. It has been known for some time in East Asian medicine that brown rice consumption has a positive effect on blood sugar and therefore, on diabetes—a condition of chronic blood-sugar elevation. However, this information has yet to be generally acknowledged in the West. In fact, an opposing view has been more prevalent—rice and grains, especially wheat, have been perceived as contributors to blood sugar imbalances,[45] and rightly so, as the grains in question have been the refined variety, which are empty foods lacking adequate minerals and other cofactors for regulating blood sugar.

Recent studies, however, are enlightening us to the value of *unrefined* brown rice. One such study finds that the coating on brown rice, the rice bran, has rather remarkable effects on lowering high blood sugar levels.[46] This healing value of rice and its bran comes as good news in a country where, according to the Centers for Disease Control, diabetes is an epidemic largely linked to the more fundamental epidemic of obesity.

In addition to reducing blood-sugar levels, rice bran is thought to be one of the most nutrient dense substances ever studied. It embodies over 70 antioxidants that can protect against cellular damage and preserve youthfulness. The discussion that follows includes a number of the more prominent antioxidants found in the coating of brown rice along with other healing nutrients.

Rice bran contains unique forms of the antioxidant **vitamin E.** These are rare "tocotrienols" that lower excesses of fat and cholesterol in the body and provide greater antitumor protection than any previously known tocotrienol form of vitamin E.[47]

The **oil in rice bran** appears to have potent antioxidant value since it neutralizes one of the most destructive and prevalent forms of oxidation, the lipid peroxides of fats and oils. In addition, the oil counteracts cholesterol excess, particularly the low-density lipoprotein variety, which can contribute to a variety of heart and vascular ailments. It also inhibits excess blood fat (in the form of triglycerides) in general.

When *fermented* and used in animal studies, dietary rice bran has been shown to bolster the vitality of the internal organs, especially the adrenals, thymus, spleen, and thyroid, which increase in mass and exhibit additional anti-stress effects.[48] Fermented rice bran is a relatively more tonifying, building remedy compared with conventional stabilized forms, which contain phytic acid, a cleansing constituent. (For those in need of fermented, more strengthening forms of rice bran that result from reduced phytic acid content, please refer to our nuka pickle section on page 571. Add shiitake mushroom to nuka pickles to enhance their immune boosting value [a shiitake/rice-bran product, "MGN-3," is described later].) In addition, sprouting or presoaking whole brown rice reduces the phytic acid in its bran as does making a fermented "sourdough" brown rice bread. Phytic acid is discussed further in the "IP$_6$" section.

Polysaccharides are complex carbohydrates of high molecular weight. The ideal type for stimulating immunity and controlling high blood sugar leading to diabetes and obesity are derived from fiber, like the polysaccharides in rice bran.[49]

Another benefit from the coating of brown rice is its calming effect, which is noted in East Asian medicine. In modern nutrition, the ability of a food to foster serenity may translate into an abundance of **B vitamins** and **trace minerals,** which rice bran contains.

Gamma-oryzanol, a formidable antioxidant, found only in rice bran in meaningful quantities, strengthens the musculature of the body while converting fat to lean body mass. It improves blood circulation to the extremities, overcomes clots and blood stagnation in general, and improves hormonal balance through regulation of the pituitary secretion.[50]

Alpha lipoic acid, a polyphenol antioxidant, promotes liver restoration, slows the aging process and converts glucose to energy.

Glutathione peroxidase (GPx) is an enzyme antioxidant that reduces mucus excesses, boosts respiratory function, and helps detoxify the body. Known to counteract the effects of aging, it is also used in the treatment of alcoholic cirrhosis, rheumatoid arthritis, multiple sclerosis, acne, and asthma.[51-53]

Superoxide dismutase, an antioxidant enzyme, is used to treat cataracts, rheumatoid and osteoarthritis, and many of the symptoms of premature aging. And there are yet other health benefits from the coating of brown rice.

Coenzyme Q_{10}, as preliminary studies suggest, treats problems of the cellular mitochondria (which are the energy sources in cells involved in protein synthesis and lipid metabolism). CoQ_{10} burns fat into energy and therefore reduces obesity. It has an affinity for the heart and is commonly used in the treatment of angina, high blood pressure, and heart disease in general. It also counteracts aging and the effects of diabetes type II by protecting mitochondrial DNA.[54,55] It has been used to treat various neurodegenerative imbalances such as Parkinson's disease and Huntington's disease.[56] Fibromyalgia symptoms may improve from CoQ_{10} ingestion—when taken concurrently with the herb ginkgo biloba.[57]

Proanthocyanidins, found in rice bran, grapes, cranberries, and other foods, are condensed tannins that are synthesized by many plants. In general, they facilitate wound healing, strengthen the arteries, veins, and capillaries, and improve blood circulation.[58] They are some of the most potent antioxidants available and thus protect against cancer and most other degenerative diseases, i.e., those marked by over-oxidation and free-radical pathology. Proanthocyanidins are additionally protective against poisons and toxins in the body's blood, lymph, and organ systems.[59]

Lecithin. This fatty substance containing phosphorus (a "phospholipid"), produced continuously by the liver, is a nutrient found in soybeans, eggs, rice bran, and other foods. From the liver, lecithin is sent via the bile to the intestines, absorbed by the blood, and distributed to diverse areas of the body. It is especially important for proper function of the brain (making up 30% of the dry weight of the brain), nerves, and cell membranes. Lecithin acts as an emulsifier for oil with water. It is composed primarily of essential fatty acids, including omega-3 and omega-6, choline (as phosphatidylcholine), and an abundance of B vitamins including inositol. Lecithin greatly helps increase absorption of fat-soluble vitamins such as vitamin A. It has been used extensively for enhancing brain activity. Though not effective in treating Alzheimer's disease, it nonetheless appears to improve attention and learning in children.[60]

This nutrient also exhibits a calming nature and thus can reduce hyperactivity.

The myelin sheath, the fatty covering of nerve endings, is primarily comprised of lecithin. Lecithin also protects against gallstone formation, high blood pressure, and cholesterol excesses. It improves memory of most types, including visual and verbal memory,[61,62] and is often quite helpful for defects in voluntary movement and muscular coordination.[63,64]

Eating too much isolated, supplemental lecithin can produce serious side effects, however, including severe abdominal pain and weight loss; it can even form large masses in the stomach, which in one case had to be removed surgically.[65] Eating eggs for their lecithin content is not recommended in cases of attention deficit, restlessness, nervousness, spasm, or hyperactivity, as eggs promote "glairy" mucus that can obstruct the liver and thereby aggravate imbalances marked with instability or erratic behavior.

Additional healing values of brown rice extracts for immune strengthening are likewise being tested. One of the most potent compounds for stimulating NK (natural killer) cells in the body is a polysaccharide composed of the hemicellulose-β extract from rice bran, which has been modified by enzymes of the shiitake mushroom.[66] One NK cell can destroy up to 27 cancer cells, taking just a few minutes for each eradication. NK cells are also noted for overcoming dangerous viruses such as hepatitis C and HIV.[67-69] This shiitake enzyme-modified rice bran extract (known as "MGN-3") can increase NK cell activity from between 100 and 500%.[70-72] Such an increase in immune response has led to some remarkable effects on nearly all pathology indicators, including tumor reduction as well as remission of disease.[73] MGN-3 is generally considered as potent as the strongest immune-modulating drugs, but with no side effects.[74] It can be used concurrently with chemotherapy and radiation to increase their benefits while simultaneously protecting against their toxicity.

Note: We do not generally recommend plant extracts that isolate active ingredients in the form of supplements unless there is an acute need. MGN-3 and other extracts are presented here to acknowledge the potency inherent in whole rice. Most often, the whole foods themselves are more effective over time for slowly and deeply building immune foundation.

IP$_6$ *(inositol hexaphosphate)* is another supplement that is frequently extracted from rice bran. Used in cancer therapy, IP$_6$ may also have applications in treating cardiovascular disease, kidney stones, and possibly even immune-system disorders like AIDS.[75,76] Although the precise mechanism for its ability to inhibit early-stage cancer is not known,[77,78] it ultimately seems to cause cancer cells to revert to normal.[79]

IP$_6$ is essentially the phytic acid in brown rice and other grains, legumes, and most seeds in general. As mentioned earlier, ingesting foods with it appears to provoke a somewhat cleansing therapy, as it is known to bind with calcium, iron, and perhaps other mineral excesses—presumably in the soft tissues of the body first.[80] Some claim that it binds with proteins and other large molecules, making them into insoluble compounds that are not readily absorbed or utilized by the body. Therefore, in the recipe section of this text, we recommend neutralizing phytic acid in grains and legumes by any of various techniques, including pre-soaking and discarding the soak water, by sprouting, by fermentation as in soybean miso and tempeh and sourdough bread, and by roasting.[81]

However, individuals with signs of *excess* (robust constitution, extroverted personality, reddish complexion [defined further on pp. 49–50]), who are embarking on a new diet of unrefined foods, may be wise to make use of the therapeutic action of phytic acid in the body to extract calcium deposits in the soft tissues, which may have resulted from overeating of poor quality dairy products and refined foods. Recalling that these calcium deposits support a number of degenerations, including vascular plaque and arthritic disorders, it is often a good idea for those in cleansing therapy, particularly for the purpose of overcoming degenerative disease, to eat phytic-acid-rich foods such as unsoaked grains and (well-cooked, but) unsoaked legumes.

Not long ago, vegetables, whole grains, and most other plant foods were thought of as mainly "fiber"—to assist in bowel functions. In the paragraphs beginning with our view of whole wheat, we dispelled the narrowness of that notion. The minerals in whole wheat, the blood sugar controlling effects of brown rice, and the plethora of phytonutrients, antioxidants, and other special features of whole rice and its bran, represent the merest sampling of the benefits available in whole foods—that we fail to receive in refined, highly processed foods. Each whole grain, including millet, quinoa, barley, rye, corn, buckwheat, amaranth, and so on, has major minerals, vitamins, and other nutrients in common as well as its own unique set of nutrients and associated healing properties.

More recently, some of the most highly regarded studies involving the phyto-chemistry of legumes (including soy), nuts and seeds, fruits and vegetables, are demonstrating that each plant food has rich stores of valuable properties. Whenever we eat refined food, whether it be white-flour foods, denatured rice and other cereals, or refined oils and sugars, we limit the opportunity to bolster our immune system, keep our blood sugar and emotions balanced, protect against degenerative diseases, maintain a trim and fit body, and in general, keep our integrated experience of life harmonious.

Many may wonder why we ever chose to refine grains, oils, sugar cane, and other foods. Clearly, refined foods are lighter, sweeter, and easier to chew, and oftentimes have much longer shelf lives. So both the consumer and producer obtain something they want.

The most vital, bitter-tasting parts of whole foods are the ones refined away, often discarded, put in nutritional supplements, or fed to animals. Yet the bitter parts include magnesium, selenium, antioxidants, and dozens of other nutrients that we need in order to avoid the stress and ills inherent in the twenty-first century lifestyle. Most of the general public fails to realize the protective and rejuvenative benefits they miss and the suffering they incur when eating denatured foods. But, considering the general lack of vitality of many people today, the time is ripe for whole-food awareness to manifest widely.

The whole grain, such as wheat and brown rice, can also serve as a metaphor. The grain's protective coating (like wheat or rice bran) can provide us with a "protective coating" for improving our immunity and health. Whereas stripping the grain of its coating, through refining essential nutrients out of these foods, strips us of valuable nutrition.

If a nutrient-starved nation can rediscover the potent value of these grains, a land of excess should soon become a land of moderation and abundant health.

Whole Foods: The Survival Imperative for the Twenty-First Century

Consider today's state of affairs: Most folks today still prefer to eat "white" refined diets, notably large quantities of foods containing white flour and white sugar. Recognizing this fact, stores of all kinds make these foods abundantly available. In fact many people who shop at a local health food store may purchase highly refined and processed foods without being fully aware of it. For example, in most health food stores one must diligently search for all whole-wheat pastas and entirely whole-grain breads. (White flour is frequently not just an ingredient but the main ingredient in many products.) A questionable practice is to make exceptionally poor-quality organic foods available as well. Examples are the foods sweetened with cane sugar sold in these stores. Most of the cane products are organic (white) sugar and various organic cane juices and cane juice powders, which are simply refined sugar—unless they are specifically labeled "unrefined"—and few are. Here the term "organic" is used to mask an unwholesome food. When consumers see the word "organic" on a product, they often believe it is a top-quality whole food. Using the highly regarded "O" word to lure consumers to buy inferior foods fools nearly everyone and is one of the slickest, most deceptive marketing ploys today.

Harder to metabolize and worse for one's health than white sugar are the refined oils. The labels of these oils often feature the words "organic" or "expeller pressed," which are indeed good processes. If the products are not labeled "unrefined," however, then they are refined and these common canola and other oils are some of the worst foods that can be eaten. (Please refer to *Oils and Fats,* Chapter 10.)

Below is a sample listing of refined foods found in most stores (including health food stores) and the quality counterparts that are recommended. (Please note that high quality foods *are* available in health/natural foods stores, but one must simply use discretion and be an educated consumer.)

Refined, Denatured Foods	**The Quality Choice**
*Refined: white sugar, cane juice, dried cane juice (often used in natural food industry), cane sugar	*Unrefined* cane juice or powder (see Resources index), barley malt, date sugar, rice syrup, whole *green* stevia powder, and *green* stevia extract

Refined, Denatured Foods	**The Quality Choice**
Tahini hulless sesame-seed spread	Sesame butter—whole sesame-seed spread
White-flour "semolina" spaghettis, noodles, and pastas	Whole-wheat spaghettis, noodles and pastas; spelt, brown rice, buckwheat, and other whole-grain pastas
White-flour wheat breads	Whole-wheat breads, whole-rye, -barley, -spelt, -oat, -corn, -rice and other whole-grain breads
* Refined oils and fats: canola oil, common vegetable oils, margarine, shortening, and virtually all oils used in restaurants in fried and deep fried foods; nearly all oils in all prepared foods in both supermarkets and natural food stores—pastries, chips, breads, soups, treats	Unrefined cold-pressed flax oil, unrefined olive oil, unrefined sesame oil and all other quality oils described in the *Oils and Fats* Chapter
Low-fat dairy products such as low-fat yogurt, milk, and cheese	Full-fat dairy products. Quality dairy is also organic and non-homogenized. Goat milk products are often superior for children and adults alike.

Note: The word "refined" rarely appears on the labels of refined cane sugars and refined oils; for quality, look for the word "unrefined" on these products.

A surprising recommendation in this text is to *avoid reduced-fat dairy products;* if you need to reduce dietary saturated fat (dairy foods are a rich source), then eat smaller amounts of dairy, or no dairy products at all. Many health-conscious people think low or no-fat dairy is better. However, dairy with its fat removed may not support the absorption and utilization of the fat-soluble vitamins D and A, which are necessary for maintaining and laying down new bone mass. Thus, calcium may go primarily into the soft tissues rather than into the bones in those who persist with reduced-fat dairy products.

Another consideration: reduced-fat foods cause people to eat substantially more food to make up for the missing fat.[82,83] In fact, it is not uncommon for today's restaurants to serve portions up to five times larger than government recommendations.[84] Our desire to overeat can stem from eating foods that are refined and therefore missing ingredients; these deficient foods can foster addiction as we are instinctively driven to overconsume them in our endeavor to obtain the missing nutrients that are never there.

In addition to refining of milk by removing fat, milk is denatured further by homogenization. The following excerpt from the Journal *Atherosclerosis* (1989; 77:251-6) coherently expresses the central issue with homogenization:

Homogenized cow's milk transforms healthy butterfat into microscopic spheres of fat containing xanthine oxidase (XO) which is one of the most powerful digestive enzymes there is. The spheres are small enough to pass intact right through the stomach and intestines walls without first being digested. Thus this extremely powerful protein knife, XO, floats throughout the body in the blood and lymph systems. When the XO breaks free from its fat envelope, it attacks the inner wall of whatever vessel it is in. This creates a wound. The wound triggers the arrival of patching plaster to seal off that wound. The patching plaster is cholesterol. Hardening of the arteries, heart disease, chest pain, heart attack is the result.

Note: For other dairy recommendations, see the *Food for Children* Chapter.

Quality: Organic Versus Genetic Engineering

Unrefined whole foods are clearly nutritionally superior to highly refined and processed ones.

However, are organically grown foods substantially better? One way that growers judge the quality of a plant is by its mineral content. More minerals imply a stronger, higher quality plant. So how do minerals in sprayed and chemically fertilized plants compare with the organic variety? There have been few reliable studies in this area but preliminary tests indicate that organic food has substantially more minerals—as much as 90% more compared with commercial foods.[85-86] This information suggests that organic foods provide better nutrition on all levels, because with better mineralization, greater quantities of vitamins and phytonutrients are found in the plant. Most people can taste the difference—richer flavor and aromas and better *"qi"* life force—in the majority of organic fruits, vegetables, and meats, compared with non-organic. *(Qi,* a term used in Chinese medicine, connotes vitality and energy.)

A great hindrance to organic farming today, though, is the proliferation of genetically modified crops. Such crops, because of serious quality concerns, are never defined as organic, but they can cross-pollinate with organic and wild plants. Once released into nature, their genetic material cannot be recalled and can pass on to all future generations. Presently the practice of cross pollination poses a grave threat to the survival of organic farming, potentially taking away the opportunity of individuals to choose to eat organically produced foods.

Genetic engineering (GE) of our food sources is creating a highly charged political and economic issue. The pure science of genetic theory appears obscured by a technology that is driven to produce GE products before the vital issues are well understood. At this point it seems that the technology is pushing the science beyond its capacity to provide quality results or adequate safeguards. The result is that organisms are being genetically engineered and produced for sale long before the risks are fully assessed.

Millions of concerned people worldwide fear the specter of a dietary future dominated by genetically engineered foods. Many refuse to blindly accept the assurances of biotechnology corporations or government bureaucrats who have personal power and financial gains at stake. The following are some areas of contention regarding genetic engineering.

Gene transfers, which are not precisely controlled processes, often disrupt the DNA sequence in an organism. These new genes can alter cell chemistry and provoke toxins and allergens that the human body has never before experienced.

The biotechnology industry promises that GE crops will reduce dependence on poison sprays and represent a solution to feeding the world's poorest countries. The reality is that GE crops have frequently been engineered by biotech companies to resist their own broad-spectrum herbicides that kill everything except the GE crop. These companies are creating markets for their own unsustainable, environmentally damaging products.[87]

People in third world countries have expressed wisdom regarding genetic engineering; the following is a sampling: Representatives of 20 African countries, including Ethiopia, have published a statement denying that gene technologies would help farmers to produce the food they needed. They think it will destroy the diversity, the local knowledge, and the sustainable agricultural systems, and undermine their capacity to feed themselves.[88] Tewolde Egziabher of Ethiopia, leading spokesperson of the African Region, rejects biotechnology as "neither safe, environmentally friendly, nor economically beneficial." Gurdial Nijar, legal adviser of the Third World Network, points out that "indigenous knowledge has fed, clothed and healed the world for millennia." The concept of patenting and owning life is antithetical to all cultures in the Third World. Furthermore, it denies the "cumulative innovative genius" of farmers over the generations. Indian leader Clovis Wapixana confirmed that it is the deep knowledge of indigenous plants and animals possessed by the Amazonian Indians which alone can sustain natural biodiversity.

Genetic engineering of food crops can involve the transfer of genes into seeds from various species, such as animals (including humans), fish, insects, bacteria, viruses, and other plants for the purpose of improving the crop. Vegetarians are often horrified at the thought of eating animal genetic material in their fruits and vegetables. Pro-GE literature informs us that genetic modification techniques are merely simpler, more efficient ways to do plant breeding. Plant breeding, however, never involved splicing animal genes into plants.

The seed production industry is being rapidly consolidated by major multinational companies with an interest in genetic engineering. Important old seed varieties that contain essential genetic diversity (our agricultural heritage) are being discontinued, lost, and replaced by new, patented GE seeds.

According to traditional Chinese medicine, the genetic aspect functions within the realm of the life essence, or *jing,* of an organism. The *jing* guides our growth and development and nurtures our spiritual awareness. Damage to the *jing* of food from the haphazard effects of genetic engineering could cause dysfunction in its sphere of influence: vitality, fertility, immunity, higher awareness, graceful aging, and hormonal function. Is it worth the risk to tamper with nature's most precious gift? On a similar topic, Charles, Prince of Wales, has had misgivings about genetic modification of food crops and questions whether science should be meddling with the "very stuff of life," saying, "I think we are tampering with something very fundamental, trying to redesign nature and re-engineer humanity in our image and not God's image."[89]

Meat, poultry, and commercially farmed fish are being fed GE feed. One way to avoid GE foods (and heal the planet) is to eat locally produced, organic whole foods; likewise, eat organic animal products and *wild* fish, not GE fish from farms. Farm fish, even if fed organic feed, easily acquire infections and are often less than vital. The effluent from fish farms often kills vegetation and other life in rivers and waterways.[90] (See "Resources" index for organizations that identify fish from ocean-friendly and sustainable fisheries.)

New and Renewed Genes

When reflecting on our own genetic makeup, we may believe that access to this gift at the foundation of biologic life should be available on a simpler level than the techniques of molecular biology.

Apparently it is. It was Barbara McClintock, Nobel Prize laureate in medicine who gave us a groundbreaking, flexible, and open concept for how genetic theory manifests in our bodies. In her words, "any organism can make any other." This can imply that "genetically determined" traits and abilities are often not determined, but rather, *influenced*. Thus the term "fluid genome" was coined.

And according to some geneticists,[91] this line of reasoning can be extended to imply that our genetic/RNA-DNA system is influenced by environment and diet and by whatever we do—even by our thoughts. If this is true, it gives us more healing avenues. Everyone has areas of imbalance that may seem hopeless. And hopelessness may arise from the thought that our imbalances may be genetically "determined." But with the vision of a highly flexible, transforming genetic process, fewer imbalances will seem hopeless. But should we wait for a biotechnology solution from genetic engineers? Rather, is there a more organic, naturally evolving process that can help us circumvent technological invasion of this most essential part of our lives?

Consider for a moment a woman who comes from a family in which most members, for several consecutive generations have had heart disease. She may decide that she is genetically predisposed to heart disease and consequently feel that not much can be done to avoid it.

An avenue of hope: Genes in this family may have become altered to promote heart disease. They may have picked up their predisposition from poor dietary influences, intoxicant addictions, or other stressors. At any one point, a person in the family with negatively influenced genes can theoretically initiate genetic renewal, and thereby remove at least a portion of the negative programming. But to do so, an integrative approach may be best, as was practiced by traditional healers in China as well other parts of the Far East.

In ancient Chinese therapeutics, the *jing* contains growth and development factors, including the genetic codes and networks (RNA/DNA). In many practices of ancient China, people would actively strengthen their *jing* with appropriate foods, herbs, and awareness practices. (Refer to *jing* topics beginning on page 360.)

One central awareness practice was reverence for ancestors. According to Chinese teachings, ancestors represent our roots and foundation, and without strengthening and purifying our ancestral connection, little or no real progress can be made. Some of the ceremonies they devised to honor their parents and other ancestors, both living and deceased, have included rituals, blessings, lighting of incense, bowing, the display of flowers and candles, and so on.

Contemporary folks may consider such rituals as purely superstitious. However, from my perspective, the conscious ritual attention we pay *to* our ancestors becomes a subconscious healing purification for the fundamental influences *from* our ancestors—our gene pool.

In the Western World, genealogy studies and ritual prayer practices, both in private and in public religious ceremonies that commemorate ancestry perhaps have a similar beneficial effect. A *daily* practice of honoring parents, grandparents, and all distant relations may have a more profound effect on our healing or genetic self-transformation over time than the customary ritual of placing flowers once a year at their burial places on Memorial Day.

In addition to food and herbal practices, living a life without extreme stress can influence how we grow and develop, and hence safeguard our genetic make-up. In fact, as discussed in the *Water Element* Chapter, nourishing our kidney-adrenal function counteracts stress and is thought to be crucial for *jing* enhancement and our future health potential.

A final practice to discuss is one of personal introspection. Breathing into the lower *dantien* (a term originating with ancient Chinese Taoists meaning "elixir field"), the area midway between the pubic bone and navel is a focal point for strengthening the kidney-adrenals as well as the *jing*. During breathing, the lower *dantien* becomes warm and aware. The mind then becomes completely peaceful as body-mind fusion engages. Such an event takes us beyond time and space, *yin* and *yang,* and we sense a fresh, clear renewal. Those in Taoist and other healing traditions of China may describe the experience as the conversion of *jing* into *shen* spirit.

I postulate that one important aspect of the experience represents better influences from ancient ancestral genetic lines coming into play in our lives, and the rejuvenation of dysfunctional genes and their DNA structural homes.

Section 2: Integrative Nutrition

Breaking the Concept Barrier

Many individuals acknowledge the value of unrefined, organic, non-genetically modified food for a variety of political and health reasons, yet rarely purchase it, even when the facts about quality and benefits are clearly known. These same individuals may place a great deal of value on their possessions. They may obtain only the best lubricants for their autos and buy fine home furnishings, while they eat the cheapest, poorest quality foods. As modern people, some of us may value possessions more than our own bodies or lives.

Looked at on purely the mechanical level, the human body, as most of us know, is magnificent, and nothing in the manufactured world can compare to it. If sensible, we would take better care of our body than any material object.

So one might ask—why is there so much self-neglect and, yet, so much focus on objects? Some of the possible answers are as follows:

First, we have little experiential awareness of what we are doing.

Second, we have been blinded by cultural conditioning to focus on objects-as-happiness, which can cause lack of respect for our own bodies and lack of compassion for others.

Third, we are not "present" in our bodies—we live primarily through a conceptual level of awareness. Thus we tend to analyze reality rather than being guided as an open channel for truth.

To illustrate this thought, I suggest the following exercise since mindful awareness can enable the kind of dietary transformation I have suggested in this book.

A Somatic Exercise

❖ What are you thinking right now?

❖ Where in your body does that thought come from?

❖ Notice as a new thought arises, how it is formed.

We often "think" we're in control, and that we "know" so very much in this Information Age.

The second part of this exercise involves questions that help us assess how much we know:

❖ Consider the process of raising your hand, as if to answer a question. Are you consciously controlling your arm, its nerves, muscles, ligaments, and tendons?

❖ How is the thought to raise your arm transmitted to your arm?

❖ When you move unconsciously, as may occur during eating, how is this controlled? (Trillions of our cells are involved in every physical action.)

❖ And most importantly, do you experience the guiding intelligence or *dharma* for these bodily processes? From ancient East Asian traditions, the *"qi"* energy that moves reality is guided by the spirit, which may be considered our highest intelligence.

As we can see, most of us are nearly totally unaware of the wondrous processes involved in our actions. What we do experience is the thinnest filament or merest fragment of reality. Yet we walk about coolly, exuding experience, as if to say—"I understand a lot—show me something new." We tend to lose our innocence and sense of wonder. We tend to live by rigid concepts rather than by direct, moment-by-moment, childlike, continually transforming, experience.

How can we return to the origin and source of reality—to the place of limitless light and renewal? Many teachings provide endless answers. However, we now explore a traditional set of priorities that can make the process flow more efficiently.

Emotional Awareness

It was Albert Einstein who suggested that one cannot easily solve a difficult problem at the level of the problem. With regard to emotional dilemmas, engaging directly with our emotions may be the least efficient approach to a resolution.

One may observe dramatic emotional healing by gaining perspective from a place of awareness so that we may be mindful of emotions, as if to gaze at them, and say, "Now I'm angry (or worried or whatever the emotion is), but it's simply like a warm breeze wafting through me." At the place of mindfulness of stuck emotional patterns, we melt the unchanging aspects of the patterns. We may still have the emotions, but we are free to watch them and even, with relaxed concentration, play with them, nudging our stuckness into healing transformation. Earlier, in the section on genetics, we gave a specific example of an ancient Taoist awareness practice (breathing into the lower *dantien*) that brought about a renewed sense of life.

For this level of mindful awareness to occur, especially to the point that it can free us from obstructed emotions, it may take a little training at quieting the mind. The focused, self-reflective mind is calm and clear. It observes with penetrating wisdom and clarity what we are presently doing. A skilled therapist can guide one in this direction. Traditional pathways to this frame of mind also exist, and involve various disciplines, the most common being meditations, contemplative prayer, yogic practices, and visualizations, as well as using a mantra (mindfully repeating valued words or sounds). It was the ancient Chinese sage Lao-tzu, who, 2,500 years ago, encouraged us with these stanzas to discover liberation:

Can you coax your mind from its wandering
and keep to the original oneness?
Can you let your body become
supple as a newborn child's?
Can you cleanse your inner vision
until you see nothing but the light?

Clearing Emotional Turmoil with Remedies from Above and Below

Awareness Practices That Quiet the Mind (Silent contemplation, meditation, self-reflection....)

↓

Emotional Turmoil (Stuck habits, depression, anxiety, panic, fear, worry, grief, insecurity, anger, resentments, addictive attachments to people, food, drugs, alcohol....)

↑

Biologic Healing (With exercise, yoga, qi gong, tai ji, appropriate whole foods, herbal therapy, acupoints....)

Three Priorities in Healing

In many ancient Eastern traditions, the first priority in the healing arts is *awareness*, a relaxed focusing of the mind, which is quite unifying and decidedly spirit-strengthening. A strong, bright spirit leads the healing process against disease—we fully grasp the nature of our current problems and have the intuition and strength to overcome them. The ideal level of awareness may occur most easily during concentrated practices similar to those mentioned above. However, any relaxing or focusing experience where we pay attention—appreciating nature or art, or playing a musical instrument—can certainly bring peace to our minds and should be encouraged when the more rigorous approaches are not suitable or acceptable.

The second priority in healing is *activity,* which comes under the "Biologic Healing" category in the chart. Certain activities blend with awareness practices. Examples include tai ji, various yoga systems, and qi gong. Other activities are likewise important. These can include manual labor, physical chores (e.g., helping the elderly or ill with housework), sports, walking, weight training, or any of the numerous exercise programs that are currently available.

According to the East Asian healing arts, exercise builds digestive fire and therefore is necessary for us to receive good nutrition from our food. Without sufficient activity, we may find it difficult to make progress in health, regardless of how good our food may be.

An important relationship from traditional Chinese medicine indicates that adequate movement, including stretching, balances the liver/gall bladder complex, which, according to mental health research, is the center for making biochemicals that influence moods and emotions in general. In support of this information, various recent studies inform us that moderate exercise makes depression and bad moods much less likely.[92,93]

Priority number three is **nutrition,** which is also listed under Biologic Healing. Coupled with exercise, nutrition represents an awe-inspiring therapy. The right type of quality food, when digested thoroughly, benefits the biochemistry of our bodies and especially that of our brain function.[94] Indeed, positive nutrition enhances the well-being of the mind in general, including how we think and feel. And if our mind is clear and self-reflective (mindful), it will help us choose ideal food, activity, and all other life patterns. From the viewpoint of East Asian healing theory, we have just completed a yin/yang, earth/heaven cycle: The mind (heaven) helps control the earthy, biologic choices, whereas the food and exercise we choose can support high level awareness. Between these two polarities are the emotional realms. From my perspective, people who improve both in personal awareness and nutrition and who are adequately active—harmonize their emotions most efficiently.

The Emotions in Harmony

When emotions are relatively balanced, we naturally sense self-respect and therefore find that quality choices in food represent the most desirable action. Moreover, we discover that inferior foods simply aren't interesting. Their energetic qualities are negative and we naturally prefer not to pollute our bodies and degrade our minds with them.

Such a relationship between food and awareness is a key to feeling complete and having emotional equilibrium. Greater awareness breaks the emotional attachment-link to food. Such simple processes are often hardest to see; we may think our emotional conundrums need a complex cure, yet by having practices that calm the mind and brighten the spirit, by being abundantly active, and choosing quality foods, we ride the emotional train to harmony!

One purpose of this text is to promote world peace in a unique and highly practical way—by encouraging the healing of our overly aggressive desires and emotions with self-reflective practices and better quality biologic choices, including food choices.

Section 3: Dietary Patterns and Directions

The Low Carbohydrate, High-Protein, Limitless-Fat Diets

A change in perception in the public mind involves the recently maligned carbohydrate, particularly in the form of grains. Carbohydrates from grains and sugars have been blamed for the extensive overweight and obesity epidemic in the United States,[95] which affects more than 60% of the adult population, according to the

Centers for Disease Control. Carbohydrates have also been held accountable for other ills, including diabetes and blood sugar imbalances in general.

Reacting to this connection between grain- and sugar-carbohydrate consumption and poor health, a minor segment of the population has moved away from protein-, fat-, and carbohydrate-rich diets to ones with large amounts of protein and fat, particularly in the form of animal meats and dairy foods. A number of high-protein diets based on animal products, with their miniscule carbohydrate in the form non-starchy vegetables, have come and gone in the past 35 years.[96] And in many cases people have lost weight.

However, thinking back to the early 1970s, I cannot recall anyone who started one of the popular low carbohydrate, protein-rich diets* who continued with it for more than a few months, although undoubtedly some adherents stayed with it much longer. It is, nonetheless, difficult to maintain a diet that contains only half the carbohydrate required for healthy functioning of the body. Carbohydrate deficiency resulting in ketosis is routinely experienced by those on the high-protein, low-carbohydrate regimens. When this happens, the body tends to burn more stored fat than carbohydrate for energy needs, which results in weight loss—as intended by the diets. Signs of ketosis may include nausea, fatigue, bad breath, constipation, muscle cramps, and headache.

Weight control is a life issue that requires sustainability rather than temporary improvement, followed by disappointment.[97] According to researchers at the University of Pennsylvania Medical School, for the majority of obese persons, reaching their ideal body weight is an unattainable goal; in fact, few people are able to maintain even modest weight losses over the long term.[98] This information affirms the perception that most "diets" are not a long-term solution to weight-loss or any of the other health benefits they promise. The diet-failure syndrome that may repeat itself a number of times can result from unbalanced eating plans that feature poor-quality foods. The dieter may wisely intuit the imbalance and stop such a plan. Another cause of failure: the plan may not support the current state of one's health or unique body type and constitution. A final cause is little or no dietary transition time to allow one to adapt lifestyle, emotions, and mentality to the new diet.

The low-carbohydrate, high-protein eating plans are marked with one well-known side effect; over 30 years of research studies all concur that high-protein consumption greatly puts one at risk for bone loss and kidney failure.[99,100]

Let's understand why such diets, which make nutrient imbalance a therapeutic feature, can be attractive.

It's well known that refined carbohydrates, either from refined-grain products, including white-flour baked goods, or from concentrated sweeteners such as refined sugar, make blood sugar levels soar.[101] When blood sugar is elevated over time, the

---

* Promoted by a Dr. Atkins in New York—who led the high-protein diet "revolution" 25 years later.

pancreas becomes stressed and may fail to produce sufficient insulin to control the sugar. Additionally, if obesity is a factor, the cells of the body tend to become less responsive to insulin. Consequently, fat is burned (oxidized) more slowly, and a portion of the sugar excess converts into fat, to be stored in the body.[102] Thus diabetes, a condition of chronic high blood sugar, regularly occurs in conjunction with obesity and overweight conditions. (Note that there are other patterns of development for diabetes.)

Obesity as a result of high blood sugar predisposes one to several illnesses; among them are infections, heart disease, and shortened life span. If we consider how most overweight and obese individuals arrive at their condition, we realize that they have eaten a standard American diet (SAD) that included a great deal of fat, protein, and refined carbohydrates. They also have been alerted by their doctors and the media to the health risks accompanying their overweight conditions and therefore are looking for a cure.

It is a physiologic fact that blood sugar can be controlled by dietary protein. And dietary fat does not directly increase blood sugar, although ingesting excesses of fatty foods, especially foods rich in saturated fat, tends to be a major long-term contributor to diabetes.[103] Nevertheless, the related conditions of obesity and high blood sugar can be at least temporarily counteracted by removing just the refined carbohydrates from the SAD. And for most people with the SAD background, simply to continue eating the regular fare of fatty, high protein animal foods— minus the carbohydrates—is far easier than a complete dietary makeover.

Quick 'n Easy Fixes

For Americans with rich dietary backgrounds, a low-carbohydrate, high-protein/fat diet is not only easy to start but provides fairly quick results as well. Most begin shedding pounds within days or, at least, weeks.

The phrase "quick and easy" applies here as it does with so many of the health fixes we have in wealthy countries: For instance, millions take antacids daily for acid indigestion; when a little tired or weak, coffee, especially with sugar, is used as an energy stimulant; stress can be somewhat ameliorated with an alcoholic drink; people smoke a cigarette for momentary sedation; and for overweight conditions, the quickest fix is liposuction; ephedrine, a potentially dangerous drug originally obtained from the ephedra plant, starts to work immediately; and a high-protein, low-carbohydrate diet is quite quick too, though it becomes less easy with time as one will eventually, and often uncontrollably, crave carbohydrates to balance massive protein intake.

The final point explains how the typical SAD diet in this country began. By loading up on protein, we fell victim to the physiologic equation: large amounts of protein in the diet require large amounts of dietary carbohydrate. (Protein and carbohydrate must be balanced for health to manifest.) And when protein is grossly overstated in the diet, one will crave concentrated carbohydrates in the form of refined sugar, sweets, pastries, polished rice, and the white-flour breads and pastas. Alcohol also enters into the equation, as it is essentially liquid sugar.

One of my students who worked in food service on a cruise ship noted that those on high protein diets would avoid the biscuits, potatoes, and rice but "drink like fishes," meaning they took in great quantities of alcoholic beverages. Eventually most people will give in to their true needs. By eating too much protein one ends up in a pathologic state. To find temporary balance, unfortunately most succumb to another pathologic extreme by over-indulging in refined carbohydrates and/or alcohol for balance. (Many alcoholics have told me they never crave sweets. They don't need sweets—they simply drink their sugar.) Another step in this scenario is drugs, both prescription and illegal drugs, and is discussed further in the Meat, Sugar, and Drug Syndrome, page 189.

The solution to the excess-protein dilemma is quite simple: Eating moderate amounts of protein balanced by carbohydrates, such as those from whole grains, legumes, starchy vegetables, and fruits. The high-protein promoters, now realizing the need for more carbohydrate, are suggesting that dieters slightly increase complex, unrefined carbohydrates after an initial minimal-carbohydrate phase of the diet.

Lacking nutritional soundness and long-term viability, even when complemented with additional carbohydrates, the high-protein diets are popular because they tend to be quick and easy remedies.

Each such remedy, nonetheless, comes with a price that must be paid for its expediency and convenience. And that price is all too often serious health challenges. In the case of any high-protein diet, the health risks include the aforementioned degenerations—osteoporosis and kidney failure; in addition, heart disease and cancer become more likely with eating too much protein and saturated fat from animal products.[104-106]

Protein Guidelines

Animal Protein Guidelines: To reduce the risks of poor health listed above, the consumption of any protein-rich animal product should be equal to or less than 4 ounces daily. Two to three ounces is often considered ideal in terms of protein utilization in the body. Occasionally, on holidays, for example, taking in 6 ounces does not normally cause imbalance. Concentrated animal protein examples: various meats, fowl, fish, and cheese.

Plant Protein Guidelines: Consumption of plant foods that are concentrated in protein and carbohydrates can safely double that of animal-protein foods: equal to or less than 8 ounces daily, with 4 to 6 ounces being ideal, and 12 ounces maximum, occasionally. Concentrated plant protein/carbohydrate examples: legumes—beans, peas, lentils, soy products such as tempeh and tofu, and the grain seeds quinoa and amaranth. Plant protein does not stress calcium reserves to the same degree as animal protein (refer to page 222). All weights above are for prepared foods.

(continued on page 30)

Protein Guidelines *(continued)*

However, the extremely concentrated plant proteins should be taken in much smaller amounts. For example, one ounce daily is a substantial quantity of nuts and seeds. Algae, valuable sources of plant protein and minerals, are available as seaweeds; see Chapter 42, for recipes with appropriate servings of various seaweeds. Other commonly available algae are the protein-rich micro-algae; dosage is normally just a small fraction of an ounce. Refer to *Green Food Products,* Chapter 16.

Combined Guidelines: To calculate a safe guideline when eating both plant and animal protein during a day, add half the weight of carbohydrate-rich protein (e.g., legumes) and the entire weight of concentrated plant proteins (e.g., nuts and seeds) to the weight of animal protein consumed. The total should fall within the animal protein guidelines above (4 ounces daily, 2-3 ounces ideally, and 6 ounces occasionally).

All guidelines above are based on studies that safeguard calcium loss versus protein intake.

Habits that Heal: Better Choices over Time

Transitioning from a SAD or other high-protein diet to recommendations in this book for proven, traditionally inspired diets represents a move toward long-term health. Such a change may involve substantial effort, but with an emphasis on moderate protein intake and unrefined carbohydrates, our approach includes dietary strategies that one can incorporate successfully over a lifetime.

One Diet for All?

Popular books on nutrition have generally put forth one diet for everyone; others have featured several diets dependent on blood type or other diagnostic aspects. This book also recommends certain basic dietary directions, such as the forthcoming Transformed Paleolithic Diet, the Plant-Based and Chinese Rural Diets, and the Integrative Food Pyramid, among others. These "diets" represent general guidelines that safeguard you against extreme choices that are unhealthful for nearly everyone. They also inform you of important overall patterns of quality foods and proportions in a balanced diet.

Therefore, rather than being precise diets *per se*, these basic guidelines are learning aids that help you, over time, to develop the flexible eating and living program that meets your unique, personal, constitutional, and daily health needs. And with the support of the assessment methods of traditional Chinese healing arts, the science of modern nutrition, and common sense, you will find appropriate food choices within these dietary directions to improve your vitality and consciousness. Thus, rather than recommending one diet, this book provides for a personal dietary and lifestyle healing process that is custom tailored to you.

The Paleolithic Diet Adapted for Today

A better alternative to a high-protein, low-carbohydrate diet is the hunter-gatherer diet of protein from lean meats with carbohydrate from ample fruit and vegetable consumption. Such a "Paleolithic" diet, assuming researchers have correctly ascertained it, has the value of being an eating tradition that some of our ancestors followed for many generations, starting at least 100,000 years ago.[107,108] Both the plants and meats in this ancient diet were wild.

There is essentially no dairy food in this simple plan, and grain and legume consumption, until the latter part of the era, was quite minimal, probably from wild seeds. Aside from the current difficulty involved in procuring wild foods, such a diet would clearly be more healthful than the modern meat-centered diets of the wealthy nations that feature highly processed foods and feedlot animals replete with chemicals, hormones, and antibiotics. Stone Age individuals, in fact, were not obese, and we may assume that this was due in part to the lack of both refined carbohydrates and poor-quality dairy and meats in their diets. Specifically, the meats they ate, being wild, would have a different mix of fats, with far more of the omega-3 fatty acids that help keep arteries clean, maintain modest body weight, and build immunity against cancer and other degenerations. (Refer to *Oils and Fats* Chapter for more information on omega-3 fatty acids.)

Certainly, one of the most important considerations of Stone Age eating patterns was the activities that accompanied them: living in an energetic, pristine environment; digging up roots and gathering berries and edible plants; cleaning and processing animal and plant foods, and walking lengthy distances on rough terrain during the hunt and when relocating.

What Can We Apply from Our Paleolithic Ancestors' Life and Diet?

The lessons of this dietary plan may prove especially useful for those in transition to a plant-based diet from one rich in meat, dairy, fats, and refined carbohydrates and lacking adequate fruits and vegetables. Detailed steps in the dietary transition process appear in *Dietary Transition,* Chapter 7. Current vegetarians may want to share the following suggestions with those who eat poor-quality, meat-based diets.

1. Regarding the quality of meats, the wild variety provides the best nutrients and *qi* energetic quality but is impractical. If many who embrace ancient diets began eating wild meats, wild animal populations would quickly become extinct. The best alternative to wild is organic, range-fed animals. Wild fish, as discussed earlier in the Genetic Engineering section, are usually, at this point, preferable to farm fish.

2. Eat whole animal foods: regarding meats, eat broken bone soup (page 295) to obtain minerals and the marrow and consume the organs (discussed further on page 135). Eating the same cut of meat over and over again, e.g., chicken

breast, can promote imbalance. Dairy foods were used very little, if at all, in Stone Age times; nevertheless, if used wisely, they can be of benefit to certain individuals and more generally, to certain races and populations. (See guidelines for using whole dairy products on page 149–151. Safe protein guidelines are listed earlier on pages 29 and 30.)

3. Careful, detailed research on intestinal contents of a mummified man indicates that some Mesolithic and Neolithic peoples ate substantial ground barley and einkorn, a primitive cereal.[109] Eat unrefined whole grains regularly but moderately, in any form, including cereals, breads, and pastas. Per earlier discussions, refined foods, including "white" wheat-flour products supply incomplete nutrition, contributing to the diseases of modern civilization.

4. Eat abundant and varied organic vegetables and fruits, particularly as a balance for animal products. The acids in these plant foods facilitate the breakdown of concentrated animal fats and proteins. In addition to the moderate inclusion of whole grains noted above, the carbohydrates in fruit and starchy vegetables such as carrots, potatoes, and winter squash supports the carbohydrate/protein balance that is missing in low-carbohydrate diets.

5. Hunter-gatherers throughout history have eaten a variety of plant seeds. Certain seeds can be recommended for their restorative properties. Try roasted pumpkin seeds (roast to eliminate dangerous *E. coli* bacteria), almonds, and ground or soaked flax meal (see directions for use on page 165). Legumes are valuable protein-rich seeds. Use them fresh—e.g., green beans, peas, and soy edamame; and dried—e.g., dried lentils and beans; also in the form of soy products such as tempeh, tofu, natto, and miso.

6. To attune with the prehistoric messages from our earth and her peoples, eat ancient foods that have not been hybridized and have remained, as a species, in essentially the same form for billions of years. Such foods are the algae, for example, the sea vegetables and micro-algae, including chlorella, wild blue-green algae *(Aphanizomenon),* and spirulina. (Please refer to *Seaweeds* and *Green Food Products,* Chapters 42 and 16.)

7. Eat wild foods that do not endanger the species. Choose with care appropriate wild herbs and plants. Wild plant examples are provided on page 215, number 2.

8. Commune with nature regularly. Mindful moments, even in a neighborhood park, can engender solace. In addition, exercise and be active outdoors to contact the *qi* vitality of plant and animal life.

Note: The limits for meat consumption suggested earlier—equal to or less than 4 ounces daily—are lower than those envisioned by some Paleolithic researchers. Regarding how accurately the Paleolithic diet has been assessed, Marion Nestle,

Ph.D., noted public health researcher and Chair of the Department of Nutrition at New York University, has commented in her studies on plant versus animal foods in human diets: "Hominoid primates are largely vegetarian [98% plant-based diets]. Current hunter-gatherer groups rely on foods that can be obtained most conveniently, and the archeological record is insufficient to determine whether plants or animals predominated."[110]

An additional goal of this book is to support the responsible use of animal products. Therefore, for numerous social, ecologic, and health reasons, the reader is encouraged to eat a mostly plant-based diet and, when possible, a vegetarian diet. Compassion should enter into our food choices too, as nearly nine billion farm animals, most of them suffering in cruel living conditions, are slaughtered yearly in the United States.[111] An additional one billion die from disease or for other reasons. If aquatic life is included, the total is 24 billion animals killed for human consumption.

If individuals need meat or fish in their diets because of deficiency, the above modified hunter-gatherer approach is vastly superior to a typical American diet that is rich in *refined* carbohydrates and contains great excesses of protein and fat.

Plant-Based and Chinese Rural Diets

Paleolithic researchers have discovered only a few subgroups of people eating highly plant-based diets during the most ancient times. We do know, however, that many peoples eating quasi-vegetarian diets have coexisted with hunter-gatherers on this and most other continents in the past 5,000 years. For example, well before the European invasion of North America, the Hopi people chose to become agrarian, to use plant-rich diets, and to center their lives in one geographic area in order to foster stability and continuity for their spiritual lives.[112] Much the same can be said for the ancient Essene desert communities in the Middle East.[113]

There have always been people on the planet who have sensed the relationship between diet and mentality. In some cases this involved knowledge of the spirit and the energetic influence of each plant and animal they were eating; and certain of these individuals have decided that living largely on animal flesh did not sustain their ideal in awareness patterns. It may be that one can avoid being overweight and be physically healthy with support from either a hunter-gatherer diet rich in quality animal foods, vegetables, fruits, and seeds, or one based on unrefined plant nutrition with few animal products. (Certainly other possibilities for healthful diets exist as well.) An essential consideration is the mental and emotional life one wants when choosing a diet, because foods, as we have discussed earlier, and will see more clearly in future chapters, directly influence our mind and emotions.

Some of our great thinkers, peacemakers, and teachers in the past 2500 years have been vegetarians or at the very least ate predominately plant-based diets. Among them have been numerous yogis and yoginis, Lao-tsu, Buddha, Socrates, Pythagoras, Jesus,[114] Nostradamus, Leonardo da Vinci, Gandhi, Einstein, and Mother Teresa. (Refer to note 114, page 685 for information that portrays Jesus as a compassionate vegetarian.)

Regarding the relationship of diet to longevity and health, today nearly all the bastions of people who live long and well eat plant-based diets, whether we observe Okinawans of Japan, Georgians (in the Caucus Mountains near Russia), Vilcabambans of Ecuador, or the Hunzas of Pakistan.[115-117]

Diets that eschew carbohydrates and focus on protein and ample fat have at least one idea that we can learn from: carbohydrates from grains, including wheat, can promote excessive weight gain.[118] Most books that decry grain carbohydrate neglect to tell us, however, that excessive weight gain will generally not occur from eating *unrefined* whole grains.

How do we know this? First, from personal experience, I have observed that virtually everyone who eats a balanced diet of whole grains, vegetables, fruits, and the right fats and protein foods, loses excessive weight. We can also consider people who eat this type of fare: Asians and in particular those on the basic rural Chinese diet. These people are generally quite trim and healthy, and although they consume 300 more calories a day than typical Americans, obesity is rare when they eat their traditional diets.[119] The explanation: ***calories burn faster when a low-fat, low-protein diet is followed.***[120,121] (Please note, however, that eating patterns are quickly changing in modern China, especially in urban areas, to include increased fat and processed-food content.)

The rural, traditional diet has even more to recommend it: those following it have reduced incidence of fatal heart disease, cancer, diabetes, and other degenerative diseases compared with those on standard American fare. One of the most important nutrition research projects—the Oxford-China-Cornell Project on Nutrition, Health and Environment that began in the early 1980's—finds support for these facts.[122] This study has extremely relevant information for those with the degenerative diseases of modern civilization. Major conclusions of the study are briefly summarized on page 35.

In this study, the health of thousands of Chinese in various areas of China was researched, and the results are on an order of magnitude that has turned conventional nutritional thinking around, if not upside down.

Often in such large-scale studies of a vast region, one would expect to find a 10 or 15% difference compared to other areas of the world. This study found a 1700% greater likelihood of a middle-aged American male dying from heart disease compared with those on a typical Asian diet.

The first thing to come to the mind of the skeptic is: Perhaps this huge percentage results from the possibility that Chinese are genetically predisposed to less heart disease. However, the study included individuals who ate rich, fatty diets similar in nutrient composition to the standard American fare and found that they had heart disease at the same rate as their American counterparts.

The total disease preventive value of the rural Asian diet has inspired many American nutritionists and epidemiologists to re-think the modern diet to provide better health.

**A Comparison: Asian and American Approaches to Diet
Based on the Cornell-Oxford-China Nutrition Surveys**

FAT

Chinese eat half the fat that Americans do

PROTEIN

Chinese eat one third less protein than Americans do

CARBOHYDRATES

Americans eat 30% less carbohydrate than people in China do

FIBER

Americans eat 70% less fiber than people, on average, in China do

HEART DISEASE—WOMEN

American women have five times the risk of dying from heart disease of Chinese women

HEART DISEASE—MEN

Middle-aged men in America are 1700% more likely to die from heart disease than men of the same age in China

- Approximately 90% of the protein consumed in China is from plant sources; 70% of America's is from animal sources.
- The nation with the lowest rate of breast cancer in the world is China.
- The lowest rates of heart disease and breast cancer in China were found where the least animal protein and the most fruit, vegetables, and grains were consumed.
- The average Chinese diet includes mammal meats just once or twice a month; poultry (including eggs) 2-3 times a week and fish, whenever available.
- American women receive twice the dietary calcium of women in China, yet have much higher rates of bone loss. Very little dairy is consumed in China.
- Along with the political, social, and economic "progress" in China, heart disease, obesity, and diabetes are on the rise in cities—as rich, greasy, fast-food diets become more commonplace.

Reference: The China Project *by T. Colin Campbell*

The task of encouraging Americans to eat more vegetables and high fiber foods (note the huge disparity in fiber between the two diets) became understood by nutritionists such as Professor Walter C. Willett, M.D., of Harvard University, who realized that the Chinese prepare their foods with more flavor. Thus Willett suggests that for Americans to learn to appreciate abundant vegetable foods, they make them more palatable with the use of certain condiments, especially cooking herbs and spices.

Spices not only add flare and flavor to vegetables, they help build digestive strength and warmth so that nutrients are better absorbed and utilized. More spice is not always better, because moderately flavored spices, especially the seed spices, can be enjoyed by most people. A few common spices and cooking herbs include: turmeric, fennel, fenugreek, caraway, dill, anise, ginger, rosemary, oregano, thyme.

Another way to enhance vegetables and whole grains is to add healthful oils. Oils can help individuals with high-fat, heavy meat eating backgrounds transition to simpler, more balanced diets. Two good oils for those needing to lose weight and to cleanse from a somewhat toxic standard diet are cold-pressed, unrefined flax oil and unrefined olive oil. These can be an ingredient in salad dressings or even directly drizzled over grains and vegetables. Please refer to Chapter 10, *Oils and Fats,* for information on oils and important quality considerations.

Plant-Only Diets

The closer you get to a plant-based diet, the better off you'll be.—T. Collin Campbell, Ph.D., professor of nutritional biochemistry, Cornell University and Director of the Cornell-Oxford-China Project.

A plant-based diet means that plant foods occupy a major part of the diet, for instance, two-thirds or more. Currently, the standard American diet is closer to two-thirds animal products. Changing this situation involves overcoming a particular bias against plants because many Americans believe vegetal foods have inferior nutrition. To test the value of plants in human nutrition, I have eaten a 100% plant-only "vegan" diet for over 30 years. I have enjoyed several benefits, particularly on the emotional and mental levels.

Are there any examples of vegans in Western history? Quite possibly, before the Great Flood of the Old Testament, but we have little evidence other than contestable references in the Bible. However, there have been millions of vegans in China over the last 1400 years. They were the Buddhists and Buddhist monks. They ate no meat, fish, or eggs. They virtually never used dairy products.[123] Buddhism is nearly extinct in modern China, and the last Buddhist patriarch in China was the legendary Hsu Yun, who lived until his 120th year in 1959.[124] He was the predecessor of my most important mentor, Hsuan Hua.

I rarely recommend long-term vegan diets to my clients because it seldom suits their lifestyle or emotional needs—it simply is not who they are. In addition, eating such a diet takes vigilance to find quality foods and to prepare them properly to match constitutional needs. However, one general use of a well-designed, client-specific vegan diet that I can recommend for a strong, robust person is a six-week or more cleansing from an overly rich, toxic diet. (Weak, frail, and deficient people should generally not follow a vegan diet.)

Various cleansing protocols are given in this text. The most detailed that can be applied for any purpose of regeneration are those found in *Cancer and The Regeneration Diets,* Chapter 32. "The Parasite Purge Program," normally followed in conjunction with the Regeneration Diets, acts not only to purge parasites but also as a basic cleansing for the internal organs and to remove toxins; directions are given in *Parasite Purge Program,* Appendix A. Both of these cleansing options normally involve highly plant-based diets, herbs, and various plant extracts, though animal products may be used in cases of deficiency and weakness.

Gentle maintenance cleansing on an ongoing basis normally entails consuming plant foods, and modern people need an abundance of these foods to overcome their rather toxic diet and lifestyle. Actually, many people endeavor to eat better, cleaner, lighter, and more healthful diets, but return to old, deep dysfunctional habits and unhealthy emotional ties with foods. Because of the high failure rates of those trying to upgrade their diets, I have found that the integrative approach to nutrition discussed earlier—one that advocates self-reflection, exercise, and gradual transition as facets of nutrition reform—has a higher rate of success.

Overweight, Immune, and Liver Syndromes: Overcoming the Origin

We now revisit an earlier topic: Overweight including obesity, according to recent data, has become a greater contributor to disease and death than the use of the intoxicants, tobacco and alcohol.[125]

Our plan for overcoming overweight (which begins on page 115) is effective and includes options that take into account the fact that those with excess weight have differing constitutions.

One health issue to address specifically in this context is that lack of mother's milk during infancy can contribute to life-long overweight issues.[126] The section that follows is helpful for anyone who has never, or was minimally (six weeks or less), breastfed. (For more on the importance of infant nutrition and breastfeeding, please refer to *Food for Children,* Chapter 11.)

Even though overweight and obesity are just one possible expression of lack of breastfeeding, such a crucial deficiency in infant feeding may influence nearly everyone adversely and have consequences beyond what is generally acknowledged in medical literature. The positive news is, with the right plan for renewal, it may be that the effects from lack of breastfeeding can be rectified.

The health of a non-breastfed person may be affected by specific nutrients she fails to receive in mother's milk. In the first days after birth, mother's milk contains a nutrient complex known as ***colostrum,*** one of the most potent immune tonics ever discovered.[127,128] Bovine colostrum, with up to 40 times the immune factors of human colostrum, is now used in human nutrition to strengthen immunity,[129] and has been shown to be effective against such autoimmune imbalances as rheumatoid arthritis, lupus, multiple sclerosis, chronic fatigue syndrome, and fibromyalgia.[130]

Colostrum has growth factors that promote healing and anti-aging responses.[131] The growth factors additionally make colostrum valuable in strengthening and building the body. It is reported to build lean muscle as effectively as many steroids—when accompanied by exercise.[132] It can also increase bone mass and renew aging skin. "Liver" and "age" spots on the skin may regress as colostrum appears to heal injured nucleic acids—our stores of RNA/DNA—thereby supporting profound rejuvenation. Further therapeutic applications of colostrum involve regenerative action for all damaged body tissues—bones, muscle, skin, cartilage, or nerve tissues—as a result of aging, surgery, or injury.[133]

Colostrum is also used for counteracting viruses and dangerous bacteria.[134] An astringent remedy, it also builds healthful intestinal flora and therefore has been a healing gift for many with severe, chronic diarrhea, including those with such parasitic infections like *Cryptosporidium parvum,* which can be deadly in persons with acquired immune deficiency syndrome (AIDS).[135]

Contraindications: Few contraindications to colostrum exist, though because of its astringency, constipation should be cleared before taking it. Allergic reaction to it is rare; even those with milk allergy usually tolerate it well.

Quality: Obtain certified organic. It is best to choose products that ensure that only excess colostrum is used and that calves always receive an adequate amount.

Colostrum and other human-milk nutrients seem to have a measurable effect. For example, receiving breast milk directly after birth and during the first 1–2 years afterwards, benefits intelligence[136] and immunity.[137,138] A central feature of immunity in general is good liver function, which indicates the ability of the liver to perform its thousands of tasks well. Two of its important immune-enhancing tasks include filtering the blood and deactivating toxins. Specifically, the liver harbors phagocytic cells that detoxify (via ingestion) many pathogenic particles, poisons, and bacteria.

In addition to colostrum, other vital nutrients in mother's milk are important fatty acids known as gamma linolenic acid (GLA). Human breast milk is the highest whole-food source of GLA. There are no other common sources although certain seeds and algae contain appreciable amounts (refer to GLA in the *Oils and Fats* Chapter). The GLA fatty acids activate liver function and enable a number of metabolic liver reactions, including production of hormone-like prostaglandins that are helpful against inflammation and tumor growth and are necessary for proper mental and emotional processes.

From this information and from personal observation, we can infer that those who were not breastfed as infants—and who therefore failed to receive the immune impetus and growth promoting activities of colostrum, GLA, and a number of other key nutritional factors in breast milk—may not have fully activated their liver functions. We next introduce rudimentary liver assessment, a useful topic for nearly everyone living in the highly developed countries, including those who have been breastfed.

Standard medical evaluation of liver health often shows little or no problem until there is gross malfunction. One rather subtle assessment method for liver function exists in traditional Chinese medicine. According to this holistic system, the liver is said to greatly influence our moods and emotions (anger, depression, manic depression/bipolar disorder, and irritability all indicate a degree of liver dysfunction), vision and eyes, tendons and ligaments, and digestion. (The liver contributes to overweight conditions when it stagnates, which slows metabolism, and also by "invading" the digestive function, thereby weakening it.) Our mental and physical flexibility, signs of stress, high blood pressure, allergies, spasms, cramps, pains and headaches (including migraine) that come and go, cancers, diabetes and large blood sugar fluctuations, arthritic disorders, chronic fatigue, fibromyalgia, and a number of forms of heart disease are adversely influenced by liver/gallbladder imbalance. For a more comprehensive perspective on liver/gallbladder signs, syndromes, and relationships to nature and diet, please see the *Wood Element* Chapter.

Because of diet and lifestyle, the liver/gall bladder complexes of modern people have degenerated greatly. Dr. Richard Schulze of Los Angeles, who taught in universities over a period of 20 years, had the opportunity to observe the condition of the viscera of numerous cadavers. According to his observations:

> Often in bodies of people over 60 the internal organs are in such a mess it is difficult for students to identify things. They smell so bad students would run from the room and even vomit. One time . . . almost every student started to vomit all over the laboratory. After that incident I always tried to get the bodies of younger people killed prematurely due to an accident so the internal organs would be more normal . . . . What was surprising to me was how many such young individuals would have fairly normal looking internal organs, but when you got to the liver and gallbladder, well it was like an alien encounter. Often the liver was shaped drastically different, swollen much larger than normal, filled with bloody fluids, pus, tumors, scar tissue and parasites. Every student was shocked to see such advanced degeneration in such young, supposedly healthy people.[139]

This description graphically depicts the liver of nearly anyone who has consistently eaten rich, greasy, highly processed foods. Those who have not been breastfed have increased risks to the health of their liver and immunity.

As we learned earlier, the liver benefits from organic plant foods, which are rich in minerals (including magnesium), vitamins, antioxidants, and various other phytonutrients. Eating vital, unrefined plant foods initiates liver cleansing and restoration, and will act as a foundation for other more specific therapies.

The program that follows accelerates liver and immune renewal, and is intended for those who received little or no mother's milk as infants. If you fall into this category but have good health, emotionally and physically, then, in all likelihood, you do not need the program.

The program is designed to function well for most constitutional types, and to initiate improvements that will make other more specific dietary and lifestyle strategies in this text more effective.

Those who *were* breastfed sufficiently and are still in need of rejuvenation, immune boosting, and cleansing can also benefit from the program. Children, either breastfed or not, when in need of stronger immunity, may benefit by following numbers 2, 3a, 3d, and 6 of the program along with dietary guidance in *Food for Children,* Chapter 21.

**Liver Renewal and Immune Boosting Program
For Adults not Breast Fed and Others Seeking Rejuvenative Cleansing**

1. Be prepared for transformation. Daily awareness practices and exercise will facilitate smooth changes.

2. Supply nutrients and compounds lacking as an infant—in order to initiate proper liver and immune function as an adult. *Note:* the following remedies also help improve liver/immune function in those who were adequately breastfed:

    a. GLA (gamma-linolenic acid) fatty acids in certain seed oils (borage, evening primrose, black currant). See dosage in Oils and Fats Chapter, page 173.

    b. Flax oil, cold pressed and unrefined, is cleansing yet regenerative to the liver and gallbladder. See dosage in Oils and Fats Chapter, page 165.

    c. Colostrum, certified organic bovine variety, a potent immune-enhancing substance. It may aggravate constipation, which should be remedied before taking colostrum. (For treating constipation, refer to pages 383–386.) Dosage: follow product directions.

3. Consume green and ancient plants with superior nutrition and life spark that cleanse and renew the liver:

    a. Chlorella has "Chlorella Growth Factor" for renewing the cells of all organs. See *Green Food Products* Chapter, pages 237–238, for dosage and usage (tablets of chlorella must be chewed up). Chlorella micro-algae, as a species, have been on the planet for over 2 billion years.

    b. Wild blue-green micro-algae *(Aphanizomenon flos-aquae)* are helpful against bad moods, sluggishness, and overweight. They are highly cleansing yet nurturing and healing to the liver. See pages 237–239 for dosage and usage. Note: If you are weak, frail, and easily chilled, then avoid these algae.

    c. Fulvic acid, an extract of ancient plant material from humic shale beds is helpful for liver rejuvenation and a superb source of "organic" minerals—those from plant tissue and bound with carbon. Dosage: Follow product recommendation.

d. Seaweeds should be used regularly in cooking for their ability to cleanse and restore the liver and gall bladder. They also mollify the effects of strong substances and therapies. See Seaweeds, Chapter 42.

4. Eat fruits which contain phytochemicals and antioxidants for renewal of liver cells:

a. Berries including strawberry, raspberry, blackberry, blueberry, huckleberry, thimbleberry, and others. Also pomegranate and grape. These fruits, in total, contain the phytonutrients ellagic acid and resveratrol, known to regenerate liver cells. Grapes additionally are a source of the substantial antioxidant proanthocyanidin, which can protect liver and other cells in the body.

b. Lemon and lime can be squeezed into water or used in food preparation on a daily basis. They are traditional "liver cleansers." Their bitter and sour flavors act to break down stagnant material in a swollen liver and gallbladder.

5. Make use of plant extracts and teas to enhance cleansing:

a. Lavender pure essential oil assists in the breakdown of toxic material in the liver, lymph and other viscera—that result from poisons in the environment and food and from old residues of hydrogenated-trans-fatty acids and synthetic polymers (from margarine, shortening, and poor quality deep-fried oils). Dosage: 1 drop daily in 1 glass water or in 1/2 teaspoon olive or flax oil, not with food. Obtain certified organic lavender oil. Note that essential oils are potent—if you experience mild repeated headaches or other minor symptoms, try taking it 3 days per week; if symptoms persist, or are extreme, stop altogether.

b. Chamomile tea: this moderate herb can help cleanse the liver and gallbladder deeply if used over time. Drink 1–2 cups per day; take in greater quantity if desired. See page 110 for herbal tea preparation.

6. Foods that fortify the body during the renewal process:

a. Broken bone marrow soup—contains stem cells of exceptional quality, which indicates the quality of nutrition in the marrow (stem cells are not viable when eaten or cooked). For non-vegetarians, this soup can support rejuvenation; builds jing essence for proper growth and development. See recipe on page 295. Use 1–3 times per week and only the bones of organic animals.

b. Royal jelly—has renewal properties similar to above soup. See page 152 for description and dosage. Take 3 or more times per week. For those who are not weak, bee pollen is better choice. See pages 151–152 for description and dosage. This elixir can be taken daily.

(Continued on page 42)

Duration of plan: at least 3 months. Use items in numbers 1, 2, 3, and 5 six days a week; use items in number 4 as often as desired. Usages of items in number 6 are listed.

Regarding the diets and therapies listed next: Choose one or a series to follow, for example, you can begin I, then continue with II after I is completed. Rebuilding the liver will take upwards of 18 months accordingto Max Gerson (about Gerson: pages 405–406; rebuilding liver: page 413). Renewal of other organs and tissues often takes at least that long as well.

Dietary Options: Integrate the above program into any of the dietary or therapeutic actions you may take below:

I. If you have signs and/or risks of parasites (pages 655–656), it is advisable to follow the Parasite Purge protocols (beginning on page 657).

II. If you prefer to initiate fundamental healing with this renewal/immune program before applying food therapies from other chapters in this book, then choose foods that appeal to you from the Integrative Nutrition Pyramid in the next section. However, to enhance the cleansing value needed for liver renewal and immune enhancement, avoid these foods in the Pyramid: peanuts, eggs, pork, shellfish, and bovine dairy products, including butter; moderate amounts of goat dairy products are acceptable—if you tolerate goat dairy. Those with wheat allergies may tolerate and benefit from sprouted wheat. Cooked whole-wheat berries and wheat sprouts are ideal wheat preparations for all others on this plan. Moderate amounts of natural leavened whole-grain breads are also healthful for most individuals (page 491). Please make note of the words "unrefined" and "whole" in the Pyramid.

III. You may follow strategies for renewing the heart and arteries (page 162–169).

IV. You may follow strategies for weight loss (pages 115–119).

V. You may rejuvenate with Regeneration Diets A, B, or C (beginning on page 407) for cancer, tumor, heart disease, arthritis, or other degenerative process.

VI. If you have signs and/or risks of candidiasis (overgrowth of candida yeasts) (pages 72–73), it is advisable to follow the Candida Plan (pages 73–77).

VII. You may use plans in this book to heal any of various other health imbalances.

VIII. You may develop a diet for your constitutional type, based on the Six Divisions (beginning on page 57) and Syndromes of Organs/Five Elements (beginning on page 303).

Many of my clients have benefited from diets and the cleansing, regenerative processes similar to those recommended above. Two of these individuals needed surgery as a result of accidents. In both cases, the surgeons noted that the livers, gallbladders, and other internal organs in these individuals were in remarkable condition—like those of young children.

Integrative Nutrition Pyramid

Consider the common food pyramid that one sees in the media. Dietitians know that fewer than 3% of the American population follow all the recommendations of the USDA (U.S. Department of Agriculture) food guide pyramid. Furthermore, studies indicate that individuals who follow a number of the pyramid guidelines may not greatly benefit in terms of health or avoidance of disease.[140] One explanation is little discernment of quality: the food guide permits major dietary contributors to diabetes and obesity—refined grain products such as white rice and white-flour breads and pastas. Another crucial area for health involves the quality of oils and fats. Just as the breads and pastas are placed in one category in the USDA guidelines without regard to quality, so too are all oils and fats. Consequently, consumers may be incorrectly led to believe that common salad and cooking oils are healthful. In reality, most are refined, rancid, and according to some researchers, the greatest dietary causes of free-radical cellular degenerations, which contribute to our most prevalent chronic diseases (discussed in the *Oils and Fats* Chapter, and elsewhere in this volume).

We should also be concerned about other health issues that the USDA guidelines fail to warn us about: hormones, pesticides, and antibiotics in typical dairy products and feedlot meats; another quality concern pertains to USDA acceptance of genetically modified foods and failure to recommend products grown using the methods of organic, sustainable farming.

Our pyramid (see below), though not intended as a complete guide to eating, provides a general pattern for healthful food selections and proportions based on the latest population studies and nutrition research. However, in order to know which foods to eat, their preparation, and other factors, one ideally puts forth some effort in learning about the different foods in the categories. In times past, such self-education was not as necessary because virtually all foods were locally grown, organic, and in a near-natural state when prepared. There were few choices. Currently, our food comes from all over this continent, indeed, from all over the planet, and much of it is ultimately processed and denatured. Although there are some advantages in having approximately 50,000 food choices available in the wealthy nations,[141] one must ferret out the quality items that support vitality.

Thus, the guide for our Integrative Nutrition Pyramid, which will help you to select an optimal food plan, is this book. The reader who endeavors to discover greater health and awareness needs to know not only the quality issues but also the properties of foods. For instance, in addition to oil quality mentioned above, we need to know more about the properties of the beneficial oils and fats. That is, which are best for cooking? Which are best for building immunity and providing anti-inflammatory activity? Regarding properties of dairy foods, who benefits from dairy products? And from which dairy products, for example, fermented (yogurt, kefir); goat, or bovine? There are also options regarding animal and plant protein choices, grains, vegetables, fruits, nuts, seeds, sea vegetables, and others.

Modern people need re-education about food. Most know little about healthful preparation of whole foods, nor for that matter, can they even identify important unrefined foods such as an oat groat or a whole-wheat berry. Separation from food extends even to growers. One time I prepared a vegetable, dried-pea soup and gave some to a farmer who had grown thousands of acres of dried peas (peas grown exclusively for drying) over a period of 30 years. I asked him what he thought it was. He had no idea. After telling him, he claimed to have never eaten food made with dried peas.

Consider your right hand. It has a front and a back that function together. The back of your hand is like knowing about food. The front, your palm, is like knowing more about yourself in terms of bodily type and function. The integration of the front and back of the hand symbolizes the close connection between the successful use of food and self-knowledge. The chapters that follow hold the keys to knowing your personal body-type assessment in simple but effective terms of traditional Chinese medicine: *excess, deficiency, hot, cold,* and other aspects of the *yin/yang* system. Available in later chapters are organ assessments that inform you on how well digestion, liver, kidneys, and various other systems are functioning and what specific nutrition they need.

The following Integrative Nutrition Pyramid features a vital ingredient in our journey towards habitual good nutrition: *awareness.* Common food charts and their implied diets are all but destined to failure when applied in the lives of people who need emotional and spiritual transformation for self-respect and clarity of mind before long-term dietary progress can be made.

The Integrative Nutrition Pyramid is not the end, but a beginning—a map that points the direction to the remainder of this text, in which we will discover through unifying modern nutrition and ancient Asian tradition how best to eat and live.

INTEGRATIVE NUTRITION PYRAMID

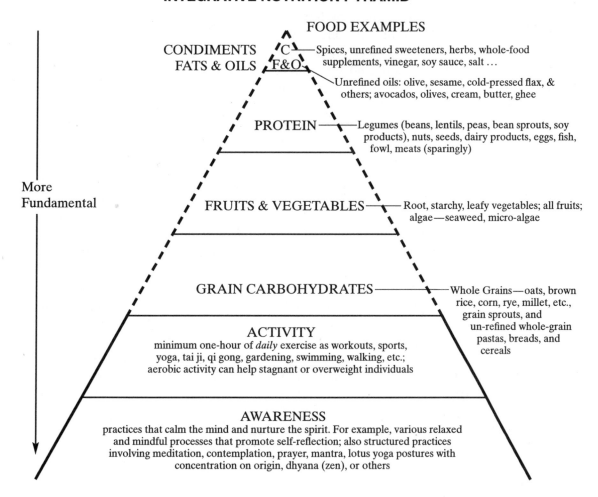

Note 1: From awareness practices we may gain emotional harmony and a foundation of integrity to put forth the discipline, commitment, and intention necessary for a long, joyful, and successful life, supported by excellent diet.

Note 2: For a more detailed listing of foods in groups, please see pages 269–270; the properties and uses of foods are given throughout this book and especially in Part V, *Recipes and Properties of Vegetal Foods;* for the recommended percentages of food groups during dietary transition, please see pages 108–109.

Note 3: Intoxicants and strong stimulants such as alcohol, coffee, tobacco, marijuana, and all illicit drugs have sought-after effects that are ultimately offset by their toxic and depleting nature. These substances will normally become less attractive as nutrition and awareness improve.

Personal Evolutionary Diets and Summary

Rather than seeking the perfect diet that is instantly available and good for all time, consider your current diet and how you might like to improve it. You may use any of the previous general eating patterns—Transformed Paleolithic, Plant-based and Chinese Rural diets, and Integrative Nutrition Pyramid—to gain perspectives on healthy dietary directions. And if you would like to initialize the process with a cleansing protocol, you may follow the Liver Renewal and Immune Boosting Program presented in the previous section. It features options for a number of therapeutic diets, including those for parasite and candidiasis purging, weight loss, heart disease, and other degenerative diseases.

As healing takes place over time, your dietary directions evolve and focus to take into account certain factors, including the seasonal influences, the type of work and activity in your life, your age, and others. With increasing awareness, intuition also plays a role in this lifestyle evolution. A major way in which your dietary evolution unfolds comes from learning about your constitutional type and corresponding nutrition based on the traditional Chinese diagnostic system in this book. Another pathway of the evolution involves knowledge of food preparation and the nature of foods. Future chapters include information on dietary transition, protein, oils and fats, sweeteners, green foods, food combining, fasting and purification, recipes and properties of foods, and others.

If you are trying to reverse a serious disease process, applying the Chinese diagnostic system can be invaluable in making an informed decision on nutrition as well as other remedies. In such cases, you may also need advice from a trusted health care practitioner.

A caution: try not to rush; avoid worry and overconcern when changing something as crucial to your well-being as your diet. As you learn more, implement the changes you are comfortable with. Let your diet evolve in ways that are harmonious—and therefore healing.

"Don't push the river."

Part I

The Roots of Diagnosis and Treatment

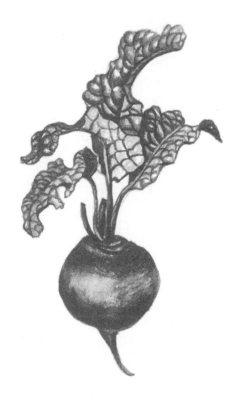

Yin-Yang and Beyond

Yin and *yang*, in essence, describe all phenomena. Some people may claim not to believe in *yin-yang* philosophy, yet these terms are merely descriptions of easily observed processes—day changing into night, youth into age, one season into the next.

The theory of *yin* and *yang* has been applied extensively in the history of East Asia, and in the last seventy years various modified versions have been used by historians and psychologists including Arnold Toynbee and Carl Jung, and by political leaders such as Mao Tse-tung and Karl Marx, who all studied Far Eastern philosophy before developing their own applications.

> Everything in creation is covered by Heaven and supported by Earth.
>
> —*Inner Classic**

History shows that if an idea or plan (such as a political strategy, economic reform, or diet) is founded on a stagnant structure that will not change with people's needs, its long-term success will be limited. Harmonious and creative adaptability is the hallmark of correctly applied *yin-yang* theory, and so we have chosen its principles to illustrate many tenets of this book. The definitions of *yin-yang* are basic and easily understood. We encourage the reader to apply them toward an awareness of the personal factors necessary for complete health.

This method of analysis has the advantage of simplifying and unifying the understanding of all things. Basically, the *yin-yang* principle holds that all objects or phenomena in the universe can be understood as limitless pairs of opposites (*yin* and *yang*) which interact according to the following principles:

The source of *yin* and *yang*, and therefore of all dualities, is that which is unified and unchanging. Even though *yin* and *yang* specify change and separation, their source is permanent: "The Great Ultimate is Unmoved," according to Shao Yung, the 11th-century Chinese philosopher. The Bible expresses this idea in the phrase, "I am the Lord; I do not change." (Malachi 3:6)

The *yang* principle is active while the *yin* is passive, yet nothing is purely *yin* or purely *yang*. The *yin-yang* symbol shows *yin* within the *yang* as the dark eye in the white fish, and conversely *yang* is shown to be contained in *yin* by the white eye of the dark fish.

Is the inside of the human body *yin* or *yang*? Simple wisdom from Chinese teachings suggests that in order to understand anything,

---

*This ancient Chinese medical classic, more completely translated as *The Yellow Emperor's Classic of Internal Medicine,* has been revered by Chinese healers for more than 3,000 years.

one must first consider its opposite. For instance, the outside of the body, including the extremities, certainly appears more active and *yang* than the inside, which is comparatively dark and still. Therefore the outside is *yang*, and the inside *yin* (represented by the dark eye in the white fish). Looking again at the inside, however, we see that it supplies much of the heat and energy *(yang)* to drive the outward processes, which is an example of *yang* within *yin* (the white eye within the dark fish). "*Yang* within the *yin*" and "*yin* within *yang*" are merely observations that things at their deepest are frequently the opposite of what they appear on the surface. Thus, the conclusion of a pattern is often contrary to what manifests at particular stages along the way. (People who are very conservative will often be liberal in their later years, or vice-versa. The flesh of a peach is delicate and soft *[yin]*, but at its center is a hard pit *[yang]*.)

As a teaching aid, *yang* has traditionally been associated with fire, and *yin* with water.

Consider "expansion" and "contraction" in the chart to the left. According to the theories of physics, most substances expand with heat and contract with cold. During the process of expansion, more heat and energy are required, and therefore expansion is *yang*. Once a substance is expanded, however, it is generally less concentrated in energy and therefore more *yin*. Most people are aware of the diminishing flavor in vegetables (such as zucchini) as they grow large; yet watery *yin* vegetables can balance overly *yang* individuals. Seeds such as grains are very concentrated, so the practice recommended in this book is to expand them somewhat by presoaking and then cooking. For individuals who are overheated (too hot and dry), completely sprouting the seeds may be appropriate. The practice of eating very expanded fruits and vegetables grown with chemical stimulants has partially balanced another extreme practice—excessive consumption of concentrated foods such as meat and eggs. Such "balancing" of extremes is typically unsuccessful over time.

Examples of Yin-Yang Pairs

Yang	Yin
Active	Passive
Heaven	Earth
Function	Substance
Outside	Inside
Mind	Body
Masculine	Feminine
Light	Dark
Time	Space
Heat*	Cold*
Energy of the body	Blood, body fluids and tissues
Excess* and acute conditions	Deficiency* and chronic conditions
Exterior* and superficial imbalances	Interior* and deep imbalances
Expansion	Contraction

* *Heat/cold, excess/deficiency,* and *exterior/interior* can be called the "Six Divisions of *Yin* and *Yang*" and are of therapeutic importance in Chinese medicine. They are explained in the Six Divisions chapters.

To understand *yin* and *yang* clearly, first look at what is, rather than evaluating the "good" and "bad." Seeking "good" and avoiding "evil" is fundamental to health, but prematurely and simplistically judging food, others' motivations, and so on can obscure the reality of a situation. *Yin* and *yang* are expressions of universal justice. They manifest over time in a perfection of balance; gradually learning to live skillfully and peacefully means recognizing this perfection.

If either *yin* or *yang* predominate, the one in excess tends to "consume" the other. For example, excess *heat* in the body dries up the fluids, creating thirst, dry eyes and skin, and a tendency to constipation. A meat-centered diet with hard physical work is the most common way to generate excess heat. Excess *yin* in the body due to the overconsumption of fluids and food can greatly diminish the body's energy and heat. Extra energy is expended in digesting an excess of food, particularly if the food is cooling.

The Principle of Extremes

> Extreme cold produces great heat, and extreme heat produces intense cold.
>
> —*Inner Classic*

When the excessive principle reaches its limit, the extreme *yin* or *yang* transforms into its opposite. This is known as the "Principle of Extremes." This principle is readily observed in warm-blooded animals, when a fever is produced in response to an exposure to cold, or when chills result from an excess of summer heat.

Other examples:

1. Extreme activity, such as hard physical work, necessitates rest.
2. If activity is very fierce and *yang* (such as in war), death (which is very *yin*) can be the result.
3. People frequently become more child-like with extreme age. Also, with advancing years, a person gradually exhibits less physical strength but, if healthy, greater wisdom. This represents the loss of bodily attachment to earth and the shifting of focus toward heaven, an example of extreme *yin* changing to extreme *yang*.
4. As internal heat and blood pressure become higher *(yang)*, a stroke resulting in paralysis *(yin)* becomes more likely.
5. Extremely energizing substances such as cocaine cause utter debility later. One also is eventually weakened by stimulants such as caffeine and refined sugar.
6. In meditation, proper concentration on a single object ultimately results in universal awareness.

The process by which phenomena change into their opposites may be described graphically with spirals, a very common pattern in the universe. These cycles of change are progressively quicker while contracting, slower while expanding. Such cycles are balanced by opposing cycles. For instance, when the national economy slows toward stagnation, cycles of emotional anxiety become ever more intense. Another pair of spirals illustrates the way in which metabolic cycles in the body take longer to fully repeat with age, with a simultaneously greater need for nutrients. For this reason, we need less quantity but more nutritionally concentrated food as we grow older.

Support and Transformation

In a normal state of health, *yin* **and** *yang* **harmoniously support and depend on each other for existence.** Support implies the balanced interplay of *yin* and *yang* and their transformation into one another at any time, not only at the extremes. For example, food in the body transforms into energy. Conversely, energy in the body, especially in the digestive organs, supports the assimilation of nutrients which build the substance of the body.

Further Examples of Mutual Yin-Yang Support in Diet and Activity

Well-cooked food<===>Cold climate

Yellow food<===>Leafy greens

Sweet and pungent food (rising energy)<===>Salty, bitter, and sour food (sinking energy)

Body heat<===>Fluid consumption

Great activity<===>Passive endeavors and rest

Chewing food more completely and breathing more deeply<===>Eating less

Minerals, vitamins, enzymes, fats, starches, proteins, and other nutrients
mutually support each other.

Transcending Yin and Yang

Every object can be subdivided indefinitely, and each subdivision can be described in terms of *yin-yang* **principles.** Even in the case of a single carrot, unlimited *yin-yang* distinctions are possible. The carrot-top greens have less carbohydrate content than the starchy root, and are also of a different shape and color. If the top is removed, we can analyze the root alone, which has an outside, an inside, and also a top and bottom. It is more contracted toward the tip; the outside and bottom are more concentrated in mineral nutrients. Regardless of how one subdivides a carrot, there are still differences in every quality, including the quality of the energy of each part. Even each cell has an orientation within the carrot and therefore a top and bottom, and an inside and outside.

With continuing subdivision (of any object), one eventually reaches the level of subatomic particles. On this level of continuous activity, the principle that all *yin-yang* relationships are in ceaseless transformation can be easily comprehended. Every object, when examined closely enough, demonstrates that all molecular and atomic patterns are either expanding or contracting, more energetic or less, or changing continuously in some other way. Therefore it is said that:

Yin **and** *yang* **are in continual transformation.** Nothing is constant, even for a moment. A state of ultimate health occurs when the moment-by-moment transformations of the body and mind are harmonious. Disease is simply the state in which changes do not happen on time, or in the right way. They may be too much or too soon, too little or too late.

To be able to see the nature of all-pervasive change, it is said that one must experience the absence of change, or stillness. In fact, this is one purpose of the *yin-yang* theory. By an awareness of the limitless changes in our life, we become attentive to consistent patterns, and then to the order in the changes. As we gain skill in understanding change, we naturally become aware of the states beyond change, which embody constant qualities. Unconditional love and compassion are examples of this. "Emptiness" in Eastern philosophy suggests unchanging experience, the disappearance of all distinctions and incomplete states of consciousness, including the ego itself.

Emptiness accompanied by a realization of perfection merits the phrase "Wonderful Existence" in Zen traditions. Without this sense of perfection, one has merely experienced the emptiness of vacuity.

To achieve a consciousness permeated with Wonderful Existence requires a balanced mind and body. This goal is achieved first through purification, then through "middle path" moral, spiritual, and lifestyle practices. "Middle path" certainly does not mean "average" practices, since the average modern person lives a stressful life that fluctuates among many different extremes. Middle-path experiences bring one to a state of balance, or the middle place at the source of all change.

Correct diet helps to achieve this balance. Centered experiences come from sincerity and the developed ability to penetrate to the essence of reality. If diet is seen as something outside of an ultimate experience, then already such thinking has separated food from awareness. If diet and all phenomena are experienced equally, then food is as good a vehicle as any for the development of a unified mind. Many food rituals are intentionally spiritual experiences. For some Christians, an elemental ritual is the recognition of common bread and wine as the substance of Christ. The original ceremony was performed by Jesus when he identified his food as his body and blood, and then asked his followers to continue this practice.

Such an identification is helpful on both the literal and symbolic levels. Literally, his remarks mean that food becomes body and blood. On another plane, where food can be regarded as a symbol of the earth (because it is generated from the soil, air, and water), it could mean that a Christ creates and spiritually directs the earth. On the most profound level, this act, repeated countless times over thousands of years, implies that the Essence of food and all things is Christ-consciousness.

Beyond *yin* and *yang* is Mind, recognizing no boundaries between food and its consumer. A Chan (Chinese Zen) phrase describes this unity: "Everything is made from the Mind alone." The direct experience of the all-inclusive Mind is what we term "ultimate health." Most of us are not able consciously to experience food as identical to ourselves because we have yet to discover our true selves. As a foundation for this, we need to establish relative and measurable health, and this is within the realm of time and space, *yin* and *yang*.

It is therefore necessary to ensure that *yin* and *yang* are accurately understood. Otherwise, we will not only find it difficult to communicate with others who study *yin* and *yang* theory, but we may also delude ourselves. Since everything that exists can be compared to and is related to everything else, there is a temptation to make capricious comparisons without fully discerning the properties being compared.

In terms of the action of foods on the body, a common oversight is to forget the time interval involved. Consider most red meats. If we compare meat with other foods such as vegetables, grains, or fruits, we see that it is high in protein and fat as well as several vitamins and minerals. According to the principles of Chinese medicine, it can be used for certain weakened conditions including a deficiency of *(yin)* fluids, blood, and substance of the body. From a modern standpoint, meat also builds the tissue and blood of the body with its high nutrient content. Therefore, shouldn't we label meat *yin?* Yes—we may label *those* aspects of red meat *yin.* However, meat also has a high caloric content, which can produce an abundance of energy, and from this standpoint meat is *yang.* And yet, if we consider the mucus buildup resulting from meat consumption (compared with most plant foods), and its acid-forming nature which can cause toxic reactions throughout the body, it is easily understood why most people now designate meat as a long-term weakening *(yin)* food if consumed in large amounts.

Since it is clear that every substance has multiple properties, it follows that there are various *yin* and *yang* designations for any food. Note the *yin-yang* food qualities in the table below, and how they can be applied, for example, to apples.

Common Yin-Yang Food Actions	
Yang	**Yin**
Warming	Cooling
Sweet, pungent	Salty, bitter, sour
Energizing	Builds blood and fluids
Ascending energy	Descending energy

In general, apples are sweet, sour, and cooling; they tonify the blood, produce fluids and energy, and have a descending action that directs energy lower into the body. Fully ripe apples are also more *yang*, since they are sweeter. Clearly, because of their mixed characteristics, it is inaccurate to define apples (or any other food) as only *yin* or *yang.* This is what we mean by the need for great accuracy in a *yin-yang* analysis.

With a little sensitivity and practice, becoming aware of at least some of the actual dimensions of the food we eat is not difficult. One may begin to notice the warming and cooling of the body, the ability of the food to build fluids (there will be less thirst and more moisture in the throat), possible diuretic value, and the effects of various flavors. One will also experience internally the *yin-yang* qualities of energy, expansion, and contraction. Food awareness is normally heightened by eating a grain- and vegetable-centered diet for at least six months; during this time one's body becomes attuned to the energy patterns of food. Except in the event of certain illnesses, the majority of one's diet should come from non-extreme foods which have more subtle flavors and actions.

A *yin-yang* analysis can also be made of personality and body types (see the table to the right); this can be invaluable in building a good general diagnostic picture of ourselves and others.

Balance should be the goal of those looking for health, since being too *yin* or too *yang* without being able to return to balance constitutes a state of disease. A modern person will often be simultaneously too *yin* and too *yang*. This is because *yin* and *yang* have not merged, due to a lifestyle more extreme than the person can integrate. When one is well balanced, it is possible to become either very *yin* or very *yang* in response to the demands of the moment, without being stranded in a simultaneous excess of *yin* and *yang*, which is always stressful. The balanced person easily expands or contracts, becomes more active or passive and at the same time remains anchored in stillness (emptiness permeated with Wonderful Existence), the place where *yin* and *yang* fuse into unified reality.

Typical Yin-Yang Qualities Applied to Human Personality and Physiology	
Yang	*Yin*
Warmer body and personality	Cooler body and personality
Dry skin and less body fluid	Moist skin and more body fluid
Outgoing	Introverted
Active	Passive
Masculine	Feminine
Positive	Negative
Focused mind	Serene
Hyperactive mentality	Unclear, dreamy
Aggressive	Timid
Angry, impatient	Fearful, insecure
Loud voice	Soft voice
Urgent	Tardy
Logical	Intuitive
Quick	Slow
Desire-filled	Complacent
Tense, strong body	Flaccid, weak body
Red complexion	Pale complexion

Most people, however, are caught in unconscious and uncontrolled *yin/yang* fluctuations. They may swing between an outgoing personality and introversion, anger and fear, strength and weakness, or other extremes, without being rooted in equilibrium; in this case the following suggestions should be helpful:

> In motion they separate; in stillness they fuse.
>
> —an ancient principle of t'ai chi

- Simply being more aware of imbalance is the first step towards becoming balanced. Once aware, focus on the qualities of balance: kindness, dependability, patience, courage, and appropriate behavior that consistently creates harmony.
- Practice disciplines that emphasize Essence, harmony, and stillness such as prayer, meditation, yoga, and t'ai chi.

- Dietary habits: avoid large amounts of extreme foods including meat, eggs, strongly flavored or refined foods, and those containing chemicals; and eliminate intoxicants, not only because of their strong nature but because their regular use muddies any hope of clear self-evaluation. In general, the dietary recommendations throughout this book support a middle-path approach.

Qi Vitality

A major functional concept from traditional Chinese medicine is *qi* (pronounced "chee" and sometimes spelled *chi*). *Qi* is similar to the term *prana* (life force) of India and is known as *ki* in Japan. A vital essence found in all things, *qi* has aspects of both matter and energy. We will refer primarily to its expression as energy, keeping in mind that energy and matter are convertible into one another. The theories of modern physics showing matter and energy to be alternate descriptions of one reality are very much in accord with the concept of *qi* and other facets of Eastern philosophy.

The *qi* concept gives us a measure for the vitality of a person, object, or state. If the *qi* of a certain food is of good quality, then the food will taste better and impart more *qi* to the individual who consumes it. In a person, good *qi* is manifested as an ability to accomplish things, lack of obstruction in the body, better functioning of the internal organs, and so on. To further understand *qi*, which itself is a *yang* quality, it is helpful to understand its *yin* counterpart—blood. Blood is *yin* and the "mother of *qi*," since the nutrients in blood support and nurture *qi*. At the same time *qi* leads and directs the blood. Furthermore, digestive and circulative *qi* must be sufficient in order for the blood to be formed and to circulate.

Whatever manifests in a person does so with that type of *qi*. Someone who is graceful, for instance, has harmonious *qi;* weak people lack *qi;* those who are strong have abundant *qi;* people with pure, clear minds have "refined" as opposed to "confused" *qi*. Thus *qi* is not only the energy behind these states of being but the intrinsic energy/substance of these states. The *qi* concept, then, provides a way to describe every aspect of life.

From a therapeutic standpoint, there are several functional aspects of *qi*. It is warming and is the source of all movement; it protects the body, flows through the acupuncture channels, and maintains the activity of the body systems and organs. Sources of *qi* in the body are three-fold: 1) from food; 2) from the air we breathe; and 3) from the essence of the kidneys, some part of which we are born with.

How well we utilize *qi* from these sources depends on how we live and on our attitudes. *Qi* is also transferred between people in interactions of every kind. The *qi* of the cook permeates the food. Exercise, herbal therapy, acupuncture, and awareness practices such as meditation are traditional ways of clearing obstructions and maximizing *qi* flow.

Qi that stagnates causes accumulations resulting in obesity, tumors, cysts, cancers, and the multitude of viral and yeast-related diseases that plague those with sedentary lives and refined, rich diets.

The *qi* of the body can be accurately measured and regulated by the diagnostic and therapeutic methods of Chinese medicine. In nutritional therapy, improving the "digestive *qi*" of the spleen-pancreas is a priority to be discussed in the *Earth Element* chapter. In other chapters we will discuss "protective *qi*" as an aspect of immunity, *qi* deficiencies of various organs, *qi* stagnation of the liver, and the practices that improve or damage *qi* in food and the body.

THE SIX DIVISIONS
OF YIN AND YANG

Since *yin* and *yang* are so broadly inclusive, a more specific diagnostic system has been a part of Chinese medicine for centuries. It is extremely rare for every imbalance in an individual to be defined as only *yin* or only *yang*. The system of the Six Divisions evolved to clarify the patterns that underlie the dynamic nature and often contradictory appearances of imbalance. When the following six patterns (three pairs of opposites) are used to describe *yin* and *yang* symptoms, we call them the "Six Divisions of *Yin* and *Yang*."

The Eight Principles

Yin	*Yang*	
Cold	Heat	
Interior	Exterior	**The Six Divisions**
Deficiency	Excess	

In this way, how *yang* a condition is depends on how hot, exterior, and excessive it is. Similarly, a *yin* condition is measured by how cold, interior, and deficient it is. When *yin* and *yang* are expressed as the summary of the Six Divisions, the result is known as the "Eight Principles."

Even though the simple names of the Six Divisions have common meanings, their definitions in the Chinese healing arts are quite specific, so we italicize them here whenever they are used in that context. Most of the definitions will still make sense according to the common usages of the names. Thus the definition of heat as a Chinese medical concept includes how one would experience heat in the body (feeling hot and dry, desiring cold fluids, and so on).

Regardless of whether a disease condition can be accurately diagnosed by modern medicine, the Six Divisions describe important dimensions of every condition: its depth *(interior/exterior)*, thermal nature *(heat/cold)*, and strength *(deficiency/excess)*. With this information, we can make basic dietary and lifestyle recommendations.

Heat/Cold: The Thermal Nature of Food and People

In traditional Chinese medicine, the two most important qualities for food-as-medicine are *heat* and *cold*. Even though these terms hardly sound significant when compared to more sophisticated medical usages, they are distilled from generations of empirical observation and, in their very simplicity, have a diagnostic value that complicated pathological explanations lack.

Heat and cold are fundamental properties in the environment, in people and everything else. When an inanimate object—a rock, for example—is subjected to the quality "cold," it becomes cold; in the presence of "heat," it becomes hot. By contrast, plants and animals in a hot environment can react to heat by cooling methods such as sweating; if they are in a cold environment, warming blood and/or fluids can be sent from their extremities to their interior. Evolution has provided a consensus "thermostat" between an organism and its environment, including for humans clothing, shelter, and food. The effects of these warming and cooling factors on people are common knowledge in the Western world, with the strange exception of food. The caloric content of foods—one of several ways diet alters body temperature—can be calculated scientifically. When used by the public, however, "calorie counting" seems to serve little purpose other than as an esoteric measure by which to practice "scientific" dieting.

The warming and cooling properties of foods actually depend on several different qualities. They change substantially with time, with the part of the plant or animal used, with the nature of meal preparation, and even with where and how it was raised and harvested.

In addition, many plants seem to have a kind of intelligence, exhibiting opposing properties as appropriate. Siberian ginseng, for instance, can lower high blood pressure or raise low blood pressure; lobelia will help discharge a dead fetus but help retain a vital one; some starchy plants (such as dandelion) will raise low blood sugar yet lower high blood sugar. Also, many foods help regulate temperature, either up or down, within certain limits.

How the *heating* or *cooling* effects of plant or animal foods change over time is also of primary importance. For example, salt is initially cooling but also an important substance in climates of high winds and exceedingly low temperatures. The Sherpas who carry supplies for climbers in the Himalayas often walk most of the way barefoot. They bring their own food—grain, salt, and perhaps a few vegetables. Even in most climates within the United States, one finds an attraction to heartier, saltier styles of cooking in cooler times of the year. The properties of salt are discussed further in the *Salt* chapter.

The Physiology of Warming and Cooling Foods

When cooling foods are eaten, the energy and fluids of the body are directed inward and lower *(yin)*, so that the exterior and upper portions of the body cool first. The flow of tree sap toward the roots in colder times of year illustrates this process.

Conversely, warming foods push the deep energy and blood up and out to the surface of the body. The hottest foods, such as cayenne peppers, cause an extreme reaction: one feels temporarily warmer but soon cools as heat radiates out of the body. This short-lived effect is not appropriate for someone who is deeply, chronically cold. Alcohol warms a person in much the same way. However, most warming foods such as dried ginger root, oats, parsnips, butter, and anchovies provide more enduring warmth. The various flavors and dynamics of foods that attune the body to the seasons are listed in the Five Element chapters.

Many theories describe the warming and cooling values of food. Some of the more widely accepted are:

1. Plants that take longer to grow (carrot, rutabaga, parsnip, cabbage, and ginseng, which takes at least six years to grow) are more warming than those that grow quickly (lettuce, summer squash, radish, cucumber).

2. Chemically fertilized plant foods, which are stimulated to grow quickly, are often more cooling. This includes most commercial fruits and vegetables.

3. Raw food is more cooling than cooked food.

4. Food eaten cold is more cooling.

5. Foods with blue, green or purple colors are usually more cooling than similar foods that are red, orange, or yellow (a green apple is more cooling than a red one).

6. Cooking methods that involve more cooking time, higher temperatures, greater pressure, dryness, and/or air circulation (such as convection-oven cooking) impart more warming qualities to food. Time and temperature combine in this way: cooking for a longer time on low heat is more warming than a short time on high heat. Depending on the degree of temperature and pressure, the usual order from more warming to less is: deep-frying or *tempura*, baking, stir-frying or sautéing, pressure cooking, simmering, steaming, and waterless cooking below boiling (212°F). "Heatless cooking" methods of breaking food down in progressively more cooling order include fermenting, marinating, and sprouting.

7. Austrian metaphysician Rudolf Steiner and others have claimed that the

amount and quality of available energy in foods depend in part on the cooking fuel. Arranged in order from the highest-quality energy to the lowest, these are: straw, wood, coal, gas, and electric. Electric cooking is not recommended, especially for people who are weak. For both subjective and scientific reasons, we find validity in Steiner's theories, particularly with regard to electricity.

Microwave cooking, a development since Steiner's time, seems to damage the molecular integrity of food, diminishing its subtle *qi*. Experiments reported in the prestigious British medical journal *The Lancet* (Dec. 9th, 1989) demonstrate that microwave cooking alters food enough to cause, upon ingestion, "structural, functional and immunological changes" in the body. The report further states that microwaves transform the amino acid L-proline into D-proline, a proven toxin to the nervous system, liver, and kidneys.

8. Manipulating food in various ways—e.g., finer cutting, pounding (as in mochi preparation), grinding, pressing (as in pressed salad), and stirring—breaks it down and releases to the body more energy and heat. Furthermore, some studies show that more finely cut food raises blood-sugar levels, which in turn strongly affect thought patterns.

9. Chewing food more thoroughly creates warmth. Even food with a cool temperature will warm if chewed thoroughly. Chewing not only breaks food down but, in the case of carbohydrates, the action of saliva initiates the release of digestive enzymes, facilitating greater assimilation and warmth. The complex carbohydrates such as grains, beans, and vegetables need to be chewed until liquid in consistency, for maximum assimilation and warmth.

10. In most areas of the world, food that provides appropriate warming and cooling properties is naturally available in animal or plant form.

*   *   *

Of all influences on food, the most important is the effect of cooking. Thus it is crucial to understand how cooking increases the warming properties of food. Heating helps break down food structure so that nutrients are more available. In moderate cooking, relatively few nutrients are lost, and those that remain are more easily assimilated. The energy of the body is less focused on digestion and can be used in other ways, such as for higher levels of thought and creativity. Also, with improved assimilation, greater availability of nutrients better sustains the warmth and other functions of the body. In major East Asian awareness practices, raw food is considered too stimulating. Moderately cooked food is recommended to help support more refined consciousness.

From traditional Chinese dietetics:

> One uses cooling foods and preparation methods for someone who is overheated, and warming foods and preparation for those who are too cold.

In order to create the appropriate warming or cooling effects, one chooses foods accordingly. Once foods are chosen, they can still be altered dramatically to fit the situation. Given a limited set of ingredients, a skillful cook can create a large array of therapeutic effects by using the various warming or cooling preparation methods.

When first learning to heal with food, one may fail to recognize the power of warming/cooling food types and preparation techniques, and overcompensate in order to correct a small imbalance. Extreme amounts of warming or cooling foods can have an effect opposite to the one intended.

Knowing the causes of thermal imbalances in the body is important in preventing them.

Heat Patterns and Their Causes

Excess *heat* in the body can be caused by too many warming foods and/or insufficient cooling foods; too much activity or work; exposure to heat or extreme climates (even a cold climate can cause excess *heat*); or obstruction of internal organs. The entire body or any part of it can have too much *heat*.

Until this point, *heat* within the body has been defined as whether or not one feels hot. There are other symptoms, although not all need be present for a *heat* condition to exist. One develops a diagnostic picture of *heat* based on the number and strength of symptoms present. (Diagnostic pictures of *cold* and the remaining qualities in the Six Divisions are developed in the same way.)

The following symptoms describe the actions of (excess) *heat* on various parts of the body. According to Chinese physiology, *heat* profoundly affects the heart, mind, and vascular system, so a good number of symptoms will affect those areas.

Signs of Heat
- Major Characteristics: Heat rises and dries fluids.
- Major Symptoms: Person feels hot, fears or dislikes heat, and is attracted to cold.
- Head (heat rises): bright red tongue, yellow coating on tongue, red face, red eyes, nosebleeds, canker sores, "rotten" smell in mouth.
- Heart, mind, and body tissues: high blood pressure, hemorrhage, inappropriate or incoherent speech, convulsions, delirium, full and fast radial pulse (six or more beats per complete inhalation and exhalation), entire body too warm (fever). The following are considered heat conditions if they are marked with redness and/or a sensation of heat: local inflammations, swellings, rashes, skin eruptions, and sores.
- Digestion and elimination (heat dries up fluids): constipation, dry and smelly stools, dark yellow or red urine, blood in stools or urine, desire for cold liquids in quantity, matter excreted (urine, feces, mucus) is forceful and urgent, mucus and phlegm are thick and yellow or green.

Suggestions for Chronic Heat Conditions

Practice listening and cultivate less aggressive attitudes. When this is successfully done, it is often much easier to desire less meat and other aggressive types of food.

> When a heat condition shows little improvement, and then meat is eaten, there will be a relapse. If too much food is eaten, then there will be residual effects.
>
> —*Inner Classic*

It is also important to eat less food and maintain ample fluid intake. Especially avoid red meats, chicken, alcohol, coffee, and cigarettes; goat's milk is recommended if animal products are to be used. Other animal products with a neutral (n) or cooling (c) energy—yogurt (c), cow dairy (n), eggs (n), clam (c), crab (c)—must be used cautiously because they may cause obstructions which aggravate *heat* conditions. Small amounts of almonds, sesame seeds, or freshly shelled sunflower seeds, although not cooling, supply important nutrients, including calcium, for the vascular system.

Cooking methods: Avoid pressure, baking, or deep-frying methods. Steam, simmer, and use more raw foods.

In addition, decrease the quantity of heat-producing foods (see examples on pages 66–67) and use more of the cooling varieties.

Cooling Foods Which Reduce Heat Signs

Fruit	Vegetable	Legumes and Grains	Other Products
apple	lettuce	soy milk	kelp and all seaweeds
banana	radish	soy sprouts	spirulina; wild blue-green
pear	cucumber	tofu	oyster-shell calcium
persimmon	celery	tempeh	wheat and barley grass
cantaloupe	button mushroom	mung beans and	kudzu
watermelon	asparagus	their sprouts	yogurt
tomato	Swiss chard	alfalfa sprouts	crab
all citrus	eggplant	millet	clam
	spinach	barley	*Herbs and Spices:*
	summer squash	wheat and its	peppermint
	cabbage (green,	products	dandelion greens and root
	purple, or Napa)	amaranth	honeysuckle flowers
	bok choy		nettles
	broccoli		red clover blossoms
	cauliflower		lemon balm
	sweet corn		white peppercorn
	zucchini		cilantro
			marjoram

Note: The following foods with a neutral energy can also be used during *heat* conditions because they will not add further warmth: rice, rye, corn, peas, lentils, and all beans besides soy and mung (listed above), and black beans (which are warming). The few common warming vegetables and fruits are given on page 66; most others are either cooling (listed above) or neutral (see "Fruits" and "Vegetables" in recipe section for their properties).

Suggestions for Acute Heat Conditions

If symptoms are acute (for instance, high fever), use mostly liquids in the form of cooling vegetable or fruit juices, broths, and herbal teas. The temperature of the beverages should not be cold, because cold food and drink weaken the body as they cool it.

Acute infections often involve *heat* and other excesses, and are discussed in the *Excess and Deficiency* chapter, page 91.

Deficiency and Heat

Fewer people today have excess *heat* symptoms than in the past. By far the most common *heat* symptom is *"deficiency-heat"* or *"deficient yin,"* produced not by an excess of *heat* but by a deficiency of the *yin* fluids and structure which provide balance for the *heat* in the body. (Recall that the *yin* aspect of the body includes not only all fluids [blood,* lymph, hormones, all secretions, intracellular fluids, etc.], but also the solid substance of the body—its bones, muscles, and other tissues.)

A person can experience this condition even with subnormal *heat* and energy, if the *yin* aspects of the body are so low that the *heat* appears relatively excessive. Nonetheless, many people who overeat rich, denatured foods exhibit signs of *deficient yin* in spite of having an abundance of fluids and ample body structure. It seems that in these cases their *yin* is of inferior quality, and functions poorly in the body. For example, their blood or other body fluids may be lacking in calcium and other cooling minerals, and their tissues may be deficient in polyunsaturated fatty acids, particularly the omega-3 variety that clean arteries and help prevent inflammation. This produces symptoms of *heat* actually caused by inadequate *yin* function.

Deficient Yin Symptoms

The classic diseases often associated with *deficient yin* are hypoglycemia, diabetes, tuberculosis, and anxiety as well as wasting diseases where there is long-term inflammation and infection from viruses, bacteria, fungi, parasites, and other pathogenic microbes. Thus, most chronic degenerative diseases eventually become marked with signs of *deficient yin*. Common symptoms of *deficient yin* include:

---

*Building the *yin* in general does not always adequately treat a blood deficiency; these are discussed in the "Blood Deficiency" section in Chapter 31.

Major characteristic: The appearance of minor *heat* signs.

Fluids: May drink small amounts of fluid often throughout the day. Dryness of mouth, tongue, cough, and breath.

Body: Tends to be thin; in extreme cases there is emaciation. A poor diet, however, may produce symptoms in any body type. Conditions of instability and erratic change (usually associated with *wind* imbalances and discussed in later chapters) are sometimes induced by a lack of *yin;* examples include vertigo, spasms, cramps, and pains that move.

Mind: Insomnia, irritability, uneasiness, worry, excess thought.

Color: Fleshy pink or fresh red tongue and cheeks, especially in the afternoon.

Heat: Low intermittent fever, palms and soles may be hot and sweaty, night sweats.

Pulse: Fast and thin.

Note: Only one symptom has to be present for *deficient yin* to exist.

Deficient yin symptoms typify the modern person—uneasy, anxious, with abundant energy that is mostly appearance; often deeper energy is lacking. This person snacks and may sip soft drinks or other beverages during the day. Relationships are filled with irritations and/or skirmishes.

What has caused the proliferation of *deficient yin?* It may be a result of the dominance of the *yang* principle and extreme heat for several generations in the industrial era. Stress, excessive noise, competition, and warming, nutrient-depleting substances such as alcohol, coffee, cigarettes, and most synthetic drugs burn up the *yin* quickly. Even overconsumption of very hot spices such as cayenne pepper and garlic can deplete the *yin*. Refined foods and those grown on wasted soils cannot build balanced *yin*. Gradually, in the offspring, the ability of the body as a whole (and the kidneys in particular) to supply sufficient *yin* fluids and substances of good quality has seriously deteriorated. *Yin* nurtures and stabilizes; it is the receptive principle, and represents the earth. The lack of quality *yin* is evident not only in people; the earth itself reflects this deficiency as high-quality sources of food and water dwindle. Actions that build a substantial *yin* foundation for an individual are the same ones that restore the planet.

Building the Foundations of Receptivity: Preserving the Yin

Cultivate practices that harmonize the active *(yang)* principle and simultaneously build the receptive, yielding, compassionate *(yin)* qualities. Awareness practices such as yoga and devotional contemplation, and activities that connect with the earth and soil such as gardening, are helpful.

Respect animals and avoid intoxicants and all refined foods. Meat, eggs, and most other animal products build the *yin* fluids and body tissues but when eaten extensively leave residues of sticky mucus. Therefore these products are questionable as primary sources of quality *yin* for the body. Refined sugar and many intoxicants offer a quick, temporarily refreshing *yin*-fix but ultimately deplete both *yin* and *yang* because of their unbalanced and/or extreme natures.

Use foods that support planetary renewal, especially unprocessed local food. Shipping, packaging, and refrigerating foods from distant origins involves an enormous waste of energy and especially petroleum resources.

Deficient Yin and Blood Sugar Imbalances

From the standpoint of both traditional Chinese and modern Western medicine, water and sugar metabolisms are interrelated and depend on the health of all the body organs, particularly the pancreas, kidney-adrenals, liver, and lungs. Protein also plays a key role in the water (*yin* fluid) and sugar balances in the body.

It is well known that protein and carbohydrates (sugars) regulate each other. As protein levels rise, so does the need for sugar in the body. A chronic, growing spiral of first taking in more proteins, followed by more sweet foods and then more protein, etc. often ends in either a low blood sugar condition (hypoglycemia), or the next and more degenerate stage known as hyperglycemia, or diabetes. As these conditions develop, the stress from the high levels of protein and sugar in the body weakens the kidney-adrenal function, which in turn decreases the distribution of fluids in the body—a *deficient yin* condition. Thus the person with insufficiency of *yin* and its accompanying fluids may have any of several minor *heat* signs such as tidal fevers, continual but small thirst, hot palms, etc. The long-term solution to the protein-sugar spiral is to use only moderate quantities of protein and sugars, such as supplied by the complex carbohydrates. (Diabetes and hypoglycemia are discussed in Chapter 29.)

Specific Foods Which Tonify the Yin

Many carbohydrates and animal products that maintain the *yin* of the body can be used therapeutically to overcome a marked *yin* deficiency, especially: millet, barley, wheat germ, wheat, rice, teff (discussed in note 7 on page 687), quinoa, amaranth, seaweeds, micro-algae (especially chlorella and spirulina), tofu, black beans, kidney beans, mung beans (and their sprouts), beets, string beans, kuzu, persimmon, grapes, blackberry, raspberry, mulberry, banana, and watermelon. In more extreme cases supplemental animal products may be helpful such as dairy products (cow's or goat's milk, yogurt, cheese, etc.), chicken egg, clam, abalone, oyster, sardine, duck, beef, or pork. It is beneficial to prepare some of the daily food in a watery medium, as in soups, stews, and congees. When allergies, degenerative diseases, or other imbalances result at least partially from overconsumption of animal products, the animal foods above may not be appropriate. In any case, herbs are highly effective for supplementing all dietary *yin* tonics; herbs for building the *yin* of the kidneys (page 357), with the exception of marshmallow root, also build the general bodily *yin* discussed here.

Cold Patterns and Their Causes

Patterns of *cold* in the body arise from lack of physical activity, eating too much cooling food, or overexposure to a cold environment; another cause is a deficit of *yang (heat)* resulting from insufficient warming food in the diet or constitutional weakness at birth.

Signs of Coldness

- *Coldness* is part of the *yin* principle and is also associated with the Water Element. Water includes the kidneys and bladder, bones, head hair, the emotion fear, and sexual function. As described in the *Water Element* chapter, these areas can be adversely affected by a *cold* condition.
- *Cold* in the body resembles ice; it is hard and motionless. *Coldness* causes contraction, so the *cold* person bends back or moves around with difficulty. Pain from *cold* can be intense and fixed. (Contraction is the body's attempt to conserve heat.)
- The major symptoms of *coldness* include chill sensations, dislike of cold, and an attraction to warmth. A person with signs of *coldness* will usually be overdressed and attracted to warm food and drinks. The complexion tends toward white. Bodily excretions will be copious and clear, such as clear urine, watery stools, or thin, watery mucus.

Specific Remedies

1. Work on fears and insecurities; become more active; avoid long hot baths; keep kidney area (in lower back), legs, and lower abdomen warm.

2. Use warming foods and methods of preparation, and fewer raw and cooling foods (see cooling food examples in "Heat" section); avoid microwave cooking. Do not eat food below room temperature, or very hot.

3. Use ginger root (preferably dried) cooked with black beans, aduki beans, lentils, or with other foods. Also use ginger, cinnamon bark or twig, cloves, basil, rosemary, and/or angelica root in teas and foods regularly. (Avoid adukis if person is thin or has *dry* signs such as dry skin, throat, and nostrils.)

4. Warming grains and seeds: oats, spelt, quinoa, sunflower seed, sesame seed, walnut, pinenut, chestnut, fennel, dill, anise, caraway, carob pod, cumin, sweet brown rice and its products such as mochi. Rice, corn, buckwheat, and rye are acceptable here, as they have a neutral energy, but the other grains are cooling, and should be used sparingly.

5. Warming vegetables and fruit: parsnip, parsley, mustard greens, winter squash, sweet potato, kale, onion, leek, chive, garlic, scallion; cherry, citrus peel, and date.

6. The most intensely warming foods are hot peppers, the hottest of them cayenne. All hot peppers (including black pepper) must be used in small pinches or they can have a strong cooling effect. In a similar but less extreme way, certain concentrated sweeteners are warming and should be used moderately (by

the teaspoon); otherwise weakening, cooling results are likely. Examples of warming unrefined sweeteners are barley malt, rice syrup, and molasses.

7. The above remedies are usually adequate; in the event that they are not, moderate amounts of animal products may help. Butter is the only dairy product that creates warmth; milk and cheese have a neutral energy. Anchovy, mussel, trout, chicken, beef, and lamb are some of the common warming animal foods.

Typical Patterns

Older people tend to be *cold;* people who are recently vegetarian tend towards *coldness* during the transition period of several months. It takes longer for a *cold* person to build warmth than for a *hot* person to lose excess *heat*. If a person is not clearly *hot* or *cold*, or if there is some confusion, then a diet balanced in warming and cooling properties according to the seasons is best.

The condition we know as "the common cold" sometimes has *cold* patterns, but since it is normally an *exterior* condition, it will be discussed in the ensuing *Interior/Exterior* chapter.

Interior/Exterior: Building Immunity

When developing a diagnostic overview, the first polarity to consider is that of *interior* and *exterior,* since these indicate the depth of the disease. An *exterior* condition is termed *yang*, and an *interior* one *yin*. Therefore an *exterior* condition has more active qualities, is often an acute condition of short duration, and affects most strongly the surface or *exterior* parts of the body. These parts include all external tissues: the skin, hair, muscles, tendons, and the orifices (mouth, nose, external ears, anus). The joints, the most external aspect of the bones, are also considered *exterior.* Knowing that an *exterior* disease lodges in these tissues tells us something about its cure—sweating (diaphoresis) is the most efficient method of driving out surface pathogens.

Conditions that manifest as *exterior* have a sudden onset triggered by external environmental influences such as wind, cold, heat, or damp; in most cases, wind combines with either cold or heat, and affects the skin, the mucous membranes of the nasal passages and lungs, and their immunity. At this point viruses, germs, or other pathogens can establish themselves, resulting in fevers, chills, joint and muscle pain. If the resulting condition is not purged by sweating or other means, then the disease will usually move deeper in stages, becoming more *interior* and chronic. If a person has extremely weak *wei qi*, the immune-energy concept of Chinese medicine, then environmental influences and pathogens can penetrate directly to the *interior* levels, without first being slowed by surface defenses.

Someone with an *exterior* condition who uses the remedies for healing an *interior* one may drive the *exterior* condition deeper. Conversely, sweating can be very dangerous for those with *interior* conditions of extreme weakness. Therefore, skill is needed to determine whether a condition is at a superficial level and easily cured, or at a deeper level requiring more time and care. We often sense intuitively whether a condition is mild or deep, but to be certain, the following definitions will help:

Signs of an Exterior Condition
- Recent condition; short duration
- Simultaneous fevers and chills
- Stuffy head, runny nose, thin coating on tongue
- Achiness, stiff neck, recent headache
- Intolerance to wind or cold

Colds, Flus, and Other Exterior Conditions

Exterior diseases first affect the body surfaces that are exposed directly to the environment—the skin and the mucous membranes of the nose, throat, and lungs. Thus the most prevalent *exterior* conditions are the common cold and flu. Contagious diseases that affect the sinuses, bronchials, and throat often have *exterior* signs in their initial stages. These and all other *exterior* diseases are usually easy to cure when they are still on the surface of the body, i.e., when they still have the above *exterior* symptoms.

The sooner one notices these conditions and takes action, the more likely their interior progress can be reversed. In order to balance such conditions, we choose spices and herbs that are expansive and reach toward the periphery of the body, and those that open (expand) the sweat glands to sweat out the *exterior* disease factor lodged near the surface. In cases where sweating does not stop the disease, it will at least greatly reduce its progress and strength. Sometimes people try to cure the common cold at its onset with strengthening, salty, or building foods such as ginseng, miso, or animal products, but these can worsen the existing condition and trap pathogens inside the body because of their strong inner-directing effect.

Suggestions for Treating Exterior Conditions
- Eat much less, and use a more simple, liquid-based diet such as vegetable or grain soup if chills predominate over the fever. If the fever predominates, fruit or vegetable juices or fresh fruits are a better alternative.
- Use sweating therapy (diaphoresis). However, sweating is contraindicated when there is emaciation, severe weakness, or lack of *yin* fluids (dryness, fast and thin pulse, fresh red cheeks or tongue, and/or night sweats). If the person is weak, with a fever and aching muscles, and perspires greatly without any improvement, such a rare *deficient* condition with spontaneous sweating implies that the ability to absorb nutrition and build protective *qi* (*wei qi* or

immunity) is low. Herbal preparations that build the nutritive and protective *qi* include teas (decoctions) of either fresh ginger root or cinnamon twig. The choices of food should be nurturing and warming (grain and vegetable-leek soups, for example).

Sweating procedure: Drink a cup or more of hot diaphoretic herbal tea, take a hot bath or shower, drink more tea, then cover in blankets and sweat. (See page 110 for ways to prepare tea.) Do not sweat to the point of exhaustion. After sweating, change damp bedding and rest.

Sweating once is sometimes enough; if not, it can be repeated twice daily until *exterior* signs lift. If baths are inconvenient, drink ½ cup of the tea every half hour until perspiring freely. When diaphoresis does not work, a deeper condition likely exists. Note: Sweating therapy is also beneficial for measles and similar infectious diseases marked by rashes. It helps bring the toxins in the rash out of the body.

Some imbalances such as chronic skin diseases and rheumatic joint and muscle diseases are primarily deep *interior* conditions with pronounced *exterior* manifestations. In these cases (discussed in later chapters), sweating therapy is still useful, but is not the primary treatment.

Common diaphoretic herbs: Yarrow, boneset flowers or leaves, elder flowers (often combined with boneset), chamomile, catnip, peppermint, desert tea* (*Ephedra viridis*), cayenne red pepper* (one of the highest botanic sources of vitamin C), ma huang* (*Ephedra sinica*), angelica*, fresh ginger root* (highly preferred over dried ginger root for *exterior* conditions). One of these teas can be drunk for the duration of the condition. A valuable folk remedy calls for adding lemon and honey (preferably raw) to the teas; use rose hips as a good vitamin C source. Fresh rose hips contain much more vitamin C than dried. The antiviral properties of garlic* can often halt a cold or flu if taken soon enough: every three hours during the day that symptoms first appear, hold, without chewing, half a peeled garlic clove between the cheek and teeth for 20–30 minutes. Move it around occasionally to avoid "burning" delicate mouth tissue. If the juice is still too strong, use an uncut clove for a longer period.

Helpful foods: Bioflavonoid-rich food such as cabbage with hearts, and green peppers with their insides. Other useful foods include parsley, carrots, broccoli, turnips, kuzu (especially good for treating a stiff or painful upper back or neck from an *exterior* condition; also useful for measles), parsnips*, horseradish*, scallions*, garlic*, lemon juice, grapefruit, and most fruits.

In some *exterior* conditions, either chills or a fever will predominate. For predominating chills, use the warming herbs and foods marked "*" for best results. When fevers predominate, or in the case of measles and similar diseases with rashes, the other herbs and foods mentioned above are more effective. If fevers and chills are of equal strength, any of the foods and herbs recommended above are helpful.

Once the acute stage and exterior symptoms pass, then gradually introduce normal foods in order to build strength. If colds, flus, and various *exterior* conditions are frequent, one is probably consuming too many sweets, salty foods, and/or excess dairy, eggs, or other mucus- and acid-forming foods (examples of these foods are in the *Fasting and Purification* chapter). In some cases colds are not easily cured, and a longer-term lung condition results, marked by strong *heat* signs, copious mucus, or other attributes. Remedies for these imbalances appear in the *Metal Element* chapter.

Signs of Interior, Deeper Conditions

Interior conditions are usually easily identified: they are all conditions that are not *exterior.* The *interior* areas of the body include all bones and internal organs, and the deeper nerves and blood vessels. *Interior* symptoms can include pains inside the body, vomiting, weakness, chronic headaches, fevers with no aversion to cold, or chills with no aversion to heat (as opposed to *simultaneous* chills and fever of *exterior* conditions), and deep or sensitive emotional states. Common examples are chronic digestive problems, mental disorders, high blood pressure, tumors, osteoporosis, diabetes, and chronic backache. *Interior* conditions in general are caused by imbalances in the emotions, weakness from birth, diet excesses or deficiencies, or the migration of an *exterior* condition to the *interior.*

After some reflection on who is afflicted by disease and to what degree, one begins to realize that nearly everyone has some sort of chronic, *interior* condition—perhaps a minor ache since youth, a problem with digestion that never quite clears up, or the predominance of a mental state such as depression, impatience, or worry.

Some chronic *interior* problems are mild; others are deep. Since it is not always obvious just how deep a condition is, some basic guidelines from traditional Chinese diagnosis are listed in the table below.

For those whose *interior* conditions seem mild, it is of course important to act quickly rather than wait and allow the condition to degenerate.

Gauging the Depth of Interior Conditions: Observation of the Spirit and Its Expression		
	Milder Condition	**Deeper Condition**
Spirit	lively	weak, defeated
Eyes	sparkling*	dull
Behavior	normal/appropriate	inappropriate
Speech/response	clear	sluggish, weak, or uncooperative
Respiration	normal	feeble, labored, or uneven

*The eyes are like a lamp for the whole body. If your eyes are sound, your whole body will be full of light.—Matthew 6:22

For more debilitating, deeper conditions, the basic recommendations appear later in Chapter 6 under "Guidelines for Treating Severe Deficiencies." Since "*interior*" is such a general category, exact therapies, diets, and medications cannot be prescribed without a more specific personal diagnosis.

Many types of chronic conditions, particularly degenerative diseases, involve impaired immunity. The next section offers important East-West insights into the immune system, along with suggestions for strengthening it.

Immunity
And the Protective Qi Concept

The model of the immune system used in the Chinese herbal and acupuncture systems presents a simple view that has proven quite functional. Whether a contagious or climate-induced condition is *interior* or *exterior* depends on the strength of one's immune system, which in turn is related to the concept *wei qi* or "protective *qi*." When the protective *qi* is strong, diseases from viruses and weather influences entering the body are completely warded off; if it is less strong, diseases may enter onto an *exterior* level and bring about a cold, flu, or other *exterior* condition; if it is very deficient, disease factors may penetrate to *interior* levels, more profoundly affecting the functioning of internal organs.

Protective *qi* is considered the most vigorous type of energy in the body. In the daytime it is mainly distributed in the skin and muscles, warming and nourishing all the outer (subcutaneous) tissues. There it circulates, opening and closing the pores and sweat glands and defending the body against outside disease factors such as the extremes of climate and the assaults of microorganisms. At night, protective *qi* circulates deeper, within the organs of the body. According to traditional teachings, it is derived from essential substances in food and in inhaled air.[1] This ancient model of protective *qi* works well with our modern concept, since both maintain that the ability to absorb nutrients and utilize oxygen is critical to immune function.

In the last generation, allergies, degenerative diseases, and other general signs of poor immunity have reached epidemic proportions. Contributing to these conditions is what is commonly known as "candida" infection.

Candida Overgrowth: Immune Inhibitor

Candidiasis, the overgrowth of *Candida* yeast-like fungi in the body, illustrates the Eastern concept of *dampness* in which there are feelings of heaviness and sluggishness, mental dullness, possible infections with yeasts and other microorganisms, and pathogenic moisture such as edema and excess mucus. Recent research shows that *Candida albicans* and several related fungi often proliferate in people's bodies in the presence of digestive and other metabolic imbalances.

It appears that candida exists in high levels in individuals with weak immune systems, although it is normal to have some candida present. A healthy digestive system has ample *Lactobacillus acidophilus* and other intestinal microorganisms which are indispensable to proper nutrient absorption. Candida has an opposite effect in the digestive tract, inhibiting proper assimilation of essential amino acids and other nutrients. What follows in candidiasis is the weakening of immunity as well as the entire organism.

The yeast does not always confine itself to the digestive tract. It slips through weakened areas in the gut lining, or can be spread from the anus into the sexual organs (especially in women), and from those areas into the blood and other body tissues. Such migrations of candida through the entire system, usually termed *systemic* candidiasis, is life-threatening if untreated, and is thought by some to be the cause of death in AIDS (Acquired Immune Deficiency Syndrome) and various other viral-related degenerative illnesses.[2] Author Dr. Kurt Donsbach,* who directs the Hospital Santa Monica in Rosarito Beach, Baja California, Mexico, which specializes in therapy for candidiasis, sees the condition as the root cause of all major diseases.

Toxic by-products of the normal metabolic processes of systemic candida stimulate the immune system's production of antibodies, and in serious yeast infestations tax the immune system to the point where it cannot respond to invading viruses or other harmful substances. Immunity ultimately breaks down, which opens the way for autoimmune diseases such as rheumatoid arthritis, multiple sclerosis, and lupus, as well as diseases of immune devastation including AIDS and cancer. Even if none of the above conditions set in, the effects of the yeast-induced systemic poisoning can cause allergic reactions to minor environmental or dietary toxins. If the condition is allowed to progress, one can become hyper-allergic, reacting to almost everything.

Candida Overgrowth Symptoms: The symptoms of high levels of candida growth may include chronic tiredness, mental sluggishness, chronic vaginitis or prostatitis, anal itching, bloating and other digestive problems, bad breath, extreme sensitivity to tobacco smoke and chemical fumes, mucus in the stools, frequent colds, craving for sweets and yeasted breads, recurrent fungal infections such as athlete's foot, and low immunity in general. Those with systemic candidiasis may suffer from any of the above symptoms and also often exhibit a scattered and unfocused mind, memory loss, and, in severe cases, mental derangements such as manic/depression and delusions; also common are allergies to many foods and environmental substances.

---

*Kurt W. Donsbach, Ph.D., D.Sc., N.D., D.C., is chairman of the Board of Governors of the National Health Federation and "has helped expose the monopolistic hold that the pharmaceutical giants and organized medicine have on the act of healing." (—from a biographical sketch in his monograph *Candida Albicans & Systemic Candidiasis*)

Dr. Donsbach is one of the most widely read contemporary writers on health issues.

Causes of Candida Problems

The yeast- and *dampness*-creating foods are those which are cold in temperature, too sweet or salty, mucus-producing, and stale or rancid. Too much raw food additionally weakens digestion, evidenced by loose or watery stools. Also included among yeast-inducing products are certain kinds of ferments, yeasted breads, alcoholic beverages, most intoxicants, and any food in excessive amounts. Complicated meals of many ingredients promote pathogenic fermentation in the digestive system, exactly what yeasts thrive on. Simple food combining (see *Food Combinations* chapter, Plan B) is required for effective yeast control.

The factor that contributes most to candida proliferation and the degeneration of digestive strength is the use of massive and/or repeated doses of broad-spectrum antibiotics. These drugs kill off all microorganisms in the digestive tract—including the favorable ones—and prepare a fertile environment for the growth of yeasts and fungi. People with chronic tiredness and other symptoms of candidiasis can often trace the source of their troubles to the use of antibiotics.

If antibiotics must be taken, re-establishing a healthy flora during and after their use can be done with acidophilus culture (available at health food stores), raw sauerkraut, chlorophyll-rich foods such as deep-green vegetables and barley-grass concentrates, and/or small daily amounts of miso soup (see "Ferments" later in this chapter for dosages). Low-level ingestion of antibiotics occurs from eating commercial meat, dairy, eggs, and poultry, since most livestock are dosed daily with antibiotics in their feed.

Women who take oral contraceptives are found to be at greater than average risk of developing candidiasis, and even though the precise etiology is unknown, it is clear that a continual unnatural stimulation of the hormonal system unbalances the same organs—the liver and pancreas—that support a healthy environment in the digestive tract.

Anxiety and worry, according to Chinese physiology, greatly contribute to *damp* excesses such as yeast overgrowth. (Other contributing factors are discussed in the *Earth Element* chapter.)

Controlling Candida with Diet

Complex Carbohydrates: Foods rich in carbohydrates must be used moderately since they are usually somewhat mucus- and acid-forming, and therefore any small excess can contribute to yeast and fungal conditions. For people without these conditions, the mild mucus-forming property of whole grains and other unrefined complex carbohydrates can be beneficial. If chewed thoroughly and not overeaten, the carbohydrates become more alkaline and less mucus-forming.

Contrary to the rules of some candida therapies, a variety of grains can be recommended—they are good sources of lignins and certain factors which inhibit yeasts and other anaerobic growth (discussed in *Cancer and the Regeneration Diets* chapter). These grains include millet, roasted buckwheat groats (kasha), rye, oats, barley, amaranth, and quinoa. Cereals such as cracked rye or barley should be freshly milled just before cooking to avoid rancidity. The lightly cooked sprouts of barley, rice, and millet, rich in digestive enzymes, are used in Chinese herbology for improving nutrient assimilation and resolving digestive stagnation. These, along with rye and quinoa sprouts, are a useful remedy for yeast overgrowth. In a candida-controlling regime, all of the above grains can account for 20% of the diet by weight. The sprouts of these grains are healthy options, and can occupy as much as an additional 20% of the diet.

The aduki bean dries *damp* conditions, and the mung bean is detoxifying, so these can be used more often than other beans. Their sprouts, and those of soybeans, are especially recommended. Beans and other legumes are easier to digest if first sprouted or if eaten only with green and low-starch vegetables (page 265). These vegetables are also among the best foods for limiting candida growth.

If the tongue coating is thick, greasy, and/or yellow, it indicates the need for cleansing accumulated mucus in the digestive tract: consume one to two ounces daily of common button or other mushrooms, about three ounces of daikon radish, or three or four red radishes.

Very sweet or starchy vegetable tubers such as yams, sweet potatoes, and potatoes are best avoided. Other starchy vegetables, including carrots, parsnips, rutabagas, and beets, may be eaten regularly. Total vegetable consumption can be 40% to 50% of the diet. Legumes (beans, peas, and lentils) and their sprouts can make up 10% of the diet.

Sweeteners and fruit: Concentrated sweeteners (e.g., sugar, molasses, maple syrup) and most fruits propagate yeast in the body and should be avoided. However, all berries, pomegranates, lemons, and limes can normally be tolerated in moderation. Additionally, the sweetener "stevia" can be tolerated. (See pages 194–195 for stevia information.)

Animal proteins: Sufficient protein is available in legumes and grains. Most milk products, eggs, and red meats have properties that promote yeast/fungus growth and are not recommended. If animal products seem necessary, fish and fowl raised without chemicals may be helpful. Also, some individuals do well with raw goat's milk, in which case the other animal products are usually unnecessary.

Ferments: Certain fermented and yeasted foods can promote yeasts in the digestive tract. This is due to a "cross-over sensitivity" between these foods and the candida yeast. However, miso, soy sauce, tempeh, and tofu are fermented foods that can be tolerated intermittently in small amounts, depending on the person. When they are cooked, the effect of the fermentation is less strong. Used correctly, quality miso and soy sauce seem to promote good intestinal flora, but they must be tested for tolerance and dosage. If there is a sensitivity, one will feel weak and tired soon after these foods are consumed in excess. Usually ½ teaspoon miso or soy sauce daily causes no problem.

Regular consumption of raw saltless sauerkraut, which can include seaweeds, garlic, and other vegetables in addition to cabbage, is highly recommended to candida sufferers. It establishes the beneficial acidophilus culture in the digestive tract. (Refer to "Pickles" in recipe section.) If such a sauerkraut is not used, then an intestinal bioculture supplement should be taken with a daily meal.

However, there are better bioculture options than the commonly used acidophilus products. Spore-based products, e.g., L. sporogenes and B. laterosporus, can replace acidophilus in almost every case and are substantially more effective. They destroy yeasts, and feed on wastes and pathogenic bacteria in the intestines while supporting the generation of acidophilus and other beneficial flora. Take either of these products on an empty stomach once daily, or twice daily when symptoms of candida are severe.

Yeasted bread, brewer's yeast, and ferments including common vinegar and alcoholic beverages are best avoided. Naturally leavened, whole-grain sourdough rye bread may be used in place of yeasted. Quality vinegar (page 205) is also useful.

Oils, nuts, and seeds: Most oils and oil-rich products such as commercially shelled nuts and seeds are rancid and a source of immune-inhibiting "free radicals," a concept to be discussed later in this chapter. Lightly roasting shelled nuts and seeds helps to diminish their rancidity; better yet, shell them just before eating. Because foods rich in oils can overwork the liver, weaken the pancreas, and cause *dampness*, we suggest that individuals with candida use nuts, seeds, avocados, oils, and other fatty foods very sparingly if at all. Flaxseed and its oil is an exception; up to one tablespoon of unrefined, cold-pressed flaxseed oil can be taken daily with a meal. (See *Oils and Fats* chapter for ways to use crushed or whole flax seeds.)

Another exception is oils rich in oleic acid. Used sparingly, these tend to inhibit candida yeasts; extra virgin olive oil is the best of the oleic-rich oils for yeast control. If oils are used in cooking, a scant teaspoon of olive can be tolerated once a day.

Other Helpful Products

Garlic has exceptional anti-viral/fungal properties and does not damage the healthful intestinal flora. Suggested dosage is ½ clove, twice a day before meals, and just after taking wheat- or barley-grass concentrates. The cereal grasses help to protect the stomach and liver from garlic's fiery quality. If raw garlic tastes too strong, garlic products rich in the anti-yeast compound "allicin" can be taken in the upper dosage range suggested by the manufacturer.

Garlic is also one of the best cures for vaginal yeasts. Yeasts in this area of the body are difficult to eradicate because they burrow through several layers of tissue, becoming intracellular parasites. As surface tissue sloughs off, a new infection can then arise. The treatment for these yeasts must be continued for at least one month. A clove of garlic, threaded through with a cotton pull-string, is inserted vaginally and left in place overnight, five nights a week for one month. If this proves to be too hot, leave another layer or two of the outer peel on the garlic. Douching with teas of garlic or pau d'arco (see below) during the day is also helpful. A douche of vinegar diluted in two parts water temporarily relieves irritating symptoms.

The herb **pau d'arco** *(Tabevulia)* excels in controlling candida. Other herbs, especially bitter ones such as chaparral *(Larrea divaricata)* and burdock *(Arctium lappa)* have been helpful. If candidiasis has arisen from overuse of antibiotics, chaparral can be taken for three weeks to draw out the residues resulting from antibiotic suppression of disease processes. (General herbal usage guidelines are listed in the *Dietary Transition* chapter.)

Green plants have abundant chlorophyll, which is purifying and stops the spread of bacteria, fungi, and other microorganisms; chlorophyll also promotes the growth of beneficial intestinal flora. Parsley, kale, collard and dandelion greens, chard, watercress, romaine lettuce, cabbage, micro-algae (spirulina, chlorella, wild blue-green [aphanizomenon]), barley grass, and wheat grass all contain significant amounts of chlorophyll. Of all the greens, barley and wheat grass are perhaps the most effective for treating yeasts; each contains hundreds of enzymes which help to resolve substances that may be toxic or difficult to digest.

For controlling candida, the cereal grasses work best as powders or tablets rather than juices, which are too sweet. We suggest up to a tablespoon (10 grams) of wheat- or barley-grass powder, or the equivalent in tablets, immediately prior to each meal. If the more concentrated wheat- or barley-grass *juice* powder is taken, the dosage is one heaping teaspoon before meals.

Kelp and other seaweeds have exceptional value in the treatment of candida overgrowth. They contain selenium and many other minerals necessary for rebuilding immunity; furthermore, the rich iodine content of seaweeds is used by enzymes in the body to produce iodine-charged free radicals which deactivate yeasts. (Before the advent of anti-fungal drugs, iodine was the standard medical treatment for yeasts.) When candidiasis is complicated with tumors or cancers, then seaweed is of additional benefit. Dosage is 3 grams of kelp tablets, taken with one meal daily, or seaweeds can be incorporated into meals. (See recipe section on "Seaweeds.") Note: Because seaweeds are cooling and cleansing to the body, they are contraindicated in emaciation accompanied by loose stools.

Salt should normally be restricted during candida overgrowth—enough can be obtained from seaweeds and other foods. However, a pinch of *whole* sea salt cooked into grains and legumes is normally tolerated. (Whole sea salt is discussed in the *Salt* chapter.)

Variables in the Candida-Controlling Diet

Healing candidiasis with diet alone is possible but takes patience and consistently good eating habits. Two dietary factors—simple food combining and adding raw saltless sauerkraut to the diet—need emphasizing because they greatly help to shorten recovery time.

For the most severe symptoms, especially advanced systemic candidiasis, the candida diet, cereal grasses, kelp, garlic, intestinal biocultures, and/or herbs may need assistance from extremely powerful remedies. For example, antifungal drugs are sometimes resorted to for reducing candida excesses. Perhaps as powerful as the drugs but safer is **citrus seed extract,** a broad-action antimicrobial, non-chemical drug proven to be highly effective against yeasts. In proper dilution it also treats vaginal yeasts as well as most external fungal infections. Individual citrus seed products vary in their concentrations, so one should follow the dosage recommended on the product. (Further uses of this extract are on page 619.)

Also powerful is safe **hyper-oxygenation** such as that supplied by sodium chlorite products. This and other hyper-oxygenation methods including hydrogen peroxide (H_2O_2) and ozone are discussed soon under "Oxygenation." If hydrogen peroxide is used orally, it is best taken with expert guidance. In very extreme cases and for quickest results, ozone injection is the most efficient; next in effectiveness is H_2O_2 injection, administered by a qualified health practitioner.

Other Treatment Options: The strength of the person should be considered in formulating a candida diet and treatment.

Weak type: frail, thin, and pale; mucus, sputum, and/or vaginal discharge is clear and watery. This person will need more cooked foods—from 75% to 90% of the total diet—and may require animal products several times a week. Cereal grasses, hyper-oxygenation therapies, and bitter herbs such as chaparral are taken sparingly or not at all. Immune stimulants such as pau d'arco, Suma, and ginseng, however, are usually beneficial, as well as the regular candida-controlling diet described earlier.

Robust type: ruddy complexion and strong voice; mucus, sputum, and/or vaginal discharge is thick and possibly yellow or green. For this person, a more quickly cleansing diet is recommended, including few or no animal products, and raw vegetables and sprouts comprising at least 50% of the diet. This type of person benefits from any of the recommended foods, herbs, cereal grasses, oxygenation methods, etc.

Most people tend to be closer to one of these types than the other, and recommendations can be altered accordingly. Also, it is important to adapt the treatment regularly to the transformations that occur during the healing process.

Treating Candida in Conjunction with the Degenerative Diseases

The program for cancer and the degenerative diseases, discussed in a later chapter, shares a number of similarities with the candida program. This is due to the fact that virtually all degenerative diseases exhibit some degree of candidiasis. However, the entire candida program needs to be followed by those with degenerative diseases when the symptoms of candida overgrowth predominate.

When this is the case, all dietary, herbal, and oxygenation methods that arrest the growth of candida ultimately promote better nutrient assimilation and thus bolster protective *qi* and the immune system. These methods for healing candida overgrowth can then be followed as the primary treatment, while other remedies for the degenerative diseases can be added, as long as they do not contradict the candida treatment principles.

Oxygenation

> We can look at oxygen deficiency or oxygen starvation as the single greatest cause of all disease.—Stephen A. Levine, Ph.D., co-author of *Antioxidant Adaptation: Its Role in Free Radical Biochemistry*

Of all nutrients, oxygen is the most essential. This element, symbolized by the letter "O," has a more fundamental nutritional role than vitamins, minerals, or any other nutrient. Everyone knows that human life ends within a very few minutes without oxygen, but not enough people are aware of the often chronic oxygen starvation of their own tissues and cells.

The body is 75% water, and oxygen accounts for 90% of the weight of water. Oxygen may be considered a *yang* force; without it, fuel in the body cannot burn for energy or heat. The red blood cells carry oxygen to every part of the body, and anemia is sometimes a result of insufficient oxygen. The *qi* of Chinese medicine has a direct relationship to oxygen; in fact, *qi* is sometimes translated as "breath." Modern perspectives on oxygen give it several functions identical to those of *qi:* it energizes the body, clears obstructions, and overcomes stagnancy. Lacking in oxygen, one feels heavy, depressed, and without vitality. Oxygen is needed for vitamin C utilization, to retard collagen breakdown, and to prevent premature aging. The person with adequate cellular oxygen has a greater capacity to be outgoing (*yang*) and socially successful; people are attracted to the charisma that comes from abundant oxygen.

Most of the oxygen we inhale is utilized by the brain and heart, and the liver also requires oxygen to rebuild its cells. Oxygen therapy greatly benefits alcoholics and others who have damaged their livers and brain functions. Once sufficient oxygen is in the system, one feels charged with life and is usually no longer attracted to intoxicants.

Another important role of oxygen is that of purifier, helping eliminate wastes in the body. Oxygen destroys germs, viruses, amoebas, parasites, fungi, and yeasts, and resolves pathogenic moisture *(dampness)* in the form of edema, mucus, cysts, tumors, and arterial plaque. Consider an easily observed example of the power of one form of oxygen: Ozone (O_3) is recognized world-wide as a treatment for purifying water by eliminating chemicals and pesticides through oxidation and by destroying all microorganisms. Ozone is a substantially better purifier than chlorine, and additionally has none of the bad side effects.

Generally, more oxygen is needed by those who are overweight, sluggish, or who have candidiasis, edema, heart disease, or viral/tumorous/infectious conditions (e.g., cancer, multiple sclerosis, rheumatoid arthritis, chronic fatigue syndrome, Epstein-Barr syndrome, AIDS).

Oxygen enrichment: The following practices help to increase and distribute oxygen in the body.

• Physical activity, regular exercise, yogic breathing exercises, and visualizations designed to circulate energy.

- Living outside of metropolitan areas. Oxygen content is normally 20% in quality air but often falls to 10% in city air.
- Fasting or undereating, and eating few animal products. Toxins in the body from overeating, poor food combining, and the uric acid of excessive meat-eating use up oxygen reserves when the wastes associated with these poor nutritional practices are metabolized. According to Chinese medicine, *qi* energy is supplied by the breath and from food. By eating less, more *qi* (and therefore oxygen) is available from the breath (a "breatharian" is one who does not eat at all). In addition, when small amounts of food are eaten, digestion is much more efficient, resulting in more *qi* than if an excess is eaten.
- Eating fresh, raw, or lightly cooked sprouts, vegetables, and fruit (fruit intake must be restricted in candidiasis), and specially cultured vegetables such as raw saltless sauerkraut.
- Adding foods to the diet which contain significant amounts of the trace element germanium, which enhances the action of oxygen in the body. Germanium foods and supplements are commonly used as cancer remedies and for immune restoration in general. Among the more concentrated food and herb sources: "turkey tails" and related shelf or punk mushrooms that grow on the sides of decaying trees; other mushrooms including shiitake, ling zhi or reishi *(Ganoderma lucidum)*, and champignon; garlic; the herbs Suma *(Pfaffia paniculata)*, ginseng, and unrefined aloe vera juice; chlorella micro-algae, and barley.

Japanese researcher Dr. Kazuhiko Asai, author of *Miracle Cure: Organic Germanium*, was one of the first to see the great value of germanium in degenerative diseases. He has developed a germanium concentrate (bis carboxyethyl sesquioxide of germanium) known as "Ge-132" or "Organic Germanium," which is now available as a nutritional supplement.

Hyper-Oxygenation

The following powerful hyper-oxygenation products help fill the incredible chasm between nutritional approaches and often-devastating drug treatments, which reach their extreme in chemotherapy. The more common concentrated oxygen therapies include hydrogen peroxide (H_2O_2), ozone (O_3), glyoxylide, and stabilized oxygen compounds such as sodium chlorite, chlorine dioxide, magnesium oxide (a preparation first developed in 1898), and electrolytes of oxygen.

The last four are the mildest and safest of the seven remedies; these stabilized oxygen compounds appear to combine greatest effectiveness with safety. All seven are beneficial for focusing the purifying effects of oxygen and destroying amoebas, viruses, and germs. They also super-oxygenate the tissues they contact and therefore bring the benefits of oxygenation, albeit somewhat artificially. Hydrogen peroxide and ozone are found in nature, but never in the concentrations now available in products and therapies; nonetheless, when an individual suffers from a deeply situated oxygen deficiency disease, the concentrated products can make sense, especially when conventional chemotherapy or other drug therapies seem too powerful because of the condition or constitution of the patient.

It must be emphasized, however, that these oxygenation treatments are more effective and have longer-term value when the entire diet is improved. In one type of ozone treatment for AIDS, blood is withdrawn, purified with O_3, then re-injected back into the bloodstream. After a series of treatments, the blood is usually free of viruses (the treatment of dozens of AIDS patients with ozone by doctors such as Horst Keif in Munich, Germany, has been very successful). Blood purity can then be maintained if a healthful diet and lifestyle are followed. (See "Resources" index to obtain more information on hyper-oxygenation therapies.)

Ozone

Perhaps the most powerful of the hyper-oxygenation methods, ozone is a remedy proven by more than fifty years of beneficial use on millions of patients in Europe. Some researchers consider it safer than hydrogen peroxide. Ozone is generally less expensive than other standard treatments for serious conditions, and its application does not require great technical skill. Unfortunately, ozone-generating machines have yet to be approved by the Food and Drug Administration for medical use in the United States. Nevertheless, approval is expected soon, and in response to growing demand, various states are legalizing the use of ozone for blood injection when administered by medical professionals.

In addition to its beneficial use in the treatment of cancer, arthritic diseases, and AIDS, ozone also has been helpful in the cure of vascular disease, systemic candidiasis, mononucleosis, herpes, and hepatitis. This list includes just a few representative conditions of microbial contamination in which ozone treatment often succeeds, particularly as an adjunct to dietary therapy. Ozone has also helped improve nervous system and brain function in Alzheimer's disease, senility, multiple sclerosis, and Parkinson's disease.

Hydrogen Peroxide in Food and the Body

Of the hyper-oxidation techniques used in the United States, hydrogen peroxide (H_2O_2) is at this time one of the most common. It is a remedy that occurs in nature: as moisture (H_2O) interacts with ozone (O_3) in the atmosphere, it picks up an added oxygen atom and falls to the earth as rain which contains an abundance of H_2O_2. Other natural sources are raw, unprocessed vegetal foods such as fruits, vegetables, grasses, and especially wild plants and herbs, mammal and fish livers, and mother's milk, particularly colostrum. A natural source of great hydrogen peroxide concentration is the renowned healing waters of Lourdes, France.

Hydrogen peroxide is also found in the cells of the body. It is created there from water and oxygen, and acts as a major defense in the immune system. H_2O_2 is produced in healthy individuals in sufficient quantity to counteract unwanted bacterial invaders.[3] Growths in the body such as yeasts, viruses, and tumors are often anaerobic, and the extra atom of nascent oxygen in hydrogen peroxide halts their spread.

Hydrogen peroxide has a vital role in every system of the body, and is essential to the metabolism of protein, carbohydrates, fats, vitamins, and other nutrients. Except for the problems that can result from its overuse, taking concentrated H_2O_2 compares with taking concentrated nutrients of any kind, including vitamin supplements. The nutrients necessary for health can normally be supplied by whole, unprocessed foods, but during a health crisis concentrated products may be needed. However, as Max Gerson found with his advanced cancer patients (refer to the "Cancer" section, page 405, for Gerson's philosophy and treatments), certain vitamin and mineral supplements made their condition worse, quite possibly because of the energy required for the metabolism of these substances. In contrast, hydrogen peroxide appears to promote energy. This may be due to its ability to destroy microorganisms that sap the body's energy with infections and low-grade fevers; it may be that H_2O_2 is one of the metabolic factors deficient in the chronically ill.

Hydrogen peroxide should not be considered a panacea. There is experimental evidence that excessive intake may inhibit enzyme systems and ignite a rash of free radicals that adversely affect immunity and damage certain cellular structures. On the other hand, peroxide adherents point to a mountain of supportive research, and claim the product to be completely safe if used according to suggested guidelines. The real criterion, of course, is whether a medicine can restore health. We have chosen to discuss this quasi-natural product because we have seen it save people from death when other methods failed.

This is not a new remedy but one that has helped thousands afflicted with virus- and yeast-related diseases over the past seventy years. Respected medical professionals have benefited from hydrogen peroxide and recommended it highly, among them heart transplant surgeon Christiaan Barnard of South Africa, who claims it cured his arthritis. It has also been reported that hydrogen peroxide is administered by the Gerson Institute clinic, which is well-known for its nutritional treatment of cancer. Dr. Kurt Donsbach (referred to earlier in the "Candida" section of this chapter) has used hydrogen peroxide extensively on hundreds of patients with unusual benefits. According to Donsbach,

> Thirty-five percent food grade hydrogen peroxide is by far the best agent for the destruction of yeast and fungal colonies I know of. Intravenous infusion of hydrogen peroxide has proven to be one of the most dramatic healing agents I have ever witnessed. Specifically for systemic candidiasis patients, you find allergies disappearing in five to ten days, and a total clearance of the yeast in twenty-one to twenty-eight days.

Part of the Donsbach treatment protocol includes adrenal cortex extract and an antiviral immune stimulant called isoprinosine, both of which are not normally available in the United States at this time. He has also successfully used hydrogen peroxide in cases of cancer, arthritis, and various other conditions of immune deficiency.

Because it is unpatentable, costs very little, is often self-administered, and can theoretically take the place of many other medications, hydrogen peroxide has few backers among the national medical associations, the drug industries, or even the vitamin and supplement manufacturers. Also, many Americans have come to associate medicine for severe illnesses with high cost, and so hydrogen peroxide therapy does not even begin to enter their concept of appropriate treatment. Yet such therapy has progressed to the level of a serious grass-roots movement; this is partly a result of years of missionary fervor by the priest Fr. Richard Wilhelm.[4]

As mentioned earlier, hydrogen peroxide may generate dangerous quantities of free radicals. However, there is good evidence that the nascent oxygen from H_2O_2 in the body combines with and *eliminates* destructive free radicals.[5] Since protection against the *possibility* of free radical damage is fairly simple with the use of antioxidants, they should be used for this purpose as well as for general immune enhancement. That is, one can increase antioxidants during oxygenation therapy to ensure against possible oxidation excesses. One of the best antioxidant food sources is the wheat- or barley-grass products discussed earlier. They promote oxygen enrichment while simultaneously providing their own antioxidant vitamins and minerals; they also contain one of the richest natural sources of the enzyme superoxide dismutase, a key antioxidant. Alternatives include the following antioxidant enzymes, often recommended in combination with hydrogen peroxide and other hyper-oxidative therapies and commonly available in one supplement: superoxide dismutase (SOD), glutathione peroxidase (GPx), methionine reductase (MR), and catalase (CAT).

Oral Application and Dosage: "Food grade 35% Hydrogen Peroxide" or diluted products containing it must be used. They are sometimes carried by health food stores, or can be mail-ordered (see "Resources" index). Standard 3% hydrogen peroxide from drug stores is *not* to be taken internally, since it contains a number of strong chemical stabilizers. In fact, some researchers claim it to be unfit even as a mouthwash, especially for those who are ill.

Note: Hydrogen peroxide must not be taken by those with organ transplants because it may boost immunity sufficiently to override the immune-suppressing drugs these people take to prevent rejection of the transplant.

Food grade 35% hydrogen peroxide must first be diluted. It combines well with pure water or aloe vera juice in $\frac{1}{2}$ cup quantities. Adding a squeeze of lemon juice to water containing H_2O_2 removes the bitter flavor. Do not mix in carrot juice, or carbonated or alcoholic beverages, because these cause an unfavorable reaction. Take on an empty stomach and not with other supplements or medicines.

Begin with one drop H_2O_2 a day for the first week. Then increase to one drop three times a day, and every three days add one more drop per dose until a level of about fifteen drops three times a day is reached. Healing reactions and discharges of toxins sparked by H_2O_2 can be extreme, so caution is urged. If an upset stomach, headache, boils, or other strong eliminative reaction occurs, it is best not to increase the dosage any further until symptoms clear. If reactions are extreme, the program can be stopped for a few days, then resumed at the last dosage level. (See "Healing Reactions" in the *Dietary Transition* chapter.) In severe candidiasis and for degenerative diseases, some individuals find that the peak effective dosage is twenty-five drops three times daily for up to three weeks; then the dosage is tapered back, at the same rate it was increased, to fifteen drops three times a day, until symptoms clear. The program can be tailored to an individual's ability to accept cleansing and renewal.

One can expect improvement in the symptoms of candidiasis after a few weeks, although complete recovery, especially in severe cases, may take four to six months. After symptoms subside, a maintenance dose of five to fifteen drops weekly (one to three drops a day for five days a week) may be needed. If commercial capsules and fluids are used containing food grade hydrogen peroxide in combination with aloe vera juice or other substances, the above protocol can be followed; these products usually list the amount of 35% food grade H_2O_2 they contain.

Intravenous and External Applications of Hydrogen Peroxide (HP)

- Intravenous and intra-arterial injection of hydrogen peroxide (hereafter abbreviated "HP") must be done by a trained physician. This method is faster-acting than oral HP and is appropriate for the most advanced cases of systemic candidiasis and degenerative conditions.

  Note: Although less than ideal, the common drugstore variety of 3% HP is acceptable for most external applications. It should not, however, be ingested or used as a mouthwash; for these purposes food grade HP must be used. To make 3% food grade HP: Add one ounce of 35% food grade HP to 11 ounces of distilled water.

- Bathing in peroxide-infused water enhances the effect of oral HP therapy, especially in yeast-induced vaginitis (add one to four pints of 3% HP to a standard-size bath tub half-filled with warm water, and soak twenty minutes).
- Externally applied gels of HP in aloe vera gel are becoming widely available. This is another way to get large quantities of oxygen directly in the blood without having to drink or inject HP.
- Those who are overcoming genital yeasts may re-infect each other during intercourse. The male genital area can be washed with 3% HP before and after intercourse to minimize the exchange of yeasts and other infections, although this is not a safe method of protection, for either partner, against infections. Women with vaginal yeasts can use a retention douche to supplement the garlic remedy given earlier: retain a solution of one-third 3% HP and two-thirds water for five minutes, once a week.
- For athlete's foot, soak feet in 3% HP once daily at night. Athlete's foot often indicates an internal yeast condition.
- For acne, ringworm, and fungal conditions in the pubic area or elsewhere on the skin, dab 3% HP on with a cotton ball; avoid getting in eyes.

- For a toothpaste, add 3% HP to baking soda until a paste is formed. Or, simply dip brush in 3% HP solution. HP inhibits decay-causing bacteria and treats gum disease.
- As a mouthwash or gargle, use 3% HP to reduce oral bacteria, heal canker sores, and stop plaque build-up. It also works well diluted by half with water.
- To remove poison sprays and parasites from the surface of produce, soak fruits and vegetables for 20 minutes in a sink full of water to which ¼ cup 3% HP is added; or use 1 tablespoon 3% HP per gallon of soak water. A quicker method is to spray 3% HP on produce, wait a minute or two, then rinse.
- Spray or water house plants with a solution of one ounce of 3% HP to a quart of water. They will become vibrant from the added oxygen.
- To purify drinking water of bacteria, add seven drops 35% food grade HP per gallon, or one pint 35% HP to 1,000 gallons. Many harmful chemicals found in water are also oxidized and effectively neutralized by HP.
- Animals with arthritis, worms, and aging diseases usually perk up with HP. Add two drops of 35% HP to drinking water daily for a ten-pound animal, and adjust the dosage according to weight for other animals. Giving pets chemical-free, quality feed is also necessary for their long-term health.

Further Insights into Immunity

Free Radicals: Immune Defenders and Destroyers

An important concept for understanding immunity is that of "free radicals." Free radicals are molecules generated by cells in the body upon exposure to toxins, viruses, germs, or fungi. They contain extra oxygen and destroy unwanted invaders through oxidation. Two common examples of free radicals are iodine radicals and superoxide. From such oxidizing substances hydrogen peroxide is created, which specifically destroys yeasts and fungi. This aspect of free radicals is a beneficial and vital part of our immunity.

For the creation of free radicals, the cells need extra oxygen, which is why exercise is important as well as the intake of foods that maximize oxygen in the body. However, after producing free radicals for their own protection, body cells themselves also become targets and must ward off the free radicals with an antioxidant defense composed of nutrients sometimes known as "free-radical scavengers." When free radicals attack unprotected cells, they disturb the action of cellular DNA, which directs key cellular activities. Cells thus damaged are no longer good conduits of protective *qi;* they stagnate and more easily become sites of cancer and growths. This kind of damage also accelerates the aging process, directly causing wrinkles and age spots and severely taxing the immune system. Thus, a major key to immunity is minimizing the need to produce free radicals, by minimizing stress and toxins in the lifestyle.

Free radicals are produced in response to the following irritants and toxins: chemical contaminants taken in from air, water, and food; radiation from any source, including positive ions from computer video display terminals; and the carcinogenic compound acetaldehyde in cigarette smoke. Acetaldehyde is also produced by the liver after alcohol consumption.

Free radicals are bound up and neutralized by the antioxidant nutrients in free-radical scavengers. Such nutrients include vitamins E, A,* C and several of the B vitamins; the minerals selenium and zinc; bioflavonoids; the amino acid cysteine, and various antioxidant enzymes, especially superoxide dismutase (SOD). If exposure to free-radical-inducing toxins is minimized, then these nutrients are adequately supplied by a varied diet of unprocessed grains and vegetables.

High natural concentrations of these antioxidant nutrients are found in wheat and barley grass, sprouts, and dark green vegetables. Those regularly exposed to elevated levels of toxins, or who have a very weakened immunity, may also benefit from antioxidant supplements.

Free radicals are also produced by oxidation in the metabolism of food and by oxidized, rancid foods. The major sources of these free radicals are rancid or overheated fats and oils, nearly always found in fried foods. All polyunsaturated vegetable oils, unless truly cold-pressed, are heated to high temperatures during processing and are virtual free-radical storehouses. Hydrogenated vegetable oils, including vegetable shortenings and margarine, are also heat-processed; in addition, their molecular structure has been distorted in other ways, so they especially stress the immune system.

Individuals with cancer and other serious immune deficiency conditions do better when all extracted oils, fats, and oil-rich products such as nuts and seeds are avoided or greatly restricted. Certain immune-enhancing oils found in foods rich in omega-3 and GLA fatty acids are an exception (see *Oils and Fats* chapter for examples and more information on oils in general).

Activity and Immunity

Either overwork or lack of exercise will result in low protective energy. It is well known that too much physical work depletes the body and that lack of activity promotes atrophy and impaired circulation. Mental overwork is as damaging as excess physical activity, since too many thoughts—especially worries—weaken the spleen-pancreas function and can cause poor nutrient absorption. (See *Earth Element* chapter for further explanation.)

Sexual Activity

Excessive sexual activity depletes the kidney-adrenal vital energy and its related essence known as *jing* (discussed further in the *Water Element* chapter). *Jing* directly tonifies life force, and when deficient, resistance to disease and adaptability to the

---

*Current research shows beta carotene (provitamin A) to be a superior free-radical scavenger and tumor inhibitor. Refer to the *Green Food Products* chapter for further properties and sources of beta carotene.

environment diminishes. Excessive ejaculation in particular reduces *jing*, draining the body's vitality. According to modern nutrition, semen contains substantial amounts of zinc and omega-3 fatty acids, which are essential to proper immune function. Excessive loss of semen, therefore, taxes the body's stores of these (and other) nutrients.

Protective Qi and Whole Foods

The protective *qi* is the body's most *yang* energy, circling vigorously about its periphery while offering protection against viruses, germs, and environmental factors. Eating too much salty food works against *qi's* outer defense of the body, since salt strongly directs energy inward. Nevertheless, except in serious cases of immune depletion, moderate use of unrefined salt can strengthen digestion and therefore ultimately support immunity.

Outer *yang* protective energy is initially supported by eating unprocessed food. The protective coating on grains and other whole foods contains valuable minerals and nutrients that strengthen immunity. For example, selenium, a key nutrient for immunity, is found in food grown on soil containing it. In grain it is located in the outer coating (bran) and germ. Consider the effect of removing such valuable aspects of grain—the bran and germ—as is often done in milling; there is a measurable loss of nutritional value.

However, what is removed in *essence* is of even greater value; a simple listing of missing nutrients cannot sufficiently describe the loss of integrity. The strength in life that comes from wholeness in general and unrefined food in particular is difficult to describe, since that perfection includes the interrelationship of all things.

Immunity: From Ultimate to Devastated

Are there historical examples of those with an exceptional immunity? The Bible attributes to true followers of Christ the quality of immunity to poisons:

> Those who believe will be given the power to perform miracles . . . to drink any poison and not be harmed.—Mark 16:17

Many remarkable examples of failed poisonings are also recorded throughout Asian history, the intended victim invariably a sage.

The immune system and its failure have become the object of acute focus since the spread of AIDS and similar conditions featured daily in the world media. Brought to public attention as a result is the correlation between a stressful lifestyle and the loss of immunity. From those treatment methods which have at least halted the advance of the disease, we have learned that a holistic approach is most effective. Awareness and attitudinal healing, lifestyle changes, activity and exercise, diet, herbs and nutritional methods, bodywork, acupuncture, and drug therapies all have been seen to play therapeutic roles. One positive outcome of our obsession with AIDS and the immune system is the growing awareness that disease affects, and can be treated from, every level of our being.

Unity and Immunity

Both Western and Eastern spiritual traditions represent attempts to indicate the unfathomable qualities of a unified reality. The onslaught in recent years of immune deficiencies and chronic illnesses, however, has caused many to question how such ideals of unity and perfection can relate to the realities of dreaded diseases, pathological acts of individuals, and the wholesale destruction of the environment. We can only conclude that if these are also manifestations of "perfection," then they must be reflections of a higher justice, resulting from past actions motivated by selfishness and excess desire.

Undercutting the Desire Cycle

Struggling with desire may increase desire. Such a cycle of conflict can be stopped, however, with selfless action, which cuts away the foundations of desire. What is selfless action? Selflessness is straightforward; it gives and serves without scheming for something in return. In this way resentments, which undermine all relationships, do not arise. At the same time, desire is held in check. Even without desire, ill fortune may still persist until past conditions, possibly from previous lives, are resolved. Since we seldom know either the real cause or the depth of our afflictions, the simplest remedy in every case is to begin now with a plan for unconditional, selfless giving. It is essential to make a firm commitment that will carry us through the difficulties inevitably encountered in profound healing.

Attitude

The single most important principle for strengthening immunity is an attitude of nonseparation in one's personal life. Such an attitude will have the greatest effect when it unifies those parts of one's life where there is greatest alienation. Courage may be required.

When separation is felt between people, it is often because of unresolved emotional issues. This can be changed through sincere forgiveness followed by unconditional gratitude for everything that happens and has happened. According to traditional Chinese physiology, getting rid of old resentments clears the liver of obstructions, which in turn permits the smooth and vigorous circulation of protective and other *qi* energies. The cliché that we hurt only ourselves with anger is in fact a physiological truth.

> Those who act with bravery and courage will overcome diseases, while those who act out of fear will fall ill.
>
> —*Inner Classic*

Once the work of resolving resentments is underway, the choices for diet and other lifestyle factors should fall into place. Without this work, one tends to eat and live in ways that support the old, unresolved patterns.

Summary of Suggestions for Building and Maintaining Immunity

1. **Activity:** Moderate regular exercise is recommended. Lack of physical activity, excess sexual activity, and overwork impair immunity.

2. **Diet:** Eat whole foods, choosing a variety from a grain- and vegetable-based diet. Moderate undereating and simpler food combinations strengthen immunity. Do not eat late at night. Avoid intoxicants, refined or chemically contaminated foods, rancid nuts and seeds, and limit oils and fats. If candida overgrowth symptoms are present, further dietary discipline (as given earlier) is necessary, and the oxygenating and yeast-inhibiting foods, supplements, and practices should also be considered.

3. **Environment:** Maintain an orderly, pleasant living and working environment. Of essential importance for those with very weak immunity is association with completely supportive people. Sunlight, clean, fresh air, and pure water strengthen immunity. If these are not available naturally, then water filters, full-spectrum lights, and air filters/ionizers are helpful. Avoid overexposure to dampness, and protect against other climactic extremes.

4. **Supplements:** Synthetic vitamins and inorganic minerals seem to work best for individuals with strong, robust signs (see *"Excess"* in following chapter), although they may benefit others also. Whole food supplements such as wheat- or barley-grass concentrates, sea vegetables, chlorella, and spirulina may be more beneficial for long-term use. Sprouts are a superb source of nutrients and can adequately supplement most grain and vegetable diets; however, they should be lightly cooked and used sparingly by individuals who are *cold*, weak, or frail.

5. **Attitudinal Healing:** This is the foundation for immunity; gratitude and forgiveness are preliminary steps. Spiritual practices such as prayer, meditation, and visualization normally support the experience of continual renewal; such practices, however, can also weaken immunity if they are used to reinforce rigid thinking and habits.

Excess and Deficiency

The final pair in the Six Divisions simply measures the relative strength of the person. Too often in modern medicine the same treatment is applied to both strong and weak alike, an oversight that undoubtedly contributes to its mixed results. A condition of *excess* is caused by too much *heat*, fluids, or other substances. Conversely, *deficiency* is due to a lack of warmth, fluids, or other substances. (These substances can be any aspect of the body and its nourishment.)

Excess

In wealthy countries, the vast majority of disease arises from excess bodily *heat* and *dampness* caused by overeating rich, greasy, highly seasoned, denatured, and/or intoxicating foods, viz., an excess of meats (especially red meats), eggs, cheese, and other dairy products; too much fried food, salt, and extremely sweet food; refined and rancid flour and oil products; chemical ingredients, drugs, and alcoholic drinks. When the body can no longer tolerate any further *excess*, it begins to malfunction, causing signs of *deficiency* to coexist with *excess*. This results in the deterioration of all organ systems in the body, as in diabetes, cancer, arthritis, and other degenerations. Some individuals do not manifest the above pattern of *excess* changing to *deficiency* because their constitutions are *deficient*. Their conditions, therefore, even though brought on by *excess*-producing foods, are basically of *deficiency*.

The treatment for degenerative disease in the West, usually caused by *excess*, has often been different from that in the Far East, where *deficiency* has long been the prevailing etiology. The Asian pattern, however, is rapidly changing to *excess* with the modernization of many areas of the Far East.

In an *excessive* condition, there is hyperfunction caused by blockages in the arteries, acupuncture meridians, or other systems. Generally the blockages stem from an extreme diet coupled with a stressful lifestyle, though some individuals are inherently predisposed to develop *excessive* conditions. When systems are blocked, the body easily generates *heat* and pressure and tends to develop such conditions as high blood pressure, constipation caused by *heat* drying the fluids, overweight, heart disease, or strokes. The main remedy for *excess* is cleansing and purging. Whatever has caused the *excess* must be eliminated. A person with an *excess* condition can take stronger treatments and more powerfully acting remedies than one who is *deficient*. As a general rule, bitter foods and herbs are used to reduce *excess*. The bitter flavor is cooling, drying (reduces *dampness*), and helps move the bowels.

It is no accident that herbology in the West has emphasized such extremely bitter herbs as goldenseal, echinacea, and chaparral; even the common chamomile, sometimes used as a social herbal beverage, is quite bitter. The idea of the "bitter tonic"* has arisen—almost a contradiction in terms—because of the great need in the West to reduce *excess*.

In a similar fashion, Western medicine has emphasized extremely powerful remedies to counter *excess* (synthetic drugs, surgery, and radiation), measures tolerated best by strong people. Even the use of synthetic vitamins, particularly vitamin C—one of the staples of Western nutrition—also reduces *excess* by helping in the breakdown of fats and cholesterol. Many important dietary treatments involve raw foods and juices, which also are eliminative.

As illustrated by the concept of *yin* and *yang*, all processes eventually reverse at their extreme; thus among the current generation we see how a preponderance of rich, building foods has finally begun to manifest as its opposite, i.e., as *deficiency*. For these persons, the Chinese tonic herbs and dietary principles prove effective. At the same time, the universal concept of balance is gaining widespread acceptance. After so many generations of building *excess*, increasing numbers of people are now attracted to dietary measures that energize yet relax, that strengthen as they support a peaceful mentality. There is no single such diet. By knowing the properties of food and the means of personal diagnosis, however, the appropriate diet can be discovered and applied in anyone's life.

In reducing *excess*, it is essential not to over-reduce. In the Chinese healing arts, one calls this practice of preserving balance "protecting the 'righteous *qi*.'" Therefore, when using raw-food diets, bitter purgative herbs, and other reducing techniques, it is important to continually monitor one's condition to avoid an uncontrolled slide from *excess* to *deficiency*.

Over the centuries, Chinese medicine has developed a remarkably simple yet accurate description of *excess*:

Signs of general *excess*: *Yang* symptoms—the person is robust, energetic, extroverted and has a normal to loud voice and reddish complexion; swellings in the body are hard and painful when pressed; breathing is heavy, the tongue coating is thick, and the radial pulse has strength.

Dietary Recommendations for Excess

As mentioned earlier, the treatment for general *excess* is reducing and purging. This is easily accomplished (at least on the level of diet) simply by avoiding the products that caused the *excess* (generally very rich, sweetened, refined, and/or intoxicating foods), and replacing them with foods that reduce or purge it: most low-fat, whole vegetal foods—sprouts (especially alfalfa), fruits, vegetables (especially leafy greens), sea vegetables, micro-algae (especially wild blue-green and dunaliella), cereal grasses, grains, and legumes (especially lima, aduki, and mung beans).

Particularly beneficial are the bitter foods—celery, lettuce, asparagus, rye, and amaranth. (More examples of bitter foods appear in the *Five Flavors* chapter.)

---

*"Tonify" implies strengthening and building-up, whereas the bitter flavor is a reducing therapy.

A sampling of *excess*-reducing bitter herbs includes the roots of dandelion *(Taraxacum officinalis)*, burdock *(Arctium lappa)*, yellow dock *(Rumex crispus)*, and rhubarb *(Rheum palmatum)* (yellow dock and rhubarb also treat constipation); and chamomile *(Anthemis nobilis)* and honeysuckle *(Lonicera japonica)* flowers. Note: It is always best to check the various other properties of herbs before using them. Other good *excess*-reducers are mushrooms, carrots, radishes, and fresh figs. If sweeteners are used, small amounts of stevia leaf or raw honey may be tolerated. One of the few oils recommended for *excess* is fresh flax-seed oil (see page 165 for dosage). The majority of the foods taken should be raw or lightly cooked.

In specific types of *excess* such as *excess heat* (discussed in the *Heat/Cold* chapter), warming foods are withdrawn and cooling foods are added. Reducing other specific conditions of *excess* such as *dampness*, *coldness*, and *wind* follows a similar process: withdraw the *excess*-inducing foods and add those that reduce. (Descriptions of the common *excesses* and their treatments are given at the end of this chapter.) In the Five Element chapters we will discuss *excesses* (and *deficiencies*) of the specific organ systems.

When acute *excesses* such as severe infections occur (signs may include rapid onset with much *heat*, redness, throbbing pain, high fever, angry boils, or very painful ear infections), the diet must be very light: fast on water, vegetable and fruit juices, and/or herbal teas; if there is hunger, vegetables and fruits may be eaten. Beneficial herbs for acute infections are the bitter, antibiotic type such as golden seal *(Hydrastis canadensis)* and echinacea (*Echinacea angustifolia* and related species). A typical formula is equal parts of these herbs combined with one-third part each of lobelia *(Lobelia inflata)* and licorice *(Glycyrrhiza glabra)*. The highly concentrated and extremely bitter citrus seed extract, a potent antimicrobial now available in most nutrition stores, may also be taken, either singly or added to the herbal beverage just before drinking. Take herbs and/or extract every 20–30 minutes in severe infections and, if possible, obtain the advice of an experienced practitioner.

> Excess causes one to forget what is proper and good, and to become careless.
>
> —*Inner Classic*

Deficiency

Signs of general *deficiency*: *Yin* symptoms—the person is frail, weak, withdrawn, with a soft voice, pale or sickly yellow complexion and weak radial pulse; lumps, if any, are soft; breathing is shallow; the tongue coating is thin or nonexistent; the pressure of touch is welcomed and improves symptoms.

Dietary Recommendations for Deficiency

In cases of general *deficiency,* obtaining balance involves building-up (for greater vigor, strength, and energy) and should proceed more slowly than the treatment of *excess*, and with greater care. The "Guidelines for Treating Severe Deficiencies" listed later should be followed if the *deficiency* is debilitating.

In addition, more "full sweet," nutritive foods are added to the diet in cases of *deficiency,* with the bitter flavor used less often. "Full" denotes the ability to tonify. With the exception of the red date used in Chinese herbalism, nearly all fruit is considered an "empty" sweet flavor which is either too cooling or too cleansing to be appropriate for weakened conditions. Most grains and legumes and many vegetables are full sweet, and their sweetness is enhanced by thorough chewing. Especially good are rice, oats, millet, barley, soy products, black beans, parsnips, rutabagas, winter squash, and small amounts of nuts and seeds.

Cereal creams and congees are used for those too weak to chew well (see "Congee" recipes). During convalescence, a daily teaspoonful of black sesame seeds cooked into a cereal tonifies *deficiency* and is helpful for constipation. Black sesame is not good, however, for individuals with a tendency to loose stools, in which case barley water decoction is a specific remedy (2 oz. of barley simmered 45 minutes in 1 quart of water). Cereals of rice, millet, and buckwheat are also useful for *deficiency*-type diarrhea.

According to the Chinese classics, such highly sweet foods as dates, yams, molasses, barley malt, and rice syrup build strength. In modern times, however, persons taking antibiotics and ingesting white sugar, denatured food, and chemicals normally have weakened digestive tracts that cannot be balanced by strongly sweet foods. This is because their *deficiency* is usually not simple but mixed with excesses of mucus, incompletely metabolized fats, yeasts, fungi, and fluids in the body, which are aggravated by extremely sweet food. *Deficient* individuals who are strengthened by very sweet-flavored foods should be cautious, since too much of any very strong flavor can be quickly weakening.

It must be emphasized that bitter foods may make the *deficient* person worse. Foods that benefit the *excessive* individual—rye, asparagus, lettuce, celery, amaranth grain, and others with a bitter aspect—should be used cautiously during a *deficient* state. If bitter herbs are required during *deficiency,* they are best combined with molasses or the herb licorice root *(Glycyrrhiza glabra).* Very often the gentle action of chlorophyll-rich foods is more suitable for cleansing during *deficiency* than bitter herbs. Chlorella and spirulina, two of the highest food sources of chlorophyll, also contain easily digestible protein—sometimes an important feature in *deficiency.*

Animal Products

The animal product best suited to most cases of modern *deficiency* is goat milk, which is sweet with a unique astringency that helps check the mucus-forming qualities typical of dairy products. If cow's milk is tolerated and of good quality, it is an ideal food for *deficiency.* (See "Dairy Recommendations" in *Protein and Vitamin B₁₂* chapter, page 150).

Other nutritive animal products such as eggs, fish, fowl, and mammal meat have been traditionally used for *deficiency,* and may help when dairy is not tolerated and vegetable products are insufficient. (A preparation method and recommended quantities for meat are given at the end of the *Protein and Vitamin B$_{12}$* chapter.)

One animal product perhaps more nutritious than any other food is royal jelly, the food of queen bees. It is commonly used for a number of weakened conditions, including senility and infant malnutrition, and to retard aging in general. It also promotes growth and mental/physical development. Royal jelly is available commercially in a variety of forms.

Deficiency Combined with Heat, Cold, and Other Factors

To balance *coldness* during *deficiency,* one adds more warming food and warming preparation methods according to the examples in the "Cold Patterns" section of the *Heat/Cold* chapter. *Deficiency* with *heat (deficient yin)* nearly always develops in those with long-term *deficiencies.* Therefore it is essential to know its symptoms when working with debility. (Symptoms, along with recommendations, were discussed earlier in the *Heat/Cold* chapter.)

Other factors important during the treatment of general *deficiency:* use fewer ingredients and simpler food combining; avoid overeating; limit raw food to slow down cleansing—cook most food until moderately well-done; and eliminate intoxicants and non-foods (refined or containing chemicals).

Equally important is the way diet is developed and how the *deficient* person is cared for. Serious and deeply situated *deficiencies* are always lengthy, chronic conditions. The debility in the final stages of degenerative disease is a prime example. Healing activity in such serious conditions accelerates when certain guidelines are carefully followed.

Guidelines for Treating Severe Deficiencies

- Treatments and therapy programs should progress at a slower rate and with greater care than for *excessive* conditions; such programs must follow a regular schedule. These guidelines are especially important for older people and those with serious conditions.
- When balancing *heat* and *cold* through diet for the severely *deficient* person, choose less extremely cooling or heating foods and preparation methods than for someone with a milder condition.
- Avoid creating a shock with a completely new dietary plan. Gradually upgrade the quality of foods the person likes, or find agreeable substitutes. Omit especially harmful foods (and all non-foods). New foods can be added one at a time according to tolerance.
- As the condition improves, if synthetic drugs and other very strong medications are being used, consider a program which gradually eliminates them with the advice of the prescribing physician.
- Appropriate herbs, mild exercise, air- and sun-baths, and acupressure/acupuncture may be helpful.

- Self-reflection and awareness practices are usually beneficial, and a severe deficiency presents a good opportunity to develop internal awareness. Relaxed meditations, affirmations, prayer, and visualizations are often appealing and a powerful factor in overcoming a healing crisis.
- Recognize the total environment. People with aversions to a particular climate such as cold or damp should avoid long periods in those environments. A person with an *interior cold* condition (and therefore an aversion to cold), for example, should not live in a cold room. Weak and *deficient* people should not be put under stress. The living space most conducive to healing is orderly, pleasant, and simple.

Even more important is the attitude of family members or friends who share the living space. When a parent is ill, recovery time improves if the children develop health and awareness practices. Likewise, it is helpful if the parents make fundamental changes when a child, no matter what his or her age, is in need of healing. This same principle operates between husband and wife, between friends, and in all other relationships. Often just the example of change by a friend or relation is more powerful than any advice.

*   *   *

The following chart summarizes all six divisions of *yin* and *yang*, along with dietary recommendations. For easy reference, two additional charts are included. The first contains a summary of the combination of *deficiency* and *heat* (*"deficient yin"*); the second (on pages 99–101) summarizes four additional climatic influences: *wind, dryness, dampness*, and *summer heat*. (These last four influences are also discussed in the Five Element chapters.)

SUMMARY OF THE SIX DIVISIONS OF YIN AND YANG

Condition	Symptoms in the Body	Dietary Suggestions
DEPTH		
Exterior (Yang)	Sudden onset and likelihood of rapid cure, e.g., common cold or flu. Simultaneous fever and chills. Affects the periphery of body—muscle and joint achiness, stuffy head and recent headache.	Use diaphoretic herbal teas (page 69) for sweating and lighter foods—primarily fruits, vegetables, and broths. During the acute phase use liquids and herbal teas only.
Interior (Yin)	All disease which is not *exterior.* Affects the interior organs. Takes longer to cure	A broad category—dietary recommendations vary according to other imbalances such as *cold,*

Condition	Symptoms in the Body	Dietary Suggestions
	than *exterior* conditions. Fever may be present without chills, or there may be a feeling of coldness (with no fever); also pain inside the body, irritability, chronic headache.	*damp*, *excess*, *deficiency*, etc.

THERMAL NATURE

Heat (Yang)	*Heat* rises, dries up fluids; person feels hot, dislikes heat, likes cool weather and cold beverages in quantity. Yellow coating on tongue, dark yellow urine, red complexion. Localized *heat:* inflamed tissues, swellings, eruptions, sores, or rashes, all marked with redness.	Use more relatively cooling food instead of heat-producing fats, meats, alcohol, coffee, spices, and other warming foods. Emphasize more liquids and cooling vegetables, fruit, and herbs (page 62); minimal or no cooking (raw, sprouted, steamed, simmered); and the cooling grains and legumes: wheat, millet, mung beans, tofu, etc. During the acute phase of *heat* use mostly cooling fluids.
Cold (Yin)	*Cold* is like ice: doesn't move easily; causes immobility and contraction; person feels cold and dislikes the cold, overdresses, and is attracted to warmth and warming food and drink.	Substitute warming foods and herbs (page 66) for cooling foods. Avoid raw and cold (in temperature) foods and minimize water intake. Increase warming methods of preparation (baking, stir fry, and sauté). Cook foods longer and with lower heat.

STRENGTH

Excess (Yang)	Robust constitution with hyperfunction—sensation of fullness, moderate to loud voice, forceful pulse, thick tongue coating, reddish complexion. Disease may be acute and progress rapidly.	Eliminate very rich, fatty, sweetened, refined, and intoxicating foods and drinks; use cleansing measures including bitter foods and herbs, raw or lightly cooked foods such as sprouts and vegetables (especially leafy greens, carrots, radishes, mushrooms), fruits, grains, legumes, fresh flax oil, and stevia sweetener. Use fewer warming foods and more cooling foods for *excess heat;* use fewer moistening/ mucus foods and add drying foods for *excess damp* conditions.

Condition	Symptoms in the Body	Dietary Suggestions
		Reduce other specific *excesses* similarly. Fast on juices and/or water during acute infections; eat vegetables and fruits if food is desired. Take bitter (antibiotic) herbs 2–3 times an hour during severe infections.
Deficiency *(Yin)*	Weak person with hypofunction —withdrawn and passive with low energy, weak pulse, little or no coating on tongue, soft voice, and sallow to pale complexion. Usually a chronic condition.	Increase sweet, nutritive foods, e.g., rice, oats, parsnips, black-strap molasses, soy, black sesame seeds, dairy; decrease bitter foods. May require animal meats. Takes greater care and patience —milder dietary therapy over a longer time. For *cold* and *deficient* conditions, add warming foods. *Deficiency* with *heat* is listed below.

DEFICIENT YIN—COMBINATION OF DEFICIENCY AND HEAT

Condition	Symptoms in the Body	Dietary Suggestions
Deficiency and Heat *(Yin* and *Yang)*	A relative type of *heat* caused by insufficient *yin* fluid metabolism; may manifest as afternoon fevers, night sweats, hot palms and soles, fast and thin pulse, insomnia, cravings for sweet flavors, continual but small thirst or hunger; thinness. Commonly seen in those with wasting diseases.	Balanced fluids and the supporting sugar and protein metabolism are built best by proper chewing of complex carbohydrates: rice, barley, millet, seaweeds, black beans, mung beans, tofu, beets, string beans, tempeh, spirulina, and chlorella are useful; dairy products, eggs, oyster, clam, sardine, beef, or pork may be helpful in extreme *yin* depletion. Avoid hot spices, alcohol, coffee, tobacco, and excesses of warming or refined foods. Use ample water in cooking, e.g., eat soups and stews regularly. Herbal *yin* tonics may be helpful (page 357).

Applying The Six Divisions

Even though the Six Divisions may occur in any combination, we will focus on the most common combinations. For a condition to exist, not all of the symptoms need to be present. To use the Six Divisions: Decide whether the condition is *exterior* or *interior.* If *exterior,* use sweating and other recommended methods.

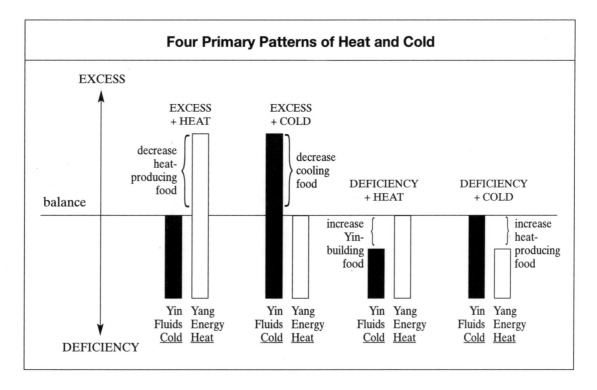

If *interior,* decide whether the condition is *heat* or *cold* and combined with *excess* or *deficiency* (four possibilities are shown in the preceding chart).

Other possibilities are variations and combinations of these four basic patterns.

In working with these patterns, it is helpful to use the concepts of *excess* and *deficiency.* For example, a person who feels cold may have either not enough *yang (deficiency* with *cold)* or too much *yin (excess* with *cold).* In the first case, more warming food is added, but cooling food is decreased carefully, if at all, because *cold* is not in *excess* (see graph). In the second case the treatment priority is to decrease the intake of cooling food; warming foods can also be added to hasten the process of reducing the *cold excess,* as discussed in the *Heat/Cold* chapter. Such distinctions cannot be made without understanding the patterns of *excess* and *deficiency.*

These patterns also shed light on the combination of *deficiency* with *heat (deficient yin).* At first, an obvious solution may be to add more cooling, *yin* foods such as water and juices. The benefits, however, are usually short-lived. Since we are dealing with a *deficiency,* too much water and cooling juices can diminish *yang* energy, which is not in *excess* (see graph). In addition, water in particular does not actively generate other aspects of the *yin,* such as the various body tissues, which are often depleted in *deficient yin.* Of course, adequate water and fluids are a necessity, but it is best to also add a number of foods such as the complex carbohydrates listed earlier in the *deficient yin* chart; these build fluids and tissues and at the same time do not overly reduce *yang* energy. Such foods produce "metabolic moisture" of their own when digested.

Further Diagnostic Foundations: The Six Influences

To diagnose the nature of an illness more thoroughly, the Six Influences—*heat, cold, wind, dry, damp,* and *summer heat*—are combined with the Six Divisions. These concepts are also developed within the Five Element chapters.

The Influences are easily misunderstood, partly because they are sometimes named the "Six Evils" or the "Six Pernicious Influences," although they have also been translated as the "Six Chi."[6] Because of the pejorative names, some who are acquainted with Chinese medicine obsessively protect themselves from even small fluctuations in the weather. Certainly an Influence such as heat or wind does not have an "evil" or "pernicious" effect until it is experienced excessively. In fact, a moderate degree of exposure to all the climates benefits health, unless the climate corresponds with one already in excess in the body (such as described in the next section).

Most people do not recognize the nature of the diseases provoked by overexposure to various climates. The Six Influences clarify the nature of imbalances that arise from too much wind, dampness, or other climatic factor. These factors can invade the body and produce symptoms similar to the climate itself—wind conditions are sudden, quick, moving, jerky. One's interior condition is a metaphor and mirror of the outward environment.

Seeing a Condition as It Is

Another misunderstanding of the Six Influences is the assumption that every condition of the Six Influences in the body must be caused by a corresponding climatic influence. This reasoning is incorrect on two counts:

1. Most *interior* conditions described by an Influence are not caused by an exterior climate, but are generated by factors of heredity and lifestyle, including diet. For example, the most typical *interior* conditions of *dampness* result from overeating rich, greasy food and from a sedentary lifestyle, rather than exposure to a damp climate. Nevertheless, any *damp* disease condition, even if caused by diet, will be made worse by overexposure to moisture in the environment. Thus, one must

especially protect against external climates that correspond with those in the body.

2. When an illness actually is brought on by a climatic influence, it may manifest in the body as a non-corresponding influence. For instance, *heat* signs of fever and inflammation in an individual are sometimes generated by exposure to winter cold. The appearance of a non-corresponding effect depends on such factors as the strength of the individual and the length of exposure. Therefore, when treating an illness with the Six Influences, *treat it according to the symptoms as they exist,* not by the climate that may have caused it. By treating the current symptoms, one also heals the fundamental, underlying imbalance in the person, including the emotional causes.

Knowing how an individual's imbalance is represented by the Six Divisions and Six Influences is a profound insight. Correct diagnosis means that the vibratory pattern of the person is identified; bringing this into balance heals the entire person. For instance, if a *damp* condition is cleared up, all *damp* excesses are also eliminated, whether they be water retention, excess weight, cysts, tumors, yeasts, and/or mucus. The person is no longer fatigued or heavy-feeling. Also, the corresponding emotional factors of anxiety and worry are resolved.

In actual practice, most conditions are combinations of both the Six Divisions and Six Influences. The three most common combinations are *heat, deficiency,* and *dryness; heat, wind,* and *excess; dampness, cold,* and *deficiency.*

In the following chart summarizing the Six Influences, *heat* and *cold* have the same *interior* symptoms and suggested diet as *heat* and *cold* of the Six Divisions. This does not mean they are identical; the Divisions are purely symptoms in the body, whereas the Influences also harbor intrinsic ties to a climatic factor. Nevertheless, in actual practice this difference diminishes and is mostly semantic. Except for *summer heat,* the Influences will be described with symptoms which correspond to the deeper, *interior* level of disease. When on an *exterior* level, the Influences are most easily purged by the methods for curing *exterior* diseases, described earlier.

DIAGNOSIS BY THE SIX INFLUENCES

Condition	Symptoms in the Body	Dietary Suggestions
Wind *(Yang)*	Arises and changes quickly, e.g., transient pain, spasm, convulsion, tremors, nervousness, dizziness, emotional turmoil. Especially affects the liver. Extremes of *wind* may cause conditions of stasis: strokes, paralysis, numbness. *Wind*	If *wind* is generated by *heat* or *deficient yin,* follow earlier recommendations for these conditions in the Six Divisions. To counteract *wind/cold,* use wind-reducers with a warming nature: oats, pine nut, shrimp, and anti-*wind* herbs such as ginger, fennel, basil, anise, and

Condition	Symptoms in the Body	Dietary Suggestions
	frequently combines with other influences to carry them into the body, as in the *wind/cold* condition of the common cold. Excess *heat* can generate wind, as oft en seen in strokes; other causes of wind are the *deficient yin* syndrome (*yin* stabilizes) and liver stagnation (page 319). Nearly always, *wind* appears in the body as either *wind/cold (wind* combined with *cold),* or as *wind/heat;* further combining with *dampness* and other influences is common.	valerian. To counteract *wind/heat,* use cooling *wind*-reducers: celery, kuzu, mulberry, strawberry, and anti-*wind* herbs such as peppermint and peony root. *Wind*-reducers with a neutral thermal nature may be used in either of the above cases: black soybean, black sesame seed, fresh flax oil, and the herbs sage, chamomile, lobelia, and scullcap. In all cases of *wind,* avoid *wind*-aggravators: eggs, crabmeat, and buckwheat. Rich foods in general often cause *wind* by promoting liver stagnation.
Heat **(Yang)**	See *"Heat"* symptoms and dietary suggestions in the Six Divisions summary, above.	
Cold **(Yin)**	See *"Cold"* symptoms and dietary suggestions in the Six Divisions summary, above.	
Damp **(Yin)**	*Dampness* creates signs of stagnation and sluggishness—the person is easily tired and feels heaviness in the body. If there is pain, it is fixed in one location. Conditions of *dampness* include edema or watery accumulations in all or parts of the body; excess mucus, tumors, cysts, parasites, yeasts such as candida, fungi, excess body weight, and a thick and/or greasy tongue coating. Affects the functioning of the spleen-pancreas, and therefore weakens digestion.	Foods which dry *dampness* are often bitter and/or aromatic. Examples: lettuce, celery, turnip, kohlrabi, rye, amaranth, aduki bean, wild blue-green micro-alga, asparagus, white pepper, alfalfa, pumpkin, vinegar, papaya, and bitter herbs: chaparral, pau d'arco, valerian, chamomile. Avoid or limit foods that promote *dampness* or mucus: dairy products, meat, eggs, tofu, and other soy products, pineapple, salt, and concentrated sweeteners.
Dryness **(Yang)**	Decreases fluids in the body resulting in dry skin, chapped lips, thirst, dry nose and throat, constipation, unproductive cough, thin body type. *Dryness* particularly affects the lungs. Often caused by the *deficient yin* syndrome.	Foods which moisten *dryness:* soy (tofu, tempeh, soy milk, miso), spinach, asparagus, millet, barley, salt, seaweed, white fungus (available in Chinese herb stores), apple,* tangerine,* pinenut,* persimmon,* peanut,* pear,* honey, barley malt, sugar cane, whole sugar (from unrefined cane juice), oyster, clam,

Condition	Symptoms in the Body	Dietary Suggestions
		mussel, pork, and pork kidney. Limit or avoid bitter foods and herbs. *These items also moisten the lungs.
Summer Heat *(Yang)*	Always an *exterior* condition that results from overexposure to extreme heat; it damages fluids in the body as well as *qi* energy; typical signs are high fever with profuse sweating, weakness, and thirst. Other signs may include shortness of breath, coughing, and wheezing. *Dampness* often accompanies *summer heat.*	Foods which protect against and treat *summer heat:* lemon, apple, watermelon, cantaloupe, papaya, pineapple, muskmelon, mung bean (in soup), summer squash, zucchini, and cucumber. For sun/heat stroke, use radish juice, bitter melon soup, or watermelon juice.

The Art of Healing

When using remedies listed throughout this book, one will often encounter such phrases as: "commonly used in the treatment of . . . ." This does not mean that "commonly used" remedies should be applied automatically. It is important to keep in mind the basic principles of *heat/cold, excess/deficiency, wind, damp,* and so on, and to recognize their dynamic natures. In this way one can discover which of the remedies are truly appropriate. Likewise, most individuals who have a certain disease described by medical science will experience it uniquely and therefore need treatments suited to their specific conditions. For example, two people with tumors in the same area of the body may have entirely different constitutions and natures. Even though both have tumors and therefore a probable *damp* condition, one person may be *deficient* with *cold* signs while the other has *excess* and *heat* signs.

Symptoms may also vary through the course of any illness. During a bout with the common cold, for example, mucus may change from light, clear, and runny *(cold)* to yellow and thick *(heat),* so that the person needs warming herbs and treatment at the outset and cooling later.

In order to adjust to changing needs, it is essential to be a creative healing artist, observing and listening on all levels, exercising care and patience, while at the same time clearly grasping the nature of the condition. The simple yet profound patterns that we have thus far developed are indispensable here. We often see the best intentions fail when people either refuse to look at underlying principles or are ignorant of them.

Intuition plays a vital role in the art of healing, but during a healing crisis there is very often fear, lack of focus, and various emotional attachments of the practitioner to the ill person, all of which cloud intuition. Diagnostic patterns such as the Six Divisions and Six Influences are invaluable aids which magnify and clarify the borders between intuition and reason, art and science, thereby securing a firm diagnostic foundation for traditional healing arts—diet, herbs, exercise, awareness practices, healing touch, acupuncture—as well as modern medical treatments.

Part II

Essentials of Nutrition

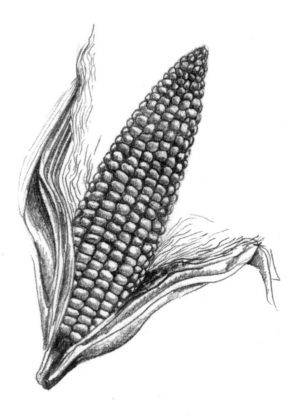

Dietary Transition

The purpose of this chapter is to assist those wishing to make a smooth transition to a better diet, including those who have previously upgraded their diets and are still in need of further improvements. This chapter offers psychological insights to help ensure success; it also maps out the patterns that typically occur in such transitions and recommends dietary measures that reduce excesses and clear up old toxic patterns.

Changes involving diet, lifestyle, and attitude will take individual pathways that depend on the person's resolve and commitment, inherent strengths and weaknesses, the difference between the previous diet and the new one, and the speed of change. Diet is an aspect of our personality. The relationship between food and personality is clearly an inexact one, since some people eat poorly and still maintain emotional integrity. A poor diet, however, will eventually undermine the strongest of minds and bodies.

Sometimes we hear that if unhealthy food is eaten, good thoughts about it will suffice to make it beneficial. There is some truth to this idea, but we have witnessed too many people with keen and sagacious minds succumb to cancer as a result of poor diet. On an ultimate level, the ability exists to alter food totally by thought, but most of us have not developed this ability. Simply put, if you know that a food is not good, don't eat it.

Wear Only One Hat

In Chinese philosophy, the practice of avoiding known evils is called "wearing one hat." A "hat" represents an action in a chain of causation. Regarding unhealthy food, the first action, or hat, can be the decision not to eat those foods. In this case, we wear only one hat. However, if unhealthy food is eaten, then this action is the first hat, and the second, third, and successive hats are how we must overcome the effects of the poor food—by suffering, by trying to change the effects with positive thoughts about the food, or by taking medicine, then by overcoming the effects of the medicine—in other words, there is a further reaction to each preceding reaction.

It is suggested that for maximum health we wear at most one hat. Each hat beyond this is an added weight, causing progressively heavier feelings and less freedom. Wearing no hat—the "zero hat" condition—is to experience the source of all change.

By following a path of correct action, we accelerate through cycles of awareness. If we are to make progress, we must unravel all negative situations stored in our bodies and minds by moment-to-moment choices of appropriate activity. The appropriate diet is highly individual, so the precise nature of this process will vary from person to person.

Those who choose a diet to impress others, to be fashionable, to gain greater power, or even to become "healthy" with no thought of sharing what was learned with others usually have a difficult transition. When one is guided by idealistic motives, such as choosing a diet because it is more humane—because it does not promote the killing of animals (vegetarian) or does not oppress Third World peoples (avoiding multinational-corporation products)—then there seem to be not only fewer problems with transition but a healthier attitude, which in turn enables better judgment regarding future dietary choices.

When a new diet is adopted, one can expect some reactions as the biochemical processes within each cell change. If the new diet is also purer, then old toxins are released, sometimes with various forms of discomfort known as "healing reactions." Such cellular changes also affect the mind and not only represent changes in the mental dimension, but are themselves the transformations of old emotional and mental patterns embedded in the RNA/DNA of the body's cells.

Healing Reactions

Healing reactions present an opportunity to go back through everything not previously resolved in one's life. We carry our entire personal histories in our bodies. Every injury that did not heal fully—whether physical, emotional, or mental—must be made right. All obstructions, toxins, aberrations, and pain must be cleared in a total healing.

The nature of a reaction indicates which phase of life is being healed. The reactions feel similar to the original disease or emotional trauma, but usually appear in a diminished form. If the reaction is an emotional discharge of anger, the feelings surrounding the discharge will remind one of anger earlier in one's life, even though the present anger may be "caused" by different circumstances. Physical discharges are also reminders of old conditions. If chronic sore throats occurred during childhood, a healing reaction could involve one or two sore throats that would eliminate any residues that accumulated from the original infection(s).

Certainly everyone wants healing reactions to be minimal or non-existent. According to traditional Japanese medicine, however, if there is no *meigan* (healing reaction), there is no cure. Most reactions involve the body's purging itself of toxins. The outward manifestations of this elimination may be severe or moderate, depending on the skill involved in regulating the process.

Examples of Healing Reactions

1. Tension or pain may occur in the upper back and neck, which may move upwards to the head, downward across the abdomen, arms, and legs, and eventually to the head top, toes, and fingers. Pain may occur in the internal organs, particularly in the liver area under the right side of the rib cage. Headache is common.
2. Vomiting may occur. Bile or various types of mucus may come up.

3. Digestive imbalances may develop: gas, cramps, diarrhea, etc.
4. Weakness, weight loss, and sensations of cold and/or heat are signs that the body is first strongly eliminating before the building and strengthening phase occurs.
5. Typical emotional reactions include unreasonable impatience, anger, and/or depression.
6. More sleep may be needed during transition, and dreams may be wild. Unusual visions, apparitions, or altered states occasionally occur.
7. Menstruation sometimes ceases but will resume when the digestion calms and the liver and kidney functions are renewed.
8. Sexual desire usually diminishes, especially in men, but eventually becomes more balanced than previously, once the kidney-adrenal function is strengthened.
9. Possible discharges include boils, pimples, rashes, body odors, carbuncles, nasal and vaginal discharges, coating on tongue, and black feces. Silver amalgam (mercury) fillings may fall out.

Most healing reactions involving pain and discharges will last less than a week, although these symptoms sometimes last longer. Since the body needs the sexual/reproductive function least at this time, the resurgence of sexual energy and menses may take the longest. It is not recommended that a woman dramatically change her diet during pregnancy, since the released toxins may harm the fetus; the shock to the system in general may also trigger spontaneous abortion. She can safely abstain, of course, from such extreme items as intoxicants and highly refined, chemical-laden products.

Chlorophyll and Dietary Transition

When toxins are discharged in the body during healing reactions, use cleansing foods to help lighten the process: vegetables, fruit, and the sprouts of seeds, grains, and legumes. If there are feelings of coldness and weakness, then cook all cleansing foods and also use less of them. When one is changing in the direction of more vegetarian eating patterns, small amounts of nutritionally rich protein food help ease the body over the shock of losing animal products. In addition, chlorophyll-rich foods are especially beneficial to discharge the residues of animal toxins, build new blood, and support cell renewal. All green vegetables can normally be emphasized during transitional healing reactions.

The regenerative qualities of chlorophyll and protein are combined in nutritious products such as cereal grass and micro-algae. For more information on these foods and possible restrictions on their use, refer to the *Green Food Products* chapter.

Foods Which Counteract Toxins

Chinese medicine recognizes certain common foods as toxin neutralizers: tofu, millet, mung beans, aduki beans, black soybeans, Swiss chard, radishes, turnips, and figs. These can be used freely in the diet during a transition and especially during healing reactions (if food is tolerated at all).

Salt and vinegar are also detoxifying, and are commonly used in both the West and East for this purpose. They are strong substances, however, and should be taken with care and primarily for digestive problems. One does not normally take straight salt, even medicinally; it should be diluted in foods or water, or taken in salt-plum products. Apple cider vinegar is mixed a teaspoon at a time in ⅓ cup of water (take undiluted for food poisoning). These products are further described on pages 204 and 205. We do not recommend the habitual use of salt and vinegar for digestive imbalances; it is better to overcome poor dietary practices instead.

*   *   *

The strongest reactions from dietary transition occur in the first six months, although major reactions can occur years later. Older or very weak people need to change dietary patterns more slowly, by replacing poor-quality foods and lessening the use of weakening foods. See "Dietary Suggestions for Vitality in the Elderly," page 366.

Recommended Proportions of Food Groups

The following proportions (by weight) in a grain- and vegetable-based diet result in nutrition that is rich in fiber, minerals, and vitamins, moderate in protein and unsaturated fat, and low in saturated fat. Populations where such a diet is prevalent experience relatively less cancer and heart disease and greater longevity.[1]

35*–60%   GRAINS: whole grains, cereals, grain sprouts, and flour products
20–25%*   VEGETABLES: green, starchy, low-starch; seaweeds and micro-algae
  5–15%*   LEGUMES: beans, peas, lentils, legume sprouts, tofu, miso, etc.
  5–15%*   FRUITS and small amounts of NUTS and OIL-RICH SEEDS
  0–10%*   ANIMAL PRODUCTS: dairy, eggs, fish, fowl, and mammal meats

The ranges given above are wide enough to accommodate most individuals except those with extreme conditions. For healthy persons with a dietary history already low in meat and dairy foods, the consumption of animal products can be little or none. Animal products in general should be used cautiously in diets of robust persons with signs of *excess,* whereas the frail, *deficient* person may require them.

---

*These percentages are appropriate for most people making the transition from a standard American diet to whole vegetarian foods. Less emphasis is placed on grain and more on vegetables, fruits, and high-protein foods.

Nuts and seeds, because of their concentrated fat and protein content, do not digest easily and should be eaten in very small quantities. A common problem resulting in digestive weakness and fatigue is the gross overuse of fruits and their juices, particularly the tropical variety.

Eating foods from the above groups in the recommended proportions is only one step toward wellness. Of equal importance are eating simple meals in healthful combinations (see *Food Combinations* chapter), not overeating, preparing and choosing high-quality foods according to one's individual constitution and condition (discussed in *The Six Divisions, Five Elements,* and other chapters), adequate exercise, and the multitude of attitudinal factors that influence our digestion and general health.

For more information on the nature and use of animal products (including dairy, meat, fish, and eggs), refer to the *Protein and Vitamin B$_{12}$* chapter. Also described therein are the many protein-rich plant alternatives to animal products, and methods for preparing meat as medicine. A plan for reducing the proportion of meat and other animal products in the diet follows.

Transition from Meat-based Diet to Whole Plant-based Diet

1. If you use refined grains, begin by slowly adding whole grains to white rice or the other refined cereals that you are used to. The greater nutrient content of whole grain reduces the desire for meat. Also avoid products that cause demineralization and loss of nutrients, such as white sugar, white breads, pastas and pastries, and intoxicants. Begin to use seaweeds; these are rich in the complete spectrum of minerals.

2. Use more vegetables with smaller amounts of meat. Soups and broths add a beneficial dispersing quality to the concentrated nature of meat.

3. First reduce your intake of red meats (or meat from mammals generally), then fowl and fish. For safe protein intake from meats and fish, see guidelines on pages 29 and 30.

4. Also reduce dairy and eggs, particularly if they are of poor quality. Many people find that substantial amounts of dairy and eggs do not mix well with a grain-based diet. (Constipation and a heavy feeling can result.) When eaten in abundance, dairy and eggs are mucus-forming, and grains are moderately so; thus the combination can cause excessive mucus accumulation.

5. To make the transition smoother and prevent binges, it is better to have small amounts of animal food regularly than large amounts occasionally.

6. Only small amounts of animal food (or in some cases, none at all) may be sufficient once a person is mentally and physically stable. Don't rush—enjoy life's changes at each stage. Changes normally come more easily with a more gradual transition. Even though notable benefits often occur within a few weeks, the full transition may take years. The process of renewal is a harmonious way of life.

*   *   *

Herbs* can aid greatly in every aspect of healing, including dietary transition. There are a number of ways to take herbs, the most common being water extractions.

Standard Herbal Preparations

Four methods of herbal preparation are given below. Herbs prepared in water are commonly called "teas," and are defined either as infusions or decoctions. Two other types of preparation include alcohol extractions or "tinctures" and encapsulated herbal powders. The herbs suggested throughout this book are to be prepared and used according to the following directions unless otherwise noted. In all dosages given below, take herbs six days a week only.

Infusions are made from dried or fresh flowers or leaves. To infuse, pour boiling water onto herbs in a non-metal teapot; cover, steep for 20 minutes, and strain to drink. Use approximately one ounce of the combined total of dried herbs to each pint of water. Herb teas can also be brewed in a thermos bottle, which will keep them warm all day and travels well, too.

Dosage: Drink ½ cup tea 2–4 times a day, between meals.

Decoctions are made from roots, bark, seeds, or stems. To decoct, simmer one ounce of dried herbs for each 1½ pints of water for thirty minutes to one hour, in a covered pot. Strain and drink. The large, hard herbs such as *dang gui* root *(Angelica sinensis)* may be simmered two to three hours, starting with two or three pints of water.

A glass, ceramic, enamel-coated, or earthenware pot is best. Do not use pots of aluminum or cast iron, or those with synthetic coatings; high grades of stainless steel such as surgical stainless are acceptable.

When a formula contains some herbs to be infused and others to be decocted, simply simmer the herbs to be decocted with enough water for all the herbs; then pour the completed decoction, still simmering, over the herbs to be infused.

Note: When decocting or infusing fresh herbs, use double the quantities given above for dried herbs.

Dosage: Same as above for infusions.

Capsules of individual herbs or whole formulas are handy when herbs are very unpleasant-tasting or inconvenient to prepare otherwise. To encapsulate herbs, powder them by grinding in a mortar and pestle, or use a seed mill, blender, or other device. Some very hard dried herbs are difficult to grind and may be available already in powder form. Also, some herbal outlets—often the same ones that sell empty capsules—will powder herbs by request. The herbal powder is then placed

---

*"Herbs" are foods with discrete, specific, and often strong properties, on the borderline between foods and medicines.

in capsules and stored in a dry place out of direct light—a dark or opaque bottle with lid works well. Herb stores often carry simple machines for putting herbal powders into capsules efficiently. They also usually offer herbs in ready-made capsules, pills, and fluid extracts.

Dosage: If capsules, pills, or tablets are used, take approximately 3,000 milligrams (3 grams) of herbs three times daily between meals, followed with water. Note: a size #0 capsule holds approximately 400–450 milligrams of herbs; a #00, 500–600 milligrams; and a #000, 650–850 milligrams. The higher milligram weights are for denser herbs, primarily barks, seeds, and roots.

Tinctures are extracts of herbs in alcohol or another medium. Like capsules, they are very convenient, and either single herbs or formulas may be tinctured. To prepare, soak each 2–4 ounces of herbs to be extracted in one pint of 60- to 80-proof alcohol such as vodka. If the herbs are lighter—primarily leaves and flowers—use 2 ounces; for heavier barks and roots, use 4 ounces. In any case, add more liquid if it is all absorbed by the herbs. Each day, shake the mixture for a minute or so. After 14 days or longer, strain off the herb-infused liquid and extract the remaining mash by twisting it in cheesecloth. Expressing the mash with a juice press, if available, is the most effective way. Store the resulting tincture in a sealed dark glass bottle. Lids with exposed metal (e.g., most canning jar lids) leach the metals into tinctures and should be avoided. Decant tincture as needed into a 1- to 4-ounce dropper bottle (available at some pharmacies and herb stores). Tinctures will maintain potency for a number of years.

Dosage: 20 drops ($\frac{1}{3}$ teaspoon) twice a day between meals, under the tongue or in a little water, herbal tea, or other liquid.

Excesses and Toxins

The discharges from healing reactions involve several common types of excesses and toxins; each has specific remedies. Chlorophyll foods and others which counteract toxins are very helpful general remedies, especially when coupled with a grain-and-vegetable diet that includes seaweeds and enzyme-rich products such as sprouts and miso. Sufficient regular exercise is essential for processing and "burning up" excesses. When reactions and discharges are especially severe or numerous, it may mean that the pace of dietary change is too fast.

In some cases, strong reactions will be difficult to avoid, regardless. Also, chronically ill people will often (wisely) venture into a more healthful dietary plan, and it is their disease symptoms rather than their healing reactions that must first be overcome. In either case, common toxins and excesses in the body are listed below, along with remedies.

Toxic Metals

People who live in industrialized parts of the world usually pick up toxic amounts of metallic elements from the air, water, and food supplies. The most common are lead, arsenic, cadmium, aluminum, mercury (also absorbed from silver-amalgam tooth fillings), and others. These toxins can remain in the body an entire lifetime, wreaking havoc with all metabolic systems until removed.

Many weakened conditions are linked to toxic metals. For example, it is suspected that an accumulation of excess aluminum may contribute to a brain deterioration syndrome known as Alzheimer's disease,[2-4] now among the five leading causes of death in the United States. Aluminum is picked up from aluminum cookware and from drinking water (aluminum sulfate is frequently used to filter municipal water and often is not completely removed). Baking powder and antacid tablets are two other common sources. The following remedies, if used in the diet 4–6 times a week for 6 months, efficiently remove toxic metals. For prevention of toxic metal buildup, these remedies may be included in the diet periodically.

Garlic	Wheat- or Barley-grass[†]
Seaweeds[†] or Algin*[†]	Mung beans (to remove lead)
Miso[†]	

Radiation

Radiation from nuclear fallout (strontium 90, cesium 137, iodine 131, etc.), X-rays, microwaves, high-voltage power lines, televisions, video display terminals (including computer monitors), all electric devices, and many other sources saturate people with radiation, causing free-radical pathology and thereby contributing to aging, cellular distortion, leukemia and other forms of cancer, birth defects, anemia, and other diseases. Whether radiation is received environmentally, for medical diagnosis, or as radiation therapy, the effects can be countered with the items marked "†" above.

Other useful chlorophyll-rich foods besides the cereal grasses are spirulina, chlorella, and wild blue-green micro-algae. Panax and Siberian ginseng are also effective. Panax is a standard ginseng grown in China, Korea, and the United States, and is used for those with *deficiencies.* Siberian ginseng *(Eleutherococcus senticosus),* its relative, is preferable to panax where no serious weakness exists.

Several other common foods help counteract radiation. The glucoside rutin found in buckwheat protects against the effects of radiation. Apples and fresh sunflower seeds contain pectin, which binds radioactive residues and removes them from the body. Lecithin and bentonite clay (very effective) also have this action. The dosage of lecithin is 1 teaspoon daily. Bentonite clay is prepared by adding 4 ounces unboiled water to 1 ounce clay. Let sit for about 8 hours, then stir and drink the clay-infused water once daily. Plenty of other fluids should be taken throughout the day. Other edible clays including French green clay may be substituted for bentonite. It should be noted that radioactive isotopes from nuclear fallout and cer-

---

*Algin, a gelatinous derivative of kelp or other seaweed, is available as a nutritional supplement.

tain medical treatments can remain radioactive in the body for days, months, or even years, depending on the isotope. Most types of radiation such as microwaves, X-rays, and electromagnetic radiation, however, simply pass through the body, causing various forms of damage in addition to that of free radical formation. Such radiation sometimes causes radiomimetic products to form in the body; though not radioactive, they mimic radioactive substances, causing similar problems. Fortunately, the above remedies also denature radiomimetic products.

Essential fatty acids are useful to initiate cell renewal after a radiation burn. One tablespoon daily of fresh flax oil supplies these fatty acids as well as vitamin A, minerals, lecithin, and other vital nutrients. Aloe vera juices or gels are useful for skin burns. An excellent external treatment in every form of radiation exposure is a bath of sea salt and baking soda. This method is used by some radioactive isotope specialists to reduce their own bodily radiation. Add 1 pound of both sea salt and baking soda to a warm bath, and soak for 20 minutes; rinse with cool water. Repeat three times a week for one month in cases of serious exposure. Another decontamination procedure is clay baths; or add clay to salt/soda baths for added effectiveness. Use 1 cup bentonite or other clay and follow the above bath directions.

People regularly exposed to elevated levels of radiation can use one or more of the above remedies daily to prevent side effects. However, prudence is urged. We know several Americans who became quite ill for weeks after the Chernobyl catastrophe in the Soviet Union—not from radiation, but from eating massive amounts of miso, seaweeds, and various supplements in an attempt to shield themselves from it. For specific incidences of contamination, recommended dosages of foods such as apples, miso, seaweeds, cereal grasses, micro-algae, sunflower seeds, and buckwheat can be the upper limits normally used in meals or as supplements. One or two remedies may be taken twice daily for three days to treat minor exposures (e.g., one X-ray diagnosis); or continue the remedies for as long as several weeks to counteract greater contamination. Ways of treating radiation and chemotherapy consistent with the cancer program are given on page 409.

Drugs

Residues in the body from either medicinal or recreational drugs are very often stored throughout a person's life in the liver, brain, and other tissues. Examples include such common drugs as alcohol, marijuana, LSD, tranquilizers, pain relief drugs, birth control pills, and antibiotics. The residues of these drugs either accumulate directly, or the reactions they produce in the body result in a buildup of toxic by-products. For example, delta-9-tetrahydrocannabinol (THC), one of a number of active ingredients in marijuana, builds up in the brain tissues of habitual users of the substance, causing long-term harmful effects.[5] (See note 22 on page 701.)

A grain-and-vegetable diet supplemented with green foods helps remove drug residues. When there has been prolonged use, an excellent remedy is the herb chaparral *(Larrea divaricata)*. To remove intoxicant and drug-related deposits with chaparral, take it only once a day for twenty days, then take one week off;

daily consumption is then repeated for an additional twenty days. Chaparral's properties can be extracted in water, but for greatest effectiveness the whole herb needs to be consumed—or it is taken in an alcohol-extracted tincture.

If chaparral powder is available, stir one heaping teaspoon in a cup of warm licorice or mint tea (to mask its very bitter flavor); do not strain but drink the powder with the tea. Chaparral powder can be made from the leaves, with a blender or mortar and pestle. The powder may also be put in capsules, or bought in ready-made capsules, tablets, or tinctures.

The herb calamus root (*Acorus calamus* and subspecies) will help restore mental damage resulting from drugs or other causes. It is used for this purpose in Ayurveda, the traditional medicine of India. (Follow standard dosage and preparation given earlier on pages 110–111.)

For treatments for alcohol and other drug abuses, see page 429.

Parasites

Various parasites infect a major percentage of the population. The most common types include pinworms, roundworms, and tapeworms, which proliferate in a mucus-laden digestive tract. One of the commonest ways to get worms is from pets such as dogs or cats living in the house. Other major causes of parasites are eating uncooked meats, fish, and sometimes raw vegetables, walking barefoot (especially in moist, warm climates), and poor hygiene in the company of infested people.

Following are some of the most common symptoms of parasites: general weakness, emaciation, voracious appetite, withered yellow look, facial pallor, bluish or purplish specks in the whites of the eyes, white coin-sized blotches on the face, anal itching (especially at night), nose-picking, fretful sleep, grinding the teeth while asleep, and cravings for sweets, dried food, raw rice, dirt (usually a symptom in children), charcoal, and/or burned food. Note: If you have a history of parasites, or are seriously imbalanced, please refer to the Parasite Purge Program in the appendix, page 654.

Many parasiticides are harsh chemicals. To clean the intestines, or as a precaution, use the following formula once a year in the late summer or spring. The foods and herbs suggested below are effective in most cases of mild infestation.

Parasite Prevention Program

1. For breakfast, chew one handful of raw rice thoroughly—eat nothing else. Other meals during the day can be normal. Whole dried corn kernels may be substituted, but must be chewed only when warm from pan-roasting; otherwise, they are too hard.

2. At a later time between meals, eat one clove of garlic and one small handful of pumpkin pumpkin seeds—lightly roasted to remove surface *E. coli.* Children and others who cannot tolerate raw garlic can usually accept minced garlic mixed with a spoonful of diluted miso; or try thin slices of garlic between slices of apple. Garlic pills can be substituted but are often less effective.

3. Two or more hours after the last meal of the day, drink one cupful of mugwort tea *(Artemisia vulgaris)*.

Follow this program for ten days, stop for seven days, and resume for a final ten days to remove parasites that have hatched from eggs after the initial ten days. Completing all three steps daily ensures a greater likelihood of success, although following any one step has been helpful in many cases.

Mucus

Common signs of excess mucus in the system are:
1. Frequent colds.
2. A history of copious dairy, meat, eggs, and white flour products in the diet.
3. Nasal, vaginal, or rectal mucus discharges.
4. Most lung and colon problems.
5. Thick coating on tongue.

To speed the cleansing of excess mucus conditions, the following "Three-F" formula replaces pathologic mucus along the mucous membranes with a thin, light, beneficial coating, while gradually renewing the entire gastrointestinal tract.

Three-F Formula

Decoct a tea of:

> One part fennel seed *(Foeniculum vulgare)*
> One part fenugreek seed *(Trigonella foenumgraecum)*
> One part flax seed *(Linum usitatissimum)*
> One part nettle leaf *(Urtica urens)*
> ¼ part licorice root *(Glycyrrhiza glabra)*

The formula is used for four weeks as an autumn tonic for the lungs, colon, and mucous membranes. (Standard dosage and preparation of decoctions are listed earlier in this chapter.) For chronic mucus conditions it is taken for longer periods of time. It is also an excellent nutritive blend during fasting.

Excess Weight

An overweight condition is best approached by seeing it as it is—just another excess or toxin to be eliminated in a successful dietary transition.

Most overweight people who change to a plant-based diet of whole grains, vegetables, and other unrefined foods can expect to lose weight. Overweight is not always caused by overeating, since there are many thin people who overeat, and some with excess weight who do not. For those who are overweight as a result of overeating, refer also to "Overeating and Aging" in Chapter 18.

Overweight conditions, like all imbalances, are supported by unhealthy attitudes. People who are obese may often find medical and other reasons to continue living and eating in ways that add weight, but once a firm decision is made to give up the weight, and a resolution is followed based on sound principles of nutrition, the result is weight loss in almost every case.

The energy in the body stored as weight comes from three sources: proteins and carbohydrates, each of which contributes four calories per gram; and fats, which yield nine calories per gram. Gaining weight from fats, therefore, is twice as easy as from proteins and carbohydrates. The great majority of fats consumed by people comes from animal products. Even "3% butterfat milk" acquires 49% of its total calories from fat, and the calories in 2% milk are 32% fat. (For weight-loss purposes, calories of specific nutrients in a product should be figured as a percentage of total calories, not by product weight, as figured by the dairy industry.)

Fats: A Major Cause of Slow Metabolism

When fats are eaten, the digestion of all food is retarded. The secretion of hydrochloric acid by the stomach diminishes with increased fat intake. Similarly, according to the "Five Element Control Cycle" of Chinese medicine, the action of the pancreas and stomach is depressed by an excessive liver, a frequent result of excessive fat consumption.

Whole Foods and Exercise

Highly processed foods such as refined sugars and flours also upset the metabolism. These devitalized foods are deficient in the vitamins, minerals, and enzymes necessary for regulating glandular secretion and proper digestion. Whole foods, therefore, are preferable. Moderate regular exercise is also essential for a smooth flow of blood and energy through the body, and for overcoming the stagnancy of excess weight. Fat and muscle are often shed at an equal rate during weight loss, and exercise helps the body maintain its muscle mass, thereby protecting the heart and other muscles from deterioration.

Guidelines for Long-Term Weight Reduction

The measures that we have seen work best for long-term weight loss include:

1. Commitment to emotional clarity with support from physical activity (ideally one-hour exercise per day) and daily awareness practice. Please refer to "Emotional Awareness," pages 24–26.
2. A balanced diet of *unrefined* foods. Please study "Whole Foods: Survival Imperative for the 21st Century," pages 17–19.

The above two steps are very effective and seldom require further dietary aids to promote weight loss. However, there are quite a few individuals who, even on a healthy regimen, lose weight only slowly or not at all. For these cases, we recommend the East Asian tradition regarding weight loss which emphasizes bitter and pungent flavors and limits sweet, salty, and sour foods. The fat content and diuretic properties of foods are also important. The following tenets, derived from Chinese and East Indian healing systems, are useful guidelines for individuals who struggle with losing weight—usually those still in transition to a diet based on unrefined grains and vegetables.

1. **Nuts, seeds, and oils:** Supporting our earlier-stated view on fats is the Ayurvedic tradition which recommends restricting not only animal fats but also those of vegetable origin. Nuts, seeds, and oils must be used sparingly if at all. Two exceptions to this tradition are the lighter omega-3 and GLA (gamma linolenic acid) oils, which increase metabolism and the rate of fat burn-off. Unrefined cold-pressed flax oil, the richest vegetal source of omega-3 oils, provides the hormonal balance necessary for a healthful body shape. Dosage: two teaspoons of flax oil are poured over food each day; or, for an equivalent amount of oil, three table-spoons of soaked or crushed flax seeds (flaxmeal) are eaten daily. The seeds help sluggish digestion. (See page 165 for flaxseed directions.) Strictly avoid hydro-genated fats (e.g., margarine and shortening) and refined oils (in virtually all com-mercial foods that contain oil, including "health foods"). These negative oils and fats as well as fluoridated water greatly hinder the fat burn-off rate.

Oils rich in GLA also prove to be highly effective for weight-reduction. The best whole-food source other than human milk is spirulina. GLA-rich oils extracted from the seeds of evening primrose, borage, and black currant are also common-ly available. 125 mg. is an effective daily dosage of GLA from any of these plants. (See *Oils and Fats* Chapter for more on GLA, omega-3, and quality oils.)

2. In the Chinese tradition, most **legumes** are classified as having a "sweet" flavor. Nevertheless, legumes have a drying, diuretic effect, and any of them except soybeans are recommended. Aduki and mung beans are especially helpful. Several cups of a decoction of aduki bean tea can be taken during the day to speed weight loss. Mung and other bean sprouts are also beneficial, and can be steamed for those with signs of *coldness* (feeling cold often or disliking the cold).

3. **Grains** also have a sweet quality, and those with a bitter component should be emphasized. These are rye, amaranth, quinoa, and oats. For weight loss, oats are ide-ally eaten in their most bitter form—raw (soaked) or roasted. The best rice to use is basmati because of its pungency. (Much of the basmati available today is refined; choose only the unrefined variety to use for weight loss.) Corn is also appropriate since it is diuretic and thus removes excess water stored in the tissues.

4. Nearly all **vegetables** are useful for weight loss, with the exception of the very watery types (zucchini, summer squash) and the very sweet ones (sweet potato and yam). The vegetables classified as having a partially bitter flavor—lettuce, celery, kohlrabi, asparagus, and scallion—are especially helpful. (Lettuce is contraindi-cated for those with eye diseases.) Eating vegetables only lightly cooked is preferable, since less cooked food adds liveliness to the usually slow, overweight person. Raw food is desirable for those with excessive appetite or *heat* signs. Those with *cold* signs should restrict raw food because it will encourage fat and water retention. These individuals need mostly cooked food.

Although sea vegetables are salty, their iodine content and wide range of min-erals and amino acids help regulate weight levels; Norwegian kelp (bladderwrack) is a specific for this purpose. Other seaweeds are also valuable; if kelp is used, it is conveniently available in tablets. The dosage is 4–6 tablets daily.

5. **Fruit and sweeteners:** Very sweet fruits (figs, dates, and dried fruit) can hinder weight loss. Also to be used sparingly are the starchy or oily fruits including banana, avocado, and coconut. The lemon and grapefruit, although their sour citric acid in itself is considered undesirable for losing weight, also contain an intensely bitter quality which more than compensates for their acidity. A daily lemon or grapefruit, eaten with its seeds, pulp and a little of the inner peel (the most bitter parts) can be an excellent weight-loss remedy. Those who have signs of *coldness,* however, should use much less lemon or grapefruit—or none at all, if chills increase with their use.

Common fruits such as apples, plums, peaches, berries, oranges, and pears tend to be cleansing, which is desirable for the overweight person; however, their acid content and sweet flavor can also prove weakening and cause *dampness* (water retention, yeast overgrowth, fatigue, sluggishness, and/or emotional heaviness). Consumption of this type of fruit should be avoided in people with these symptoms.

Two sweeteners can be recommended during weight loss. The first is *raw* honey; by "raw" we mean honey that has not been heated in any stage of its processing, and when used in liquids such as tea, not heated above 130°F. Raw honey has a pungent effect when metabolized, which is desirable for losing weight; even so, it is a powerful substance and should only be used in small amounts. The second sweetener is stevia leaf ("honey leaf"). (See *Sweeteners* chapter.) All other natural sweeteners tend to encourage weight gain. Avoid chemical sweeteners altogether.

6. **Animal products:** Avoid rich, weight-promoting food such as eggs and bovine dairy including butter; reduce meat consumption although wild fish and free-range fowl may benefit those with weakness. Goat dairy normalizes body weight so has value for both over- and under-weight persons.

7. **Spices and seasonings:** These play a valuable role in a weight-loss program. However, salt and products high in salt must be restricted in overweight conditions, since they tend to promote the accumulation of moisture in the body. When salt is used in cooking, it must be applied sparingly, ideally in the form of unrefined whole salt. Likewise miso, soy sauce, salt plums, pickles, and other salty products need to be used minimally and should be of quality unrefined salt. When there is edema (water retention/swelling), omit salt from the diet altogether.

All pungent foods promote energy circulation and increase the metabolic rate. Notable examples are the herbs cumin, ginger, cloves, spearmint, fennel, anise, and cayenne. A person with *heat* symptoms, however, should avoid these warming pungents and should use neutral or cooling ones instead: peppermint, chamomile, kohlrabi, turnip, radish, taro, and white pepper.

8. Most **bitter herbs** are beneficial since they reduce moisture in the body, purify the blood, and take out *heat* toxins sometimes associated with excess weight. Particularly useful are:

Burdock root: Decoct the dried herb, or eat the fresh root (raw or cooked). This common root is found growing in most areas of the United States; it is also available in Japanese food stores as *gobo,* and can often be obtained through large food/produce stores by request. Most herb stores carry dried burdock root. Eaten in quantity, raw or cooked, this mildly bitter herb is a virtual cure-all for conditions of *excess*, and significantly purifies the blood while reducing fat and regulating blood sugar.

Other useful bitter herbs are **dandelion root**, **chamomile** (also pungent), **yellow dock root** (laxative), and **bupleurum root** (also pungent), known as the common Chinese herb *chai hu.* In addition, bupleurum is beneficial for treating all prolapsed conditions (prolapsed uterus/intestines, hemorrhoids etc.). Chinese **green tea** is also very useful for weight loss. Other types of tea including bancha twig can be substituted, and have a milder action.

Alfalfa can promote weight loss, and because of its drying action it is also classified as having a bitter flavor even though its actual taste is pleasant. Alfalfa is eaten fresh or as a cooked green in various dishes, or in the form of sprouts. It may also be consumed as a tea infusion, or taken as tablets. For information on the decoction of alfalfa seeds and instructions on sprouting methods, see "Sprouts" in recipe section.

A traditional Western wild green that helps reduce fat is **chickweed**. It is commonly available as both a garden weed and a dried herb, and should be decocted.

The bitter herbs and greens listed above should be safe for overweight people; however, since they are cooling, they are not appropriate for those with pronounced signs of *coldness.* Further properties of most of these herbs can be looked up in many standard herbal texts.

9. To relax and heal the stomach and regulate appetite at the beginning of meals, take wild blue green alga (2 grams) or cereal grass powder (4 grams). (For usage directions and suitability for your health status, refer to *Green Food Products,* Chapter 16.) Micro-algae as well as bee pollen contain specific nutrients that can moderate body weight. Taking 1–4 grams of wild blue-green micro-alga (ideal to counteract depression) or 10 grams of either spirulina or bee pollen will usually eliminate blood-sugar imbalances and cravings, and may be substituted for snacks or missed meals.

10. Sunshine strongly stimulates hormonal centers and promotes weight loss.

Emotional/Psychological Discharges

Throughout the process of purification, the individual can be expected to have a number of healing reactions arising from the residues of past experiences. The cells of the body—in particular those of the brain and liver—are actively encoded with every emotional or mental issue that has not been resolved. After all, "everything characteristic of a human—size, shape and orderly development from infancy to death—is recorded by an arrangement of molecules and DNA."[6] This arrangement, on whatever level it is embodied, is always going to reflect the path of the person throughout life.

When a balanced diet and lifestyle are followed, the cells of the body relax and eventually normalize. As cell and tissue distortions are released, the repressed emotions that accompanied them are also released and begin to surface. In Biblical times, these releases were called "demons" and still could be, for the demons that plague us are our psychological projections generated by unresolved issues or ambivalence toward our unfolding paths.

From the perspective of Chinese healing arts, smooth emotional interactions rely on the health of the liver. The modern person's liver is usually enlarged to at least twice what its size should be if healthy, for it can store pounds of undesirable material. This material consists of residues from excess consumption of meat and other animal products, from environmental toxins, and from overeating in general.

When one starts the process of purification by eating better-quality food in smaller quantities, the liver and body in general begin to discharge excesses that have been carried for years. Simultaneously, many rigid mental perceptions of reality begin to dissolve. Because of the emotional and sometimes physical pain involved, most individuals will unconsciously stop this process by eating more of the products being discharged; that is why those particular foods are craved at this time. Such a pattern is observed in alcoholics, where the pain from alcohol withdrawal subsides if even a small amount of alcohol is consumed. Few people consider food and household-medicine addictions to be of this nature; we have witnessed, however, extreme processes of withdrawal from refined sugar, meat, drugs (especially tranquilizers), nicotine, coffee (caffeine), and other common foods and medicines.

More common than the physical pains of any withdrawal are its psychological and emotional symptoms. Making it through withdrawal can of course be greatly aided by purifying, cleansing foods which assist in the discharge of toxins on all levels. But even with these foods as aids, the most significant factor for achieving success in dietary transition will be the willingness to face whatever comes up, to learn from it, and to resolve it. This attitude of discipline and perseverance eases emotional distress while allowing the body to continue to purify new areas, until one eventually attains the spontaneity and innocence of a child.

Purification is not solely a physical or emotional matter; it entails purification of the mind, which ultimately includes inner development, attention, and wisdom. In nearly all cultures, fasting is accompanied by prayer or similar rituals. Very few of us have ever thoroughly purified ourselves or developed higher faculties of awareness, but individuals who have accomplished both have a unique quality: they are able to accept difficulties that others find intolerable. This capacity is an indication that they have worked through major emotional obstructions and experienced deep discharges. A Zen phrase describes the recipe:

> "Sweet mind, bitter practice
> Sweet practice, bitter mind."

A number of popular teachings now available emphasize that very little needs to be done to achieve penetrating awareness. On one level these philosophies are accurate, since ultimate awareness is inherent in our nature and cannot be "bought" by our efforts. Before one can experience the ultimate, however, deep purification is needed, if only to prepare the body and mind for increased levels of consciousness. Quick and easy enlightenment is not likely.

Summary of Suggestions for Easing Emotional and Mental Discharges

1. Accept whatever happens as the perfect medicine for the situation.
2. Maintain a daily practice for improving awareness and focus.
3. Allow all emotional issues to resolve completely (however painful the process).
4. If the emotions are strongly obstructed, focus on clearing the liver (see the liver-related areas of the *Wood Element* chapter) and become more involved in creative movement and exercise.

Transition Patterns

Common Causes of Difficulty During Transition

1. Arrogance: Alienation which occurs as a result of negative judgments on the diets of family and friends. Feeling that a good diet makes one "superior."
2. "Missionary Complex": Attempts to convert others to a better diet without first having substantial personal experience and background. A successful example is more effective than convincing arguments.
3. Attempting to make whole vegetarian food taste as rich as meat, dairy, and eggs. This is usually done by the use of unhealthy quantities of salty and oily products; high-salt examples are miso, soy sauce, pickles, umeboshi salt plum, and sea salt. Products high in oil are nuts and seeds and their butters; oils, and margarine. The combination of salty and oily high-protein foods is rich-tasting, for example, sesame butter/miso spreads and sauces. However, only small amounts can be taken without upsetting the liver and causing digestive problems.
4. Feeling protein-deficient because of uncertainty about the value of plant-based protein, and then overcompensating with too much protein in the form of beans, legumes, tofu, nuts, or seeds. Digestive upset can result from combining too many foods in an attempt to obtain the government standard or some mental concept of "complete protein."
5. Not fully recognizing and letting go of destructive habits—consumption of alcohol, cigarettes, coffee, marijuana, sweets, etc.
6. Failure to chew food thoroughly will cause some of the above problems; one does not feel satisfied eating partially masticated vegetarian foods and will

seek balance with extremes of sweets, proteins, oils, and/or excessive amounts of food. (See "The Art of Chewing," page 252.)

As one's diet is improved, one realizes that how food is prepared and eaten is at least as important as the quality of the ingredients. This perception is not forced or merely poetic; it is part of an evolutionary process in which the mind becomes able to mirror reality accurately. As we mature in our food consciousness and cultivate better dietary habits, the common difficulties of dietary transition will provide their own resolutions.

A new diet does not promise health automatically, but if carried out correctly and in the right spirit certainly supports and is an essential force in the total healing process.

Disease arises from inaccurate and rigid views of reality. A dietary transition is a remedy for rigidity since it brings change and the opportunity to melt, on both a physical and emotional plane, fixed and painful parts of one's personality. With perseverance, such transformations become a gradual immersion in a sea of unending renewal.

Water

Water is the most abundant nutrient in the body, comprising two-thirds of the body's mass. Some people make a real effort to obtain unadulterated food but neglect to seek water of similar quality. When a person is *deficient*, has a weak immune system or a degenerative condition, water free from toxic residue is important. In some cases, it actually seems to be the decisive factor between recovery and further degeneration.

Every type of water has a unique quality. Rain water tastes lighter; well water is more mineralized; river, lake, and spring water each bear qualities encountered in their journey. If a river has rapids or a waterfall, its water is enlivened. Spring water may filter through thousands of feet of clay or mineral beds. Water can have a greater or lesser intrinsic energy *(qi),* just as we do. Once water is polluted with chemicals or combined with various other wastes, its life energy is diminished. Finding a high-quality source of water is becoming a difficult task in the modern world. As rain water falls through the atmosphere, it encounters the thick band of pollution that now encircles the Earth. It picks up smoke, dust, germs, lead, strontium 90, minerals, and a host of chemicals. A generation or two ago, rain water was considered a good source of drinking water. Now we can no longer recommend drinking unfiltered rain or snow water. This suggestion is based not only on scientific data about atmospheric pollution but on the testimonials of many who have had adverse reactions.

Mountain Streams and Country Wells

Mountain streams and country wells have long been considered good sources of water. In some cases this still may be true, but if a stream originates from melted snow, rain water runoff, or springs that don't filter water well, then it probably carries even greater pollution than rain water, since air contaminants settle and concentrate in the ground.

Country wells are often in close proximity to zones of chemical agriculture and livestock. Surface water combines with the residues of poison sprays, fertilizers, and animal excrement, then seeps down into the ground. If the route through the earth to a well's aquifer does not purify water, then it will be unsafe to the degree that there are poisons in the area. A major toxin in farm wells is nitrates from various farm chemicals, which convert to highly toxic carcinogenic nitrites by heating, microbial action, or contact with certain metals. According to toxicology researchers, nitrites create "free radicals" which neutralize enzymes in the human body and can cause virtually every deficiency symptom and contribute to every degenerative disease. Herbicides, defoliants, pesticides, and soil fumigants are some of the other chemicals that may be present.

Recycled Water in Cities

There is a 40% chance that the next water you drink will have passed through someone's sewer or an industrial conduit filled with wastes, poisons, and bacteria.[1]

Water supplies from larger lakes and rivers are subject to all the pollutants found in streams and shallow wells. In addition, they often contain other forms of pollution from industrial and municipal discharges. A trend in large American cities is the recycling of used water teeming with bacteria and contaminated with human excrement and chemicals. How thoroughly this water is cleaned before recycling is debatable. Most cities add chlorine to disinfect water, and two-thirds now add sodium fluoride for tooth-decay prevention.

Chlorination

Once out of the tap, chlorine evaporates; many people draw chlorinated water and let it stand at least thirty minutes. Unfortunately, chlorine combines with any organic substances that may be in the water to form chloroform, a poisonous cancer-causing chemical which does *not* evaporate.

When chlorine is regularly ingested, it destroys vitamin E in the body,[2] and its presence is closely linked with vascular disease.[3] It will also destroy beneficial flora in the intestines. Chlorine is considered a hazard even on the surface of the body. The Environmental Protection Agency has warned that prolonged swimming or bathing in chlorinated water contributes to skin cancer.

Fluoridation

Fluoridation of drinking water is one of the most insidious practices in America. Even if fluoride were not a controversial chemical, should everyone receive some people's medicine? Perhaps in the future tranquilizers and mood alterants will be put into community water. Is drugging an unstated motivation behind fluoridation? Fluorite, a naturally occurring compound of calcium and fluoride, is already used as a formidable tranquilizer in traditional Chinese medicine;[4] and Prozac™ (Fluoxetine Hydrochloride) a modern antidepressant, is based on the fluoride molecule. Judging from the intensity of the battles that rage, and the tremendous pro-fluoride support coming from some factions in the government, there must be something behind fluoridation besides merely promoting healthy teeth. Otherwise local and federal governments could easily advocate free fluoride pills for children whose parents consented (it is presumed that the teeth of children benefit most from fluoride). This would cost less than city-wide water-treatment installations.

Originally, decay-prevention tests with fluoride were carried out with *calcium* fluoride, yet *sodium* fluoride and fluorosilicic acid are the chemicals added to city water supplies. These chemicals are toxic by-products of the aluminum and fertilizer industries, often highly contaminated with lead and arsenic, and were expensive to dispose of until cities were persuaded to put them in the public water for tooth decay prevention. Up until this time, the primary use of fluoride was as rat poison. After approval for city water, the price of sodium fluoride shot up 1000% almost overnight.

Many tests have been performed with fluoride; some indicate improved teeth while others show a worsening effect. As a result of research in Europe, fluoride treatment of water is now illegal in Sweden, Denmark, and Holland. Germany and Belgium have discontinued their fluoride experiments on the human population, and France and Norway have never found sufficient evidence to warrant water fluoridation. In truth, most tests are difficult to interpret since the mineral content of the water itself is one of the deciding factors. If there is adequate calcium in water, fluoride will form calcium fluoride, which may be of some benefit. Nevertheless, studies indicate that fluoride *per se* is one of nature's principal aging factors.[5]

Undesirable Properties of Fluoridation

- Inhibits proper functioning of the thyroid gland and all enzyme systems.[6, 7] This makes weight reduction more difficult and is thought to be partially responsible for the abnormal height of some young people, as well as a contributor to very broad bottoms.
- Damages the immune system. Serious disorders that may first arise are sclera derma, lupus, and various forms of arthritis. Ultimately, the likelihood of cancer and other degenerative conditions is increased.[8]
- Fluoride in public water is usually in quantities of one part per million.

According to principles of homeopathic medicine, this concentration of fluoride can be a potent pathogen when used regularly.

Fluorine in Food

Fluorine and its compounds in food are entirely different from chemically produced sodium fluoride. Once an element is extracted from the soil and incorporated into plant life, its properties change greatly. Fluorine compounds in food, for instance, have important nutritional functions. The combination of organic calcium and fluorine creates a very hard surface on teeth and also in the bones. That is why, when there is tooth decay, we assume a fluorine shortage. Also, fluorine helps protect the entire body from the invasion and proliferation of germs and viruses.

Fluorine in food is volatile and evaporates with cooking. (Chemically fluoridated water, in contrast, loses no fluoride with heat.) One of the most concentrated sources of fluorine is goat's milk. Other sources are seaweed, rice, rye, parsley, avocados, cabbage, and black-eyed peas; herbs high in fluorine include juniper berries, licorice, lemon grass, bancha tea twigs, and other tea plants.

Other Chemicals

A number of other chemicals are intentionally added by some city water departments to stabilize the action of water and keep pipes from rusting.

The following statistics help illustrate the magnitude of the pollution in the United States:

Chemical production: 70,000 chemicals are now in commercial production, and the Environmental Protection Agency (EPA) has listed 60,000 of them as either potentially or definitely hazardous to human health.

U.S. industrial waste: 300 million tons of waste are generated by industry annually; the EPA estimates that 90% of this waste is improperly disposed of.

Much of this waste finds its way, either directly or indirectly, into our air, water, soil, and food supplies. Since pollutants are increasingly concentrated in the higher species, it is all the more important for us to use the best food and water available.

Our Personal Waterways

The various fluids in our body, including blood and lymph, carry many of the same wastes but in greater concentrations than exist in the water, air, and food chain. From this perspective, the reason for a general lack of vitality among modern people is obvious: the liver and kidneys—the body's waste filters—are saturated with chemical and waste poisons and the imbalanced nutrients of devitalized food. The kidney-adrenals supply energy for the entire body, and it is the work of the liver to regulate this energy (see the *Water Element* and *Wood Element* chapters). If these organs must work continuously to clean toxins from the body, they have little energy left for normal healthful activity.

A survival imperative for people in the early twenty-first century is to support efforts to purify and heal the Earth and its people. The grim alternative is epidemics of diseases related to toxic overload, resulting in immune failure and serious mental and physical degenerations.

In this age, most water used in food preparation needs to be purified. Exceptions may be water from wells or springs known to be of exceptional purity, or any underground sources that have been tested and found free of poisons and dangerous minerals. The contamination of water with artificial toxins is only part of the problem. Well water, for example, in an area with no chemical farms or sprayed forests may still pick up toxic natural aluminum compounds in its aquifer.

Filters and Purifiers

The term "purifier" denotes a government-regulated standard which specifies that "purified" water is very nearly only pure water; a water "filter" removes at most the suspended material and leaves all minerals and other substances (including possible toxins) that are water-soluble.

Activated charcoal filters can remove most of the wastes and other toxins that are not water-soluble. The major water-soluble dangers are nitrates, nitrites, and sodium fluoride. If these are not present, a filter can be very useful if its filtering ability is high, it does not accumulate bacteria, and it is renewed or replaced promptly when its filtering capacity is exhausted.

Modern *reverse-osmosis purifiers* are now being used by some institutions as an alternative to distillers. These membranous units take out just about all toxins, gases, and minerals, leaving nearly completely purified water. At one time very expensive, they are now price-competitive with quality charcoal filters and often are less than distillers. Their drawback is that they discharge several gallons of waste water for each one they purify.

Water distillers claim to do what nature does—evaporate water, leaving behind all residues—then condense the vapor as 100% purified water. However, municipal water often contains hydrocarbons, which have a lower boiling point than water, and a "fractional" valve system must be used to let off the hydrocarbon gases that otherwise end up in the distilled water. If fractional valves aren't supplied, then the better units often run the distilled water through a final-stage charcoal filter.

Purified water from reverse osmosis purifiers or distillers, chemically similar to what rain water used to be before pollution surrounded the Earth, will still not have the life-energy of rain water. To improve it, leave the purified water in an open glass container for a day or so, exposed to sunlight if possible.

Purified Water as Cleansing Agent

These purified waters are helpful to those with conditions of *excess* and those who need cleansing. If substantial amounts of animal products are eaten, then purified water is important. People afflicted with gout, rheumatism, and arthritis especially benefit from purified water, since it dissolves toxins and foreign deposits in the body.

If *deficiencies* exist, or cleansing is not specifically called for, remineralize purified water by stirring in a scant ⅛ teaspoon per gallon of whole salt or kelp powder.

Filtered Water

Activated charcoal-filtered water will still contain its water-soluble minerals. If pure demineralized water is not needed, and as long as the original water does not contain water-soluble toxins such as sodium fluoride and nitrites, then charcoal-filtered water is the best alternative to natural water from a pure source.

Another option for removing sodium fluoride is to stir briskly one teaspoon calcium powder per gallon into charcoal-filtered fluoridated water. The fluoride will combine with the calcium to form calcium fluoride. This may not be harmful in small doses, but if it is not wanted, let it settle to the bottom of the container and use the water off the top. (Dr. Bronner's Calcium-Magnesium Powder is commonly used for this purpose.)

The Meat and Water Connection

In countries with high levels of meat consumption, the medical profession advises people to drink plenty of water. Eight or more glasses per day is often recommended. For most people who eat an abundance of meat, we agree with this recommendation. Large-scale meat-eating can overload the body with uric acid and other wastes, and water helps flush them out. Also, the concentrated nature of meat needs the dispersing nature of water to balance it. When the obstructive and inflammation-producing quality of flesh foods is neutralized with water, then there is less attraction to dispersing agents such as alcohol and most other intoxicants.

The land areas and waterways of meat-consuming populations are befouled by the livestock industry in a homomorphic way reminiscent of the residues of meat-eating in the body. Although an incomprehensible amount of water is either polluted or consumed by the manufacturing industry, even this figure palls before the total for the livestock industry. Meat production uses more water than the rest of the nation combined.[9]

Sixty percent of *all* United States cropland is used to grow feed and fodder for animals, and over half of the nation's water consumption is drawn by irrigators onto these crops. In the process, the corn, oats, milo, alfalfa, and other animal feeds are highly sprayed and chemically fertilized. These chemicals wash down into the rivers, lakes, and underground aquifers, causing more water pollution than any other industrial source.[10] Also, the slaughterhouses often dump animal blood and parts into major waterways. In recent years the Missouri River has been so clogged in stretches with hair and balls of fat that it is difficult to paddle a canoe across.

Thus, in the United States, the purity and supply of water is seriously undermined by agriculture as a result of excessive meat eating. When people eat a higher percentage of vegetarian food, far less water is wasted since fewer crops need to be grown. Superb nutrition can be obtained from a very small amount of grain, legumes, and other plants compared with what is used for livestock.[11]

Personal Water Consumption

> Eat when hungry, drink when thirsty.
>
> —Zen maxim

Perhaps the most important principle regarding personal water consumption is listening to the wisdom of one's own body, and drinking according to thirst.

If large amounts of water are consumed for reasons such as hard work or internal heat, this is best done at least thirty minutes before or one hour after meals. Otherwise digestive enzymes and secretions are diluted, and food nutrients are not effectively extracted. When water is taken with meals, it is best that it be only a few ounces and warm, possibly in the form of soup or herbal tea at the end of a meal.

The optimal water intake for individuals varies widely, and a person's requirements can be far different from one day to the next. Although thirst is the most important indicator of need, not everyone is in touch with his or her own thirst. Just as our natural instinct to breathe deeply can be blunted by polluted air, many people no longer drink enough water because of its impure nature. This is usually not a conscious choice. When good water is available, the natural instinct to drink it must often be relearned. Most though certainly not all people should increase their fluid intake, but to recommend a healthful amount for everyone is impossible.

Key Factors that Influence Personal Water Needs

Water requirements are lessened by	Water requirements are increased by
Sedentary lifestyle	Physical activity
Consumption of fruit, vegetables, and sprouted foods	Consumption of more meat, eggs, or salty foods
Cold, deficient conditions	Fever, *heat,* or *excess* conditions
Cold or damp climates	Dry, hot, or windy climates

Major Properties of Water: relaxing, moistening, soothing, cooling, and dispersing.

The above key factors and properties as well as the following signs of excess/ insufficient water consumption can help guide water intake and stimulate revitalization of one's instincts.

Excess or Insufficient Water Consumption

The bulk of water intake for primarily vegetarian people can be obtained from food. Vegetables and fruit are often more than 90% water, and most other vegetarian foods, such as grains and legumes, are more than 80% water when cooked. Soups, broths, and teas are nearly all water.

Too much water from any source can cause sensations of coldness, and weaken the digestion and the energy of the whole body. This view is supported by Chinese healing traditions, which state that an excess of water depletes the "digestive fire" of the spleen-pancreas and hinders the kidney-adrenals' ability to provide warmth and energy *(yang qi)*. This applies especially to cold water or foods. When too much of these are taken, one tends to be attracted to animal products in an attempt for balance, rather than to fruits and vegetables.

Insufficient water consumption causes toxicity of the body as well as constipation, tension, tightness, overeating, dryness, and kidney damage. *Heat* symptoms such as inflammations, fevers, and feeling too warm can also occur.

Although those on a rich meat diet usually have insufficient body fluids, it is also common among vegetarians who eat large quantities of salty food, little or no soup or tea, and food such as grains cooked in minimal water.

The amount of water in the diet will significantly influence long-term health. The health of the body and its internal functioning also determine how efficiently water is utilized and distributed. Foods which influence the *yin* of the body, discussed in the "Deficient Yin" section (page 65), also modify fluid metabolism.

Protein and Vitamin B$_{12}$—The Plant and Animal Kingdoms as Sources

Amino Acids

Protein literally means "primary substance," an accurate description since all the tissues of the body are built and repaired with protein. Amino acids, the building blocks of protein, are key factors in most of the processes and functions of the body. The antibodies of the immune system, most hormones, the hemoglobin of red blood cells, and all enzymes have protein as their basic component.

Until very recently, nearly every standard source of information on nutrition, whether in schools or in texts and articles, emphasized the need for adequate protein and cautioned that total vegetarians may easily become deficient in protein, and also in vitamin B_{12}. Because of this widespread concept, many concerned vegetarians use protein supplements, eggs and dairy, or extra amounts of legumes, brewer's yeast, miso soy paste, seeds, and nuts combined with quantities of grain to ensure abundant and "complete" protein nutrition. Often the net result is not only a bloated condition but a reduction in actually usable protein.

The root cause of this concern is misinformation that protein of plant origin is deficient in certain amino acids and "incomplete" for humans. The recommended vegetarian solution has been to combine various forms of plant protein—for instance, a grain and a legume—in order to obtain an amino-acid pattern that is "complete."[1] These ideas for protein-combining and the standards for completeness go back to experiments done on rats in the early part of this century.

At that time it was discovered that rats flourished on protein with amino-acid patterns similar to those found in animal products (e.g., cheese or eggs). It was assumed then that those same patterns would be required for humans, and therefore a standard amino-acid profile was developed (for people) based on an ideal for rats. This profile has been the basis for judging the quality of all vegetable protein for many years. More recently, however, the World Health Organization has developed a protein standard ("PDCAAS") that takes into account human protein needs. This standard validates plant protein sources yet suggests that a higher amino acid profile is better—which does little to allay the mania surrounding protein. Knowledge of the following research can help reduce the insecurity and uncertainty that often coexist with protein obsession.

About forty years ago, careful experiments were designed with methods more advanced than those for rats, to measure protein requirements for humans.[2] These tests indicate that nearly all the complex carbohydrates, such as those in a whole grain, bean, or potato, have amino-acid profiles adequate for human protein needs. This means that when energy needs (calories) are satisfied by a *single* complex carbohydrate, protein requirements are also fulfilled.* Of the twenty or so amino acids currently known, those that cannot be synthesized in the body and must be obtained from food are called *essential* amino acids. For years it was claimed that humans needed certain dietary proportions of the ten essential amino acids found to be beneficial for rats. It is now commonly accepted that the adult human requires only eight essential amino acids.**

One often reads that an essential amino acid is missing or low in a given food. Virtually every unrefined food from the vegetable or animal kingdom has not

---

*Carbohydrate metabolism is not efficient in infants until 18–24 months of age. See *Food for Children* chapter.

**This information is now found even in widely read periodicals such as *Reader's Digest:* an article on rice appeared in the August 1985 issue stating that rice is a complete protein, containing "all eight" essential amino acids.

only all eight essential amino acids, but all twenty commonly recognized amino acids; therefore saying they are "missing" is inaccurate. "Low" levels of amino acids nearly always means low compared to a standard of "complete" protein based on animal products as the ideal for rats. As an example, according to this standard, the amino acid pair methionine-cystine is commonly identified as the lowest found in foods and is therefore called a "limiting amino acid." According to the limiting amino acid (LAA) theory, the amount of protein available in food is limited to the level of the lowest essential amino acid; by this reasoning, if methionine-cystine in a certain food measures up to only 30% of the standard amino-acid profile (Estimated Amino Acid Requirement—EAAR), then just 30% of the profile amounts of the other amino acids in that food are considered usable by the body. Even if a better protein/amino-acid standard based on human needs were used, the concept of an LAA is still questionable, since it has been found that a pool of stored amino acids in the body is available to complement the amino acids in recently ingested food.[3] However, methionine-cystine is consistently considered an LAA in many foods because of the unusual amino-acid profile it is judged against—a profile based on the great need of rats for methionine-cystine to sustain their full-body growth of hair, which is profuse by human standards.

The benefit of this past misunderstanding of human protein needs is that we are aware of a wider variety of options. To obtain vegetable protein resembling that of meat, one may choose a grain and a legume (bean, lentil, or pea) in a ratio of approximately two parts grain to one part legume. Using seeds or nuts with grains also increases the amino-acid spectrum. Pregnant and lactating women, very young children, hypoglycemics, people under psychological or physical stress (anxiety, grief, infections, surgery), recovering alcoholics, recent vegetarians, and those with protein deficiency generally benefit from higher-profile vegetable protein— but not always. Some people do not efficiently digest legumes and grains, or similar combinations, taken at the same meal. (See *Food Combinations* chapter.) For these individuals, the foods can be alternated—grains at one meal, legumes at the next—and the amino acid pool mentioned above will complement both the grain and the legume with its amino-acid reserves.

In the last few years the search for high protein levels in low-fat sources has led researchers into many new areas of nutrition, and especially to chemically processed yeasts and other microorganisms that appear and taste somewhat like meat. This search goes on, regardless of the information indicating that most people's protein requirements are satisfied by a simple vegetarian diet based on whole grains. If you are a vegetarian or ever considered becoming one, you probably lost track of how many times you have been asked, "But where do you get your protein?" Most people do not view protein rationally. The word is stereotyped and issues forth mindlessly as a synonym for quality nutrition, health, meat, and other animal products. This mega-protein mania symbolizes the consciousness of a society based on continuous growth, as protein is the body's builder.

Except for the special protein needs mentioned earlier, those who crave animal products and believe they need more protein are usually craving the total matrix of nutrients available from animal tissue or milk. The similar structures of animal and human cells make possible the quick exchange of energy and nutrients that gives many meat eaters a certain sense of being well-nurtured, without which they feel deprived. Such an exchange, rather than consisting of just protein, is in reality the emotional and physical sense of having consumed a large concentration of minerals, vitamins, enzymes, fatty acids, amino acids, sugars, and other nutrients. This initial experience, nevertheless, is often short-lived because only a certain portion of meat is digestible. When meat is overconsumed, the remaining portion—part of which easily becomes a toxic mucoid substance known as *ama* in Ayurvedic tradition—contributes to heavy mucus conditions that make one sluggish and attracted to stimulants such as coffee, refined sugar, and alcohol. Discussed in other areas of this text are the connections between meat overconsumption and obesity, heart disease, bone loss, and many degenerative diseases. Therefore, when using meat, using it sparingly is the key to its positive qualities.

In fact, fresh, properly prepared meats and eggs are considered very nutritious for the body (but not necessarily healthful for the mind) by most medical traditions in the East. They are usually prescribed only in small therapeutic doses, for example, two to three ounces per day in a broth. Large amounts of such a concentrated product can have an opposite and weakening effect, as described above, and any amount may have negative mental consequences, depending on the person's sensitivity and ethical alignment. (At the end of this chapter are some optimum preparation methods for meat.) As a general principle, when there is severe deficiency, it has been considered acceptable—even by many who have moral objections to taking animal life—to use as medicine any plant, animal, or other product that the earth offers as long as it does not harm people.

Many medical specialists, from both the East and West, believe that the modern person needs to eat animal products to help overcome the stresses of contemporary life. There is some truth to this opinion, but much of the stress that meat-eating people experience is a *result* of the toxic by-products of too much meat, which can obstruct the body's functions and therefore the mental processes. A grain- and vegetable-based diet tends to be relaxing, even tranquilizing,* yet energizing. Also, within the plant and mineral kingdoms are products that may be stronger than meat in some important properties, which can strengthen an individual against the pressures of life perhaps even better than meat, with far fewer toxic residues. Miso-seaweed soup is a prime example of a protein, vitamin, enzyme, and mineral food that is, in fact, so strong that we caution against its overuse. Miso offers nutrients particularly effectively because they have been predigested in the bacterial action of fermentation.

---

*Eating complex carbohydrates maximizes the concentration in the bloodstream of the amino acid L-tryptophan, which is manufactured in the brain into the "calming chemical," serotonin. Most people feel calmer within half an hour of a carbohydrate snack, if foods concentrated in protein and fat are not eaten with it.

Attraction to Meat and Animal Products

The common desire of people to eat meat in excess, and for vegetarians to want protein similar to meat, stems from a false sense of need. According to Nevin Scrimshaw, Ph.D., head of the Department of Nutrition and Food Science at the Massachusetts Institute of Technology and an acknowledged leader in the field of protein and human nutrition research:

> Individuals can and do, if they can afford it, consume two to three times their estimated protein requirement. . . .
> —from the Ninth Annual W.O. Atwater Memorial Address, 1977.

That protein requirements are routinely exceeded in wealthy countries is demonstrated by the fact that nearly everyone has symptoms of excess protein consumption: acidic blood, calcium deficiency, and a tendency to carcinogenic and other degenerative diseases. Studies show that the diets of Americans generally exceed the Federal government's Recommended Daily Allowance for protein by 100% for men and 40% for women.

When given the opportunity, most people will not only take in too much protein but will opt for rich foods in excess of their needs. Even many vegetarians who eat whole food have discovered ways to make extremely rich dishes that overrun nutritional requirements.

The average Western diet contains more than 50% animal products. (In the United States, this figure is over 60%.) Many of us have built our tissue, nerves, bones, and viscera with these products. This diet has attained the momentum of many generations. To make the dramatic change to a completely vegetarian diet can be shocking, to say the least. It takes the body a certain amount of time to learn what to do with some vegetable products or, for that matter, with any food to which it is not accustomed. How long the transition takes depends on a person's background and inherent strengths and weaknesses. For people from societies with traditionally low levels of meat consumption—parts of Latin America, Ireland, the Far East, or among certain agriculturally based Native American cultures—the process can be less of a physiological strain.

Yet cravings for animal products are deeply rooted. If protein and other requirements are easily met by vegetarian products, why do people crave meat? Is it because meat is a food their bodies recognize? Our observation in working with people attempting to totally abandon animal products is that often they will return to these products for a combination of physical and psychological needs. Animal products greatly support certain deep emotions* and feelings of identification of

---

*Animal products only *support* a particular mentality; they do not compel any behavior. The tendency of meat in particular to support certain behavior is delineated in Ayurvedic medical tradition: commonly available meat is one of the *tamasic* foods, and when eaten, "the mind easily fills with dark emotions, such as anger and greed."

the individualized self (ego). Until the ego is sufficiently developed, it is impossible and even undesirable to move beyond it. Unfortunately, it is all too easy to become fascinated with various levels of the ego—our personal desires for possessions, power, sensuality, and emotional stimulus. Rich foods like meats that become obstructive if overeaten support stagnant ego positions and attachments. Ego development, however, cannot be maintained or halted by any class of food itself, but merely occurs more easily, smoothly, and harmoniously with vegetal foods.

Cravings for meat also result from deficiencies; some people who are nutritionally lacking can quickly extract needed nutrients from animal tissue. (Using meat for deficiencies is discussed later in this chapter.) To stop the cruel use and killing of sentient beings and the eating of their flesh is a laudable goal, but it must be accomplished in ways that actually work. For most people, a gradual approach is best.

It is surprising how few people, having eaten animals their entire life, have actually considered the essential nature of animals. One traditional East Asian view teaches that an animal comes into being as a precise manifestation of cause and effect, with attributes determined by how it existed in previous realms or incarnations. Examples of special attributes include the speed and cunning of the leopard, and the grace and sensitivity of deer. Each animal also is saddled with negative attributes: the extreme attachment of the goose to its mate, the desires of the pig, the shyness of the rabbit, or comparable traits. When we eat an animal, all the various forms of its consciousness, as well as its physical substance, are assimilated into our own. One is normally not aware of this until animal product consumption is stopped for several months and then resumed.

The Food Chain

Animals are generally considered to have less or incomplete awareness compared with most humans, but they are nonetheless conscious, sentient beings. Buddhist teachings[4] and the tenets of certain other religions have long posited that taking the life of another creature carries a karmic effect proportional to the concentration of sentience in that creature.

According to this hypothesis, it follows that the taking of lower forms of animal life for human consumption is preferable to the taking of higher forms. The current vogue of eating fish and poultry is a better choice than consuming pork and beef, from this point of view. Personal investigation and intuition, of course, also play a role in this decision.

Does nutritional science support this theory? Excess dietary fat and cholesterol have been targeted as primary causes of heart disease, diabetes, breast cancer, colon and prostate cancer, to mention only the major degenerative diseases. Fish and fowl, however, have a high percentage of polyunsaturated fat which, in contrast to the highly saturated fat in red meat, tends to help the body eliminate excess cholesterol. This is particularly true of the fish rich in omega-3 fatty acids (discussed in the *Oils and Fats* chapter).

Further down the food chain, animals generally have a progressively smaller concentration of pesticides, heavy metals, and other contaminants. For various reasons, different cultures and religions prohibit or encourage the consumption of certain of these "lower" animals or their parts. A holistic principle, for example, maintains that if one is to eat animal products, it is best to use the whole animal. Traditional peoples usually ate the bones, tripe, and tails of the larger animals, as well as many other parts we now discard; these practices remain in the diets of some people still linked with their cultural backgrounds. An advantage of eating the less-evolved animals is that the whole animal seems more homogeneous, and therefore can be more nearly consumed in total. Examples are anchovies, sardines, clams, and oysters (nearly everything but the shell), snails, eggs and caviar, insects (in many cultures), and the microorganisms of fermented food.* One might well be *less* horrified at killing an insect and eating it than taking the life and eating the flesh of a very developed animal such as a pig or sheep.

In dealing with ferments, we should note that there is no such thing as a pure vegetarian (or vegan**) because of the consumption of microorganisms in all food, particularly in the ferments. However, the assimilation of this lower order of life is far preferable nutritionally and morally to taking the life of higher forms. Nutritionally this is true because fermented foods and micro-algae are often on par with—or better than—products from more highly evolved animals. Morally, the lower forms are preferable because of the way most livestock are raised. Even committed meat eaters who disagree with a karmic effect from killing animals might change their thinking if they knew how the animals they eat were fed, treated, and slaughtered. More damning than anything that can be said is a visit to the feedlots, slaughterhouses, and chicken farms where flesh food is produced.

Vegetarians

How do we know that a completely vegetarian diet promotes strength and endurance? We can of course see its living results in deer, horses, and many other herbivorous animals, and human examples, even in the West, are plentiful. There have been pure vegetarian traditions among the Hindus, Buddhists, and Taoists for twenty-five centuries, involving millions of people. Many such traditions exist in India, but since dairy products are widely used there, the best vegan examples are the previous generations that occupied large areas of China where consumption of dairy was nearly nonexistent. (Modern China has few vegetarians, although

---

*Food technologists are now using various microorganisms such as bacteria, yeasts, and fungi to weave textured products that uncannily mimic meat or chicken.

**Vegan (pronounced vej´un, or vee´gun) is a person whose diet includes no animal products.

many Americans call themselves "vegetarian" with a diet containing more fish, eggs, dairy, and fowl than eaten by the typical Chinese.)

An interesting record of the life of Kwan Saihung, one of the last highly trained Taoist adepts of China, is preserved in the book *The Wandering Taoist*.[5] His advanced level of martial arts and meditation training from childhood was supported by a pure vegetarian diet with the Zengyi-Huashan sect in a large Taoist mountain community. Chicken and fish were raised only for those who were sick. Extensive herbal therapy strengthened members of the community to help develop their skills in the healing arts and awareness practices.

Vitamin B$_{12}$ and the Modern Vegetarian

Since the Western diet is based on meat, the typical Western body has become habituated to a certain type of nutrition. Most high-quality animal products are characterized by abundant protein and also by vitamin B$_{12}$, the nutrient many medical doctors claim to be most difficult for vegetarians to obtain. Vitamin B$_{12}$ is produced only by microorganisms. When it is found in at least trace amounts—in air, water, the herbs *dang gui (Angelica sinensis)* and comfrey root *(Symphytum officinale),* mushrooms, the leaves of certain vegetables (especially parsley and turnip greens grown in highly composted soil), and traditionally fermented products (e.g., the tempehs produced in small, less-than-sterile Indonesian shops)—it is specifically because such foods and substances contain B$_{12}$-producing bacteria.[6–10]

Among healthy people, large amounts of vitamin B$_{12}$ are manufactured by beneficial bacteria in the colon, and smaller amounts appear in the saliva and throughout other parts of the gastrointestinal tract.[11] There is, however, some controversy as to whether enough of this B$_{12}$ is actually absorbed. Since the colon and the digestive tract in general are often among the least healthy areas in people, we suggest that vegetarians make certain that sufficient vitamin B$_{12}$ is included in their diets.

Properties of Vitamin B$_{12}$: Required for red blood cell formation and normal growth; important for fertility and during pregnancy; builds immunity and treats some degenerative diseases (often administered in therapy for cancer, AIDS, osteoarthritis, and multiple sclerosis); used therapeutically in many mental and nervous disorders. More recently it has been used to energize the body and counteract allergens.

Enough vitamin B$_{12}$ can be stored in the liver to last three to six years, so a deficiency may exist for several years before it becomes apparent. Even so, deficiency surfaces within a few months in the many people who have poor liver function or do not assimilate the vitamin well.

Signs of Vitamin B$_{12}$ Deficiency: The classic symptom is the development of pernicious anemia, resulting from interrupted red blood cell production. It is now known, however, that there are a number of nervous, mental, and emotional disorders linked to B$_{12}$ deficiency that sometimes occur *without* blood deficiency signs.[12] The earliest signs of B_{12} deficiency are weakness, listlessness, fatigue, diarrhea, depression, and indigestion. Other signs are paleness, numbness in the fingers and toes, heart palpitations, anorexia, shortness of breath, infertility, and mental imbalances including faltering memory, moodiness, apathy, paranoia, hallucinations, violent behavior, personality changes, and other derangements. These conditions may appear in varying degrees; generally the elderly experience them more severely.[13]

As the deficiency progresses into the latter stages, the protective myelin sheaths on the nerves and brain deteriorate, resulting in a diminished sense of weight and balance in the lower extremities, tingling skin, further memory degeneration, loss of sensory and mental sharpness, visual impairment, and urinary and fecal incontinence. The tongue is an indicator of serious B_{12} deficiency. It becomes red, shiny, and smooth, and is sometimes ulcerated. In the final stage before death, irreversible paralysis and brain damage occur.

Symptoms of vitamin B_{12} deficiency do not always show—they can be masked by the B-complex vitamin folic acid. Folic acid and B_{12} have certain similar functions, and each requires the presence of the other in many of their activities.[14] While folic acid alone *seems* to alleviate symptoms of B_{12} deficiency, an insidious process is actually underway as damage from insufficient B_{12} continues in the nervous system, with fewer outward symptoms. Most at risk in folic-acid masking are those who are B_{12}-deficient but otherwise take in a quality diet with abundant folate: grains and vegetables—especially leafy greens, legumes, and sprouts.

Pernicious anemia was fatal in the past, but can now be halted with injections of vitamin B_{12}. Studies in Sweden confirm what few physicians knew until recently: pernicious anemia can also be very successfully treated with large oral doses (1,000 mg. daily) of B_{12}.* Anyone, vegetarian or omnivore, with weak digestion—whether from a poor constitution, faulty nutrition, or an imbalanced lifestyle—can become deficient in vitamin B_{12}. In addition to poor digestive absorption, there are other specific factors that deplete the body of vitamin B_{12}:

1. Birth control pills and antibiotics
2. Intoxicants (alcohol, cigarettes, coffee, and all others)
3. Stress from any source, especially from injury, surgery, or trauma
4. Liver diseases and chronic illnesses.

The foremost cause of vitamin B_{12} malabsorption is the stomach's gastric juice losing its "intrinsic factor," a mucoprotein enzyme that makes the uptake of B_{12} efficient (about one percent of ingested B_{12} is absorbed even with no intrinsic factor according to the study cited above). Intrinsic-factor manufacture diminishes with age; it can also be destroyed by stomach surgery, parasites, or bacterial excess in the gastrointestinal tract. Most often, intrinsic factor is lost through "autoimmune

*Lederle, Frank, M.D. Commentary: "Oral Cobalamin [vitamin B_{12}] for Pernicious Anemia: Medicine's Best Kept Secret?" *Journal of the American Medical Assn.*, pages 94–95, January 2, 1991.

reactions," when the immune system produces antibodies that attack the body's own tissues. Autoimmune reactions commonly attack the intrinsic-factor-producing areas of the stomach. Oral vitamin B_{12} supplements must include intrinsic factor (usually procured from animals) for cases of B_{12} deficiency induced by lack of intrinsic factor. Vitamin B_{12} injections are the most common medical treatment for this condition.

Plant Sources of Vitamin B_{12}

Vegetarians in the West have relied for a generation on three food sources thought to contain ample vitamin B_{12}: fermented foods, algae, and yeasts.

Fermented Foods

These include miso, soy sauce, tempeh, pickles, amasake, nut and seed yogurts, and sourdough (naturally leavened) bread. It has been commonly thought by vegetarians that all fermented food contains at least traces of B_{12}. This assumption tends to be true in Third World countries where sanitation is poor and B_{12}-rich bacteria proliferate, especially in fermented products. People rarely show a deficiency of the vitamin in these locales. On the other hand, in most Western countries where sanitation is strongly enforced by law, food producers usually maintain nearly sterile shops. Even though cleanliness is of unquestionable value in food processing, its does halt the natural propagation of vitamin B_{12} in ferments.

Tempeh, a currently popular cultured soy product with origins in Indonesia, has some of the highest B_{12} content of any food (up to 15 micrograms of the vitamin in a 100-gram serving). When tempeh was introduced in America in the 1970s, it was generally produced by cottage industries, and B_{12} levels often ran a respectable four micrograms. As demand grew, tempeh was made in larger batches, causing the bacteria-to-culture ratio to drop; in addition, new tempeh machines and facilities were designed to be cleaned more easily. By the late 1980s, most tempeh contained absolutely no B_{12},[15] even though manufacturers still listed high levels on the labels. When more recent test results became known, some companies took their B_{12} listings off the containers, while others began inoculating the tempeh with bacteria that produce the vitamin.

Most other fermented foods produced in modern facilities, such as miso and soy sauce, are likewise virtually devoid of B_{12}, even though various publications over the years have recommended them as valuable sources. One truth in these inaccurate recommendations is that fermented foods, because of their vital digestive enzymes, may very well be an aid in the absorption of B_{12} from other sources and stimulate B_{12} bacterial growth in the intestines.

Algae: Micro-Algae and Seaweeds

Scientific tests have shown a number of algae to be excellent sources of B_{12}. In fact, micro-algae such as spirulina, chlorella, and wild blue-green *(Aphanizomenon flos-aquae)* were once considered the highest food sources of vitamin B$_{12}$. The tests that confirmed these levels were microbiological, the same procedure recognized by the United States government. In the last few years, however, there are indications that these tests can be inaccurate, since they measure certain analogues to B$_{12}$ as well as the vitamin itself. B$_{12}$ analogues, which do not have the properties of real vitamin B$_{12}$, appear to a large extent in micro-algae, and they may be responsible for a majority of the readings for B$_{12}$ levels.

Another testing method known as "radioassay" indicates that B$_{12}$ in micro-algae generally exists at only 20% of the value of the microbiological tests;[16] the remaining 80% are sometimes considered to be B$_{12}$ analogues. If only 20% of the supposed B$_{12}$ in micro-algae were true B$_{12}$, they would still be excellent sources. But when taken to counter B$_{12}$ deficiency, the micro-algae do not seem effective,[15] which leads to speculation that the analogues somehow interfere with the uptake of true B$_{12}$ in the body.[17]

This information is at first baffling, since spirulina and other micro-algae are excellent remedies for most cases of anemia, and B$_{12}$ is essential for building red blood. Most cases of anemia, however, are not merely a result of B$_{12}$ deficiency alone; it may be that the massive amounts of chlorophyll, iron, protein, and other nutrients in micro-algae overcome anemia. In our personal experience, we have observed many people who have taken various micro-algae regularly for a decade or more, and when other sources of B$_{12}$ are included in the diet, B$_{12}$ deficiency does not arise. This suggests that the analogues in micro-algae do not interfere with other B$_{12}$ in the diet.

Certain *macro*-algae—nori, wakame, and kombu seaweeds—are sometimes touted as having significant B$_{12}$ content, but these have also not been effective in halting B$_{12}$ deficiencies.[15] Perhaps owing to the presence of analogues in greater quantity than the true B$_{12}$ contents, algal sources of B$_{12}$ may not be bioavailable, i.e., they do not seem to satisfy the body's requirement for vitamin B$_{12}$. However, when B$_{12}$-producing bacteria is inoculated into a food product such as tempeh or brewer's yeast, it can be highly effective.

Nutritional Yeast

Nutritional yeast (a.k.a. brewer's yeast and various other names) has been a nutritional cornucopia and B$_{12}$ standby for vegetarians for more than thirty years. The B$_{12}$ in yeast is either included as an additive at the end of its manufacture, or else the yeast is grown in a B$_{12}$-enriched medium. The latter method is best because it incorporates the vitamin into the living food. (Some nutritional yeasts do not contain vitamin B$_{12}$; to be sure, check the list of nutrients on the container.)

Yeast does not contain large amounts of B$_{12}$ analogues, and its B$_{12}$ level is consistent, independent of cleanliness factors. However, yeast is exceptionally rich in certain nutrients, and deficient in others that are needed for balance. The high phosphorus content of yeast, for example, can deplete the body of calcium; thus some yeast manufacturers now add calcium also.

Another problem with yeast is its very nature: microorganisms of this sort tend to induce unhealthy amounts of candida-type yeasts in the body, especially in individuals who are susceptible to candida overgrowth, or *dampness* in general.

When buying nutritional yeast, the better grades are "primary" yeast, produced specifically as a food supplement. This kind is usually grown on molasses or sugar beets, is pleasant-tasting, and does not require further processing. Most yeasts, however, are a by-product of the brewing industry, grown on hops, grain, and malt. They pick up alcohol and various chemicals, and develop a bitter flavor. They are then processed to remove any bitterness, which lowers the general nutritional quality.

Vitamin B_{12} During Pregnancy and Lactation

Since vitamin B_{12} builds immunity and promotes growth of the nervous system and body in general, it is essential during pregnancy and nursing. To grasp the B_{12} requirements of a fetus, consider that the newborn, compared to the mother, has over twice as much B_{12} in its blood, and that the placenta contains more than three times as much of the vitamin.[14] Yet vitamin B_{12} is one of the most commonly deficient vitamins during pregnancy and lactation.[18] Pregnant and lactating vegetarians in particular need to be certain they are getting enough.[19] Children born to mothers low in the vitamin run a high risk of retarded mental and physical development and weakened immunity.

Mothers who only occasionally consume B_{12} put their breast-feeding infants at risk of becoming deficient. The mother can recycle B_{12} stored in her body for her own purposes; she may feel healthy and so (falsely) assume that her milk is completely nourishing. Unfortunately, there are indications that only vitamin B_{12} ingested *during* the formation of milk will go into the mother's milk; B_{12} stored in the mother's body does not.[20] This means that for a nursing infant to receive B_{12} in its milk regularly, the lactating mother must take in B_{12} regularly.

A Margin of Safety for Vegetarians

The majority of high vitamin B_{12} sources are animal products. This is as it should be, since it is often suggested that those who use animal products require much more B_{12} for immunity and quality blood formation in the highly acidic mucoid environment created by abundant meat, dairy products, and eggs.

In India, Indonesia, and most other Third World areas, vegetarians obtain B_{12} from bacterial cultures and tiny organisms which populate their food, especially the fermented foods. In the more technologically advanced areas of the West, the vegetarian choices for B_{12} sources are minimal, so the one supplement we generally recommend to the pure vegetarian is B_{12}. Nevertheless, taking vitamin B_{12} in pill form is not always welcomed by vegetarians as a long-term solution to the B_{12} dilemma. Ideally, solutions will be found to provide significant amounts of

B_{12} cultures in whole-food products.

Most health agencies worldwide agree on a B_{12} requirement of one to three micrograms (mcg.)* per day for adults. When sources of B_{12} are purchased, however, their labels often list the amount of B_{12} compared with a standard called the U.S. Recommended Daily Allowance (U.S. RDA), which is six micrograms of B_{12} daily for individuals twelve and older. When we contacted Food and Drug Administration authorities on this issue, they stated that it is a twenty-year-old standard originally developed only for packaging and labeling purposes, and has not been updated because of the expense involved for food manufacturers. They also claimed that this standard is not to be used for any other purpose, and that the government position on nutritional needs is reflected by an entirely different set of standards known as the Recommended *Dietary* Allowances (RDA), which is monitored by the National Academy of Sciences. The current adult Recommended Dietary Allowance for B_{12} is two mcg. daily; the RDA for young infants is 0.3 mcg. per day, and for children, 0.05 mcg. per kilogram of body weight until they reach the adult RDA of 2 mcg.; the standard for pregnant and lactating women is 2.2 and 2.6 mcg. per day, respectively.

Therefore, when buying vitamin B_{12} foods or supplements, the percent of B_{12} in the U.S. Recommended *Daily* Allowance should be tripled to give the percent relative to the Recommended *Dietary* Allowance. For example, a product in which a serving contains twelve mcg. of B_{12}—listed as 200% of the adult U.S. RDA for vitamin B_{12}—would supply 3 x 200% = 600% of the Recommended Dietary Allowance. Excess levels of B_{12} are not thought to be a problem, however, and a dangerous amount of the vitamin has never been established. (Injections of 1,000 mcg. and more are used therapeutically.)

Vegetarians (including those who eat small amounts of organic eggs, fresh fish, or other high-quality animal products only occasionally) should take supplements if they want to meet the RDA for B_{12} without having to rely on brewer's yeast or some other inoculated food each day. Nearly all B_{12} supplements are non-synthetic and are not derived from higher animal sources; they are produced from bacteria. For convenience, one fifty-mcg. supplement can be taken each week. Also, it is helpful to use some enzyme-rich foods such as miso, unpasteurized sauerkraut and pickles, and sprouts to maximize the spawning and uptake of B_{12} in the digestive tract. Multiple vitamin and mineral supplements which contain B_{12} may not be a good source of this nutrient, since the combination of minerals in them can cause B_{12} analogues to form.[16]

Idealists who use no animal products and believe that their vitamin B_{12} needs will be supplied by the flora of their intestines and by minute amounts found in certain organic vegetables and ferments are sometimes right. However, there have

---

*Note that the unit of measure for vitamin B_{12} is the microgram, just one millionth of a gram and a thousandth of a milligram. This is one of the smallest measures used for any nutrient.

been enough instances of B_{12} deficiency among strict vegetarians—particularly vegan children—to warrant caution. We suggest that the initial deficiency symptoms be kept in mind.

Also recommended for all vegetarians are B_{12} tests, easily available from most health clinics and medical doctors. The most common test involves sampling the B_{12} levels in the blood, but this test is not entirely appropriate for vegetarians because a healthy vegetarian requires relatively low levels of B_{12} in the blood. However, if blood levels go much below 200 picograms per milliliter, then there may be cause for concern; World Health Organization research has established that B_{12} levels below this are known to lead to deficiency symptoms.

If a reading dips below the 200-picogram barrier, one should see a qualified health advisor in order to determine the best way to rebuild B_{12} to safe levels. When B_{12} is close to the 200-pcg. level, to determine whether it is adversely affecting physiological processes, then the test for UMMA (urinary methylmalonic acid) may be advisable. UMMA is a chemical that increases when B_{12} is insufficient for proper functioning of the body.

A need for special testing arises when the psychiatric symptoms of B_{12} deficiency listed earlier are present—apathy, memory loss, moodiness, and paranoia—but the serum B_{12} levels are adequate and there are no indications of anemia. Such a condition is especially prevalent in the older segment of the population[21] and sometimes is a sign of B_{12} malabsorption due to lack of intrinsic factor. This kind of deficiency is commonly misdiagnosed,[22] but must be halted before it deepens.

To ensure an accurate diagnosis, take the Schilling test, which measures the intrinsic factor and thus the ability of the body to absorb vitamin B_{12}. Although a rather involved procedure, it reveals problems with B_{12} assimilation even when blood tests for anemia and B_{12} are normal. This use of the Schilling test is rare but invaluable, since it also alerts one to the early stages of pernicious anemia, in which symptoms are more easily overcome.

The standard use of the Schilling test over the last thirty years has been to confirm the suspicion of pernicious anemia based primarily on blood tests.

Further Protein Perspectives

Following the primarily vegetarian guidelines suggested in this book provides more than twice the World Health Organization (WHO) minimum protein standard of approximately 5% of calorie intake. An 8% level is close to the protein and calorie guidelines suggested by the National Research Council. It is interesting to note that mother's milk derives 5% of its calories from protein and serves as sufficient nutrition for infants at a time when growth and development are at their peak.

The WHO and other standards, which use a ratio of protein calorie value to total caloric intake, are based on the insight that protein needs vary directly with energy needs.

Protein and Vitamin B$_{12}$ Sources

Protein in grams* per 100-gram (3½-ounce) edible portion
Vitamin B$_{12}$ in micrograms shown in parentheses ( ) by foods containing it.

Plants

Fruit — Protein (g)

	Protein (g)
All fruits	.2–2

Vegetables

Carrots	1
Cabbage	1
Cauliflower	3
Broccoli	4
Kale	4
Parsley (t)	4
Brussels sprouts	5

Grains

Rice	7
Barley	8
Corn	9
Rye	9
Millet	10
Buckwheat	12
Oats	13
Hard red wheat	14
Spelt	15
Amaranth	16
Quinoa	18

Nuts and Seeds

Filberts	13
Almonds	19
Sesame seeds	19
Sunflower seeds	24

Legumes (dried)

Aduki beans	22
Dry peas	24
Lentils	25
Soybeans	35

Ferments, Algae, and Yeast

Ferments — Protein (g)

	Protein (g)
Rejuvelac (t)	0
Non-pasteurized pickles (t)	1-4
Amasake	3
Soy sauce (Shoyu or Tamari)	6
Tofu	8
Sourdough bread	10
Nut or seed yogurt (t)	9-15
Miso (t)	15
Tempeh (t)	20

Algae**

Seaweeds (dried)

Agar agar /Kanten	2
Hijiki (t)	6
Kombu (3)	7
Wakame (5)	13
Kelp (4)	16
Alaria (5)	18
Dulse (7–13)	22
Nori (12–70)	35

Micro-algae

Chlorella (25+)	55
Wild blue-green (40+)	60
Spirulina (40+)	68

Yeast

Nutritional yeast (6–47)	50

Animal Products

Dairy — Protein (g)

	Protein (g)
Milk, whole (.4)	3
Yogurt (.6)	3
Cottage cheese (.6)	14
Cheese (1)	25-31

Fish

Oyster (18)	9
Clam (49)	14
Herring (10)	17
Cod (.5)	18
Bass (1)	18
Abalone (1)	18
Anchovy (7)	19
Mackerel (12)	19
Sardine (10)	24
Tuna or bonita (2)	29

Meat and Eggs

Eggs (1)	3
Fowl (.5)	16–24
Beef, other red meats (2)	17-21
Beef heart (11)	20
Beef kidney (31)	20
Beef liver (59)	20
Chicken liver (23)	21

*Since these figures are based on 100-gram samples, they also represent the percentage of protein by weight. Tempeh, for example, is 20% protein by weight.

(t)A trace of vitamin B$_{12}$ is sometimes found in these products, depending on how and where they are produced.

**Even though the seaweeds and micro-algae are listed as having appreciable amounts of vitamin B$_{12}$, they appear to be unreliable sources; studies have suggested that their B$_{12}$ is not bio-available.

If refined sugar products, alcohol, and other non-foods are added to the diet, calories increase dramatically, which is why people are drawn to very concentrated forms of protein to maintain the protein:calorie ratio. Vegetarians who eat large quantities of sugary foods—fruit juice, soft drinks, sweets, etc.—may become attracted to animal products.

There is currently a great deal of interest in high-protein foods. However, those foods listed in the preceding table with protein values above fifteen grams should normally be taken only in small amounts. Urea, a product of excess plant or animal protein consumption, leaches calcium from the body through its diuretic action. Without sufficient calcium, bones weaken and the nerves and heart atrophy (see *Calcium* chapter). Also, an excess of any kind of high-protein food causes the body to become saturated with uric acid, which significantly weakens all its functions, especially that of the kidneys. Gout and kidney stones are two possible consequences.

If one chooses meat as a major protein source, excess urea, uric acid, fatty deposits, and mucus are likely results. Thus, when needed for overcoming weakness, meat is best used as a supplemental rather than major source of protein. Moreover, the present toxin level in commercial meats is appalling. Many animals are saturated with environmental toxins as well as residues from daily antibiotics and growth hormones in their feed. In 1985, because of unspecified contamination, eleven U.S. meat companies were banned from importing into Europe by the European Common Market.

If animal products, including dairy and eggs, do become necessary as protein and other nutrient sources, we strongly suggest that the animals be naturally raised on organic feed.

Protein Deficiency

In the past, in countries where famine was widespread, one often heard of efforts to "fill the protein gap." What was commonly considered protein deficiency is simply general malnutrition[23]—a lack of *all* nutrients. As soon as a sufficient quantity of calories is available in virtually all traditional diets, "protein deficiencies" vanish.

Protein deficiency, however, is still possible in those with sufficient caloric intake. Examples are the individual with alcoholic liver damage,[24] the young weight-conscious bulimic woman, the person who lives on pastries, candy, and soft drinks, the pure fruitarian, and the vegan who a) does not chew food well enough (meat eaters do not have this problem since meat protein assimilates whether or not it is chewed); b) seldom eats grains, legumes, nuts, or seeds; c) greatly over-eats; or d) eats many highly processed sweets and other non-foods.

Also at risk are completely vegetarian children[25] who are weaned early and take in no dairy products, and neither chew food well nor have their food prepared properly (food for young children needs to be mashed or ground up).

Signs of Protein Deficiency

True protein deficiency is reflected in many facets of body maintenance and development:

- Body tissues deteriorate, leading to hemorrhoids, weak muscles and nails, hair loss, slow healing of wounds, and a general lack of energy and strength.
- Mental concentration and emotional stability degenerate.
- Immune response suffers, leading to allergies and infections.

The following suggestions are not only for the protein-deficient individual but for anyone who wants to utilize protein efficiently.

Improving Protein Utilization

1. These recommendations are based on the relationships of internal organs to emotions as described by traditional Chinese medicine. They involve strengthening the digestive functions of the liver and pancreas by making attitudinal and lifestyle adjustments:
   a. Harmonize work; rest when weary; and exercise regularly.
   b. Avoid stressful and worrisome situations.
   c. Do one thing at a time, mindfully.
2. Avoid all intoxicants and refined foods. Especially harmful is refined sugar. Also avoid excesses of concentrated sweeteners and coffee. Limit fruit intake if protein deficiency is severe.
3. Chew food thoroughly.
4. Large amounts of protein-rich foods are not necessarily better; small amounts, taken more often, usually have a more beneficial effect.

The Higher Sources of Vegetable Protein

Legumes, very rich in both starch and protein, become more digestible when prepared with mineral-rich sea vegetables (as described in the recipe section) and if they are chewed well and eaten at most once a day in ½-cup to one-cup quantities. Soybeans, rich in protein and starch as well as fat, are very difficult to digest and are not advisable unless sprouted or fermented, as in tempeh, soy sauce, or miso, or processed as in tofu or soy milk. Tofu is cooling and weakening if overeaten; it must be well-cooked for those with *deficiency*. Tempeh is also cooling but less so than tofu, and has a higher protein content. Protein powders are usually far too concentrated and often contain soy and other proteins in not easily digestible forms.*

Nuts and seeds offer valuable concentrated protein and fats but must be consumed only in small amounts, to avoid liver problems and especially smelly flatu-

---

*Soybeans contain stachyose, a complex indigestible sugar that is transformed to a digestible form by sprouting or fermentation in tempeh, miso, and soy sauce; stachyose is removed in the process of making soy milk and tofu.

lence. Excessive use of tahini (hulled sesame butter), nuts, seeds, and their butters, out of preference for their meaty taste, is a common practice among vegetarians. Skillfully prepared as condiments, they digest better while contributing moderate amounts of protein. However, since these products are often rancid, it is safest to make your own nut and seed preparations. For more information, see "Nuts and Seeds," "Condiments," and "Rejuvelac and Yogurt" recipes.

Grains contain more protein than most people realize. Trying to make grain protein more "complete"—more like that of meat—will diminish the actual protein available to some people with sensitive or weak digestion. For someone with digestive problems, combining only grains and vegetables at any one meal, or only legumes with leafy green vegetables, may help. (See *Food Combinations* chapter.)

Greens, Provitamin A, and Protein

Green vegetables benefit the liver (see *Wood Element* chapter), the organ where subtle protein metabolic processes take place. Vitamin A, or the carotene (provitamin A) from which the body synthesizes it, is essential for the correct use of protein by the body. Provitamin A is highly concentrated in blue-green microalgae such as spirulina, and is also abundant in green and yellow vegetables. Excellent green leafy sources of provitamin A are kale, parsley, and watercress, and turnip, collard, beet, mustard and dandelion greens.

Yellow vegetables with significant provitamin A content include carrots, sweet potatoes, and winter squash, although the starchy quality of these plants can interfere with digestion of very high-protein foods such as legumes. Starchy plants are best eaten at another meal with any other vegetable or grain. For those who have good digestion without protein deficiencies, the starch-protein issue is not so important, although eating the highest-protein foods first in a meal still significantly aids digestion and reduces flatulence.

The high-fat and/or high-protein grains such as kamut, oats, spelt, quinoa, and amaranth may be most suitable for Westerners who are used to high-fat animal protein. The amount of protein in quinoa and amaranth is in the same range as that in most meats; when combined with another grain, their amino-acid/protein profile is higher than meat or any other animal product. In addition, quinoa is rich in fat and calcium. Oats and kamut, also rich in fat, are recommended for those with nervous disorders or blood sugar imbalances. To decide which grains are most suitable, please refer to their properties in the recipe section.

Fermented foods supply protein and other nutrients in a more easily digestible form as a result of predigestion by bacteria or other micro-organisms. Once the fermentation is complete, the micro-organisms remain in the food, contributing protein and, under the right conditions, vitamin B_{12}. Fermenting completely changes the character of foods. Starches transform into sugars and alcohols, giving ferments an expansive quality in the body.

Added salt controls the fermentation in miso, soy sauce, and pickles. The grains and soybeans in miso and soy sauce are joined through bacterial action, and the result usually causes no problem for those who normally cannot tolerate starch and protein together.

One needs to take care when obtaining protein from these products. Amino acids abound from the wedding of soy and grain, enhanced by the amino acids of the bacteria. The protein is within a living medium that assists its absorption, and therefore small but adequate amounts of protein can be assimilated very easily. Such proteins are best consumed in small amounts. Since the processing of miso and soy sauce takes from several months to two years, the fermentation is quite advanced. When eaten in moderation, these foods foster healthy intestinal flora. However, excessive use of ferments such as miso have been known to feed *Candida albicans* and similar yeasts. (See "Candida" section, page 71)

The **algae** known as seaweeds have a broad range of protein content, in addition to a remarkable ability to combine with other vegetables, grains, and legumes. Not only do they contribute valuable protein and other nutrients, but in general* their mineralization is superior to that of any other plant or animal food.

As a result of the drastic depletion of our soil by modern agricultural methods, food grown in it today contains fewer minerals and other nutrients than in past years. Seaweeds can supply many of these missing nutrients, especially trace minerals. In conditions of overall *deficiency,* minerals must be present before other nutrients will be effective. Seaweeds are so concentrated in minerals that they are normally used as a supplementary item in recipes to provide a mineral foundation for better utilization of protein and all other nutrients.

Highest Sources of Protein

The **micro-algae** have been a relatively new source of nutrition in the mainstream of industrial civilization during the last thirty years, although they have been used by certain traditional peoples in Latin America, Africa, and elsewhere for millennia. They will become increasingly important throughout the planet if other food supplies dwindle. Already spirulina cultivation projects are underway in various parts of the world, particularly where there is malnutrition. (See *Green Food Products,* Chapter 16, for more nutritional information and dosages.)

Spirulina, chlorella, and wild blue-green (*Aphanizomenon flos-aquae*) micro-algae are the richest whole-food sources of protein, provitamin A, and chlorophyll. Some forms are thought to contain every nutrient required by the human body, although certain nutrients are present only in minute quantities. Micro-algae vary in nutrient content, depending on the variety and the way they are cultivated. Ordinarily, a food primarily either builds the body up or cleanses it. Judging from their protein levels, these micro-algae are building foods, yet they are also good cleansers and purifiers because of their chlorophyll content.

---

*The commonly used seaweed gel agar-agar is an exception, containing a relatively small amount of minerals and protein.

> The origin of Heaven and Earth is based on the principle of the middle path.
>
> —Shao Yung, 11th-century Chinese sage.

Protein and Brain Function

The micro-algae are generally used to help attain high levels of physical and mental health and to increase energy. When a wide range of amino acids is plentiful in the body, an ample amount will be available to manufacture brain chemicals. There is much new research into the effects of nutrition on intelligence, including studies of both natural products (such as lecithin, herbs, nutrients, and micro-algae) and a variety of synthetic substances.[26] Not enough is known to make a clear evaluation of the long-term effects of either of these; however, one is nearly always safer with nutrients in the matrix of whole foods. In our experience, most individuals with great intelligence, clairvoyance, and/or wisdom have not relied on super-nutrition or strong substances, but lived simply, in moderation and balance.

Nevertheless, there are stages in life during which powerful nutrition can be helpful: spirulina and other micro-algae are beneficial at times of stress, since protein supports growth and repair functions. Similar qualities are helpful during developmental transitions such as dietary change, new activity patterns, and difficult mental or emotional phases.

Micro-Algae and Meat: A Comparison

According to standard nutritional tests, the digestive absorption of the protein in spirulina and chlorella is four times greater than that in beef.[27, 28] Since they contain about three times more protein than beef, greater absorption means that twelve times more protein is available from the algae than from the same weight of beef.

Protein Equivalence: One Teaspoon Spirulina = One Ounce Beef

Calculation: Three grams (one teaspoon) of powdered spirulina (or chlorella) is equivalent to (3 x 12 =) 36 grams beef, which is more than one ounce.*

If two or three teaspoons of micro-algae are taken daily, this is the protein equivalent of two to three ounces of meat, which is our recommended quantity for the medicinal use of meat mentioned earlier. But it is important to remember that high protein levels come at the expense of calcium. Studies show that when

---

*In such equivalency calculations, Net Protein Utilization is normally applied (NPU of beef is 67%, of spirulina, 57%). This factor, however, rates proteins based on the amino-acid profile developed in animal studies, a profile assumed to be ideal for humans. As mentioned earlier, we disagree with this standard. If applied in this case, however, to demonstrate its effect, one would deduct 15% from the equivalence (NPU of spirulina is [$^{57}/_{67}$ x 100% =] 85% of the beef NPU), making the protein of 3 grams of spirulina equivalent to (36 gm. beef minus 15% =) 30.6 grams of beef, still more than one ounce.

daily protein intake goes beyond seventy-five grams—a boundary easily crossed with either a standard American or a high-protein vegetarian diet—most people lose more calcium in their urine than they absorb from their food.[29]

Sources of Animal Protein

Dairy products are used by vegetarians more than any other animal product. Provided that one is not allergic to dairy, the best-quality products supply protein, vitamin B$_{12}$, and other nutrients of great benefit for those who lack protein or have *deficiencies* in general. According to Chinese medicine, (quality) milk builds *qi* vitality, the blood, and the *yin,* which includes the fluids and tissue of the body. Therefore dairy consumption specifically benefits thin and weak people with a tendency toward *dryness.* However, these same teachings indicate that milk can be hard to digest by those who have mucous problems or weak digestion (see *Earth Element* chapter). Milk that is pasteurized, homogenized, and filled with chemicals is much more difficult to digest properly, even by those with strong digestion.

Milk has a bad reputation among many modern Western health advisors because most people already have an overabundance of mucus and are overweight as a result of their excessive consumption of meat, sugar, fat, and dairy. Furthermore, having lived all their lives on these highly mucus-producing foods, many have developed digestive weakness and are consequently allergic to dairy. Inherent in some allergies is an inability to digest milk sugar (lactose). "Lactose intolerance" is prevalent among Asians (80% of the population is lactose intolerant), Africans/Black Americans (70%), Mediterranean peoples (60%), Mexican-Americans (50%), and anyone whose ancestors did not consume dairy foods.

When there are allergies or intolerances to dairy, the obvious remedy is to avoid these products. We rarely see adults in the United States or Europe who need to consume *more* milk products, although this is true of a few of the many children being raised with no dairy.

Dairy and Mucus Conditions

When mucus-related problems exist—such as discharges from the nose or other parts of the body, frequent colds, asthma, allergies, sinus problems, tumors, cysts, constipation, colon trouble, profuse growth of *Candida albicans,* excess weight, or thick tongue coating—dairy users may wisely consider consuming better-quality and/or fewer dairy products. When other strongly mucus-forming foods are also present in the diet, mucus problems can become severe. Lack of exercise can also be a major factor, since the heat of physical activity normally burns up watery mucoid accumulations.

For further discussion of the following suggestions, refer to the various "milk" and "dairy" sections in *Food for Children,* Chapter 21.

Dairy Recommendations

1. Use full-fat certified raw milk and milk products. Avoid low-fat dairy. Goat's milk and its products are generally preferable.
2. Soured and fermented products are superior for everyone over seven years of age. Common examples are yogurt, kefir, cottage cheese, buttermilk, and soured milk.
3. Anyone with lactose intolerance characterized by abdominal cramps, gas, and diarrhea after dairy ingestion will usually do better with the fermented products above, although in some cases dairy must be avoided altogether.
4. Nursing children should have mother's milk. Neither animal milk nor commercial formula is an *adequate* substitute.
5. If pasteurized milk is used, bring to a quick boil and then cool, to complete the breakdown of protein chains. If raw milk is not digested well, especially by people with signs of weakness and *deficiency*, try this quick-boil method for them as well.

Homogenized milk is not recommended; it allows the enzyme xanthine oxidase to enter the vascular system and scar it, setting up ideal conditions for fatty deposits in the arteries.

Soured Milk Preparation: To make soured milk, warm one or two cups of raw milk to body temperature in a pan of water, then stir in a tablespoon of buttermilk or yogurt as a "starter." Allow it to sit and coagulate in a consistently warm place (70 to 80°F) for 24 hours. Two tablespoons of this soured milk can be used as a starter for the next batch.

Is Milk-Drinking Natural?

Among all wild mammals, milk is reserved for the newborn, and no other animal drinks another animal's milk. However, this does not mean that the adult human is necessarily wrong to use dairy; we do many things unique to our species. It is our feeling that milk products should not be a main feature in any diet beyond the infant stage, but are best used as a supplement, provided they are well tolerated and of good quality.

The Ethical Issue

One important issue concerning most commercial milk is the way in which the animals are treated. In India, where milk is considered a pure or "Sattvic" food, cows are cared for with gentleness and respect. Regardless of the motivation for this treatment, the end result is that the milk is of high quality, since the cows are calm, content, and well-fed on unsprayed grasses and plants. In America and other parts of the West, dairy cows are given hormones, drugs, and sometimes chemically laden feed. When they stop producing, they are routinely slaughtered. Thus, by using most commercial dairy products, one is also supporting the meat industry.

Another dairy-meat connection is of therapeutic importance: many lacto-vegetarians have not used flesh foods for years and do not welcome that influence in their bodies and lives. But, according to our observations, dairy products prevent the cleansing of residues of meat consumption from earlier in one's life. In order to discharge these residues, one must stay completely free of dairy for a minimum of six months—some health practitioners estimate several times this long.

Goat's Milk

This "retaining" property of dairy applies to all animal milk, although most of the preceding discussion on dairy has referred to commercial cow's milk. Goat's milk, however, has different properties. Those with excess mucus would still want to be cautious in the use of goat's milk, but it forms far less mucus than cow's milk.

Goat's milk is frequently considered an exception to many problems with dairy. Goats are usually healthy and clean and therefore are not normally given regular doses of antibiotics or other drugs. The fat structure of their milk is much more digestible than that of cow's milk; since it is already naturally homogenized, goat milk does not have to be mechanically homogenized. Also, it is likely to be available raw. Because goats that graze freely enjoy a large variety of leaves, grasses, and herbs, their milk contains rich amounts of nutrients not found in cow's milk. For all of these reasons, goat's milk is universally prescribed as a superior product for many types of deficiency, from youth through old age. When animal-product nutrition is needed, raw goat's milk is usually a good choice.

Pollen and Royal Jelly

Bee pollen, the food of the young bee, is a rich source of protein and vitamin B$_{12}$. Considered one of nature's most completely nourishing foods, it contains nearly all nutrients required by humans. About half of its protein is in the form of free amino acids that are ready to be used directly by the body. Such highly assimilable protein can contribute significantly to one's protein needs. Pollen also contains substances not yet identified. These may contribute to its remarkable properties, which cannot be fully explained by the effects of its known nutrients.

Pollen is considered an energy and nutritive tonic in Chinese medicine; cultures throughout the world use it in a surprising number of applications—improving endurance and vitality, extending longevity, aiding recovery from chronic illness, adding weight during convalescence, reducing cravings and addictions, regulating the intestines, building new blood, preventing communicable diseases such as the common cold and flu (it has antibiotic properties), and helping overcome retardation and other developmental problems in children. It is thought to protect against radiation and to have anti-cancer qualities. Pollen and raw, unprocessed honey (which contains pollen) are remedies for many cases of hay fever and allergy. (For bee products to help with hay fever, they must be taken at least six weeks before pollen season and then continued through the season.) Before taking a full dose of pollen, test for a possible extreme allergic reaction by ingesting just one pellet.

The optimal dose of pollen varies with individual needs. For allergy prevention, for example, 6 grams daily in the form of tablets, capsules, or loose pellets (about a teaspoonful) is often sufficient. Athletes seeking strength and endurance may ingest 10–15 grams or more daily.

When eating bee pollen, consider that a 6-gram dose takes one bee, working eight hours a day for one month, to gather. Each bee pollen pellet contains 2,000,000 flower pollen grains, and a teaspoonful contains 2.5 billion grains of flower pollen.

Royal jelly, a food of infant bees and the sole food of the queen bee, is made by nurse bees who chew pollen and mix it with secretions from glands in their head tops. Like bee pollen, royal jelly is an energy and nutritive tonic, but to a far greater degree. It is useful in all of the above applications for pollen, but has a stronger effect on the glandular system, and is considered strengthening for the reproductive systems of both men and women. Royal jelly has also been used effectively in the treatment of malnutrition in children, arthritis, leukemia, severe *deficiencies* and wasting diseases. Further uses are given in other sections (see index). It is available in many forms including capsules, freeze-dried powder, and preserved in honey. Because of its potency, a normal dosage is just 100–400 milligrams daily.

Pollen and royal jelly may also be taken by those in need of rich animal nutrition who prefer to not eat meat.

It is wise to be aware of the tremendous energy expended by bees in making pollen grains and royal jelly, and to use these nutritional elixirs mindfully.

Eggs, Fish, Fowl, and Mammal Meats

If, after a serious effort to use them, vegetarian, dairy, and bee products are not effective against deficiencies, then other animal products such as eggs or meat may be needed. Each animal product has unique properties and its own level of evolution. Note: "Neutral" thermal nature in the following discussion means that the food has neither a warming nor cooling thermal nature.

Eggs: If we start with the lower-order animals as sources of food, perhaps the least evolved is the egg, which represents a single cell (even fertilized eggs remain a single cell if they are kept refrigerated). Many people seem unaware that an egg is a flesh food, albeit undeveloped.

Properties and uses of chicken eggs: Neutral thermal nature; "sweet" flavor; blood and *yin* tonic. Eggs have an "ascending direction," which influences energy and fluids to move higher in the body. Thus they can be used curatively in cases of diarrhea and to secure the fetus when there is a tendency to miscarry. They are also useful for calming a fetus with excess movement. Since eggs moisten the upper body, they are sometimes helpful for dryness of the lungs, throat, and eyes; because of their ability to nurture the blood and *yin* (includes the fluids and tissues of the body), they may be appropriate for the person with a *dry,* thin, anemic constitution.

However, eggs can also create a thick type of mucus; for this reason, consumption of eggs often causes imbalance, especially for the sluggish, overweight person or others with *damp*-mucus symptoms.

The protein content of common chicken eggs is moderate, and substantially less than that of meat; it is somewhere in the neighborhood of the high-protein grains such as oats and hard red wheat. Some nutritionists, however, praise the quality of the protein in eggs, since its eight essential amino acids have a consistently high profile. From this perspective, eggs are one of the best animal products for protein deficiency, except for the major drawback of their extremely sticky mucus-forming quality which can eventually obstruct the gall bladder, slow the functioning of the liver, and leave deposits throughout the body. A related viewpoint from Chinese medicine claims that eggs can contribute to *wind*, manifested in liver-related conditions such as vertigo, strokes, nervousness, spasms, and paralysis. Thus, eggs are contraindicated in *wind* conditions.

Since the allergenic potential of eggs is among the highest of any food, some people metabolize eggs much better than others. For those who are not allergic to them and have no mucous problems, eggs are recommended above meats in cases of insufficient protein and other deficiencies. The standard commercial eggs are best avoided since the hens that lay these live in sterile, mechanical environments and are fed various drugs. The eggs they produce often have little or no vitamin B$_{12}$ and are lacking in virtually every other nutrient.

Eggs are considered one of the most concentrated of foods. Ovo-vegetarians commonly use them in soups or casseroles, a practice that disperses their richness and is beneficial for those who require small amounts of potent animal product.

The number of salmonella-infected eggs has been on the rise in recent years, according to information from the Centers for Disease Control concerning a report in the April, 1989 *Journal of the American Medical Association*. The *Salmonella eneritidis* bacteria causes adverse reactions in humans: diarrhea, cramps, vomiting, and fever. In infants, the elderly, and those with weakened immunity, death can result. To avoid salmonella, keep eggs refrigerated, discard dirty or cracked eggs, and thoroughly cook eggs and recipes containing them.

Meat (fish, fowl, and mammals) as protein: Thus far, several properties of meat have been discussed, including its impact on consciousness. On the positive side, from a strictly nutritional standpoint, meat contains high levels of protein, certain vitamins, and an abundance of minerals and trace minerals. But meat is high in fat content, is often laden with toxins, hormones, and antibiotics, and when eaten routinely in large amounts, produces copious dense mucus, urea, and uric acid. Meat and other animal products had been the main source of protein in the West for most of the last century, but this practice is now being seriously questioned.

More than its protein level, the single most important nutritional feature of meat is its cell structure, which, as mentioned earlier, is similar to ours. The nutrients absorbed from meat are rapidly and easily transformed into tissue and blood—thus the rush of energy from meat-eating. Small amounts, then, can be used therapeutically to strengthen those with *deficiencies,* although meat is not always tolerated, in which case, its use should be discontinued.

Choices—When Animal Foods Are Necessary

The properties of the various animals and their parts have been the subject of long-term study in both Chinese medicine and Western nutrition and physiology. Following are some of the traditional principles to aid in choosing animal products:

1. Summary of previous suggestions: Try to use the least-evolved animals. The sequence of eggs, fish, fowl, red meat is a basic evolutionary pattern to follow. From a nutritional and holistic standpoint, if animals are to be eaten, use as much of the animal as possible. There are many fish and shellfish examples; a Japanese one is the use of tiny dried whole fish such as *tazukuri, chirimen iriko* (anchovies), and *chuba iriko,* commonly part of soup and condiment recipes.

2. Choose animals according to traditional relationships. In the Five-Element theory of Chinese medicine, specific human organs benefit from certain animals: Liver—poultry; Heart—sheep; Spleen-Pancreas—cattle; Lung—horse or fish; Kidney—pig. Simply being in contact with the animal that benefits a weakened organ can sometimes be helpful. Whether through food or friendship, one receives various qualities of an animal's nature. Sedentary people, for example, benefit from active animals.

3. Use animal parts according to their correspondence with the parts that are imbalanced in the human. This is the ancient medical principle of "like heals like." For example, animal kidney is commonly used for human kidney deficiency. In general, the "variety" or organ meats are more concentrated in nutrients than muscle meats, and therefore tonify *deficiency* more efficiently. Common variety meats are liver, kidney, heart, tongue, brain, and "sweet breads" (glands of calves or lambs). Precaution: certain variety meats, especially liver, will normally contain high toxin levels unless the animal was raised organically.

4. Choose animal foods according to specific therapeutic properties such as their warming/cooling/drying/moistening/tonifying/reducing attributes, the healing value of their flavors, and their ability to treat specific disorders. Such properties appear below in descriptions of various animal products.

In the following sampling based on the Chinese healing arts, most of the animals—especially the mammals—are inappropriate for those with *excess* conditions. Beef, for instance, may be used for low backache or diabetes if there is weakness and *deficiency,* but *not* if there are signs of *excess* such as a strong pulse, loud voice, robust personality, and reddish skin color.

When the term *"yin"* is used in describing actions of foods on the person, it refers to the fluids and tissues of the body (as discussed in earlier chapters); thus the phrase "nurture the *yin*" means to build up the fluid metabolism and the structure of the body, its flesh, tendons, bones, and other parts as well as the person's practical, grounded nature. "Spleen-pancreas" in the following list represents the Chinese idea of "spleen," which corresponds somewhat with the pancreas and its effects on digestion, and is explained further in the *Earth Element* chapter.

Properties and Common Uses
of Fish and Meats[30, 31, 32]

clam*   *Thermal nature:* cooling. *Flavor:* salty. *Properties:* Moistens *dryness,* nurtures the *yin,* facilitates proper body fluid distribution, and aids in resolving *damp* conditions such as excess mucus and sputum, edema, and vaginal discharge (leukorrhea); also is used in the treatment of excessive vaginal bleeding, hemorrhoids, and goiter.

mussel*   *Thermal nature:* warming. *Flavor:* salty. *Properties:* Strengthens the liver and kidneys; improves the *qi* energy and *jing* essence; builds the blood; often used for kidney/*jing* deficiencies such as impotence and low back pain; also treats excessive vaginal bleeding, intestinal blockage, abdominal swelling, goiter, and vertigo.

oyster*   *Thermal nature:* neutral. *Flavor:* sweet and salty. *Properties:* Nurtures the *yin* and builds the blood; especially useful for syndromes involving deficiencies of the *yin* and/or blood such as nervousness, dryness, and insomnia; also helpful for treating indecision. Contraindicated in skin diseases.

crab*   *Thermal nature:* neutral. *Flavor:* salty. *Properties:* Nurtures the *yin,* moistens *dryness;* used for bone fractures and dislocations, poison ivy, and burns. In quantity, it has a toxic effect. Contraindicated in conditions of *wind* (strokes, nervousness, spasms, etc.) and during *exterior* conditions such as the onset of the common cold.

shrimp*   *Thermal nature:* warming. *Flavor:* sweet. *Properties:* Enhances the *yang* (warming, active) principle and increases *qi* energy; overcomes *wind* conditions, increases lactation, discharges mucus, and eliminates worms. Contraindicated in skin diseases marked with redness and inflammation, and in spermatorrhea.

carp   *Thermal nature:* neutral. *Flavor:* sweet. *Properties:* Promotes proper body fluid distribution, increases lactation. Used for edema, jaundice, insufficient lactation.

herring   *Thermal nature:* neutral. *Flavor:* sweet. *Properties:* Moistens *dryness,* has anodyne effect (relieves pain), detoxifies the body, treats general *deficiency.* Contraindication: skin eruptions.

---

    * Many fish, especially shellfish, now contain dangerous quantities of chemical toxins and heavy metals that reduce immunity and reproductive capacity. If you use fish, particularly for overcoming *deficiency,* it is best to obtain those from the least polluted waters possible, preferably near large, pristine land areas. See Resources index for organizations that identify which fish are from sustainable fisheries.

sardine   *Thermal nature:* neutral. *Flavor:* sweet and salty. *Properties:* Nurtures the *yin*, increases *qi* energy; fortifies the sinews and bones; acts as a mild diuretic; facilitates blood circulation. Caution: excessive amounts cause mucus accumulations and *heat* conditions.

whitefish   *Thermal nature:* neutral. *Flavor:* sweet. *Properties:* Promotes proper body fluid distribution; strengthens spleen-pancreas function (used to treat indigestion); improves appetite.

mackerel   *Thermal nature:* neutral. *Flavor:* sweet. *Properties:* Improves *qi* energy and dries *damp* conditions; especially useful for obstructive *damp* diseases such as rheumatism.

chicken   *Thermal nature:* warming. *Flavor:* sweet. *Properties:* Acts as a *qi* energy tonic; specifically affects the digestion (spleen-pancreas and stomach); increases the *jing* essence and improves the condition of the bone marrow; aids lactation. Is often used when the following conditions result from spleen-pancreas imbalances: anorexia and poor appetite in general, edema, diarrhea, diabetes, excessive urination (as in diabetes), vaginal hemorrhage, vaginal discharge, weakness following childbirth. Contraindicated in diseases that involve *heat, excess,* or *exterior* conditions. Avoid the common commercial chicken raised with chemical-, hormone- and antibiotic-laden feed.

chicken liver   *Thermal nature:* warming. *Flavor:* sweet. *Properties:* Strengthens both the liver and kidneys; helpful in treating impotence, childhood *deficiency* and malnutrition, blurred vision, tendency to miscarry, and urinary incontinence.

lamb   *Thermal nature:* warming. *Flavor:* sweet. *Properties:* Increases *qi* energy, internal warmth, and lactation; improves blood production. Has a general relationship to the integrated "heart-mind" concept of ancient Chinese medical theory. Used in the treatment of general weakness, kidney and spleen-pancreas deficiencies, anemia, impotence, low body weight, and pain in the lower back. Contraindicated in *heat* conditions and hyperlipidemia (high blood fat). Commercial lamb is typically given fewer antibiotics and drugs than other red meats, and often grazes on unsprayed grassland.

lamb kidney   *Thermal nature:* warming. *Flavor:* sweet. *Properties:* Strengthens the kidneys, enhances the *yang* principle, increases the *jing* essence and improves the condition of the marrow. Useful in *deficient* kidney conditions such as low backache, fatigue, hearing loss, sterility, diabetes (especially if kidney-related), weak legs, painful knees, excessive urination, and urinary incontinence.

beef   *Thermal nature:* warming. *Flavor:* sweet. *Properties:* Strengthens the spleen-pancreas and stomach, builds the blood, increases *qi* energy, and strengthens the sinews and bones. Used in the wasting stage of diabetes; treats insufficient *yin* and/or blood manifesting in *dryness* and emaciation; also used for general weakness, low backache, and weak knees. Contraindications: nephritis and hepatitis.

beef kidney   *Thermal nature:* neutral. *Flavor:* sweet. *Properties:* Strengthens the kidneys and treats kidney-related conditions such as impotence, lack of sexual drive, low backache, weak knees and bones, and hearing difficulty.

beef liver   *Thermal nature:* neutral. *Flavor:* sweet. *Properties:* Strengthens the liver; commonly used in the treatment of eye conditions such as blurred vision, night blindness, glaucoma, and optic nerve atrophy (in Chinese medicine, the eyes are related to the functioning of the liver).

pork   *Thermal nature:* neutral. *Flavor:* sweet and salty. *Properties:* Specifically affects the kidneys, spleen-pancreas, and stomach; moistens *dryness* and nurtures the *yin.* Used to treat those with thin, dry, nervous, and weak constitutions; also used for dry cough, constipation, and the wasting stage of diabetes. Defatted soup of pork is drunk for dry cough and constipation. Contraindications: obesity, diarrhea, hypertension, conditions of yellow mucus (mucus with a *heat* condition), or stagnant *qi* energy—the latter often resulting in conditions such as tiredness, stress, pain, spasm, or paralysis.

pork kidney   *Thermal nature:* neutral. *Flavor:* salty. *Properties:* Strengthens the kidneys and improves bladder function; moistens *dryness.* Used in treating kidney deficiency signs such as lower back pain, spermatorrhea, deafness as a result of aging, and night sweats.

pork liver   *Thermal nature:* neutral. *Flavor:* sweet and bitter. *Properties:* Builds the blood and strengthens the liver; benefits the eyes. Used in the treatment of weak vision, night blindness, pinkeye; also used for edema.

The methods of meat preparation that reduce toxicity and maximize therapeutic effects are listed below. It is not our intention to promote the consumption of animal products; however, we have seen cases in which they helped overcome *deficiencies* during illness or dietary transition. From the perspective of compassion, animal foods that involve the taking of life should be used solely as medicine for weakness, and only when other approaches are unsuccessful.

Meat Preparation for Deficiencies and Dietary Transition

Even though we do not list recipes which include meat, the following techniques improve the digestibility of all meats, including the red meats, poultry, and fish:

1. Use small amounts—two or three ounces at one daily meal.
2. Acid marinades help break down fats and protein chains—slice meat in thin pieces and marinate for 30 minutes or longer in any of the following solutions:

> apple cider vinegar, diluted in two parts water
> lemon juice
> wine
> tomato juice
> beer
> other strongly alcoholic beverages, diluted in two parts water

3. Cook into a soup or broth with ginger root. Ginger helps rid the body of the acids and toxins from meat. Marjoram may also be used in cooking to help the liver digest the fats in meat.
4. The vegetables that best aid in the digestion of meat protein and fat are the green variety, especially leafy greens; also sulphur vegetables such as cabbage, broccoli, onion, and garlic. These vegetables can be cooked with the meat or otherwise included in the same meal.

Oils and Fats

Fats, including oils, are a very important part of every diet (oil is fat in a liquid state). Reducing or eliminating animal food and dairy products in the diet usually results in a desire for more vegetable-quality fat and oil to satisfy the taste and give a feeling of satiety.

Some people need more fat than others. In cold climates, a diet high in fat is superior to a carbohydrate diet for supplying deep, internal heat.* Fats digest more slowly than other foods. They produce body fat for insulation, for protecting the vital organs and holding them in place. In addition, they are necessary for the assimilation of the fat-soluble vitamins, namely vitamins A, D, E, and K.

Nevertheless, many health problems can be related to excessive and poor-quality fat intake. Fats make up 30–40% of the American diet. Although several national health organizations recommend 20%, a balanced vegetarian diet will often contain about 10% fat, based on caloric intake. Within limits, appropriate con-

---

*Both proteins and carbohydrates yield four calories per gram, whereas fat provides nine calories per gram.

sumption of fat, like any nutrient, varies with the individual. In general, it is the upper limit that is overstepped. A high-fat diet promotes tumors, cancers, obesity, heart disease, gall bladder and liver disorders, and may contribute to diabetes, among other degenerative conditions.[1, 2, 3]

Other fundamental problems generated by mental/emotional imbalances may surface when oils and fats are consumed excessively: cravings, sensual over-stimulation, cloudy mentality, weakened vision, emotional attachments, promiscuity, and inflammatory extremes such as anger, fits, and arthritis. Most problems involving pain, spasms, and cramps also can ultimately be traced to excess dietary fat. These maladies are due in part to the impact of fats on the liver.* Since the energy released in the body from fat combustion is more than twice that of any other nutritional source, it is easy to see why fats can cause excesses and inflammations. To help remember the effect of too much fat on the mind, one can associate the sticky, filmy quality of fats with an unclear and grasping (attached) type of consciousness.

It is healthier for most people to cut down their fat intake slowly. If one's liver is used to large amounts of fat, a sudden drop may cause a temporary feeling of dissatisfaction, which may lead to subsequent overindulgence. As soon as one reduces fat consumption, the liver will start to cleanse itself and eventually the body will stop "wanting" so much. But the desire for fats is carried a long time. They are stored by the liver from early childhood, and it may take several years to get over a "fat tooth."

Cutting down on salt helps reduce the desire for fats, as does a diet of whole foods.

The Nature of Fats

A key to knowing how much fat should be consumed is understanding the nature of fats according to traditional East Asian wisdom: fat consumption supports the *yin* principle and creates a sense of security, heaviness, and a slowing, grounding influence. Fats build the tissues, enhance the fluid metabolism, and direct nutrients into the nervous system. Then the predominately *yin* aspect of fat gradually changes into a *yang,* physically energizing, and warming quality. This is why fats, whether from oils, nuts, seeds, or animal products, are so highly valued—people like to feel secure, to slow down, and to have ample energy and warmth.

From a therapeutic standpoint, those who benefit most from a moderate amount of fats are thin, dry, nervous, unproductive, or lacking a strong sense of connection

---

*The liver plays a central role in fat metabolism. In traditional Chinese physiology, it is also the seat of the emotions and strongly influences the eyes, tendons, and ligaments; furthermore, the liver acupuncture meridian passes through the head and around the surface of the genitalia. Pain and spasms ensue when the liver loses its ability to support smooth *qi* flow (see *Wood Element* chapter for further correspondences).

with the earth. In fact, in several Asian traditions, herbs prescribed for the flighty, dry type of person are mixed with an oil such as sesame.

Precautions: Fats and oils should be used sparingly by those who are overweight, slow, mentally or emotionally heavy, materialistic, overheated (manifested by red face, bloodshot eyes, yellow tongue coating, some kinds of high blood pressure, a tendency to feel too hot), or who have *damp* symptoms (candida yeast overgrowth, edema, tumors, cysts, excess body weight). These cautions, however, do not apply to the use of omega-3 and GLA oils, to be discussed later in this chapter.

These traditional profiles of fats and their healthful application are a very useful guide, particularly when combined with the following perspectives of modern nutrition.

The Saturated Fat/Cholesterol Connection

Some oils contain "omega-3" fatty acids, which can help reduce the effects of harmful fat and cholesterol accumulations (fatty acids are the components of fat that define their flavor, texture, and melting points). To grasp the value of omega-3 and other dimensions of oils, it is important to know more about the interrelationship of fats and cholesterol in the body.

Animal products are generally high in both saturated fats and cholesterol (a fat-related substance necessary for good health). Cholesterol is either manufactured by the body or consumed in animal products. Within the body, it is found in the brain and nervous system, liver, blood, and to a small degree in other body tissues. It is used to form sex and adrenal hormones, vitamin D, and bile, which is needed for the digestion of fats.

Clearly, a major cause of too much cholesterol in the body is its overconsumption, but there are others: saturated fats in the diet greatly increase the manufacture of blood cholesterol; other contributing factors are stress, cigarette smoking, and consumption of coffee and refined sugar. Chronically elevated blood cholesterol leads to arteriosclerosis (hardening and thickening of the arteries) as well as other circulatory problems including heart disease, high blood pressure, and risk of excessive clotting.

Twice as many people die from arteriosclerotic disease (heart and blood-vessel disease) as from all cancers combined. According to Dr. William Castelli, director of the landmark Framingham Heart Study,[4] cholesterol levels are a direct measure of heart disease: "For every one percent you lower your serum cholesterol, your subsequent heart attack rate lowers by two percent." Consider that we are born with serum cholesterol levels of about 70 mg/dl, and from age one through seventeen our average is about 150 mg/dl, which is the level for 75% of the world's adult population.

Heart disease is very rare at 150 mg/dl. Even though medical texts in the recent past generally assigned the cholesterol danger level at 250 mg/dl, the bulk of heart attacks strike people in the 200–250 mg/dl range, according to the Framingham study and other recent data.

Saturated Fat and Cholesterol in Common Animal Products

Saturated fat calories as a percent of total sample calories; cholesterol in milligrams per gram of sample

Animal Product	Cholesterol	Fat	Suggestions for Minimizing Saturated Fat and Cholesterol Buildup
Egg yolk	6.0	24%	Avoid or greatly limit foods highest in saturated fat and cholesterol—eggs and butter. Note that saturated fat in organ meats is relatively low. The extreme fat and cholesterol in eggs is offset somewhat by the lecithin they contain, although it is still thought that eggs can add significantly to arterial plaque.
Whole egg	5.5	19%	
Chicken liver	4.4	9%	
Beef liver	3.0	9%	
Butter	2.2	63%	
Lobster	2.0	9%	
Shrimp	1.5	4%	
Chicken heart	1.3	16%	
Clam	1.2	10%	
Crab	1.0	9%	
Colby cheese	.96	46%	Avoid cheese or use it sparingly; even though it is not a commonly known fact, cheese is high in cholesterol and is one of the richest foods in saturated fat (saturated fat causes blood cholesterol to rise).
Milk, dry	.96	30%	
Mackerel	.95	11%	
Swiss cheese	.93	42%	
Feta cheese	.89	50%	
Herring	.85	9%	
Chicken (dark meat)	.81	19%	
Sardine	.71	23%	Most red meats, including those listed here, contain moderate cholesterol but large amounts of saturated fat —avoid or use them sparingly. The fish and light-meat chicken in this group are relatively low in saturated fat; the fish contain omega-3 oils and are therefore one of the safest animal products. Fat levels are reduced by trimming the separable fat in meat such as roasts and steaks, by removing the skin of fowl, and by cooking methods such as broiling. "Select" grade of red meat contains less fat than the "prime" or "choice" cuts.
Ground beef	.67	35%	
Pork bacon	.67	34%	
Tuna	.65	13%	
Salmon	.60	20%	
Haddock	.60	1%	
Lamb chops	.59	42%	
Chicken	.58	15%	
Ham	.57	16%	
Porterhouse steak	.57	39%	
Trout	.55	11%	
Oysters	.50	12%	Several fish—haddock, halibut, cod, and scallops—are among the animal products with the least saturated fat and cholesterol. The percentage by caloric value of saturated fat in dairy indicates its true contribution to body fat and is especially useful since milk and other dairy products are commonly used in nearly every meal of the modern American diet.
Halibut	.50	1%	
Cod	.50	1%	
Scallops	.35	1%	
Milk, cow	.13	30%	
Yogurt	.13	30%	
Milk, goat	.11	34%	

Anyone with a high-fat dietary background should have cholesterol levels checked. If the level is above 200 mg/dl, it is time to take preventive measures.

Vegetable foods—grains, land and sea vegetables, fruits, legumes, nuts, and seeds—contain no cholesterol and are generally low in saturated fat. (The few common plants rich in saturated fat are listed later in the "Saturated Fats" section of this chapter.) Certainly the simplest dietary route for reducing a fat and cholesterol problem is to increase foods of plant origin and decrease those from animals. Omega-3 fish oils are an exception, although even these may be replaced with certain plant oils. But which plant products lower fat and cholesterol most efficiently?

Cleansing the Heart and Arteries

Specific nutrients that reduce cholesterol and saturated fat in the blood and arteries are lecithin, vitamins E and C, and niacin. These nutrients function efficiently in cleaning the arteries when taken in whole food. Lecithin is found in most legumes, especially soybeans. Both soybeans and mung beans are recommended by Chinese medicine for cleansing arteries, although nearly all beans, peas, and lentils are beneficial. This is partly because legumes are a good source of choline, a lipotrophic agent that controls fat metabolism; choline is also a primary component of lecithin.

When *heat* symptoms occur with arterial problems, the cooling qualities of soy and mung bean sprouts are useful. These sprouts are commonly found in grocery stores and markets with well-stocked produce. (See "Sprouts" in recipe section.) Sprouts are also an excellent source of vitamin C, as are cabbage, parsley, bell peppers, and citrus. Eating the white insides of peppers, the core of cabbage, and a little of the pulp and inner peel of citrus provides bioflavonoids, which work synergistically with C to strengthen blood vessel walls.

Plant fiber, particularly that in whole grains, helps to reduce fat in the blood and prevent hardening of the arteries. Because of this now-widespread knowledge, many people have started to include extra fiber in the diet in the form of bran. Too much isolated bran, however, can be unhealthy in other respects (see *Metal Element* chapter). Eating the whole grain with all of its fiber and other nutrients intact produces better results than eating the bran alone. Most helpful for cleansing the arteries are the grains with a slightly bitter flavor: rye (an old European remedy for reducing arterial plaque), quinoa, amaranth, and oats, but all other whole grains are helpful for this purpose. Unprocessed grains are also an excellent source of niacin, and they all contain the freshest type of vitamin E in their oils.

The Omega-3 Effect in Heart Disease, Immune Deficiency, Brain Development, and Malnutrition

If saturated fat and cholesterol are not eliminated from the diet, or if the process of lowering cholesterol is too slow, then the consumption of omega-3 fatty acids is useful. EPA (eicosapentaenoic acid) and DHA (docohexaenoic acid), two primary examples of omega-3 fatty acids, are plentiful in fish. The omega-3s, particularly EPA, are often added to the diet to clean the circulatory system of cholesterol and fat deposits. Specifically, these and other omega-3s reduce blood viscosity, lower lipid levels, reduce clotting, lower blood pressure, and help prevent ischemia (the damage to body tissue that results from interruption of blood flow; examples are strokes and heart attacks). Thus the omega-3 oils not only minimize circulatory disorders but also encourage blood flow to tissues damaged by lack of circulation.

DHA and Brain/Nerve Renewal

DHA and EPA mutually support each other in the function of vascular renewal. DHA also plays other vital roles. It is a major structural component of the brain,[5] and is found in the retina of the eye and in sperm.

DHA appears to be essential to brain development and growth, ultimately affecting learning ability.[6, 7, 8] Fifty percent of the brain's DHA is formed during the fetal stage; the remaining fifty percent accumulates in the first year or so after birth. Evidence that many women have low levels of DHA[9] suggests that their infants may be deprived of full mental development. Studies indicate that mother's milk can be an adequate source of DHA for infants, and that DHA levels are increased most quickly by ingesting preformed DHA, such as that found in fish and fish oil;[10] foods rich in alpha-linolenic acid (examples given later) also increase DHA levels. One reason modern mothers may be deficient in DHA is the widespread consumption of common polyunsaturated vegetable oils. Most of these oils contain primarily linoleic acid, which can inhibit the formation of DHA from alpha-linolenic acid.[11] This is especially the case since most vegetable oils are rancid and refined.

DHA and Other Fatty Acids in Malnutrition

Since laboratory research on the subject of omega-3 oils is not abundant in the area of malnutrition and resultant brain damage, we spoke to someone with extensive experience in treating the malnourished. John McMillin, Ph.D., of Edmonds, Washington, worked for more than fifty years in hunger camps in devastated areas of the world, beginning as an assistant to his father in the late 1930s. Involved with the rescue of starving Jews in the concentration camps after World War II, he later worked with the famished in Africa, South America, and East Asia.

Early on, the McMillins discovered that both spirulina and fish are very helpful in cases of extreme malnutrition. Fish could usually be procured locally, and spirulina was harvested from certain waterways where it grew profusely, such as Lake Chad in Africa. In Peru, the McMillins inoculated lakes with spirulina as early as 1941. Part of the problem with starvation is that eventually the desire to eat is lost. Certain plant and fish oils, according to Dr. McMillin, help stimulate the appetite more quickly than any other remedy he has found.

Dr. McMillin now identifies the EPA/DHA omega-3 fatty acids in fish, as well as alpha- and gamma-linolenic acid (an omega-3/omega-6 pair in spirulina), as critical to his success in reviving famished people and renewing brain function. When fish gruel and spirulina are given, remarkable reversals of learning disability may occur, particularly in malnourished children. When asked if other meats may be substituted, Dr. McMillin claimed that if beef or other red flesh meats are given too early, their saturated fats will cause spasms which literally tear the fragile digestive tracts of starving people. However, he suggested that beef or other mammal liver can be used with some success, since its saturated fat content is fairly low and it contains substantial omega-3s and gamma-linolenic acid. This is particularly true if the animal is range-fed, which is often the case in poor countries.

It may be that spirulina alone is sufficient for treating less severe cases of malnourishment, as indicated from research in Mexico and China with children weakened from an inadequate diet.[12] This makes sense if we consider that various omega-3-rich micro-algae are the probable source of the omega-3 oils in fish.

In the developed countries where nutrient starvation takes place as a result of excessive refined food, intoxicants, and a glut of animal products, micro-algae such as spirulina, wild blue-green *(Aphanizomenon flos-aquae),* and chlorella, used in conjunction with unrefined vegetable foods, are helpful in healing the many prevalent disorders of the nerves and brain.

Sources of Omega-3 Fatty Acids

Fish with the highest amount of EPA/DHA omega-3s are salmon, mackerel, and sardine; other good sources are herring, anchovy, pilchard, butterfish, lake or rainbow trout, and tuna. Obviously, one way of obtaining omega-3 nutrition is through fish consumption; seven to ten ounces of fish per week should be sufficient. An alternate form of omega-3 is in capsules of the fatty acid derived from fish. Stores carrying supplements usually stock these capsules.

Another source of omega-3 is alpha-linolenic acid, which is a fatty acid found in the oils of certain plants. The advantage of vegetable oils is that no animal must die to produce it for humans. There are also fewer contaminants in vegetable oils—dangerous levels of pesticides and PCBs (polychlorinated biphenyls) are often found in fish oil. For cases of malnutrition where omega-3 action is required in large amounts for brain-nerve deficiencies, the fish oils are more effective,[13] since alpha-linolenic acid is converted by the body slowly into EPA and DHA.

Recommended sources of alpha-linolenic acid include flax seed (53% of its oil is composed of alpha-linolenic acid), chia seed (30%), hemp seed (20%), pumpkin seed (15%), rapeseed (10%), soybean and its products such as tofu and tempeh (8%), and walnut (5%). Dark green vegetables—kale, collards, chard, parsley, and the cereal grasses (wheat- and barley-grass products)—are additional good sources. This is because all green (chlorophyll-rich) foods contain alpha-linolenic acid in their chloroplasts.

Thus the milk of cows that feed on grass or the meat from range-fed beef or wild herbivorous animals has important quantities of omega-3 fatty acids not found in feedlot animals. Lamb is one of the few commonly available range-fed meats raised without hormones or daily rations of antibiotics. Goats and sheep too nearly always browse on wild grasses and herbs, so the dairy products from these animals are generally of superior quality. At cheese shops one will often find six or seven European and American cheeses made from sheep and/or goat milk. The varieties made from raw milk preserve certain key nutrients and are therefore more wholesome. See the *Protein and Vitamin B₁₂* chapter for the properties, ethical uses, and preparation of animal products.

Plants that grow in cold climates are relatively more concentrated in omega-3s; these include hard red winter wheat and cold-climate nuts, seeds, grains, and legumes. Omega-3 fatty acids are sometimes compared with antifreeze, since they keep the blood relatively thin and circulating well in cold weather—yet a number of clinical trials indicate omega-3s never cause or provoke hemorrhage.[8]

Except for rapeseed, all of the above omega-3-rich plant foods are available in grocery, health, or herb stores and may be eaten regularly by those with circulatory disorders from elevated levels of cholesterol and fat. The fish and fish oils can be added to the diet by people with an extreme need for preformed DHA/EPA oils; raw milk products from free-ranging goats are widely tolerated; dairy of similar quality from sheep or cows and meats from grass-fed animals are most appropriate for *deficient* and weakened individuals. In those with elevated blood fat, even the highest-quality mammal products must be taken in small amounts and prepared properly since they still have a substantial saturated fat and cholesterol content.

Using food high in alpha-linolenic acid also makes sense as a preventative measure for nearly everyone, since most people are severely deficient in it, even in the absence of circulatory problems. It is estimated that the quantity of omega-3 oils consumed by modern Westerners is one-fifth the level found in traditional diets.[14]

When therapeutic doses are necessary, one may use fresh flax-seed oil which has been processed at low temperatures without exposure to oxygen or light, and refrigerated at all times. This oil is becoming widely available in stores carrying unrefined foods. Commercial linseed (denatured flax-seed) oil must not be used—it is highly refined and may cause more harm than good.

Dosages of flax products: four tablespoons of ground flax seed (flaxmeal) with meals once daily; or four tablespoons of soaked flax seeds once daily (soak in water four to eight hours and strain; then, because of their slippery nature, they must be chewed thoroughly without any other food in the mouth); or one tablespoon of fresh flax oil taken with meals once daily. Dosages for acute disease processes or during the early phase of healing chronic conditions can vary: generally at least double the above dosage by taking more at one time and/or by taking it more than once a day. *Excessive* individuals (strong body and extroverted personality, reddish complexion, thick tongue coating) typically require a larger dose than those without these signs. Flaxmeal should be freshly ground (seed or coffee mills work well), or bought in a tightly sealed container and refrigerated. The seeds and meal lubricate the intestines, and thus are useful for treating constipation.

Further Benefits of Omega-3 Oils

In the 1950s, biochemist Johanna Budwig and cancer researcher Max Gerson independently discovered the virtues of using the omega-3 oils for cancer and other degenerative diseases. In applications of this kind, it appears that plant-source omega-3 oils such as those in flax seed work as well as the fish oils. Gerson discovered that tumors dissolved much faster when flax oil was added to his cancer treatment regimen. Since that time, the omega-3 oils have been used for immune enhancement on a cellular level to fortify membranes of healthy cells while simultaneously destroying tumor cells.[15]

In addition to treating cancer and heart disease, the immune-bolstering capacity of the omega-3s makes them useful in AIDS, osteo- and rheumatoid arthritis, and other degenerations involving poor immunity; additional applications include kidney disease, ulcerative colitis, depression, bronchial asthma, hives, psoriasis, enlarged prostate, and migraine.[8, 16, 17, 18, 51] These uses are explained in part by the "prostaglandin" (hormonal) theory of fatty acids, which appears later in this chapter.

Heart and Artery Renewal

Very often, circulatory problems yield quickly to diet and lifestyle modifications. With a history of chronic high blood pressure, fifty-three-year-old John Dukeminier attended a two-week training seminar taught by the author at the Heartwood Institute near Garberville, California. The course involved eight hours of daily practice in Zen Shiatsu acupressure, t'ai chi movement, meditation, and instruction in principles of diet and traditional Chinese medicine. The food served at the Institute included a variety of whole cereal grains, legumes, vegetables, fruit, nuts, and seeds. Also included were salad greens such as lettuce, celery, and sprouts. Mr. Dukeminier had been attempting to lower his blood pressure for two years using herbs and relaxation methods, but with imperceptible results. However, after three days at the Institute, his blood pressure plummeted and he no longer needed his medication. Also, a long-standing abnormality in his pulse, noted by his physician, normalized after twelve days. He lost weight and felt more fit than he had in years.

Numerous similar results have been achieved by those who embark on a healthier lifestyle and diet, although part of the dramatic change in the above case was a result of the therapeutic advantage of day-long acupressure, t'ai chi, Taoist breathing and visualization techniques, Pure Land mantra (chanting), and Zen meditation.

Nevertheless, just through a diet based on whole grains and vegetables in conjunction with mild daily exercise, nearly everyone can expect significant vascular renewal within a few weeks. From a report in the *Journal of the American Medical Association,* most heart by-pass operations would be unnecessary with as few as thirty days of a high-fiber, low-fat diet.[19] Other research indicates that over 97% of those who take medication for high blood pressure no longer need it after simple dietary changes similar to those suggested here.[20]

Summary of Dietary Options for Heart and Artery Renewal

Foods Which Remove Arterial Residues of Fat and Cholesterol

Nutritional Features

LEGUMES
Very effective: Mung* and soybeans, and their sprouts; also tofu, tempeh, and most other legumes such as peas, beans, and lentils.

Lecithin: found in all legumes, but especially both yellow and black soybeans. **Vitamin C:** abundant in legume (and all other) sprouts. **Vitamin E:** rich in soybeans and all bean sprouts. **Niacin:** legumes and their sprouts are good sources. **Omega-3 Oil:** an important nutrient in soybeans.

GRAINS
Whole grains, especially rye, oats, and amaranth; also rice, sprouted wheat (preferably hard red winter wheat), and buckwheat.

Niacin: in all grains, especially brown rice. **Vitamin E:** in all grains, especially sprouted wheat. **Rutin:** in buckwheat—strengthens arterial walls.

VEGETABLES AND FRUITS
Pungent foods: radish,* horseradish,† hot peppers,†c and the onion family† (garlic,* onion, leek, scallion, shallot, chive); leafy greens: cabbage,c spinach, carrot greens, mint leaf, nasturtium leaf, dandelion greens, kale, wheat and barley greens, broccoli, parsley;c also asparagus, bell pepper,c rose hip,c tomato,*c citrus,c celery,* banana,* persimmon,* seaweeds,* chlorella, cucumber, and mushrooms.

Vitamin E and Omega-3 Oil: in beneficial amounts in the green leafy vegetables; in cabbage, vitamin E is richest in the outer leaves, which are often removed from commercial cabbages; asparagus and cucumbers are also rich in E, and chlorella contains a significant quantity of omega-3 oil. **Vitamin C:** those vegetables and fruits marked with superscript "c" are good sources.

NUTS AND SEEDS
Almond, hazelnut (filbert), flax seed, chia seed, pumpkin seed (lightly roasted to remove surface *E. coli*), poppy seed, walnut, and sunflower sprouts.

Vitamin E: in all nuts and seeds, but especially in almonds and hazelnuts. **Omega-3 Oil:** concentrated in flax, chia, and pumpkin seeds as well as walnuts. **Lecithin:** very rich in sunflower sprouts and greens, which are an ideal form of sunflower, since commercially shelled seeds are usually rancid.

ANIMAL PRODUCTS
Fish: sardine, salmon, mackerel, and other deep/cold-water fish. Raw honey* and bee pollen.

Omega-3 Oil: these fish are a valuable source. Raw honey is the only sweetener that reduces fatty accumulations in the vascular system.

(continued on next page)

Summary of Dietary Options for Heart and Artery Renewal (continued)

HERBS

Hawthorne berry* (very useful), dandelion root, burdock root, chaparral, peppermint (for heart palpitations and for strengthening the heart muscle), cayenne pepper,*†c ginger,† rhubarb root (also for constipation), yarrow, chamomile, motherwort, and valerian. A typical and effective combination: equal parts of yarrow, ginger, hawthorne berry, and valerian. (Herbal preparation and dosages are described in the *Dietary Transition* chapter.)

---

* Foods that specifically treat hypertension.
† Pungent plants to be avoided in cases of *heat* signs.
c Foods rich in vitamin C.

Notes

Taken in total, the above foods contain virtually all nutrients necessary to human nutrition. The features listed are only those commonly known to cleanse and rebuild the arteries and heart—lecithin, vitamins E and C, niacin, and omega-3 fatty acids. Fiber also belongs on this list but is not included here because it occurs in different forms in all plants, and is obtained in sufficient quantity and combinations simply by eating a variety of plant foods.

When the diet includes a wide sampling of the above foods, nutritional support is available for rebuilding the entire vascular system, and problems such as hypertension (high blood pressure) should diminish.

Certain pungent- and bitter-flavored herbs and foods are often used for cleansing the arteries and heart. Pungents and other warming foods should be avoided or used carefully by those with *heat* signs such as a red face or deep-red tongue color. Those with *wind* signs, especially a tendency to a stroke or dizziness, should avoid buckwheat and use all warming foods with caution.

It must be remembered that the known nutrients are only one dimension of food, and that many of the most effective healing foods act in ways that cannot be fully explained or, in some cases, they have no nutritional explanation whatsoever.

The above program has several major effects from the perspective of Chinese medicine: it removes mucus and stagnant *qi* and blood; it directs cooling *yin* fluids to the liver; and it detoxifies the system. The program is best suited to the robust person with at least some signs of *excess* (strong radial pulses, strong voice, thick tongue coating, and/or outward-oriented personality). In Western medical terms, these dietary features generally help the person with a high cholesterol rating and a rich dietary background.

Anyone undertaking this program can benefit from the information on heart imbalance found in the *Fire Element* chapter, which offers a picture of the importance of mental and spiritual awareness to heart and vascular renewal. Those who are frail, weak, pallid, or have other signs of *deficiency* will benefit from the "Syndromes of the Heart" section in the *Fire Element* chapter. Understanding specific heart syndromes will complement the suggestions in this present chapter.

Polyunsaturated Oils and the Essential Fatty Acids

Polyunsaturated oil contains "essential" fatty acids, those that the body is unable to provide. There are two essential fatty acids—linoleic acid and alpha-linolenic acid (note the subtle spelling difference between "linoleic" and "linolenic"). Arachidonic acid is in reality a third essential fatty acid that most people have in excess. Based on experimentation with animals, it has been thought until very recently that linoleic acid, the most common fatty acid, was converted into arachidonic acid (AA) as needed during human fat metabolism, but we now know that most humans are virtually devoid of the enzyme delta-5-desaturase, which makes that conversion possible.[21] This metabolic peculiarity may have occurred in modern humans who eat great quantities of animal products, the richest and principal source of AA. When delta-5-desaturase is not needed to create AA, the body may stop producing this enzyme.

Pure vegetarians concerned with possible AA deficiency may eat nori seaweed, an adequate source. Peanuts are another source (see page 533 for information on using peanuts). For the vast majority of people who eat plenty of animal products, the major concern with fatty acids is not how to get more AA, but how to get better-quality linoleic acid and more alpha-linolenic acid.

The essential fatty acids may be viewed in terms of their effect on blood clotting. Linoleic and arachidonic acid are "omega-6" fatty acids and encourage blood clot formation, whereas we know that alpha-linolenic acid, an omega-3 oil, reduces clotting. The ideal is to achieve a balance between omega-6 and omega-3 fatty acids.

Functions of Essential Fatty Acids: Promote healthy, youthful skin and hair; support proper thyroid and adrenal activity and thus bolster immunity and are required for normal growth and energy; promote healthy blood, nerves, and arteries; and are crucial in the transport and breakdown of cholesterol.

Deficiencies in the Essential Fatty Acids: Can lead to skin disorders such as eczema and dry, scaly skin; other common imbalances are dry hair and loss of hair, nail problems, gallstones, irritability, liver problems, varicose veins, susceptibility to infections, low body weight, infertility, and retarded growth.

Since the use of vegetable oils is so widespread, it would seem that a lack of essential fatty acids would seldom occur—but many oils contain rancid forms of these fatty acids. All polyunsaturated vegetable oils contain two or more double bonds on the molecular level that easily accept oxygen (thus leading to rancidity). Monounsaturated oils contain only one such bond per molecule, and saturated oils none.

As polyunsaturated oils oxidize and become progressively more rancid, they create free radicals in the body, which foster aging and weaken immunity. Except for truly cold-pressed, fresh flax and other similarly processed oils, we recommend that extracted polyunsaturated oils not be used (see "The Dangers of Polyunsaturated Vegetable Oils . . ." later in this chapter). However, when polyunsaturates are eaten in the context of whole, unprocessed food, they are preserved within the food and are usually in their freshest, most beneficial form, and contain an appropriate balance of omega-3 and omega-6 fatty acids.

The following chart shows how abundant sources of unsaturated fatty acids are (unsaturated fatty acids include both mono- and polyunsaturates; but only the polyunsaturates contain essential fatty acids). Nuts and seeds are the highest sources of unsaturated fatty acids. To avoid the rancidity of oxidized fatty acids, eat them freshly shelled. Because they are so concentrated in fats, nuts and seeds are difficult to digest, and are best eaten in small amounts. See "Nuts and Seeds" in the recipe section for their properties and preparation methods.

Unsaturated Fat Sources

as a percentage of total calories

Nuts and Seeds		Grains, Legumes, and Fruit	
Almond 71%	Pumpkin/squash seed 59%	Avocado 64%	Oats 9%
Flax seed 74%	Sesame seed 65%	Buckwheat 4%	Olive 73%
Hazelnut 62%	Sunflower seed 63%	Corn 5%	Quinoa 11%
Pecan 77%	Walnut 68%	Garbanzo 9%	Rice, brown 5%
Pine nut 58%		Millet 5%	Rice, sweet 5%
		Miso 9%	Soybean 31%

The oils in the above foods are 50–90% essential fatty acids with the exception of the foods highest in monounsaturates: olive and avocado are only 6% EFA, while almond is 16% and sesame 31%.

In cases of modern essential fatty-acid deficiency, flax seed and its freshly pressed oil may be one of the best specific remedies because they contain both the essential fatty acids in the proportion and form most people need most: an abundance of alpha-linolenic acid (omega-3) and non-rancid linoleic acid.

The Prostaglandins: An Insight into the Essential Fatty Acids

Much of the effect of the essential fatty acids is a result of their conversion into hormone-like substances in the body known as prostaglandins (PGs). Prostaglandins, now the subject of some of the most exciting and intensive research, are thought to play a role in the regulation and function of every organ and cell in the human body. Their wide-ranging effects help explain the multitude of diverse properties of the essential fatty acids.

There are many different PGs; the most relevant according to current research are those of the "E family." There are "series" (subgroupings) within the "E" and all other PG families which depend on the fatty acid source; these series are denoted by subscripts. For example, the nutritional value of alpha-linolenic acid and its transformation into EPA and DHA was discussed earlier. However, much of the action of EPA and DHA is a result of their conversion into an "E" family of prostaglandins denoted by the subscript 3: PGE_3.

Gamma-Linolenic Acid (GLA) and PGE_1

GLA, a fatty acid synthesized in the healthy body from linoleic acid, converts into a PG of the "E" family but is denoted by the subscript 1. PGE_3 and PGE_1 both have the heart- and artery-protecting values discussed earlier. In addition, they both exhibit a wide range of other functions. The following remedial actions apply specifically to PGE_1, but many are also omega-3/PGE_3 actions listed in previous sections. Even though these two oils ward off many of the same diseases, each has separate functions in the body. Therefore, nutritionists now often recommend ample intake of both GLA and omega-3 sources.

Actions of PGE_1 Against Disease

- Required for proper functioning of the immune system—activates T-cells, which destroy cancer and other unwanted substances in the cells of the body.
- Inhibits cell proliferation and normalizes malignant or mutated cells—thereby promotes cancer cell reversal.[22]
- Effective against inflammatory conditions such as eczema and arthritis as well as auto-immune diseases including rheumatoid arthritis. Drugs commonly prescribed for these diseases, however, deactivate PGE_1. In addition to its own anti-inflammatory action, GLA/PGE_1 controls the release of stored arachidonic acid, thereby further reducing potential pain and inflammation. (The pain- and inflammation-inducing effect of excess arachidonic acid is discussed in the next section.)
- Protects against various forms of heart and vascular disease including stroke, heart attack, and arterial deterioration. PGE_1 is a vasodilator, controls blood pressure, and inhibits blood clotting, a major cause of thrombosis, strokes, and heart/artery disease.
- Regulates brain function and nerve impulses; clinical trials show GLA to be helpful in the treatment of schizophrenia.[23]
- Often alleviates the "dry eye" (Sjogren's and sicca) syndrome—the inability to create tears.[24]

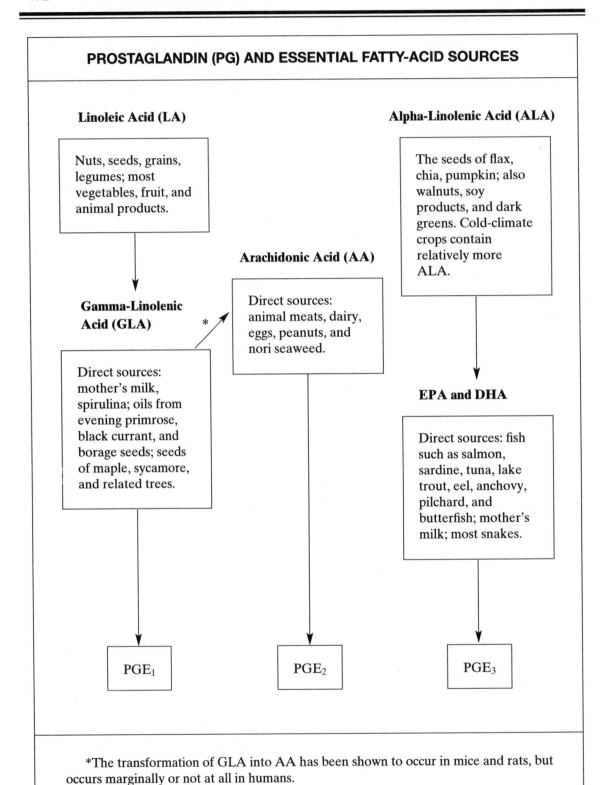

PROSTAGLANDIN (PG) AND ESSENTIAL FATTY-ACID SOURCES

Linoleic Acid (LA)

Nuts, seeds, grains, legumes; most vegetables, fruit, and animal products.

Gamma-Linolenic Acid (GLA)

Direct sources: mother's milk, spirulina; oils from evening primrose, black currant, and borage seeds; seeds of maple, sycamore, and related trees.

Arachidonic Acid (AA)

Direct sources: animal meats, dairy, eggs, peanuts, and nori seaweed.

Alpha-Linolenic Acid (ALA)

The seeds of flax, chia, pumpkin; also walnuts, soy products, and dark greens. Cold-climate crops contain relatively more ALA.

EPA and DHA

Direct sources: fish such as salmon, sardine, tuna, lake trout, eel, anchovy, pilchard, and butterfish; mother's milk; most snakes.

PGE$_1$

PGE$_2$

PGE$_3$

*The transformation of GLA into AA has been shown to occur in mice and rats, but occurs marginally or not at all in humans.

- Is a "human growth factor"—stimulates growth that has been retarded.
- Alcohol use temporarily raises PGE_1 levels dramatically, but depression occurs afterward (hangover), which is cured by GLA/PGE_1. Alcoholics are deficient in PGE_1, as alcohol leads to failure of the body to produce it.[25, 26] Thus GLA reduces cravings for alcohol; it also helps restore liver and brain function in alcoholics.[27]
- Regulates the action of insulin and is therefore beneficial in diabetes; appears to minimize damage to the heart, eyes, nerves, and kidneys in all forms of diabetes.[28–30]
- Multiple sclerosis (MS) is thought to result in part from linoleic acid not being converted to PGE_1.[31, 32]
- Prostate problems, premenstrual syndrome (PMS), cystic mastitis (breast lumps), brittle nails, and hyperactivity in children all commonly result from a deficiency in PGE_1.[33, 34]
- Speeds up the metabolism in those with stagnancy and obesity. Is often used to assist weight loss.[35]

Note: Certain nutrient deficiencies, intoxicants, synthetic drugs, excess saturated fat, and other conditions limit the production of PGE_1.[36] A detailed list of these factors is found at the end of the chart on page 176.

The sources from which GLA is derived are plentiful: linoleic acid, which converts into GLA under the right conditions, is the most abundant polyunsaturated oil in nuts, seeds, grains, and other plants. Clearly the conversion from linoleic acid to GLA is often inadequate in those with vascular disease and other conditions listed above, so these individuals can take GLA directly. The richest whole-food sources of GLA are mother's milk, spirulina micro-algae, and the seeds of borage, black currant, and evening primrose. The extracted oils of these seeds are widely available as concentrated sources of GLA. The dosage is the amount of oil that provides 150–350 mg GLA daily. Dosages near 150 mg are appropriate for persons who eat a primarily vegetarian diet of unprocessed foods, and who also include a substantial source of omega-3 fatty acids such as flax oil in the diet. A standard 10-gram dosage of spirulina provides 131 mg of GLA; seed oils can be added to increase the GLA total. Most of the original research on GLA was done on evening primrose oil, so some of the beneficial results may have been due to other qualities of this plant.

Vegetarian Diet and the Fatty Acids

The essential fatty acid arachidonic acid (AA) has several effects counter to those of both gamma- and alpha-linoleic acid. In the following discussion, it is helpful to remember that excess AA in the human body arises primarily from one source—the consumption of animal products.

Arachidonic acid causes production of prostaglandins of the type PGE_2; in excess, they can produce pain and inflammation, and encourage blood to clot.

AA also releases in the body substances known as "leukotrienes," which act beneficially to heal wounds and injuries but in excess are thought to provoke breast lumps and inflammations such as arthritis. The inflammation of rheumatoid arthritis is considered a direct result of excessive leukotrienes. Other leukotriene-related conditions are asthma, dermatitis, rhinitis, psoriasis, and lupus (systemic lupus erythematosus).[37] AA/PGE_2 also stimulates cell division and proliferation, which, when taken to an extreme degree, can be directly linked to cancer and tumors.

Aspirin and various steroid drugs block the production of PGE_2 and therefore reduce clotting, pain, and fever. Aspirin in particular is now used to protect the heart, and for the pain of arthritis and other maladies. However, aspirin also blocks the production of the beneficial PGE_1, so that when it is used for arthritis and heart disease, the inflammation and deterioration of tissue from leukotrienes continue. A healthier choice than aspirin is to increase the production of PGE_1 as well as PGE_3. Two important reasons for this are: 1) PGE_2 production is limited by increases in either PGE_1 or PGE_3; and 2) Both PGE_1 and PGE_3 have their own anti-inflammatory action and many other valuable properties.

The effectiveness of PGE_1 and PGE_3 is most easily increased by first decreasing all animal product consumption (except for fish in certain cases) and then avoiding the factors that limit the production of these PGs. Adding GLA and omega-3 foods to the diet is also helpful. As mentioned earlier, grass-fed animals and their dairy products are relatively higher in omega-3s, but they are still very concentrated in AA/PGE_2. Thus mammal products should be excluded from the diet of those with excess PGE_2 problems such as pain and inflammation; an exception is the cautious use of animal products when these individuals are frail and severely *deficient*.

From the standpoint of the essential fatty acids and the prostaglandins they create, it is easy to see why a vegetarian diet of unrefined whole foods is so effective at relieving painful and inflammatory disorders such as arthritis, in cleansing the heart and arteries, and as a support in the prevention and cure of many degenerative diseases, including cancer. In fact, much of the story of disease in the modern world can be related to excessive arachidonic acid and deficient alpha- and gamma-linolenic acids. Not only does overconsumption of AA from saturated fat and cholesterol-rich animal products set the stage for sinister disease processes, but it directly inhibits the generation of the invaluable prostaglandins from GLA and omega-3 oils.[38, 39]

The Original Diet

The stories and lessons from the Old Testament of the Bible are often metaphors to be adapted and then applied to the reader's life. According to the Old Testament, God gives man the dietary prescription for the Garden of Eden, and it contains no animal products. This same prescription might wisely be followed by those wanting a firm basis upon which to build life patterns leading beyond pain and suffering.

Summary of Fatty-Acid Uses

Symptom	Fatty-Acid Recommendations
General essential fatty-acid deficiency dry, scaly skin dry and falling hair retarded growth infertility gallstones liver problems varicose veins infections irritability "flightiness" and nervousness	Improve quality of all oil sources; switch from refined, rancid, and hydrogenated oils to unprocessed plant sources of essential fatty acids—whole grains (unmilled, freshly milled, or sprouted), legumes and their sprouts, fresh nuts and seeds, dark green vegetables and micro-algae. Use oils rich in both linoleic and alpha-linolenic fatty acids such as flax-seed, pumpkin-seed, and chia-seed oils. Note: Use these oils *only* if they are recently cold-pressed and unrefined.
Vascular system problems strokes heart attacks arterial hardening and deterioration high blood pressure high blood cholesterol stress migraine	The following fatty acids are beneficial: 1. Alpha-linolenic acid (an omega-3): Use seeds or fresh seed oils of flax, chia, and/or pumpkin; soy foods, dark- green plants, cold-climate crops. 2. Gamma-linolenic acid. Produced in the healthy body from linoleic acid, which is found in the essential fatty-acid sources listed above; available directly from spirulina, and oils of borage seed, black currant seed, and evening primrose seed. 3. EPA and DHA in fish, especially tuna, sardine, salmon, anchovy, or fish oil.
Brain/nerve damage or incomplete development from famine, disease, or lack of DHA during fetal development.	Especially DHA from fish or fish oil; also GLA (and other nutrients) in spirulina; and to some extent, the alpha-linolenic acid sources in (1) above.
Diseases of inflammation arthritis (all types) eczema, psoriasis, hives colitis, bronchial asthma	Especially alpha-linolenic acid sources in (1) above; gamma-linolenic acid (GLA) and EPA/DHA sources in (2) and (3) above are also beneficial.
Diseases of cell proliferation breast cysts tumors cancers	(same as above)
Other conditions poor immunity, AIDS, MS kidney disease, enlarged prostate	(same as above) *(continued on next page)*

alcoholism, addictions
schizophrenia, depression
premenstrual syndrome
obesity

GLA-Blocking Factors: The following factors interfere with the metabolism of GLA and/or its transformation into the prostaglandins, particularly PGE_1:

Trans-fatty acids, the synthetic fats in margarine, shortenings, and refined and highly heated oils (above 320°F)

Alcohol and tobacco

Radiation including low-level radiation such as from appliances, etc.

Aspirin and most other synthetic drugs

Carcinoid processes—cancer and other free-radical activities

Saturated fats and cholesterol in excess

Aging

Excessive arachidonic acid from overconsumption of animal products

Deficiencies of vital nutrients, especially vitamins B_3, B_6, C, and E, zinc and magnesium. These nutrients are all well-supplied in a diet based on unprocessed grains, vegetables, legumes, nuts, seeds, fruits, and seaweeds. In extreme cases, extra care must be taken to obtain adequate vitamin C; excellent food sources are listed in the earlier section "Cleansing the Heart and Arteries."

Dietary Plan for the Garden of Eden: In the book of Genesis, Chapter One, verse 29, God tells man what he should eat: "See, I have given you every herb [plant] that yields seed which is on the face of the earth, and every tree whose fruit yields seed; to you they shall be for food."

At about the time the Old Testament was being written, Gautama Buddha of India taught in the *Shurangama Sutra*: "Beings who want to enter samadhi must first uphold the pure precepts (avoid killing, false speech, thievery, intoxicants, and sexual misconduct). They must sever thoughts of lust, not partake of wine [alcohol] or meat...."[40] As explained in the Sutra commentary, alcohol in general causes loss of concentration, and wine and meat are considered aphrodisiacs.

Eating Better-Quality Fatty Acids

As emphasized earlier, the essential fatty acids in the modern diet are lacking in omega-3/alpha-linolenic acid aspects, and are of poor quality in the omega-6/linoleic acid aspects. Consequently, the products of these fatty acids, including DHA/EPA, GLA, and their respective prostaglandins, are not adequately present for health to flourish. This explains why using common vegetable oils, which are usually rancid, refined, and filled with toxic "trans-fatty acids" (discussed later in "Refined Oils" section) as a result of high-temperature processing, rarely solves essential fatty-acid deficiency. Even when there are good short-term results, the long-term use of poor-quality oils compromises immunity and leads to a greater likelihood of degenerative disease. Very often, simply eating fatty acids from a diet rich in "plants that yield seed"—grains, legumes, vegetables, fruits, nuts, and seeds—while avoiding denatured vegetable oils will improve a person's overall fatty-acid picture, even when *total* fatty acid consumption is less. In essential fatty-acid deficiencies or to hasten healing, oils carefully extracted from plants or fish may be included. To avoid needless killing, we suggest that fish be used only when other methods are inadequate.

Saturated Fats

These lipids are derived primarily from animal products such as cheeses, butter, eggs, and meats, although a few plant products—coconut, peanut, cottonseed, and palm kernel—contain substantial amounts. Saturated fats are considered "heavy" and are solid at room temperature, whereas monounsaturated oils are liquid at room temperature but solid in the refrigerator. Polyunsaturates are liquid even at refrigerator temperatures.

Because of their relatively dense nature compared with unsaturated oils, the therapeutic uses listed earlier in "The Nature of Fats" section should be closely observed with saturated fats. They are the most stable of all fats and have the fewest rancidity problems, and maintain their integrity better than other cooking oils (a recipe for clarified-butter cooking oil is included on page 183). For those who regularly consume animal products, the saturated fats are often a problem, since these fats and the associated cholesterol can eventually obstruct the arteries and cause heart failure. For long-term total vegetarians (vegans), moderate amounts of saturated fats from plant sources generally pose no threat.

Monounsaturated Oils

As cooking oils, these strike a balance between saturated fats and polyunsaturated oils, and exceed both in at least one nutritional aspect. They do not cause cholesterol to accumulate as do saturated fats, and they do not easily become rancid, as do polyunsaturates.

Monounsaturated oils have another unique feature: they do not deplete the blood of high-density lipoproteins (HDL), which pick up cholesterol from the arterial walls and transport it to the liver, where it is broken down into bile acids and flushed from the body. At the same time, monounsaturates reduce low-density lipoproteins (LDL), which cause cholesterol to be deposited in the arteries. Polyunsaturated oils also reduce LDL; unfortunately, they decrease HDL by an equal amount.

A significant illustration is seen among Mediterranean populations who consume an abundance of olive oil, the oil highest in monounsaturates. These people eat an unusually high-fat diet, yet have a low incidence of heart disease.

The degree to which oils are monounsaturated is determined by the amount of oleic acid present; virtually all of the monounsaturate content of common oils is in the form of the fatty acid, oleic acid.

Monounsaturated forms of traditionally polyunsaturated oils are now available. Plant breeders have developed new strains of sunflower and safflower, two of the most popular oil plants, with largely monounsaturated oils. These oils can be identified by their labels, which list them as "high in oleic acid" and/or "monounsaturated." Rapeseed oil, esteemed in ancient India and China, is now also being offered widely in a monounsaturated form called "canola."

All oils contain all three types of lipids (saturated, monounsaturated, and polyunsaturated), but in varying percentages. They are usually classified according to which type predominates. For example, descending in the following chart, the last oil that can be termed "monounsaturated" is sesame.

Proportions of Fats in Common Cooking Oils

Oil	Mono-unsaturated	Poly-unsaturated	Saturated
Olive	82%	8%	10%
Oleic* sunflower	81%	11%	8%
Oleic* safflower	75%	17%	8%
Avocado	74%	8%	18%
Almond	70%	21%	9%
Apricot kernel	63%	31%	6%
Peanut	60%	22%	18%
Canola (Oleic* rapeseed)	60%	34%	6%
Sesame	46%	41%	13%
Corn	29%	54%	17%
Soy	28%	58%	14%
Sunflower	26%	66%	8%
Walnut	23%	63%	14%
Cottonseed	18%	52%	30%
Palm kernel	16%	1%	83%
Safflower	13%	79%	8%
Coconut	6%	2%	92%
Clarified butter	5%	30%	65%

*More recently developed oils, as discussed above, that are higher in oleic acid (and therefore more monounsaturated) than the regular variety of these oils.

Types of Oils
Unrefined Oils

These are mechanically (expeller-) pressed only, under relatively low heats of approximately 160°F; in some cases they are filtered once to remove the residues. They retain their original taste, aroma, and color, and sometimes appear cloudy. Unrefined oils retain their vitamin E content, which tends to preserve the oil from rancidity and also reduces free-radical damage in the body that can easily occur from consumption of the polyunsaturated portion of any oil. Like other unrefined foods, unrefined oils contain numerous nutrients not found in the refined variety; without the complete range of naturally occurring nutrients, oils lack vitality (see "Refined Oils" section later). *Regardless of the oil used, it should be unrefined.* If it is truly cold-pressed, this is another positive feature for monounsaturated oils, and a requirement for the production of health-promoting polyunsaturated oils. Of all the information printed on a bottle of oil about its processing, "unrefined" is the most important, because no refined oil *of any type* should be ingested. Do not be tricked into thinking other processes mean that the oil is unrefined. For example, only a small percentage of all "expeller-pressed" oils are unrefined.

Cold-pressed and Expeller-pressed Oils

In the recent past, "cold pressed" was often a misleading label employed as a marketing aid to confuse customers. It has been known for generations in the vegetable oil industry that heat damages oil. The lower the processing temperatures, the better the oil. Nearly all oils, including most of those formerly marketed as cold-pressed, have been heated for commercial extraction; the primary exceptions are the highest grades of olive and coconut. More recently, flax and several other oils are being truly cold-pressed in the absence of light and oxygen, with special low-volume presses. Even so, the incorrect use of the term "cold pressed" has had at least some meaning in previous years—cold-pressed oils were generally expeller-pressed, which distinguished them as superior to oils extracted by chemical solvents. Although an accurate phrase, "expeller pressed" does not guarantee the highest quality—most expeller-pressed oils are also refined, as described below.

In the last few years, major vegetable oil distributors decided on self-regulation, dropped the misleading phrase "cold pressed," and replaced it with "expeller pressed" or similar terms. Far less than 1% of all oil is actually processed at temperatures considered "cold"; some companies have suggested a reference point of 100°F, or about body temperature, as the temperature below which an oil may be termed "cold pressed." Many firms that now use the term "cold pressed" in this more accurate way also list on the container the maximum temperature the oil reaches during processing.

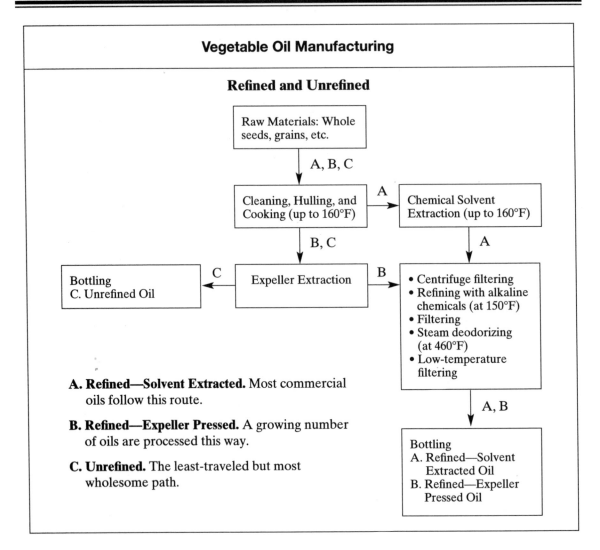

Refined Oils

There are two types of refined oils. The most common are solvent extracted at high heat with harsh chemicals such as hexane. They are bleached and chemically treated to ensure a colorless, tasteless oil with a long shelf life. The taste of rancidity has been removed, but the harmful effects remain. (This is a metaphor for most of our food industry.) A smaller but growing percentage of refined oils are expeller- rather than chemically extracted; at least these contain no traces of chemical solvents. Nevertheless, these oils are subjected to several steps beyond extraction, involving high heat and alkaline chemical solutions.

In contrast to unrefined oils, both expeller- and solvent-extracted refined oils have been depleted of certain vital nutrients, including lecithin, chlorophyll, vitamin E, beta-carotene, calcium, magnesium, iron, copper, and phosphorus.

The temperatures reached in the refining process often exceed 450°F—far above the temperature at which the unsaturated fatty acids transform into a synthetic fat called "trans-fatty acids." (Trans-fatty acid formation begins at 320°F.) Earlier we discussed the effect of trans-fatty acids in preventing the healthful transformation of fats in the body into immunity-building fatty acids and prostaglandins. Recent research indicates that these synthetic fats raise cholesterol levels in the arteries much the way saturated fats do.[41, 42] Thus trans-fatty acids not only increase the likelihood of a variety of metabolic disorders including arthritis and cancer, but also contribute to heart disease. In the United States, 95% of trans-fatty acid ingestion is from eating margarine and shortening.[43]

Once refined, these and all other oils typically form more trans-fatty acids during frying or baking when temperatures exceed 320°F. An even more serious situation arises when oil is repeatedly re-used for deep frying, as is the case in many restaurants. After two full days, other greatly toxic compounds form when the fatty acids in the oil start to break down and combine with one another into synthetic polymers (large chains of molecules—the synthetic variety are commonly found in products such as the most durable car waxes).

The overwhelming majority of vegetable oils are highly refined. In fact, the bland taste and unclouded look of these oils is what people have come to expect. The rich flavor of unrefined oils is a new taste for most of us, even for those who use primarily whole foods.

Many people believe refined oils to be inherently superior because of their clear, golden color. A Chinese woman once came to us for a consultation. She had suffered from stomach ulcers since leaving mainland China. Her diet seemed quite balanced but included a fair amount of oil in wok-fried food. We asked what kind of oil she used, and she was proud to say that ever since leaving China, first for Taiwan and then the United States, the quality of oil had been exceptional, because it was "pure"—not cloudy with a strong aroma—like oils on the mainland. We suggested she return to unrefined oils and take an herbal decoction of marshmallow root and licorice root for a couple of weeks; her ulcers soon healed and did not return. This story illustrates a common attitude about refined oil that is supported by international high-budget advertising images in the free-market areas of both East and West.

The Danger of Polyunsaturated Vegetable Oils, Margarine, and Shortening

Many people have changed from using animal fats like butter and lard (high in cholesterol and saturated fat) to using highly refined polyunsaturated vegetable oils free of cholesterol and low in saturated fat. Their intention has been to prevent arteriosclerosis, heart attacks, and strokes, which are often precipitated by high blood fat. According to demographic and case studies, individuals who consume polyunsaturated vegetable oils in quantity, especially in the form of margarines and shortening, have a greater risk of heart attack and cancer.[44, 45] Instead of preventing disease, as claimed by advertising, these oils seem to make the situation worse. In animal studies, the intake of these oils promotes cancer even more readily than does saturated fat consumption.[46, 52]

Margarine and shortening, furthermore, contain hydrogenated polyunsaturated vegetable oils. Hydrogenation is an extremely harmful process that creates an immune-damaging synthetic fat, a type of trans-fatty acid described earlier that—to the dismay of confirmed margarine users—has also been found to actually elevate blood cholesterol. Most margarines made from soy and safflower oils and sold as "natural" are also hydrogenated and just as harmful as any other margarine. However, margarines made by other processes are now becoming available. One such process involves using gelatin and/or lecithin as emulsifying agents for suspending both saturated and unsaturated fats in a gel. Even though some of these margarines contain preservative chemicals, colorants, and other questionable ingredients, they are to be preferred over hydrogenated margarines. These margarines are identified by checking the ingredients for the absence of "hydrogenated" or "partially hydrogenated" oils; they are often sold in certain supermarkets and health food stores. Perhaps their biggest drawback is the denaturing and/or rancidity that occurs when refined polyunsaturated oils are an ingredient, although we expect to see better-quality versions with unrefined, monounsaturated oils available soon.

While making regular, biweekly Chinese pulse diagnosis, we have on several occasions been able to guess, from a rapidly worsening reading in the liver/gall bladder position, that a client recently began daily consumption of conventional margarine. In each case the margarine had been purchased at a health food store.

Clarified Butter as Cooking Oil

Butter is a better choice than margarine and most refined oils. A unique feature of clarified butter *(ghee),* which is butter with the milk solids removed, is a healing property not found in other saturated fats. According to Ayurvedic teachings, clarified butter enhances the *ojas,* an essence that governs the tissues of the body and balances the hormones. Ample *ojas* ensures a strong mind and body, resistance against disease, and is essential for longevity. Clarified butter promotes the healing of injuries and gastro-intestinal inflammations such as ulcers and colitis.

The ability of clarified butter to support physical and mental renewal has been substantiated to some degree by science. According to Rudolph Ballentine, M.D., clarified butter contains butyric acid, a fatty acid that has antiviral and anti-cancer properties, and which raises the level of the antiviral chemical interferon in the body. Butyric acid also has characteristics found to be helpful in the prevention and treatment of Alzheimer's disease.[47]

Ojas, like the *jing* essence of the Chinese, is depleted by excess sexual activity. By improving the *ojas,* clarified butter can benefit those who have damaged their immunity with sexual overindulgence.

Ayurveda also describes clarified butter as one of the finest cooking oils; it increases "digestive fire" and thereby improves assimilation and enhances the nutritional value of foods. Made by heating butter and skimming the foam off the top, clarified butter is actually the best way to use butter for sautéing, stir frying, and similar cooking needs. Covered and stored in a cool place, it will keep without going rancid for a few weeks. Because pesticide residues from modern cattle feed concentrate in butter fat, it is best to obtain butter derived from organically raised cows.

Clarified Butter Preparation: Heat two pounds of sweet (unsalted) butter in a saucepan until boiling, then adjust heat to maintain a slight rolling boil. The foam that collects on top will condense and thicken, and should now be skimmed off. After 12–15 minutes, when boiling stops and a frying-oil sound begins, quickly remove from heat and allow to cool for a minute or two; then pour the clarified butter into a non-plastic container such as glass or pottery. The sediment in the bottom of the pan and the skimmings from the top are milk solids and can be used creatively in or on any food. Makes approximately one pound of clarified butter.

Olive/Butter Spread: When using regular butter as a spread, its saturated fat and cholesterol content can be diluted by making it into "olive butter": blend softened butter with equal parts of olive oil, then refrigerate to keep solid. Lecithin granules mixed into olive butter keep it solid at room temperature (quantity of lecithin is one-half the weight of the butter). This spread has less cholesterol-raising effects than butter because of the monounsaturated properties of olive oil. Flax oil may be substituted for olive to make "flax butter." It should be kept refrigerated and in a sealed container when not in use to protect its delicate omega-3 oils.

The following guidelines refer to oils available on the market today. In the last few years, an intense and long-overdue interest in oil quality has developed. Undoubtedly, the major forces in the oil market will begin to respond to the demands of the consumer, and we can now look forward to an ever-increasing variety and availability of wholesome oils.

Oil Guidelines

1. Since all oils are extracted and hence are less-than-whole food, none are recommended for daily use except when taken medicinally. Suggested maximum (extracted) oil consumption in one day: a) None or very little for the person who is overweight or has *damp* conditions such as sluggishness, tumors, candida yeast overgrowth, etc. However, these individuals can take omega-3 and GLA oils according to earlier recommendations; b) up to one tablespoon for the thin, dry person; c) for people with no particular imbalance, at most only one teaspoonful, since all oil requirements are normally satisfied with a varied diet of whole foods.

2. Many of our recipes are adaptable to cooking with or without oils, and several methods of oil-less cooking are presented. When using oil for frying, we suggest the oil-water sauté method to prevent overheating the oil while still capturing the flavor of oil sauté. (See recipe section for "oil-less" and "sauté" methods.)

3. When purchasing an oil, first choose among those labeled **unrefined**. All other oils will almost certainly be refined, although they are never labeled as such.

Unrefined oils are currently carried almost exclusively in stores that specialize in health food products and unrefined foods.

4. In general, avoid the common polyunsaturated oils such as **corn, sunflower, safflower, soy, linseed/flax,** and **walnut**. Avoid even the unrefined versions of these oils unless they are recently pressed and stored without exposure to heat, light, or air. All such **fresh, cold-pressed polyunsaturated oils** may be used as medicinal oils or as essential-fatty-acid sources in food preparation, but they must not be used as cooking oils. The shelf life of these oils is about three months, *if* they are kept cool. Fresh, cold-pressed polyunsaturated (and monounsaturated) oils are available in some stores or by mail-order (see "Resources" index). Examples of these polyunsaturated, **omega-3-rich oils are: flax seed, chia seed, hemp seed, pumpkin seed, soy, and walnut**, with flax by far the most concentrated source. Soy oil has the disadvantage of being difficult to digest and is regarded as slightly toxic by traditional Chinese medicine.

5. For general use in cooking, the **unrefined monounsaturated** oils generally are more healthful than the polyunsaturated oils. They are also recommended above saturated ones such as clarified butter or coconut oil, for individuals who have too much stored fat and cholesterol—most of those who eat substantial amounts of animal products. People in this group include some ovo-lacto-vegetarians.

6. The monounsaturated oils we recommend most highly are unrefined **olive** and **sesame**. These oils fulfill the following important criteria: a) a long history of safe, healthful use; and b) very easily extracted, they can be pressed at the lowest temperatures. Other monounsaturated oils include **almond, canola, avocado,** and **apricot kernel**. These oils are nearly always sold in a highly refined state. They are, however, sometimes available unrefined by mail-order or through whole-food stores. Canola oil is often recommended to consumers because of its low saturated fat content (6%), its omega-3 fatty acids (10%), and its monounsaturated properties. At this point in time, canola oil is most often derived from genetically modified plants, although organic varieties are sometimes available. This popular oil is virtually always refined or at least partially refined and thus lacking in nutrients essential for proper metabolism. Refinement additionally harms its omega-3 content. As unrefined oil, it tastes distinctly bitter and few people can tolerate it. Thus there is little incentive to produce quality, unrefined canola oil. In general, avoid this oil.

7. Two other unrefined monounsaturates given high marks by recent research are *oleic* **sunflower** and *oleic* **safflower**—both of these appear relatively resistant to deterioration, making them far superior in this respect to their polyunsaturated (non-oleic) counterparts (see "safflower oil," number 11 below).

8. **Olive** oil is perhaps the most trusted vegetable oil and has been consumed with healthful results for thousands of years. The quality of olive oil varies widely. The top three grades are rated by maximum allowable acidity:

		Maximum Acidity
First grade	Extra Virgin	1%
Second grade	Fine Virgin	1.5%
Third grade	Current Virgin	3%

These grades are worth the extra cost because they usually represent a first pressing, at lower temperatures and without chemicals, although sometimes they are refined. The unrefined variety will be more nutritious and flavorful. Olive oil labeled "pure" is frequently solvent-extracted at high temperatures and may include a minor percentage of virgin oil added for flavor.

9. Like olive oil in the West, **sesame oil** has been traditionally favored in the Orient. Even though sesame oil is 46% monounsaturated, it is nearly equally (41%) polyunsaturated. This would normally mean that the large polyunsaturated fraction of sesame oil could easily become rancid. Fortunately, rancidity is kept in check by "sesamol," an antioxidant naturally present in the oil. This discovery concurs with dietary teachings of ancient India, which rate sesame as one of the most stable of all oils.

Sesame oil has a number of uses as a remedy. It lubricates *dryness,* working as an emollient when applied to dry and cracked skin; it also relieves constipation from dry stools, if a few drops are added to food during cooking. For faster results in more serious conditions, take one to two tablespoons on an empty stomach to induce bowel movement. (Sesame oil is contraindicated during diarrhea.) Sesame oil also detoxifies. It destroys ringworm, scabies, and most fungal skin diseases— apply once daily until the condition is relieved. It is a superior massage oil for sore muscles and the pain of rheumatism/arthritis.

10. When high temperatures are involved in cooking, especially above 320°F, one of the most stable oils is **clarified butter**. Those who wish to avoid animal products may try **palm, palm kernel,** or **coconut oils.** These oils, as well as clarified butter, are often found in stores that carry East Indian foods, although they are beginning to appear more frequently in natural food stores. All of these highly **saturated fats** are relatively stable, but are most safely used by those who have low fat/cholesterol backgrounds—generally, long-term vegetarians or vegans.

11. **Safflower** has been acclaimed by advertisers and some health professionals because it contains the largest polyunsaturated fraction (79%) of common oils. To reverse such recommendations, made over a score of years, is not easily done; nonetheless, safflower oil has few desirable properties. Not only does safflower have the rancidity problems (discussed earlier) inherent in polyunsaturated oils, it provokes ill health according to both Ayurvedic medicine of India and our own experience, regardless of the quality or freshness of the oil. Only **oleic-rich safflower oil** has the properties of a monounsaturated oil which promote *balanced* cholesterol reduction and relatively slow deterioration. Though it is apparently superior to regular safflower oil, it is still too soon to recommend the oleic variety unconditionally.

12. **Cotton-seed oil** should not be ingested because it contains the fatty acid

cyclopropen which causes toxicity in the liver and inhibits normal essential fatty acid metabolism. Since peanuts and cotton crops are typically rotated on the same land, and cotton is one of the most heavily sprayed cultivated plants, the soil and the peanuts later sown on it can become contaminated. Peanuts regularly host the mold *Aspergillus flavis,* which produces the cancer-causing substance aflatoxin within the nut and its oil. *Organic* **peanut oil** should be used to avoid toxic sprays; it also is less likely to contain aflatoxin because the organic peanut is hardier and less subject to *Aspergillus.* (See "Nuts and Seeds" in the recipe section for other properties of the peanut.)

Beneficial aspects of peanut oil: a) Has a monounsaturated to polyunsaturated ratio of three-to-one, and substantial saturated fat (18%); it is therefore stable enough to cook with, and is commonly used in quick wok frying at high temperatures. b) Has exceptional healing value in most cases of bursitis, even severe cases when an arm cannot be raised because of shoulder pain. The peanut is rich in two B vitamins—biotin and niacin—that help with fat metabolism and circulatory problems, respectively. To use peanut oil for bursitis, rub the affected area liberally with the oil at least twice a day. A teaspoon of the oil can also be poured on food. Very often pain will diminish within a few days. Once the oil treatment is stopped, pain will usually return unless other factors in the diet and lifestyle have been altered. The peanut oil remedy was discovered during a clairvoyant reading by the late Edgar Cayce.[48]

13. **Castor oil** is a medicinal oil. It is most commonly used as a powerful laxative. (Take 1–2 tablespoons at bedtime for this effect.) Castor oil is also used with great benefit externally, in a poultice, to dissolve and draw out cysts, tumors, warts, growths, and other toxic accumulations. It also has an emollient effect and will help soften and remove scars. For these purposes, soak a wool flannel cloth with castor oil and apply one or more times daily to the affected area for one or two hours. For increased effectiveness, put a protective layer on the poultice and apply heat directly on top of it with a hot water bottle or heating pad. (See "Resources" index for a source of cold-pressed castor oil.)

Storage of Oils

Proper storage of oil keeps it from rancidity. The less saturated an oil, the more quickly it becomes rancid; thus polyunsaturated oils oxidize most quickly. When oil starts to taste rank and bitter, it should of course no longer be used.

Both heat and air speed the deterioration of oil. Keep oil in a closed container at a temperature of at most 65°F, preferably lower—the ideal is 38–45°, or normal refrigerator temperature. Most oils that are more highly monounsaturated than sesame—olive, oleic sunflower, and oleic safflower, for example—tend to solidify at very cool refrigerator temperatures if they are unrefined. This does not present a problem if the oil is used primarily for sautéing, frying, and similar applications. Simply refrigerate the oil in a wide-mouth jar, then spoon it out and melt it in the warmed pan. Remember that all saturated oils/fats such as clarified butter contain at least some polyunsaturated portion, and therefore these too should be kept cool.

The effect of light on oil, which is far worse than air, rapidly alters the unsaturated fatty acids into free-radical chains.[49] Store oil in the dark, or in opaque containers.

Oil readily combines with most types of plastic to form toxic plasticides. A common practice in some stores is to sell bulk oil from large plastic containers. The taste of such oil is lifeless, especially compared with the same oil kept in glass. However, certain specialty oils such as fresh, cold-pressed flax oil may be bottled in completely non-reactive plastic. When such plastic is used, it is usually so stated on the label (if not, to be certain, ask the manufacturer).

Those who "must" use common polyunsaturated oils or any kind of refined oils can partially counter effects such as accelerated aging and damaged immunity, as well as further deterioration of the oil, by adding vitamin E to the oil once each month. Use about 300 I.U. of vitamin E per pint. It is also wise to supplement the diet with vitamin E when regularly consuming these kinds of oils.[50] Fresh, cold-pressed polyunsaturated oils, described in number 4 above, kept cool and in the dark since pressing, need no further protection with vitamin E.

Living Without Extracted Oils

During a summer healing camp in Idaho, we decided to cook entirely without oils. We made sauces and salad dressings with seed "yogurts." Campers made their own chopped nuts and seed meals to sprinkle on vegetable dishes. This provided variety to the simple grain-and-vegetable fare. There were no complaints about the lack of oil. Everyone felt satisfied and enjoyed the lightness of the meals. Since then, the majority of those people have used much less cooking oil, and several have done well with none whatsoever.

How to Prepare Baking Pans Without Oil

- Dissolve lecithin granules in warm water (use equal parts). Brush pans lightly with lecithin water, as with oil. Lecithin burns easily, so avoid heats over 350°F.
- Wet pans and sprinkle with corn meal or flour.

Sweeteners

We gain a fresh perspective on sugars and the sweet flavor in general by comparing an Eastern traditional view on sweets with present-day Western attitudes toward nutrition.

Actions of the Sweet Flavor

According to:

Traditional Chinese Medicine*	**Modern Physiology and Nutrition**
1. Enters the spleen-pancreas	1. Sugars activate insulin production by the pancreas; in the form of whole food, they activate the pancreatic enzyme amylase.
2. Ascending, outwardly dispersing, and	2. Sugars influence and fuel the process of the brain. Hyperglycemia (excess blood sugar) promotes a scattering, disorienting effect. Sugars dilate blood vessels, causing blood to move to the periphery of the body.
harmonizing	Deficient blood sugar levels are known to be a cause of irritability, dizziness, headaches, and other disharmonies; also, with enough of certain amino acids such as tryptophan in the brain, insomnia, depression, and pain diminish, while harmony predominates. Balanced blood sugar levels maximize tryptophan sent to the brain.
3. Removes *coldness*	3. Carbohydrate and sugar combustion promote warmth.
4. Tonifies; is proper food for *deficiency* and weakness	4. Sugars (from unrefined carbohydrates) are fuels for the muscles, nerves, and brain and are the principal source of energy for all bodily functions.
5. Moistening	5. Quality sweet flavor in the form of unrefined complex carbohydrates forms a thin, healthy mucus coating on the mucous membranes. Excess sweet food or that of poor quality promotes unhealthy mucus and moist conditions, favoring the formation in the body of yeast and fungi including *Candida albicans;* such food also causes watery swellings (edema).
5.1. Lubricates dryness in the mouth, throat, and lungs	5.1. The most effective cough syrups, drops, and throat lozenges are traditionally made in a sweet base (ideally from honey, licorice, etc.).
6. Excess makes bones ache	6. Excess sweet food retards calcium metabolism and initiates skeletal problems including bone loss and arthritis.
7. Excess makes head hair fall out	7. An excess of sweet food acidifies the blood, destroys B and other vitamins, depletes the body of minerals—all of which cause unhealthy hair, among other problems.

Note: In very early chronicles of Chinese medicine, the sweet flavor was usually defined in terms of whole food such as nonglutinous rice, dates, and mallows.

*The effects 3, 4, and 5 are present in many but not all sweet foods. For example, numbers 3 and 4 do not apply to the majority of fruit, which is generally not the proper food for *deficiency, coldness,* and weakness.

Excess Sweet Syndromes

Chinese medicine counsels one against an excess of any flavor. From the viewpoint of Western nutrition, the action of too much sweet flavor can be explained by the following principle: Carbohydrate metabolism regulates protein metabolism, and vice versa. If too much sweet flavor (carbohydrate) is eaten, especially in the form of refined sugars, then protein needs increase. (For most individuals, grains and legumes have a balanced amount of protein and carbohydrate.) As the use of concentrated sugar increases, one may desire a more concentrated protein and will often find it in animal products; if this cycle accelerates, a meat and sugar syndrome is a common result—i.e., excess quantities of both are consumed. Such a syndrome causes obstructions in the body and mind. Tranquilizers, pain-relieving drugs, and intoxicants are often then employed for an immediate, but temporary, clearing of obstructions. The entire cycle is commonly called "The Meat, Sugar, and Drug Syndrome."

Another sweet syndrome may develop when a person is deficient in protein relative to sugar. In this case, the controlling function of protein on sugar metabolism decreases, and if protein is not increased in the diet, there is a desire for more and more sugary foods. This pattern is seen in primarily vegetarian diets containing denatured proteins and lacking in minerals such as the white rice/white sugar/soft drink-based diets in many parts of modern Latin America. It is also seen among vegetarians who eat the refined-food diets of meat-eating areas— less the meat. Another cause of this sweet syndrome is when wholesome vegetal foods dominate the diet but are eaten chaotically in horrendous combinations and without adequate chewing. (See "Improving Protein Utilization" in the *Protein and Vitamin B12* chapter.)

Use and Misuse of Sugar

Sugar is a major life force and our bodies need it as fuel to feed the ongoing fire of life's process. The sugars in whole foods are balanced with the proper minerals. The energy obtained from breaking down and assimilating these sugars is of a constant and enduring nature.

When natural sugar is refined and concentrated, the life force is dispersed and the natural balance upset. Refined sugar passes quickly into the bloodstream in large amounts, giving the stomach and pancreas a shock. An acid condition forms which consumes the body's minerals quickly. Thus calcium is lost from the system, causing bone problems. The digestive system is weakened and food cannot be digested or assimilated properly. This leads to a blood-sugar imbalance and to further craving for sugar.

Refined sugar delivers high energy and enables one to keep working, but unfortunately, it is addicting and contributes greatly to disease and unhappiness. While in very small amounts it can be used as medicine, in large amounts sugar leads instead to obesity, hypoglycemia, diabetes, high blood pressure, heart disease, anemia, immune deficiency, tooth decay, and bone loss; it contributes to herpes, yeast infections, cancer, pre-menstrual syndrome, menstrual problems, and male impotence; it weakens the mind, causing: loss of memory and concentration, nervousness, shyness, violence, excessive or no talking, negative thought, paranoia, and emotional upsets such as self-pity, arguments, irritability, and the desire for only sweet things in life.[1–5] This last consequence is the author's personal observation that those who fail to accept the appropriate and often-difficult challenges in life usually consume an excess of sweet food, which fuels their laziness.

Satisfying the Sweet Tooth

- The best source of sweetness is a diet of whole vegetal foods that are chewed well to bring out their natural flavor and sweetness. All complex carbohydrates such as grains, legumes, and vegetables become sweeter the longer they are chewed. Cravings for sweets will gradually go away, and simple balanced meals provide this satisfaction.

- Be wary of so-called "natural" sweeteners such as fructose, brown sugar, and turbinado sugar. They are nearly as refined and concentrated as white sugar and have similar effects.

- Balance your *yin-yang* intake. Salty foods such as sea salt, pickles, miso, and soy sauce strongly direct energy lower in the body and thereby create a craving for sweets, which have an ascending nature. Most animal foods—meats, fish, and cheese—are high in protein, and as discussed earlier, should be used sparingly to avoid sugar cravings.

- If you do consume meat regularly other than for overcoming a frail and *deficient* condition, then for balance eat salads, radishes, mushrooms, potatoes, wheat or barley grass products, and fruit instead of sugar. Also very useful are the recommendations which follow.

- Sweeten desserts with fruit, fruit juices, rice syrup, barley malt, stevia, unrefined sugar (unrefined cane juice powder), maple syrup, molasses, or amasake.

- Eat sweet vegetables (beets, Jerusalem artichokes, carrots, winter squash, sweet potatoes, parsnips) for dessert or in desserts. Raw carrots are especially helpful for sugar cravings. We find some recent studies to be correct which indicate that certain vegetables, particularly carrots, effect a blood sugar rise faster and for a longer time than refined sugar, but to a less extreme level.

- Use sprouts or sprouted products such as Essene bread—sprouting changes starch to sugar. Micro-algae predigest certain of their own starches into sugars; they are also excellent sources of easily digested protein for quickly regulating sugar metabolism: spirulina, chlorella, and wild blue-green are highly effective in reducing sweet cravings.

- Eat something sour, pungent, or spicy to diminish cravings.

- Cravings can be caused by hyper-acidity, which often results from lack of exercise or eating too quickly, too much, or an excess of meats and refined foods. In that case, have some raw or lightly cooked vegetables or a glass of bancha tea with lemon, or even do something which doesn't involve eating. Exercise or breathe deeply until the cravings subside.

Prepare meals at home to avoid sugar in restaurants and manufactured food. Read labels. Sugar and chemical sweeteners are in almost everything—breads, cereals, salad dressings, soups, mixes, cured meat, canned food, bottled drinks.

Reduce the intake of sugar slowly and use some discipline and self-reflection to take you smoothly through the withdrawal symptoms of tiredness, anxiety, and depression. Suddenly dropping sugar usually results in a desire to binge.

People who stop eating sugar nearly always experience higher spirits, emotional stability, improved memory and speech, restful sleep and dreams, fewer colds and dental problems, more endurance and concentration, and better health in general.

Honey

Some people are aware that white sugar is one of the worst foods and are replacing it with equally large amounts of honey. Honey is highly refined by bees and has more calories than white sugar. It is much sweeter and is assimilated directly into the bloodstream very quickly. However, honey does contain some minerals and enzymes and thus does not upset the body's mineral balance as much as sugar.

For centuries honey has been used as medicine. All types of honey, both raw and heated, work naturally to harmonize the liver, neutralize toxins, and relieve pain. Its warming/cooling energy is neutral. In addition, pasteurized or cooked honey moistens dryness and treats dry or hoarse throat and dry cough. Both raw and heated types of honey are useful for treating stomach ulcers, canker sores, high blood pressure, and constipation and can be applied directly to burns. Honey's sweet and antitoxic properties are used to break the cycle of alcoholism (alcohol is a sugar); give honey by the spoonful during a hangover when more alcohol is craved. Honey's harmonizing effect is also beneficial when a person is overworked, having menstrual problems, or is exhausted from salty and rich foods.

For those whose diet is primarily grains and vegetables, a small amount of honey is normally adequate. For most purposes, dilute one to three teaspoons of honey in warm water or mix with other food to reduce its strong effect. Heat-processed honey should not be used by people with copious amounts of mucus. Raw, completely unprocessed, unheated honey is preferable; it has the ability to dry up mucus and is helpful for those with *damp* conditions including edema and too much weight. Raw honey is not recommended for infants, as explained in the *Food for Children* chapter.

The science of Ayurveda has long claimed that the beneficial properties of honey are lost when heated. Raw honey can be obtained from some grocery and natural food stores, or from beekeepers.

Comparison of Sweeteners

Chemically Processed Sweeteners

Sweetener	*Composition*	*Source*
• White sugar	99% sucrose	cane and sugar beets
• Raw sugar	96% sucrose	cane and sugar beets
• Brown sugar	98% sucrose	white sugar with molasses added
• Corn syrup	96% sucrose	processed from corn starch
• Blackstrap molasses	65% sucrose	by-product of granulated sugar (contains minerals)

• Fructose, xylitol, and sorbitol can be made from natural sources, but it is too expensive, so they are refined from commercial glucose and sucrose.

Naturally Processed Sweeteners

Sweetener	*Composition*	*Source*
• Unrefined sugar	82% sucrose	unrefined cane juice powder
• Maple syrup	65% sucrose	boiled-down sugar maple tree sap
• Sorghum molasses	65% sucrose	cooked-down cane juice
• Barbados molasses	65% sucrose	cooked-down cane juice
• Rice syrup and barley malt	50% maltose	fermented grains—less destructive to the body's mineral balance
• Honey	86% glucose-fructose combination	nectar from flowers processed in the stomach of bees
• Fruit juices	10% sucrose	fruit
• Fruit syrups and date sugar	70% or more sucrose	fruit—far more concentrated and sweeter than fresh fruit
• Amasake	less than 40% maltose	fermented rice

Note: In addition to the above percentages, rice syrup, barley malt, and amasake also contain small amounts of glucose; the fruit sweeteners contain fructose as a minor percentage; and unrefined sugar contains substantial amounts of glucose and fructose—a combined average of eleven percent of its total composition—making it 93% simple sugars.

Sugars such as sucrose in the form of whole food have little negative effect on the body, but in the refined state these sugars can upset the blood-sugar balance.

Comparative Sweetness of Sugars		
Based on fructose = 10 reference units		
Sugar	*Sweetness*	*Natural Source*
Fructose	10	fruit and from sucrose sources such as corn (sucrose is composed of fructose and glucose)
Sucrose	6	fruit, tubers, seeds, grain, sugar cane
Glucose	4	fruit, grain, plants
Maltose	2	malted whole grains
Lactose	1	milk products

Recommendations

In the last few years, many sweeteners have been promoted with claims for their health benefits. One such sweetener is fructose, which is substantially sweeter than white sugar but does not tax the pancreas to make insulin. Others are synthetic sweeteners that have no calories.

From our viewpoint, any food that is highly processed and taken out of its whole-food environment of minerals, fibers, vitamins, and enzymes is already limited in nutritional content. Also, despite claims that a certain sweetener is a wholesome product, an excess of the sweet flavor *from any source* upsets the protein/carbohydrate balance, weakens the kidney-adrenal function, and depletes minerals, among other effects.

The Grain Malts

Our recommendation is to use the least concentrated, least sweet, and most nearly whole-food sweeteners. From the above information, these are the products with maltose, since they are only one-third as sweet as white sugar (sucrose) and are not highly processed. The rice and barley grain malts are primarily maltose and are easily available, even in granulated form. In addition, amasake—another product rich in maltose—is becoming much more widely available because of demand for its subtly balanced sweet quality. It has the added advantage of being easily prepared at home (see "Amasake" in recipe section).

At least half the composition of these grain-based sweeteners are nutrients found in whole grains; they also contain good percentages of complex sugars, which take much longer to digest than the simple variety. This smooths out the blood-sugar peaks and valleys associated with the consumption of highly refined sweeteners.

Unrefined Sugar—Unrefined Cane Juice Powder

For those accustomed to the easy application of white sugar, the syrups such as honey, molasses, and rice syrup may seem inconvenient at first; even granulated barley malt, with a consistency of table sugar, is spurned as too bland by those who have yet to wean themselves from sugar's shocking sweetness. A relatively healthy alternative for these individuals is granules of unrefined, dried cane juice, which has existed in certain tropical areas for 5,000 years. It is made by simply evaporating the water from whole sugar cane juice. This type of whole sugar, although nearly as sweet as its sinister cousin, refined white sugar, has a full array of other subtle flavors like any whole food. It is not to be confused with brown sugar or various kinds of raw sugar; it has far more mineralization and other nutrients to help prevent tooth decay and the plethora of diseases brought on by all refined sugar.[4, 6, 7] Called *gur* in India, dried, unrefined cane juice has been difficult to export because of fermentation resulting from its moisture content. In recent years drier, nonfermenting products are being produced in the West for the first time. (See "Resources" Index.) A typical 150-gram sample of these cane juice granules contains 1.1 grams of protein, 1,600 I.U. vitamin A, 50 mg. vitamin C, 20 mg. each of vitamin B_1, B_2, and B_3, 165 mg. calcium, 50 mg. phosphorus, and 40 mcg. chromium. *None* of these nutrients occur in white sugar. Unrefined sugar also offers more than twenty times as much iron and zinc as white sugar. (The other naturally processed sweeteners listed above also possess a full complement of nutrients.)

Several food producers are acutely aware of the advertising advantage of no longer listing "sugar" as an ingredient. Now they still put in refined sugar but list it as "dried cane juice" or "cane juice." However, when dried cane juice is highly refined, it is simply another name for refined white sugar. To be certain of a whole-food product, choose *unrefined* dried cane juice.

Stevia

Stevia rebaudiana, a small plant that grows throughout Latin America as well as parts of the southwestern United States, is becoming much sought-after for its sweet leaves and flower buds. It has been used for a hundred years as a sweetener in South America and now has wide commercial value in Japan, where it is put in everything from soft drinks to soy sauce. With thirty times the sweetness of sugar, yet with negligible calories, this herb is expected by Japanese researchers to be the main natural sweetener in the future.

Because stevia is a whole herbal food, it contains other properties that nicely complement its sweetness. A report from the Hiroshima University School of Dentistry indicates that stevia actually suppresses dental bacteria growth rather than feeding it as sugars do. Other studies have shown a beneficial relationship between stevia and the regulation of blood sugar levels. For instance, no signs of intolerance appeared in 24 cases of hypoglycemia.[8] Similar results occurred with diabetic patients.[9] In fact, no harmful effects have yet been reported. Japanese and Latin

American scientists have discovered other attributes of stevia including tonic, diuretic properties; stevia also treats mental and physical fatigue, harmonizes digestion, regulates blood pressure, and assists weight loss.[10]

Stevia is increasingly available in the United States as a powder or liquid extract in stores that carry natural foods. The sweetening power of stevia is great—one to three drops of the extract sweetens one cup of liquid. The powdered leaf can be made into a simple extract by mixing one teaspoon in a cup of water and allowing it to soak overnight. Stevia's sweet flavor is not affected by heat; thus it can be used in teas and other beverages, canning fruits, and baking all kinds of desserts. Its use in desserts, however, does not add the richness or moisture of most high-calorie sweeteners; likewise, it doesn't appear to have the same *damp*-producing quality in the body and therefore is potentially a good sweetener for the over-weight person or those suffering from mucus, candida, edema, or other signs of *dampness. Note:* Obtain only the green or brown stevia extracts or powders; avoid the clear extracts and white powders, which, highly refined and lacking essential phyto-nutrients, cause imbalance.

Lactose and Fruit Extracts

Lactose from milk is not an ideal sweetener because it is a refined product to which many people have an intolerance.

Fruit juices can be recommended because of their availability and the rela-tively low sweetness their watery composition provides. When they are concen-trated into fruit syrups, however, their sugar content becomes very high. In contrast to the grain ferments, the fruit juices and syrups are much further from being whole foods, i.e., from having the multiple nutrients of whole foods. Because large quantities of sprays used on most commercial fruits are concentrated into the fruit syrup, it is wise to use the organic varieties of these sweeteners.

Fruit juice and amasake are the two sweeteners that can normally be consumed alone as beverages. This feature is important since sweeteners do not combine well with other foods—unpleasant digestive fermentation can occur.

Using Sweeteners with Awareness

One can easily be blinded by quality and forget quantity. A little refined sweetener can be more balancing than too much of a better one.

Even though a grain-and-vegetable diet does not promote a regular need for concentrated sweeteners, there are times for celebration that call for sweets and their strong harmonizing, ascending, and dispersing qualities.

Sweet food has become such an everyday occasion in the United States that we have lost our gratitude for its special nature. Much effort has gone into an entire industry of creating sweeteners: growing crops that are then transformed through extraction, ferment, heat, or other means into a purified substance worthy of mindful use.

Salt

In the past fifty years a controversy has raged in the West around salt. Most of the evidence is in, and it shows salt to be a true culprit. However, the salt being tested is not the whole salt used for millennia by traditional peoples but the highly refined chemical variety that is 99.5% or more sodium chloride, with additions of anti-caking chemicals, potassium iodide, and sugar (dextrose) to stabilize the iodine.

We see the rising tide of information against salt as a warning about the overuse of refined salt. Modern salt reminds one of the state of such other highly processed substances as refined white sugar and the white breads, pastas, and pastries. Unfortunately, relatively few people are informed about the denaturing of real salt.

Salt has the most "grounding," descending activity of any substance used as food. It can greatly influence all the rest of food preparation. In the Ayurvedic tradition, the active quality of salt was emphasized as markedly strengthening one's energy—to the point of hostility if overused.

As with most extreme substances, salt has a dual nature, and it oscillates between its aspects in the human body. Its *yin* nature represents the earth, and thus salt can be used to bring a person "down to earth," or to give food an earthy, more substantial quality. It strengthens digestion and contributes to the secretion of hydrochloric acid in the stomach, an "Earth Element" organ (see *Earth Element* chapter). In the outer dimensions, salt enables one to focus more clearly on the material realm. Excess salt, in fact, is thought in Chinese folklore to encourage greed.

At first, salt is cooling. It directs the energy of a person inward and lower, the appropriate directions in cooler weather. Most people are familiar with this pattern as it occurs in nature: plants such as trees send their sap deeper within and downward in cold weather. The *Inner Classic* advises the use of cooling foods in the winter and warming foods in the summer. The appropriate foods for winter, according to this theory, would encourage exterior cooling, to concentrate the warmth in the *yin,* interior, lower body areas. Salt has this action, and this may be the reason it is classified as warming by Ayurveda.

Consistent with its *yin* quality, salt also stimulates the kidneys, which then promote fluid metabolism and a moistening effect beneficial to dryness in the body. This tonic action on the kidney fluids is especially helpful in the winter, when dryness from the heat-producing activity of the body is at its height and fluids are needed for balance. At the same time, the purifying properties of salt detoxify poisons. Thus a little salt can help counteract poisoning from poor-quality foods and unhealthy food combinations. When the blood is impure (indicated by symptoms such as skin eruptions), salt can be used externally, since its extended internal use for purification is thought to "injure the blood," making the complexion luster-less and the muscles weak.

Another paradoxical aspect of salt is its ability to soften some areas of the body and tighten others. For instance, salt softens hardened lymph nodes, glands, and muscles. It also promotes bowel action. Abdominal obstructions and swellings can be "softened" or dissolved by salt according to traditional Chinese instructions; yet salt may create pressure in other areas such as the arteries. Because salt has an affinity for water, a large percentage of sodium settles in the vascular fluids of the body. As this sodium attracts more fluids, the pressure in the vascular system can rise. This is one reason salt is contraindicated in cases of high blood pressure. Since most instances of high blood pressure not only involve arterial problems but are also closely related to excesses of the liver, very small amounts of whole salt—ideally in the form of seaweeds—can help detoxify the liver, once poor-quality and fatty foods are eliminated from the diet and the blood pressure is out of the danger zone.

Reactions to salt, as with all powerful substances, vary greatly from one individual to the next. Edema (excess fluid retention) can occur with just a few grains of salt if an individual has a tendency to retain fluids; in other cases, even large amounts of salt will not affect an individual. Problems arise when too much salt is consumed for one's own tolerance level—especially salt in its refined form.

In the past, salt tablets were recommended in the summer to replace salt lost by athletes or others who sweat heavily. This practice is used far less today, since we now know that relatively more potassium and water are sweated out, leaving the tissues with higher concentrations of sodium. A sodium/potassium balance must be maintained to sustain health. Salt in the body should eventually be replenished, but with the accompaniment of potassium, water, and/or food. Thus the person who works hard and sweats will generally use more salt but also needs even more juices and other potassium-rich nourishment. The role of potassium, and its sources, are discussed a little later in this chapter.

From the viewpoint of Chinese medicine, salt benefits the kidneys. But its overuse damages them, leading to emaciation, weakened bones and blood, and deficiencies of the heart and spirit. Modern physiology has demonstrated that an excess of salt interferes with the absorption of nutrients and depletes calcium, whereas appropriate salt usage enhances calcium absorption and nutrient utilization in general. It is now understood that the uptake of calcium depends on the health of the kidney-adrenal function, and that calcium metabolism is of essential importance for the health of the nerves, muscles, heart, vascular system, and bones.

This close agreement between traditional and modern knowledge reinforces our awareness of the effects of salt overuse. Most current guidelines for daily salt consumption recommend about 3,000 milligrams, while the average American takes in 17,000 mg., or about 3½ teaspoonfuls of highly refined salt each day. This gross overuse of salt illustrates the tenet that when a food is not balanced (such as salt that has been refined), people have a tendency to overeat it.

Common refined sea salt has been stripped of nearly all of its sixty trace minerals. Perhaps the body craves more in an effort to capture the wholeness that it instinctively knows should be there. Salt cravings will usually decrease sharply once whole, unrefined salt is used for a few weeks.

All salt originates from the sea. Ancient dry salt beds tell us where oceans once were. These salts are usually lacking in some minerals found in sea salt, since they have been leached by rain water for thousands of years. They have built up various other minerals depending on the geology of the surrounding land. Whole salt from the sea has a mineral profile most similar to that of our blood.

In order to obtain this salt, one must usually seek it out. Salt labeled "sea salt" at health stores is typically the refined pure white variety. Whole natural sea salt is slightly grey and will be in larger crystals, granules, or a powder. Brands currently available throughout most of Western Europe and America are Lima and Celtic (from Brittany), Muramoto and "Si" (from Mexico), and Maldon (from England).

Recommendations for salt consumption vary greatly. Consider the fact that many communities and areas of the world in both historic and recent times have used no salt other than that found in food. At the same time, other peoples have relied heavily on unrefined salt for thousands of years.

Sodium, one of the major elements in salt, is found in good quantities in many foods including eggs, seafood, all meats, kelp and other seaweeds, beets, turnips, and greens such as chard, spinach, and parsley. Since deficiencies of sodium are very rare, especially in areas where animal products are consumed, why would salt ever be needed or craved in a diet?

It may be because of its action in the body. Salt has the most descending characteristics of any substance we eat. It relates closely to our root *chakra,* the lower foundation area of the body. The key emotional quality of this *chakra* is security, without which smooth social interaction and other vital activities fail. We mentioned earlier the relationship between salt and the kidneys. A similar proposition in Chinese physiology states that the kidneys rule the emotions fear and insecurity. Our desire for salt may reflect an internal wish for a more emotionally safe foundation, particularly in a modern society characterized by tremendous change and uncertainty. The anchor of security provided by salt is something to be highly valued. However, too much of an extreme substance such as salt causes its properties to reverse—kidney damage, fear, rigid legs and pelvis are all symptoms of a poor emotional and physical foundation resulting from excess salt.

Since World War II and the advent of chemical farming and food processing, the soil and food of much of the world have been depleted of minerals and other nutrients. Our food, whether of vegetable or animal origin, is not only deficient in nutrients but also full of pollutants and farm chemicals. The science of modern nutrition teaches that minerals are a basis for the formation of vitamins, enzymes, and proteins. A craving for salt is perhaps a craving not only for the many minerals normally associated with unrefined salt but for some of the same minerals that are lacking in chemically grown food.

As important as the mineral content of salt is its purifying effect on the vast array of toxic residues in food and the environment. These toxins, which contribute to scattered consciousness, can be neutralized in a variety of ways. Salt has the unique ability to produce a quick mentally centering effect to counter the scattered consciousness caused by toxins, as well as to aid in general detoxification. According to the *doctrine of signatures,* an ancient principle still used in herbology and other forms of biologic medicine, a plant or substance will sometimes

> Salt . . . is a grounding crystal that takes us down into the body/mind where well-centered concentration of matter attracts a clear perception of its opposite: Spirit (non-matter).
>
> —Jacques De Langre, in *Seasalt & Your Life*

have a visual appearance which suggests its use. Salt has a crystalline structure, which suggests definition and clarity. From our observations, salt promotes a lucid, grounded, centered experience. The *Inner Classic* supports this view, telling us that salt in moderation strengthens the heart and mind.

Most disease processes involve an acidic blood condition. (See *Fasting and Purification* chapter for examples of acid/alkaline foods.) In addition to the building foods such as meats and grains, the majority of intoxicants and highly processed foods are acid-forming. Salt, on the other hand, alkalizes and thus is craved by those whose systems are overly acidic. This property of salt is one reason people heavily salt their meat, since meat strongly acidifies the human body. Similarly, adding a touch of salt to the cooking water of grains restores balance to these acid-forming foods. The consequence of salting already sodium-rich foods such as meats, however, is all too often an extreme sodium excess in the body.

Despite the positive aspects of salt—its clarifying, alkalizing, purifying, and centering qualities—there is still a great potential for its misuse. When people give up high-sodium, high-protein, rich, greasy foods and yet still have the same mental set of desires, they will often turn to salt, together with high-fat and protein vegetarian items, to support those desires. In the last generation many new vegetarians, especially those who use Japanese products, have overused very salty products such as soy sauce, miso, umeboshi (salt plums), and gomasio (sesame salt), as well as sea salt, so that they consume far more sodium in their diet than when they ate animal foods. And until recently, nearly all of these salty products were made with refined salt. In several American soy factories and a few traditional shops in Japan, wholesome ingredients including whole sea salt are now being used in high-quality misos and other similar products. Yet quality products made with care are still rare, and must often be mail-ordered or specially requested at stores.

Because of their background of relatively little meat consumption, the Japanese have apparently been able to thrive on a diet filled with a great variety of salty products. Even so, their use of salt has been excessive; they are prone to all of the calcium depletion symptoms which damage the heart, arteries, nerves, bones, kidneys, and muscles. In addition, the Japanese also have the highest incidence in the world of stomach ulcers and cancers, which, according to modern physiology, are conditions that are aggravated by excessive salt intake. We find that the stomach and heart governor* acupuncture meridians tighten like a bowstring in those who take in too much salty fare.

As we all know from experience, consuming too much salt produces thirst. If salt intake is high and physical activity is also enough to sweat the excess out, then this produces one type of balance. A more common way to balance excessive salt is to use dispersing, relaxing beverages such as certain teas, juices, soft drinks, and alcoholic beverages. It is surprising how many vegetarians who use salt extensively turn to beer and other alcohol-based drinks, which all too easily results in a salt-alcohol interdependence akin to the Meat, Sugar, and Drug Syndrome discussed in the previous chapter. According to Chinese medicine, the energy of concentrated sugars including alcohol rises and expands outward in the body; this action balances the extreme sinking, contracting quality that results from overuse of salt and other high-sodium foods.

Of course, we strongly recommend against the precarious balancing of extremes. The obvious solution is to use less salt and, when craving beverages with refined sweets or alcohol, to substitute quality sweet drinks such as licorice-mint or honey**-ginger tea, amasake, and carrot or cherry juice. This process merely substitutes a better quality of sweet for the poor-quality sugars. (Pungent herbs such as mint or ginger can be included since they too have an expansive effect and raise energy to the higher portions of the body.)

In addition to simply balancing the salty flavor, sweet food has another beneficial role—it reduces the desire for excess salt. (This action is described by the control cycle in the *Five Elements* chapter.) Of course, more subtle sweet foods can be used for controlling salt cravings as well as maintaining long-term sugar balance. These are the complex carbohydrates, whose complex sugars break down gradually, helping to stabilize blood sugar levels.

The Sodium/Potassium Relationship

Potassium is a mineral that naturally balances the metabolic action of sodium. On the cellular level, potassium resides on the inside of cells while sodium permeates the fluid on the outside and between the cells. When the potassium/sodium ratio is at equilibrium, the body's water and acid/alkaline balance is stable and the nerves and muscles function properly. When there is deficient potassium relative to sodium, neuromuscular function decreases—the body becomes weak, muscles

---

*Among other functions, the heart governor relates to the health of the heart and arteries and influences blood circulation.

**As described in the *Sweeteners* chapter, honey is a Western folk remedy for alcoholism. Traditional Chinese medicine claims it neutralizes toxins in the body.

lose their tone, and reflexes become poor. Rarely is there a relative excess of potassium compared to sodium, but this condition is seen in some fruitarians and others with very low-sodium diets.

Unlike sodium, potassium promotes upward and outwardly expanding energy. Thus the potassium-excess personality may seem to be floating, not rooted, and unproductive in terms of material accomplishments. In such a person, even the digestion—which indicates a person's relationship to products of the earth—may have what is called "counter-current energy.*" Nutrients are not extracted or properly absorbed, and in severe cases vomiting occurs, which symbolically follows the ascending nature of excess potassium. (Large doses of warm salt water can also cause vomiting because of the toxic nature of excess salt.)

Because sodium usually is in excess, potassium has a curative role. For example, if blood pressure is high because of excessive salt intake, one of the first remedies in Western allopathic medicine is to use potassium supplements while restricting salt.

All potassium-rich foods can be used to balance conditions that result from excess salt consumption. High concentrations of potassium are found in every vegetable and especially in green leafy vegetables, all types of potatoes (with skins), soy products, millet and other grains, and legumes; also in bananas and most other fruits.

Virtually all whole, unprocessed plant and animal foods (with the exception of shellfish such as crab and lobster, which have substantially more sodium than potassium) contain more potassium than sodium. The ratio in meats averages about seven times more potassium. Grains, vegetables, legumes, and fruits usually offer ten times to several hundred times more potassium, and yet the average American is said to be deficient in potassium. In addition to high salt use, this is a consequence of the over-consumption of refined, highly processed foods. The processing of whole wheat into white flour, for example, removes 75% of the potassium. Coffee, alcohol, and refined sugar contain little or no potassium and are known to deplete the body of its potassium stores; they are, therefore, particularly poor choices for balancing sodium, although diuretic liquids in general help work salt out of the body.

There is no standard potassium/sodium ratio to recommend. By eating whole foods, however, one usually receives adequate but not excessive potassium. A little salt will supply sufficient sodium; it can be cooked into or combined with foods in such a way that it magnifies the flavor of the food without making it taste salty. If the salt can be tasted, too much has been used (unless it has been purposely added for specific medicinal goals). When someone has a very strong need for salt, what would normally be considered oversalted food will taste bland or even sweet.

---

*A term in Chinese medicine also translated as "rebellious *qi*."

As the most primitive life forms began to evolve in the salty ocean, they developed the ability to create cells that concentrate potassium. Many metabolic processes of lower forms of life occur without oxygen, while the more evolved forms utilize oxygen and also more potassium. A unique feature of tumor tissue is a "primitive" sort of carbohydrate metabolism that occurs in the absence of oxygen. One conclusion from this, borne out by the work of Max Gerson (discussed in later chapters), is that tumors and cancers diminish with increased potassium and decreased sodium in the diet. This lends some credence to the use of high-potassium food as a remedy for these conditions; however, serious diseases such as cancer have also responded well to a balanced use of sodium and potassium foods.

The craving of salt by modern people, especially those in large cities, is explained in part by the centering quality of sodium in a fragmented environment, and also by the fact that salt is an antidote to all forms of radiation. Thus it is understandable why salt beds have been considered as storage sites for nuclear waste. Every electrical or electronic item gives off radiation, from car generators to house wiring to the megawatt television and radio stations. This sea of radiation, now commonly referred to as "electric smog," is thousands of times stronger in big cities than in the countryside, and its effects are sensed, consciously or not, by everyone.

It seems that in this modern age of scattered thought and electromagnetic permeation, whole salt used appropriately can help put us in touch with our ancient, basic, biologic foundations.

Salt Summary

1. Salt's primary action is cooling; a moderate amount is beneficial to the kidneys, which in turn can better regulate body fluids and moisten conditions of *dryness.* The moistening property of salt is especially appropriate in the winter, when the body tends to dry out. Increasing salt increases the need for more fluid intake.

2. Salt counteracts toxins in the body and is used to neutralize the effects of impure food or poor food combinations. When the blood is toxic, as indicated by skin eruptions, salt can be used externally (see "Common Remedies" below).

3. The direction of salt's action is inward and downward, appropriate for fall and winter. This descending quality provides an "earthy" experience, and gives food this same quality.

4. Salt strengthens digestion and can soften or remove abdominal swellings and intestinal obstructions, and help move the bowels. This softening property can also reduce hardened glands, muscles, and lymph nodes.

5. The alkalizing quality of salt helps balance beans, peas, grains, meats, and other acid-forming foods or acidic conditions.

6. Whole sea salt is slightly grey-colored and contains many minerals and trace minerals. Most "sea salt" sold is highly refined.

7. A salt metaphor: the crystalline nature of salt is said to translate into clarity in its user. The *Inner Classic* states that salt tonifies the heart/mind.

8. Salt relates to the simplest life forms in an oceanic environment and can beneficially connect us to our primitive origins. Excess sodium or insufficient potassium, however, may foster primitive anaerobic cell growths such as tumors and cancers.

Excess Salt

Excess salt is known to be a cause of high blood pressure, ulcers and cancer of the stomach, edema, fear, cravings, kidney damage, diminished absorption of nutrients, and calcium deficiency, resulting in weakened bones, nerves, muscles, and heart. Early signs of excess salt intake are unusual thirst, dark urine and complexion, clenched teeth, and bloodshot eyes. Salt cravings may be an attempt to balance:

- the use of refined salt, or a lack of minerals in the body;
- acidic blood conditions or toxicity (including radiation);
- chaotic environment;
- expansive food and drink (alcohol, refined sugar, soft drinks, etc.);
- weak digestion or low hydrochloric acid secretion; or
- fear and insecurity.

Insufficient Salt

Symptoms are sometimes seen in those on salt/sodium-restricted diets: diminished strength and sex drive, intestinal gas, vomiting, and muscle atrophy. (These symptoms may also arise from many causes other than lack of salt.)

Potassium for Sodium Balance

Potassium and sodium should be in dynamic balance in the body. An excess of one depletes the other, and it is usually sodium that is over-used in the diet. Salt is the highest food source of sodium. Healthy choices for balancing salt or sodium include the following:

1. Potassium-rich foods: vegetables—especially leafy greens, legumes, grains, fruit, and herbs.

2. For strong alcohol and sugar cravings resulting from excess salt or sodium-rich foods such as meat, substitute very sweet potassium foods: rice syrup, honey, amasake, figs, yams, etc. These will not only produce a better-quality balance to salt/sodium than alcohol and refined sugar, but will also control further salt cravings.

Steps Toward Moderate Salt Use

- Balanced salt usage is highly individual. Except when used therapeutically, salt should enhance, not dominate, the flavor of food; if food tastes salty, too much salt is being used.

- Most recipes and canned and packaged foods contain too much salt.
- Use whole salt in moderate amounts, cooked into food. Instead of salt, periodically substitute high-sodium foods: kelp powder and other seaweeds, beets and their greens, celery, chard, parsley, spinach, and kale.
- Avoid table salt. Sesame salt can be used instead. It is listed in the "Condiments" recipes. Highly salty items such as miso and soy sauce also need to be cooked into (or well-combined with) food. Use pickles and other salty condiments sparingly.
- Salt lost through sweating because of heat or work is best replaced with food and drink containing moderate sodium and abundant potassium. Salt tablets are no longer considered a healthy way to replace sodium.
- Salt use is naturally greater in the cooler seasons and climates. For seven days each spring, it is advisable to avoid all salt in order to purge any excess that may have accumulated during the cool season, and to renew the ability to appreciate subtle flavors.

Use of Salt in Common Remedies

Abdominal pain and/or bloating from poor food combining or poisonous or rancid food—eat ½ or more umeboshi (salt plum), or drink a little salt water. Prepare the latter by pan-roasting salt until brown, then mix 1 heaping teaspoon salt per cup of warm water; drink up to ¼ cup. Salt plum or salt water can be taken several times an hour for this purpose. **Bleeding, inflamed gums**—brush teeth and gums with fine sea salt twice daily. Also helpful for purulent (pus-containing) gums. However, salt is not for regular use as a dentifrice. It is too abrasive and according to research appearing in the *Journal of Periodontology* (Nov. 1987), extended use may cause erosive lesions of the gums. Better dentifrices, recommended in this text and by many dental hygienists, are hydrogen peroxide and baking soda. **Sore throat**—gargle hot salt water every hour. **Skin inflammation, eruptions, itching, poison ivy or oak**—wash area in salt water.

Condiments, Caffeine, and Spices

Condiments and Chemical Ingredients

Certain strong condiments and chemical ingredients—distilled vinegar, commercially ground pepper, MSG (monosodium glutamate), baking soda, and baking powder—irritate the stomach and cannot be converted into good blood. However, good quality vinegar and black pepper and standard baking soda have several healing applications.

Vinegar

Distilled vinegar should not be used internally since it is highly demineralizing. Quality vinegars for internal use contain more of their own minerals; even so, these are potent and should be used sparingly. The best types of vinegars are organic, naturally brewed, unfiltered and unpasteurized versions of apple cider, (brown) rice wine, white wine, and umeboshi. As a folk remedy in America, apple cider vinegar has been used for many types of disorders.[1] However, when chronic conditions are benefited by vinegar as the sole remedy, one must usually continue to use vinegar, or the condition returns. This leads to a kind of vinegar dependency, which can be overcome if the diet and other pertinent factors in the lifestyle are improved.

Properties and Uses:
- Vinegar is warming. It creates a temporary warming circulation of energy *(qi)* in the body and removes stagnant blood. It can quickly alter emotional stagnation as well, particularly in children—bad moods will usually disappear a few moments after taking vinegar.
- The sour and bitter flavors of vinegar reduce accumulations in the liver and abdomen resulting from a rich diet. Lemon juice helps in this manner to some extent but is a cooling and more moderate remedy. People who feel toxic and sluggish during a transition from a refined-food and meat-centered diet to one of whole vegetal foods can profit from a little vinegar or lemon. For this purpose, use 1 teaspoon vinegar or a quarter lemon squeezed in water. This remedy can provide relief while toxins are being released.
- Vinegar neutralizes poisons in the body and is good for food poisoning. Take ¼ teaspoonful every fifteen minutes until relieved. One of the best applications for vinegar is in cases of nausea from eating old foods, overly fermented foods, or too many combinations. For these conditions, follow the dosage below.
- Vinegar relieves *damp* conditions such as edema, overweight, excess mucus, and athlete's foot. Soak feet daily in vinegar to help clear up athlete's foot.
- Vinegar stops bleeding. Use in the treatment of nose bleed, spitting up blood, and for fainting due to blood loss and anemia after childbirth.
- Vinegar removes parasites and most worms that live in the digestive tract; soak raw salad vegetables in a dilute vinegar-water solution to remove parasites (see "Salads" in recipe section for directions).
- Vinegar overcomes the toxic effect and pain of insect bites or stings. Apply to the area repeatedly or use a vinegar compress until there is relief.

Dosage: except where specified differently above, sip ⅓ cup of water mixed with 1 teaspoon of apple cider vinegar two or three times daily; for increased effectiveness in the cases of nausea, bad moods, and dietary transition, stir 1 teaspoon of honey into the vinegar water.

Contraindications: weak digestion marked by loose, watery stools; general *deficiency* (frailty); muscular injury or weakness, including rheumatism.

Black Pepper

This spice is ideal for general prevention. Unfortunately, most commercial ground pepper is roasted and is therefore an irritant rather than a stimulant. To make fresh ground pepper, use a peppermill and whole peppercorns.

Properties and Uses:
- Black pepper is warming; it stimulates a warming flow of energy in the body. It specifically warms the abdomen and is used in the treatment of diarrhea and watery stools.
- Black pepper is diaphoretic—opens the pores for sweating and is helpful at the onset of the common cold.
- A very hot/pungent flavor such as black pepper benefits the lungs and helps protect against simple viral infections such as colds and flus.
- It counteracts food poisoning and indigestion.

Application: use several times a day for the acute conditions. Freshly ground black pepper can be stirred into soups, herbal teas, or added to food.

Mustard

Properties and Uses:

Very warming, pungent, stimulating, and diuretic. It strengthens digestion, particularly "cold digestion" (loose or watery stools and chills or other *cold* signs); and resolves white or clear lung phlegm. Use the seeds in a tea decoction or the whole or ground seeds (dry mustard) in food.

Baking Powder and Baking Soda

Most baking powder contains aluminum salts which accumulate and may cause deterioration of brain cells. Health stores carry baking powder without aluminum. Even so, baking powder and baking soda both are chemicals which deplete baked goods of the B vitamins thiamine and folic acid. These compounds also create a type of alkalinity in the body that eradicates vitamin C.[2] The sourdough natural leaven process described in the recipe section is nutritionally superior for all leavening purposes.

An excellent use of baking soda is as a dentifrice. Its highly alkaline properties neutralize plaque acids and eliminate the bacteria that cause tooth decay. Even more important, baking soda helps stop the major cause of tooth loss—gum infection and inflammation such as gingivitis and pyorrhea—better than most commercial toothpastes. These traits and its non-abrasive quality make it a safe and effective toothpowder for regular use. This old-time remedy is becoming widely used in European dentifrices, and several brands featuring it are now available in the United States.

Baking soda is useful in the treatment of athlete's foot: dust feet liberally in the morning and then put on cotton or wool socks. It also provides relief from the itching and burning of poison oak or poison ivy: mix baking soda with water into a paste and dab on the affected areas, or add two pounds of baking soda to bath water and soak at least one-half hour. For bee stings, apply a wet paste to draw toxins and reduce pain.

Sodium bicarbonate (baking soda) injected in the bloodstream has been a standard treatment since the 1920s to reduce lactic acid in the blood of heart attack patients. However, the July 1989 issue of the *American Journal of Medicine* reported human experiments that confirmed earlier animal trials involving sodium bicarbonate in the blood: blood flow decreased, the body's oxygen use fell 25%, and lactic acid levels in the blood actually rose. These negative effects also occur to some extent when food which contains baking soda is absorbed into the blood.

Monosodium Glutamate

Small amounts of the flavor-enhancer monosodium glutamate (MSG) have been shown to cause nerve and brain damage in young laboratory animals.[3] Its heavy-handed application in Chinese and other East Asian restaurants has been alarming; fortunately, there are a growing number that no longer use it, or will withhold it upon request.

The Caffeine Products

Caffeine is clearly the most prevalently used stimulant in the world. Coffee, tea, chocolate, cocoa, many soft drinks, diet pills, aspirin, various analgesics used for migraine headache and vascular pain, and even some herbal preparations contain either caffeine or very closely related substances. Examples of such caffeine-like substances are theobromine in chocolate and cocoa and theophylline in tea. When caffeine and similar compounds are taken in excess, any of several symptoms usually result: anxiety and nervousness, insomnia or light sleep patterns, various types of heart disease, stomach and intestinal maladies, and moodiness. When consumed regularly, as little as two cups of coffee can initiate these symptoms. Children who exhibit hyperactivity are often victims of diets rich in chocolates and cola drinks.

Coffee

Properties and Uses: Coffee is warming, stimulating, and diuretic. It has a bitter/sweet flavor and is a purgative. Through the ages, the stimulant quality of coffee has been used to wake people up after sleep as well as from alcohol intoxication and narcotic overdose. It has also been considered a mental stimulant. As a folk medicine, coffee has been prescribed in the treatment of snakebite, asthma, jaundice, vertigo, and headache. When a rich, greasy, heavy diet is eaten, coffee helps stimulate the user through periods of sluggishness from toxic overload. Coffee also purges the bowels in individuals who are commonly constipated from such a diet.

An ideal use of coffee is as an external remedy. A poultice of wet grounds will speed the healing of bruises and insect stings. Perhaps the safest internal use of this strong purgative-stimulant is the coffee enema in cases of asthma and cancer (described in Chapter 32: *Cancer and the Regeneration Diets*).

Dangerous chemicals are used in the production of coffee: poisonous herbicide and pesticide sprays in its cultivation, petroleum-based solvents in its decaffeination, and other chemicals in making it instant; in addition, the oils in coffee easily go rancid once it is ground. Therefore, organic, whole coffee beans, which can be freshly ground as needed, are preferable. If a decaffeinated coffee is desired, choose the types that are steam processed.

Coffee drinkers are at risk of developing specific diseases. A meta-analysis of thirty case studies suggests that coffee drinkers increase their likelihood of developing urinary tract and bladder cancers by twenty percent.[4] Coffee consumption during pregnancy increases the rate of miscarriages and birth defects.[5] Coffee intake has been shown to be directly related to pancreatic cancer and heart attack—the more coffee consumed, the greater the likelihood of these conditions.[5,12] Even moderate coffee drinking of two daily cups or more raises cholesterol.[6]

The acid in coffee eats away the villi of the small intestine, reducing their effectiveness in supporting nutrient assimilation—most heavy coffee drinkers are deficient in calcium and other minerals. Thus the acids in coffee may cause as much problem as the caffeine. To aid in restoring a coffee-ravaged small intestine, use nettle leaf *(Urtica urens)* tea, two or more cups daily, for at least six weeks. De-acidified ground coffee is most commonly available in supermarkets. Coffee makers which use a cold-water method to remove the harmful acids are also available from kitchen supply stores. However, coffee that is nearly as acid-free can be made without special equipment.

Acid-free Coffee Extract:
- Add one pound of freshly ground, organic coffee to eight cups water in a glass bowl.
- Place the mixture in a cool dark corner and allow to soak approximately sixteen hours.
- Filter off the liquid extract through a coffee or fabric filter into a glass jar that can be tightly closed.
- The extract is concentrated, and 1–2 tablespoons added to eight ounces of hot water yields one cup of de-acidified coffee.
- Store the extract in the sealed jar at refrigerator temperatures; it will keep for two weeks. If de-acidified coffee is taken in daily one-cup doses, there will usually be no problems in the robust and healthy individual.

Withdrawal from coffee is difficult for many. Perhaps a gradual withdrawal is best, as it is with most intoxicants. When coffee is stopped abruptly, headaches and constipation result, as well as drowsiness. Drinks made from barley- or wheat-grass-juice powders help detoxify in any withdrawal program. These are also beneficial for constipation, although laxative herbs and foods may be necessary for a few days (check the index for examples). In addition, nourishing and satisfying grain-and-root coffee substitutes are available in natural-food as well as most grocery stores. A remedy which calms a nervous mind during withdrawal: a couple of cups of carob tea daily (mix one or more teaspoons carob powder into a cup of hot water). Carob is also effective for this purpose when taken as an ingredient in food.

As a further consideration, keep in mind that the political/moral issue of coffee involves large plantations in Latin America where profits stay in the hands of a few corporate land owners. The land where this coffee is grown could be used more wisely to produce wholesome foods for the desperately poor and hungry people in many of these areas. Much the same can be said regarding banana and other large plantations where the crop is exported to wealthy nations while the Latin American soils are depleted and the masses go hungry.

Tea

According to the Chinese herbal classic, the *Pentsao,* common black or green tea has several uses, some of which are health benefits.

Properties and uses: Brightens the eyes, clears the voice, invigorates the constitution, removes flatulence, opens the acupuncture meridians, illumines the spirit, improves the digestion, relieves thirst, and is cooling, diuretic, and astringent. As a digestive aid, tea also has a special solvent property that cuts the fats and oils from a rich meal. For its health-promoting benefits, tea should not be strongly steeped, but lightly infused.[7] One method is to pour boiling water through the tea (a tea strainer works well for this). In China, when tea is too strong for an individual, a traditional way to modify it is by adding more hot water to that person's cup. The second infusion of the tea leaves is often the most appreciated for its subtlety because the tannic acids in the tea do not overpower the infusion. Much of the negative value of tea will not exist in this milder version.

In medicinal uses, tea is usually strongly brewed by simmering the leaves for thirty minutes or more. Tea is traditionally used in both the East and West for cases of diarrhea as well as poor digestion from either acute or chronic inflammations (gastritis or enteritis). For these conditions drink one teaspoon of strong tea several times a day. Tea is also helpful as an aid in curing dysentery, and its astringent property dries up herpes and poison oak/ivy outbreaks—for these skin conditions use a wash of concentrated tea or apply a poultice of tea leaves that have been soaked in hot water. For the mildest tea with the least caffeine and most minerals, use the branches of certain tea plants. These are marketed under names such as "bancha twig tea" or "kukicha." The minor amount of caffeine in this kind of tea offers mild stimulation and helps in the digestion of a meal centered on complex carbohydrates such as grains, legumes, and vegetables.

Spices

- Cinnamon, cloves, coriander, ginger, nutmeg, and cardamom all have expansive, drying, warming qualities which reinforce the expansive aspects of sweet foods while reducing their moistening aspects. Foods which generally digest better with the addition of these spices include yams, sweet potatoes, winter squash as well as any other very sweet fare, particularly desserts and cooling fruit dishes. Adding pinches of these spices to highly mucus-forming foods—milk, yogurt, kefir, sour cream, and other dairy—also greatly improves digestion, especially in the *cold* or *damp* individual.

- Green leafy spices (oregano, basil, thyme, bay, etc.) have aromatic powers that lighten up dark beans and heavy sauces.
- Seeds grow in clusters and seem to engender a sociable quality. Caraway or dill seeds add zest to breads, soups, and cabbage and beet dishes.
- Coriander, cumin, and ginger combine well with bean dishes to diminish problems of flatulence. This root-and-seed combination adds a strengthening quality to the diet. Fresh ginger is used to help break down high-protein foods such as meats and beans and lessen the effect of uric acids in the body from eating these foods. Other uses for either fresh or dried ginger include nausea, vomiting, morning sickness, menstrual cramps, suppressed menstruation, bronchitis, aches, and spasms. Dried ginger feeds the properties of foods and herbs to the lower extremities—the colon, kidneys, ovaries, sexual organs, and legs; it also treats motion sickness, and is most convenient in the form of capsules or a tincture for this purpose. Ginger should not be used when signs of *heat* are present.
- Garlic and cayenne are good remedies for *exterior* conditions such as the common cold. For example, a garlic-cayenne soup would have antiviral, antibiotic, and diaphoretic (sweating) properties at the onset of a cold. Cayenne is one of the highest botanic sources of vitamin C. Garlic and the rest of the onion family are extremely pungent and dispersing. They help overcome stagnant *qi* energy and thereby help balance the obstructive effect of excess meat or other dietary extremes. They also control the growth of putrefactive bacteria caused by eating animal products, overeating, and combining food unwisely. However, their pungent aspect disperses mental concentration. Once one is beyond the early stages of a healthful vegetarian diet, the regular need for these plants normally decreases. Thus they are listed in many recipes in this text as options, to be used by those who need them during periods of dietary transition or illness. Other specific properties for the onion family appear later under "Vegetables" in the recipe section.
- Turmeric, an Indian spice, has important healing properties. Curcumin, the primary ingredient which gives it its yellow color, has anti-inflammatory and antioxidant qualities and protects the liver from toxins.[8] It also lowers cholesterol and inhibits the replication of HIV-1.[9,10] In subjects with rheumatoid arthritis, dietary curcumin (available as a nutritional supplement) improved flexibility and reduced joint swelling.[11] Turmeric is warming and bitter; it is used to improve protein digestion, reduce uterine tumors, decongest the liver, dissolve gallstones, increase ligament flexibility, and reduce menstrual pain. Dosage: $\frac{1}{4}$- to $\frac{1}{2}$-teaspoon daily, as a spice or taken in capsules.

Vitamins and Supplements

The urge to take supplements of vitamins and various other nutrients is a response to the way modern people live. Supplements are usually taken to replace what is lost through poor dietary practices and an irresponsible lifestyle. Most Americans want to know what to "take" to solve health problems instantly.

A first principle in healing is discovering not what to add, but how to eliminate the cause of disease. In dietary healing, this means to remove negative foods (such as intoxicants and chemical ingredients) and poor food habits.

The next priority is to replace inferior products with those of quality. For example, whole grains should be substituted for refined grain products, unrefined monounsaturated oils for rancid oils, and organic foods for the sprayed variety. Next it is important to know how to supplement any existing deficiency with strengthening and tonifying remedies. The supplementation of deficiency is generally more successful in the long term when whole foods are given, not just separate nutrients in a pill. In the event an excessive condition exists, it should be reduced after any weakened, deficient areas have been reinforced. Ironically, as we shall see later, synthetic vitamin "supplements" are sometimes better at reducing excess than supplementing deficiency. If negative and inferior foods are removed from the diet according to the first two priorities above, then steps 3 and 4 (supplementing and reducing) tend to occur as a consequence, and there is far less need for supplementation with vitamins, minerals, enzymes, and isolated nutrients.

Even though it is clear that supplements have merit, it is questionable if they are ever truly necessary when diet is optimal. Supplements are used both for prevention and for overcoming imbalances and disease. People who choose supplementation as a means to prevent disease and maintain health often give the following reasons for their choice: Lack of proper nutrition in food, stress from an extreme lifestyle, and toxins in the food and environment. Prevention is increasingly being measured in terms of immune system vitality. A sampling of nutrients known

---

Dietary Priorities

1. Eliminate negative foods
2. Replace inferior foods
3. Supplement deficiency
4. Reduce excess

Dietary Abuses that Destroy Nutrients in the Body

Faulty Habits
overeating
hurried eating without chewing properly
eating late at night

The Use of . . .
All intoxicants:
  caffeine—coffee
  nicotine—tobacco
  marijuana
Rich, greasy, highly seasoned food
Refined foods:
  refined sugar
  white-flour foods
Chemical additives in food and water
Antibiotics and most synthetic drugs

to strengthen immunity includes zinc, selenium, and the vitamins A, C, E, and B complex. Limitless approaches abound to using these and all other nutrients; detailed vitamin and individual nutrient therapies are not included in this book.

However, it is important not to lose sight of the nature of supplementation in relation to food. For instance, can individual, often-synthetic nutrients be made to act like whole food? Is food itself an effective supplement?

How well nutrients work when they are synthetically derived is questionable. Even "natural" vitamin supplements are usually more than 90% synthetic.

Vitamins within plants and living organisms are organized into extremely subtle and complex patterns composed of many other nutrients. Such patterns cannot be duplicated except in a living environment. Thus, vitamins in whole food are often immeasurably more effective than the synthetic variety; furthermore, the life force in whole foods is absent in synthetic vitamins.

Those attributes which are measurable tell us that nutrients in food may be far more active. For example, 70 mg. of vitamin C ingested in the form of parsley or broccoli (one cupful) may strengthen immunity more effectively than 700 mg. of synthetic vitamin C. Studies indicate that only 10% of synthetic vitamin C is absorbed; in contrast, the absorption and utilization of vitamin C in these green plants above are maximized in the context of beta-carotene, chlorophyll, enzymes, minerals, and other cofactors.

Since supplements containing only synthetic nutrients have neither the integrity nor value of whole food, some supplement manufacturers now create a base for vitamins and other nutrients out of such highly nutritional substances as wheat grass, herbs, yeast, and spirulina. By having an abundance of whole-food nutrients in the presence of synthetic ones, they hope that a synergetic effect will occur and that all the cofactors necessary for efficient metabolism will be present. Taking supplements at mealtime will offer some of these same benefits. Another manufacturing approach is to incorporate synthetic vitamins and non-organic* minerals into a living yeast base through a process of fermentation. In this way the vitamins and minerals become part of a living food and therefore metabolize more completely. According to our observations, these approaches to supplements are more effective, especially for *deficient* or relatively balanced people.

In the case of *excess* conditions that result from a very rich diet coupled with a strong constitution, synthetic vitamins may be temporarily helpful as a means of reducing the excess. If a person has a history of eating too much concentrated food (for example, eggs and meat), the excess is partly stored in the liver in the form of protein, fat, minerals, vitamins, and other nutrients. Synthetic vitamin C, taken in large amounts, may help balance this condition. Since vitamin C utilizes numerous other nutrients to carry out its activities and many of these nutrients will be in the liver, it reduces possible excesses there. This theory whereby excess is reduced

*"Non-organic" in this usage means not organized by plant or animal life. A non-organic mineral will usually be derived from mineral deposits in the earth.

by vitamin C is supported in part by the well-known action C has in reducing blood fat and cholesterol.[1]

The reducing action of synthetic substances is not confined to synthetic nutrients. Primary examples are the synthetic additives to food, such as synthetic sweeteners, preservatives, flavor enhancers, and colorants. Excess in the body is also reduced by alcohol and vinegar, which can be thought of as strong solvents, exemplified by their common usage as marinades to break down meat. In fact, all refined food has the characteristic of reducing certain types of nutrients in the body while adding others and creating imbalance as a result of incomplete digestion. Thus many individuals become obese yet mineral-deficient from eating too many carbohydrate foods containing refined sugar and white flour.

Until recently, the human species has known only whole food. When refined food or synthetic substances are consumed, the body robs itself of nutrients to make these products appear complete. In all but the most *excessive* conditions, this reducing process ultimately leads to *deficiencies.*

Synthetic supplements can upset balance in other ways. When many separate components of food (e.g., multivitamins) are taken, the liver can become confused in its metabolic role, with disharmonious effects differing from person to person. The risk is less in those with a strong liver. If those taking supplements regularly refrain at least one day of the week, possible side effects from the complex, non-integrated, and often-synthetic nature of supplements are minimized. This is true of all medicines and strong nutrients, since when the body rests, it renews its ability to respond. (There are exceptions when medicines *must* be used daily. If you are taking prescribed medication, consult with the practitioner before attempting the above plan.)

Supplemental Vitamin C

Because vitamin C has been the subject of such controversy over dosage levels and its effects, we have chosen to present three claims surrounding this nutrient. The proponents of vitamin C (ascorbic acid)—those who state that not nearly enough C is ingested by modern people—often support their recommendations with the following claims. After each claim are remarks and evidence suggesting other valid viewpoints.

Claim: Humans, unlike many other mammals, have lost their ability to synthesize vitamin C in their bodies.[2-4] *Remark:* Research by Japanese scientists has demonstrated that vitamin C *is* generated from healthy human intestinal flora.[5]

Claim: The ideal daily intake of vitamin C is often determined to be the amount just before diarrhea is induced by the vitamin.[6] *Remarks:* For many individuals, this intake of ascorbic acid will be more than 10,000 milligrams. There is evidence that vitamin C taken above the 1,250-mg. level on a daily basis reduces chromium uptake[7] and mobilizes calcium from the vitreous and scleral complexing within the collagen matrix of the eye[8]—thus excess vitamin C seems to reduce the availability of calcium. Vitamin C ingestion above 1,500 mg. appears to antagonize gut uptake of copper, thereby reducing superoxide dismutase (SOD), a copper-dependent enzyme that is a "free-radical quencher" and essential for proper immunity.[9]

Claim: Ancient humans ingested large amounts of vitamin C from natural sources—perhaps several thousand milligrams daily—and therefore the modern person needs a similar quantity.[10, 11] *Remarks:* More recent estimates place the daily consumption of vitamin C by Paleolithic man at 400 mg.[12] This level is easily exceeded by modern people who emphasize fresh vegetables, fruits, and sprouts in the diet.[10] When these reducing, cleansing foods become the majority of the diet, daily vitamin C intake will often surpass 1,000 mg. Chromium, a mineral which is greatly deficient in the contemporary diet, is one measure of correct vitamin C dosage. Chromium uptake is enhanced when vitamin C consumption falls between 400 and 1,250 mg. daily.[7] Above this level, as noted above, chromium decreases. Since large quantities of highly active vitamin C along with its associated metabolites can be obtained from one's diet, it may be that supplemental C is really never necessary when the diet is optimal. Therefore, in the conditions listed below which benefit from vitamin C supplementation, it is assumed that the diet contains insufficient C.

People who eat a meat-centered diet of overly processed foods may well benefit from a gram (1,000 mg.) or so of ascorbic acid daily. Individuals with serious illnesses, especially with *excess* and *heat* signs (such as those observed in high blood pressure/heart disease victims) seem to benefit from very large amounts of C, sometimes more than ten grams, but these levels need to be monitored and adjusted regularly. In addition, the various nutrients that are depleted by high levels of C should be added. Large amounts of vitamin C may also be valuable for certain chronic immune disorders including some forms of cancer, because of the vitamin's antioxidant properties. Certainly the antihistamine value of C is generally beneficial at the outset of the common cold or flu, and C has been shown to reduce the severity of symptoms from these and similar *exterior,* acute conditions.

In those who are fairly healthy and eat a wholesome vegetarian diet, we have seen diarrhea occur from just 300–500 milligrams of ascorbic acid. A low tolerance to the synthetic form of the vitamin may indicate:

1. Ample C is already in the diet—perhaps it is even being synthesized by healthy intestines;
2. The reducing action of C, especially the reduction of fats and cholesterol, is not utilized by this physiological type; and
3. A highly responsive body/mind, sensitized with whole foods, tends to reject any isolated and synthetically derived nutrient.

There are seemingly endless other considerations when a decision is made to take vitamin C or, for that matter, any other nutrient. Similar questions on dosage, application, and safety arise for each known nutrient. For example, vitamin E reduces blood clotting and improves immunity. But ingestion above 1,000 I.U. daily promotes clotting and suppresses immunity.[13] Other immunotonics such as vanadium and zinc impair immunity when consumed at high levels.[14, 15]

Supplements as Medicine

The therapeutic use of individual vitamins and other nutrients for serious disease conditions requires uncommon skill and experienced guidance. A system still in its infancy, nutrient supplementation is nevertheless helpful in many instances, most often during the first few months until a healing diet has been followed long enough to bring substantial improvement. Exceptional doses of nutrients are often involved; when such therapies are used in conjunction with quality whole-food nutrition, less supplementation is required. If food habits are not simultaneously improved, then massive supplementation must usually be maintained; otherwise any gains acquired from the nutrients will be lost.

Unfortunately, such use of supplements can have a sinister side: improvement often reaches a plateau after a few months, and then a slow slide back towards the original imbalance begins. To avoid this scenario, one can simply plan to *gradually* discontinue the supplements as other improvements in diet and lifestyle take hold. Any sharp reduction in long-term supplementation can have bad results. When the body has become accustomed to large amounts of certain nutrients, a slow withdrawal over several weeks is best; it allows the organs of digestion to shift from isolated nutrients to absorbing and metabolizing the nutrients from foods. The fact that mega-dosing with nutrients can have at least some positive short-term benefits is not a sufficient recommendation for its use. At this time there is no evidence that those who improve with such a program would not improve even more efficiently with an ideal diet of whole foods.

Supplements for Prevention

Human studies indicate that *long-term* supplementation with isolated vitamins such as A, C, E, and beta-carotene neither cures nor prevents serious diseases, including cancer.[17,18,19,20,21] Clearly, the safest route for prevention is to avoid nutritional extremes and to use food of the highest quality available. Unprocessed, unsprayed, organically grown food is vastly superior to supplements (and chemically raised food) in nutrition, taste, and vital energy, and is becoming increasingly available in the United States and Europe. Beyond food, the concepts of attitude, lifestyle, and immunity are essential, as discussed in Chapters 5 and 52.

Vital Alternatives

Alternatives to commercial supplements for prevention are the especially concentrated sources of nutrition:

1. Use suitable herbs. Those such as parsley, alfalfa, nettles, Siberian ginseng, and gota kola build resistance to disease.

2. Gather wild foods—these can have very high potency: dandelion greens and roots, pigweed, lamb's-quarters (a species of pigweed), fiddleheads, burdock, and watercress. Dry some of these for the off-season.

3. Use seaweeds, the highest plant source of minerals. Minerals in seaweeds (and any plant) are much more easily assimilated than minerals in supplements,

which are often from non-living sources. By rotating various seaweeds through a diet, all minerals, including the trace minerals, are made available. A good variety of seaweeds is suggested in the recipe section.

4. Include some very concentrated sources of vitamins, bioflavonoids, and/or chlorophyll, such as wheat or barley grass. The cereal grasses are simple to grow, or use them in the form of commercial juice powders and tablets. (Note: before the advent of synthetic vitamins, wheat grass tablets were considered a superior supplement based on hundreds of scientific studies and were carried by virtually every pharmacy in America by the year 1945.) Other sources include bee pollen and flower pollen (available straight from flowers and in products), and micro-algae such as spirulina, wild blue-green *(Aphanizomenon),* and chlorella. These micro-algae and the above cereal grasses are important sources of one of the most overlooked nutritional deficiencies—the omega-3 and gamma-linolenic (GLA) fatty acids.

5. Sprouts, popular among the Chinese for thousands of years, are an exceptional source of easily assimilated vitamins, enzymes,* chelated minerals, free fatty acids, and amino acids. They are alkaline-producing, cleansing, and most varieties are cooling (but less so when lightly steamed). Sprouts are most appropriate in the spring and in warmer climates. Excessive use may weaken digestion. Smaller amounts should be eaten in the winter and by those with *cold* and *deficient* conditions.

6. Fresh vegetable and fruit juices are another way to concentrate vitamins and enzymes. Taking juices in large amounts can weaken digestion and is most suitable for the robust person or during diseases marked with *excess* signs (strong pulse, ruddy complexion, thick or yellow tongue coating, etc.). Juices composed of the entire fruit or vegetable, which therefore retain all the fiber, edible peels, and pulp, include the plant's complete "phytochemical" makeup, and provide the total spectrum of nutrients (see note 16 on page 691 for a discussion of phytochemicals). Such "whole-food" juices can be made with specialized electromechanical processors, although hand mills preserve food's oxidizing enzymes better and make sauces rather than juices. Dehydrated whole-food juices that are concentrated into powders, tablets, or capsules are also available. When processed carefully at low temperatures, they retain some the plant's least stable vitamins and enzymes. Less vital than fresh fruit and vegetable juices, they nonetheless provide a balanced source of nutrients. Other ingredients such as cereal grasses, micro-algae, seaweeds, and herbs are frequently concentrated into complex whole-food products.

---

*Enzymes are a protein-vitamin-mineral complex that provides a natural "chelated" bond with minerals as well as a protein base for vitamins, making the vitamins and minerals highly assimilable. Specifically, chelation represents a bond between a mineral and a protein structure such as an amino acid. This bond protects the mineral from forming compounds with other substances in the digestive tract that inhibit its availability. However, if the bond is too strong, the mineral is never absorbed. It is thought that enzymes, which are highly concentrated in sprouts, form an optimal chelation.

Calcium

In East Asian healing traditions, calcium and mineral-rich substances such as oyster shell, fluorite, gypsum, calcitum, and fossilized bones of animals are taken as medicine for their cooling, relaxing, calming, and moistening dimensions. Thus, these kinds of substances typically appear in formulas for insomnia, thirst, nervous anxiety, and various over-*heated* conditions. In Chinese physiology, the "*yin* fluids" that calm the spirit, relax the liver, and moisten the lungs are undoubtedly infused with calcium and other minerals, and as such relate to the Western practice of using calcium foods to benefit the nerves and heart.

In most American minds, the primary benefit of calcium in the body is to build and strengthen the bones. The Chinese, however, ingest oyster shell—a calcium supplement used in the West—for its sedative and cooling value, not for maintaining bone mass. Instead, bone problems are treated by improving the kidney-adrenal complex at the level of its *jing* essence and by enriching the *yin* fluids with various foods and herbs that build the structural aspects of the body—some of which contain very little calcium. (See *Water Element* chapter.) In fact, several remedies for nurturing the kidneys appear in this chapter as specific bone-building, calcium-fortifying substances. Interestingly, recent developments in modern nutrition point more in this direction than toward supplementation with pure calcium compounds. This chapter offers an expanded approach to the concept of calcium deficiency and shows which foods are most effective in the cure of so-called calcium disorders.

For years, calcium has been a well-advertised nutrient in the United States because it is thought that people are generally more deficient in calcium than any other mineral. Yet despite all the talk about the importance of calcium, very little is said about the factors essential for effectively absorbing and utilizing it.

All the minerals in the body are in a delicate, dynamic balance. If a deficiency in calcium exists, other minerals will also be out of balance. Thus, the recommendations in this chapter to increase calcium absorption will also improve the effective use of all minerals in the body.

Exactly how minerals should be balanced internally is a biochemical puzzle which scientists reinterpret and question from year to year. For example, the ideal ratio of calcium to magnesium in the diet was once thought to be two-to-one. More recently, researchers have advocated a one-to-one ratio, and now some are asserting that magnesium intake should be twice that of calcium.[1] This last ratio corresponds more closely to the natural ratio in a grain-and-vegetable-based diet. In fact, a favorable mix of all known nutrients essential for calcium absorption is found in a balanced whole-food diet.

Calcium in the American diet is perceived as almost synonymous with the use of dairy products. Unfortunately, dairy foods are generally not of good quality, and perhaps this is one reason that Americans, who consume large amounts of dairy (25% of the average diet), still have widespread calcium deficiency problems such as arthritis and osteoporosis. It may be that dairy has been wrongly characterized as a cure-all for calcic disorders. In China and areas of Southeast Asia, where dairy consumption is minimal, arthritis and bone deterioration are not the major health problems that they are in the wealthy countries of the West. Evidence points to certain cofactors of calcium metabolism as the problem: calcium absorption requires adequate dietary magnesium, phosphorus, and vitamins A, C, and D. In fact, without certain of these nutrients, it appears that calcium cannot be absorbed at all.

The Magnesium Connection

It is common knowledge that vitamin D is essential for efficient calcium utilization. In response to this information, the dairy industry has fortified nearly all available milk with synthetic vitamin D_3.

For many years, magnesium also has been recognized as valuable in calcium absorption, but its absolute necessity has been underscored in several recent human experiments. In one, calcium and vitamin D were abundantly supplied while magnesium was withheld; all subjects in the experiment except one became calcium-deficient. When magnesium was reintroduced in the diet, calcium levels rose dramatically.[2]

The Hormonal Activity of Magnesium

Calcitonin is a hormone which increases calcium in the bones and keeps it from being absorbed into the soft tissues. Magnesium stimulates calcitonin production and therefore increases calcium in the bones while drawing it out of the soft tissues. Many forms of arthritis are characterized by excess calcium appearing in the soft tissues while skeletal calcium is lacking.

A magnesium-rich diet of whole foods is generally a cure for these types of osteoarthritis as well as most forms of calcium deficiency. The food groups in order of their magnesium content are: the dried seaweeds, including wakame, kombu, kelp, hijiki, arame, and most others; beans, including soybeans and their products; also mung, aduki, black, and lima beans; *whole* grains, particularly buckwheat; also millet, wheat berries, corn, barley, rye, and rice. Nuts and seeds, especially almonds, cashews, filberts, and sesame seeds, are good sources of magnesium, as are the high-chlorophyll foods—wheat- or barley-grass products and microalgae such as spirulina, wild blue-green *(Aphanizomenon),* and chlorella. Even though the chlorophyll foods are normally consumed in small amounts, they contain as much magnesium as the beans, and their impact on the body's magnesium levels can be significant if they are eaten regularly. The chlorophyll itself in these foods is also beneficial for calcium utilization, as we shall see later. Animal products—dairy, eggs, and meat—and fruit contain the least magnesium of common foods. Most refined foods are also lacking in magnesium; for example, only 8% of the magnesium remains after the milling of wheat berries into white flour.

One other food, with the highest magnesium levels of any food besides sea-weeds, should be mentioned—chocolate. It seems that most "chocoholics" have a magnesium-poor diet and crave chocolate to improve the calcium status of their nerves and bones. Unfortunately, chocolate is only rarely available in healthful forms; usually found in candy, cakes, and other sweets it is mixed with refined sugar, hydrogenated fats, and other denatured (non-) foods. In recent years, some chocolate products have appeared which contain wholesome ingredients. Nonetheless, chocolate is extremely rich in oxalic acid and contains theobromine, a caffeine-like substance. If used habitually, chocolate inhibits healthful overall mineralization of the body.

The Relaxing Effect

While calcium contracts the muscles, magnesium relaxes them. Thus calcium-blocking drugs are given to help stop vasospasm in heart disorders and headaches. However, some practitioners simply recommend additional dietary magnesium for the same purpose; since giving magnesium can be as effective as the calcium-blockers,[3] it is clearly a more desirable remedy because it has no side-effects.

Of all drugs ingested, the majority are taken to overcome stress and neuro-muscular tension. Alcohol, the most widely used of them, acts temporarily to depress anxiety and relax muscles. Certainly a much healthier alternative to the possibility of addiction to tranquilizers, alcohol, or even chocolate is plenty of magnesium-rich foods in the diet—whole grains, beans and legumes, vegetables, seaweeds, nuts, and seeds.

Chlorophyll: Regulator of Calcium

Photosynthesis, an extremely complex and poorly understood process, takes place in plants in the presence of sunlight and results in the formation of chlorophyll. All plants touched by sunlight contain chlorophyll, but the green plants are by far the most concentrated sources.

At the center of the chlorophyll molecule is magnesium. Most green plants are also valuable sources of phosphorus and vitamins A and C, important cofactors for calcium absorption, as mentioned above. The other nutrient necessary for proper calcium metabolism is vitamin D, the "sunshine vitamin." Fortunately, chlorophyll foods act as a form of stored sunshine, performing like vitamin D in the body to regulate calcium.

Very often those who receive the least sunshine and therefore need green foods most are invalids, office

> Many of the benefits man gets from the sunshine he can get from greens. Anyone in the city should especially think of greens as a means of getting sunshine to the body.
>
> —Dr. Bernard Jensen, from *Health Magic Through Chlorophyll*

workers, and people living in the core of a metropolitan area.

In fact, because of the ability of chlorophyll foods to regulate calcium in the body, those who consume dairy in quantity and are also truly healthy nearly always eat plenty of green vegetables. The plants richest in chlorophyll—the micro-algae and cereal grasses—were cited earlier as good sources of magnesium. Green plants also have the greatest concentration of calcium of any food; because of their magnesium, chlorophyll, and other calcium cofactors, increasing the consumption of green plants often is a simple solution to calcium problems. However, three common greens are high in oxalic acid, which tends to counteract their ability to supply calcium. These are spinach, chard, and beet greens.

Three Calcium Soups

A traditional European recipe for calcium replenishment is the "green and grain" soup of barley sprouts and kale. The barley must be whole, not "pearled," in order to sprout. Vitamins A and C (the two calcium cofactors that are low in unsprouted seeds) are greatly increased in the sprouting process. This soup is simmered just ten minutes. Soaked barley can be substituted for sprouted barley, but must be cooked much longer, until the barley is soft. In this case the kale is added toward the end of the cooking process. (Soak whole barley at least eight hours, then discard the soak water.) This soup is also suitable for those who are convalescing as a result of chronic health problems.

Another calcium soup is based on the traditional Chinese principle that the kidneys, part of the Water Element, rule the bones. Since ancient times, beans have been assigned a role in the regulation of the kidneys. Seaweeds are also a tonic for the Water Element. A soup of beans cooked with seaweed is considered beneficial for the kidneys, and therefore for the bones. (For a method of using seaweeds with beans, see "Legumes" in the recipe section.) This particular Eastern prescription corresponds with modern nutrition: we know that seaweeds are the food group highest in both magnesium and calcium, while beans are also exceptionally concentrated in both these nutrients.

A third calcium soup follows the logic of "like heals like." Any bones from organically raised animals are broken, then cooked into a soup with acid vegetables to extract the marrow and various minerals. This soup is described further in *Food for Children*, Chapter 21. A similar idea is to include in a soup whole fish such as sardines or anchovies. This practice accords with the principle of using foods as whole as possible. These fish, of course, also have available nutrients for calcium renewal when served in other ways.

Therapeutically, these three soups are listed in ascending order by their effectiveness; the bone and whole-fish soups are the most useful for the seriously *deficient* (frail, weak, pale) individual. In order to minimize animal products in the diet, these soups can be replaced with the other calcium-building soups once the *deficiency* is resolved.

The Similar Calcium Needs of the Older Woman and the Female Athlete

The older woman is most at risk of becoming calcium-deficient. Caucasian women in particular are eight times more likely than men to develop osteoporosis; after age thirty-five, women lose bone tissue three times faster.[4] These problems are explained in Chinese medicine by the fact that the supply of minerals to the bones depends on the vitality of the kidney-adrenal function and its ability to produce rich *yin* fluids, a function that diminishes with age. Also, women draw on the *yin*, moistening, cooling, and nurturing elements such as calcium and the feminine hormones more intensely than men as a support for their relatively more *yin* nature as well as for childbearing.

In addition to the problems of nutrient malabsorption that accompany old age in general, the postmenopausal woman often develops hormonal imbalances which worsen the outlook for calcium retention. To counter glandular imbalance and the associated calcium loss, doctors have in recent years prescribed the hormone estrogen, derived from animals in forms such as Premarin™ (from PREgnant MARe urINe). When used in large amounts, estrogen has been known to increase the likelihood of cancers of the breast, ovaries, and uterus. However, even when taken in relatively small amounts for slowing calcium loss and balancing hormones, studies indicate a dramatic increased risk of strokes, heart attacks, and breast cancer.[5] Millions of women take estrogen partly because of earlier information that it would also provide protective effects against heart disease. Recent research discredits this information. Eating a wholesome diet accompanied by exercise provides a safe, effective alternative to estrogen therapy.

The woman who exercises for long periods of time often has a calcium problem similar to the older woman. Moderate exercise prevents calcium loss, but in women an excess of strenuous physical activity sets the stage for calcium loss at about the same rate as in postmenopausal women.[6] To halt rapid calcium loss, the female athlete must follow calcium-conscious practices even more carefully than others.

Other options exist for improving hormonal balances. One is the regular use of herbs as a food supplement. The Chinese herb *dang gui* root *(Angelica sinensis)* is so effective at regulating hormonal imbalance that it will often completely relieve hot flashes and other symptoms of menopause. In China, women commonly use *dang gui* as a food, putting a root into soup. The root is very hard in the dried state, and the same root can be made into an herbal decoction several times by cooking in water for half an hour. When the root becomes entirely soft, it is customarily eaten as a vegetable with rice. This white root has the aroma of celery and is particularly beneficial for the pale, *deficient,* anemic person with a tendency towards poor circulation and signs of *coldness.* It should not be used when there are *heat* signs such as inflammation, fever, or redness; it is also contraindicated in cases of diarrhea or a swollen abdomen due to excess mucus, tumors, or other *damp* obstructions. One of the most common Chinese herbs used in the West, *dang gui* is available through most herb and health food stores in several forms, including convenient tablets. Small amounts (500–700 mg. in tablets, or one cup of tea) can be taken three to five times per week as a prevention against calcium loss due to hormonal deficiency.

A plant known to directly stimulate the production of estrogen is the Brazilian herb "Suma™" *(Pfaffia paniculata [Martius] Kuntze).* Suma has safe estrogenic activity because of its store of sitosterol, a compound which increases the natural estrogen of the body without stimulating an excess. Suma falls in the category of an adaptogen: It enhances immunity and enables one to adapt more easily to stressful experiences. The general tonic properties of Suma are useful in such conditions as fatigue, anemia, impotence, tuberculosis, bronchitis, diabetes, and cancer. For boosting estrogen production, Suma can be taken according to the guidelines for *dang gui* listed above.

The older woman should limit her consumption of the typical feedlot variety of muscle meats, since these contain excessive arachidonic acid, the precursor to the inflammatory prostaglandin PGE_2, which can upset the feminine hormonal system in general. (Of course, even too much range-fed meat causes calcium loss for other reasons to be discussed soon.) Dark green vegetables such as kale, collards, wheat- and barley-grass products, seaweeds, and micro-algae all inhibit the production of prostaglandin PGE_2.

The following chart shows the degree to which calcium abounds in the vegetable kingdom. As a group, the calcium-rich plant foods are also the best sources of the previously mentioned cofactors of calcium metabolism. Thus, it is not surprising that vegetarians often have greater bone mass than meat-eaters.[7]

Further reasons vegetarians have stronger bones and fewer calcium deficiencies in general:

a. The digestion of meat results in acids which must be neutralized by calcium and other alkaline minerals.

b. Flesh protein contributes to a phosphorus/calcium ratio in Americans four times greater than desirable. Even though phosphorus is essential to calcium utilization, too much phosphorus depletes calcium.

c. Sulphur, concentrated in meat, limits calcium absorption.

d. Meat is rich in saturated fats, which combine with calcium to form a soap-like compound that is eliminated by the body.

Listed on the right side of the chart on the next page are the substances that tend to reduce calcium utilization, and conditions that require extra calcium.

Excess calcium, which usually occurs from over-supplementation with calcium pills, can result in loss of other minerals in the body, especially iron, zinc, and manganese. Simultaneous over-consumption of calcium and vitamin D pills can cause calcium deposits on the bones and in the tissues, especially those of the kidneys. These excessive conditions can be passed on to the fetus during pregnancy. Although we don't know to what extent the proper use of supplemental calcium directly adds to bone mass, at the very least it has a calcium-sparing action which

Calcium Sources, Inhibitors, and Requirements

100-mg. (3½-ounce) edible portions

Food	Calcium in Milligrams
Hijiki*	1,400
Wakame*	1,300
Kelp*	1,099
Kombu*	800
Brick cheese	682
Dried wheat grass or barley grass	514
Sardines	443
Agar-Agar*	400
Nori*	260
Almonds	233
Amaranth grain	222
Hazelnuts	209
Parsley	203
Turnip greens	191
Brazil nuts	186
Sunflower seeds	174
Watercress	151
Garbanzo beans	150
Quinoa	141
Black beans	135
Pistachios	135
Pinto beans	135
Kale	134
Spirulina	131
Yogurt	121
Milk	119
Collard greens	117
Sesame seeds	110
Chinese cabbage	106
Tofu	100
Walnuts	99
Okra	82
Salmon	79
Cottage cheese	60
Eggs	56
Brown rice	33
Bluefish	23
Halibut	13
Chicken	11
Ground beef	10
Mackerel	5

Calcium Inhibitors

1. Coffee, soft drinks, and diuretics
2. Excesses of protein, especially meat
3. Refined sugar or too much of any concentrated sweetener or sweet-flavored food
4. Alcohol, marijuana, cigarettes, and other intoxicants
5. Too little or too much exercise
6. Excess salt
7. The *Solanum* genus of vegetables—tomatoes in particular, but also potatoes, eggplant, and bell peppers contain the calcium inhibitor solanine.

Times of Increased Calcium Requirements

- During periods of growth:
— in childhood and adolescence
— during pregnancy and lactation
— during rapid mental/spiritual growth
- With age:
— older people assimilate less calcium
— women especially have greater needs after menopause
- In the presence of:
— heart and vascular disease, including hypertension (high blood pressure)
— bone disorders, including bone deterioration, easily fractured bones, arthritis, and tooth-and-gum problems including pyorrhea
— most nervous system disorders

*These sea vegetables are now available in most whole-food stores. In this chart, their calcium content is based on dried samples. (To prepare, see "Seaweeds" in the recipe section.)

indirectly preserves the bones: the cooling value of calcium mentioned earlier counteracts the hot and acidic substances in a Western diet—coffee, alcohol, cigarettes, and uric acid as a result of meat consumption—so that calcium is not withdrawn from the bones for this purpose.

Recommendations for Increasing Calcium Absorption

1. Get sufficient vitamin D from sunshine. The ideal daily sunshine exposure to ensure adequate vitamin D for proper calcium absorption is 20% of the skin of the body exposed for thirty minutes at sea level. Many people expose only their face and hands (5% of body surface) in the cooler seasons. The majority of contemporary people spend most of their daylight hours inside working. For these individuals to obtain adequate vitamin D from sunshine, several hours should be spent outside on days off. The use of full-spectrum indoor lighting is also helpful. The chlorophyll foods, as discussed earlier, are essential for those receiving insufficient sunshine. Sunshine through clouds is also effective, but requires longer exposure. Prolonged exposure to the sun at midday should be avoided.

2. Eat calcium-, magnesium-, chlorophyll-, and mineral-rich foods, especially grains, legumes, leafy greens (including cereal grasses and/or micro-algae), and seaweeds. Avoid the calcium inhibitors.

3. Exercise regularly and moderately to halt calcium loss and increase bone mass. Convalescent people need to walk or at least stand daily if possible. Bones need to bear weight and exert force against gravity to prevent loss of calcium, as was confirmed by studies of astronauts in gravity-less space.

4. Calcium supplements can be helpful, especially if the basic diet is poor, and can help halt the development of severe calcic disorders such as arthritis, deterioration of bones and teeth, and heart disease. For maximum assimilation from calcium supplements and to minimize the danger of calcium accumulation in tissues, include plenty of green vegetables in the diet. In addition, these supplements are best taken with either a very high-mineral food such as alfalfa or kelp tablets, or in conjunction with a mineral supplement. The mineral supplement should contain at least calcium, magnesium, potassium, iron, zinc, copper, selenium, iodine, chromium, manganese, boron, and trace minerals. The minerals in "multivitamins" are usually insufficient for this purpose.

Individuals with a history of kidney stones should consult their physician before taking calcium supplements. If the diet is not improved while supplements are taken, noticeable changes may take place only very gradually over several years.[8] The dietary and herbal remedies suggested in this chapter should initiate marked improvement within a few months.

5. Presoak grains and legumes before cooking to neutralize their phytic acid content, which otherwise binds the zinc, magnesium, calcium, and other miner-

als in these foods. See the recipe section for details of this method.

6. Use oxalic acid foods sparingly—rhubarb, cranberries, plums, spinach, chard, and beet greens—as they also bind calcium.

7. If dairy is used, the fermented kinds digest most easily: yogurt, cottage cheese, buttermilk, kefir. Goat's milk products are preferable. (See "Dairy Recommendations" in *Protein and Vitamin B₁₂* chapter.) Avoid skim milk—it is devoid of fat and enzymes necessary for proper calcium absorption.

8. If there are signs of kidney-adrenal weakness such as weak legs and knees, low backache, loose teeth, ringing in the ears, and unusual head-hair loss, specific kidney tonics may be indicated. (See description of deficiencies of kidney *yin, yang,* and *jing* in the *Water Element* chapter.)

Accelerated Calcium Absorption Through Silicon

Calcium disorders often arise in old age, a period in life when nutrient absorption decreases. Nevertheless, many younger people now have arthritis, heart diseases, extreme dental deteriorations, and other diseases typically associated with aging. Normally, when magnesium, chlorophyll foods, and other calcium cofactors are abundant in the diet, calcium absorption is excellent. However, if calcium deficiency conditions are present, dietary silicon can be helpful in accelerating absorption.

Silicon, found in all plant fiber as silica (SiO_2), is essential for efficient calcium utilization and for increasing bone strength. It is an integral part of all connective tissues of the body, including the blood vessels, tendons, and cartilage, and necessary for their health and renewal.

French chemist Louis Kervran also believes that additional silicon is an efficient way to improve calcium metabolism, but for a previously unsuspected reason. Kervran, at one time a Nobel Prize nominee, has advanced a highly controversial theory called "biological transmutation,"[9] a process by which minerals in all living organisms transmute into other minerals through the action of enzymes. This theory is particularly difficult to prove because the purported process of transmutation only occurs in living organisms, not in test tubes.

If biological transmutation is ever accepted as fact, it should have an impact on the life sciences, including nutrition, greater than the theory of relativity had on physics, for it would describe the physiological mechanism whereby a simple (balanced) diet supplies ample quantities of all nutrients. According to Kervran, each element in the body can transmute; manganese, for example, transmutes to iron, and silicon to calcium. By eating a diet high in manganese and silicon, a person consumes more potential iron and calcium than by actually taking iron and calcium supplements.

Whether biological transmutation can be proven or not, we have had excellent results applying these principles. In one case, a woman in her seventies took the silicon-rich herb horsetail in a tea for several months. When she went to her dentist, he was amazed to find that a number of small cavities had filled in. Horsetail (a.k.a. shavegrass) actually has the "signature" of looking like jointed bones and is regularly prescribed by herbalists for broken bones and other skeletal disorders as well as connective tissue problems. Horsetail is one of the most primitive plants; it is near the border between the plant and mineral kingdoms, and it readily offers its store of minerals if decocted in a tea. (It also contains a poisonous enzyme, thiaminase, which is easily neutralized by simmering in water for ten minutes.) When using horsetail products in the form of pills and capsules, purchase only those that are specially processed to be non-toxic. Horsetail is also a diuretic and astringent herb and should be ingested in small quantities (see formula below).

Mineral-Rich Formula

An herbal formula for improving teeth, bones, arteries, and all connective tissue, and for strengthening calcium metabolism in the body:

1 part Horsetail *(Equisetum arvense)*

1 part Oatstraw *(Avena sativa)*

1 part Kombu seaweed or Kelp powder

⅓ part Lobelia *(Lobelia inflata)*

Simmer each 1 ounce of formula in 1 pint water for 25 minutes and drink ½ cup two or three times a day. At the end of every three weeks, stop using the formula for one week. Those with bone and connective-tissue weaknesses can expect noticeable renewal from taking this formula during one entire season of the year, ideally in winter. At the same time, it is important to follow the calcium-preserving suggestions listed earlier.

Alfalfa is another highly mineralized herb and a time-honored remedy for bone disorders such as arthritis. Its ample silicon is balanced with a very wide range of trace minerals, and its enzymes aid in the assimilation of these and other nutrients. Alfalfa seeds and leaves can be made into a tea, and its sprouts and tablets are available in most food stores. See "Sprouts" in the recipe section for information on decocting and sprouting alfalfa seeds.

Silicon Foods

When one eats whole foods chosen from grains, vegetables, legumes, and fruit, there is rarely a problem with insufficient fiber or silicon, a major component of fiber. The milling of bran from grain extracts 90% of the silicon, and close to 100% of the silicon is removed in the refining of sugar. Thus the major dietary sources of silicon are the unrefined vegetable foods. As we have seen earlier, these foods, taken as a whole, are also excellent sources of calcium and its cofactors such as magnesium.

For individuals who are rebuilding connective tissue and the arterial and skeletal systems, those foods highest in silicon should be emphasized: all lettuce, especially the Boston and bib varieties, parsnips, buckwheat, millet, oats, brown rice, dandelion greens, strawberries, celery, cucumber (silicon is richest in the peel), apricots, and carrots. When these foods are included in the diet, the above "Mineral-Rich Formula" becomes even more effective.

Balancing Sweet Foods and Maintaining Calcium

An additional benefit of the silicon-rich foods containing large amounts of chlorophyll is that they balance sweet foods. An excess of highly sweet products—even of quality foods such as honey, rice syrup, and most fruits—acts as a calcium inhibitor and promotes the growth of pathogenic bacteria and candida-type yeasts in the digestive tract. (Even minor amounts of refined sugar can have these effects.) Chlorophyll/silicon plants can help balance the consumption of very sweet food: chlorophyll slows the spread of unhealthy microorganisms while silicon encourages calcium absorption.

Two common green vegetables with ample silicon are celery and lettuce; these also combine well with fruit according to food-combining principles. An important property of celery and lettuce is a mildly bitter flavor, which enables them to dry *damp* conditions such as mucus or yeast in the body.

Both vegetables are especially beneficial if eaten before and/or after the consumption of any very sweet food. Try chewing sticks of celery after a dessert. Most people experience a far milder reaction to the effect of the sweet flavor; the body feels less heavy, and the sensation in the mouth is not sticky-sweet but clean and refreshed.

Excess sweets should not be eaten in any case, and the above suggestion is recommended for use on special occasions celebrated with sweet festive foods of high quality.

Green Food Products

Highest Sources of Chlorophyll, Beta-Carotene, Protein, and Other Nutrients

The power of green plants in healing has been recognized throughout history. Many indigenous peoples—and all mammals except modern *Homo sapiens*—live primarily on grasses and green plants in times of disease.

In the past thirty years, a number of green-food supplements have become popular. These all have one obvious property in common: chlorophyll, the substance that makes plants appear green. Actually all plants, even citrus fruits, contain at least some chlorophyll; the greater the amount of chlorophyll, the greener the plant. To understand green foods it is important first to grasp the nature of chlorophyll and the color green.

In color therapy,* green is sometimes referred to as the "master color," which benefits all conditions. One always has the option of choosing green when uncertain about the best color for correcting an imbalance; green can be used both for reducing and sedating excesses and for strengthening weaknesses. Green, the color associated with spring, is primarily characterized by the power of renewal. According to the principles of Chinese medicine, it has healing value for the liver. In various metaphysical and ancient Vedic teachings, the green ray correlates with the heart *chakra* located at the center of the chest.

Diagnosing and treating the heart and the liver by use of the green color makes sense in the West, where a rich diet often overburdens the liver, which in turn can weaken the heart and arteries. (This relationship between the heart and liver is discussed in the "Five Elements" chapters.)

When used in a meal, green plants provide a refreshing, vital, and relaxing presence. This visual intuition is accurate, since the green hue corresponds to the fundamental properties of chlorophyll. These include the ability to purify, quell inflammations, and rejuvenate, as indicated below.[1–13]

Properties and Actions of Chlorophyll

Purification	Anti-inflammation	Renewal
Stops bacterial growth in wounds, and anaerobic yeasts and fungi in the digestive tract.	Counteracts the following inflammations: sore throat pyorrhea gingivitis stomach and intestinal inflammation and ulcers all skin inflammations arthritis pancreatitis	Builds blood Renews tissue Counteracts radiation Promotes healthful intestinal flora Improves liver function Activates enzymes to produce vitamins E, A, and K
Deodorizes: eliminates bad breath and body odor.		
Removes drug deposits and counteracts all toxins; de-activates many carcinogens.		
Halts tooth decay and gum infection (when used as a tooth powder).		

---

*Color therapy uses color from light or in materials to augment healing. It is applied in a variety of healing arts, as well as by psychologists and businesses to motivate specific behavior patterns.

In addition, chlorophyll benefits anemic conditions, reduces high blood pressure, strengthens the intestines, relieves nervousness, and serves as a mild diuretic.

The ability of chlorophyll to enrich the blood and treat anemia may be due to a similarity in molecular structure between hemoglobin (red blood cells) and chlorophyll. Their molecules are virtually identical except for their central atom: the center of the chlorophyll molecule is magnesium whereas iron occupies the central position in hemoglobin. Thus chlorophyll is sometimes called "the blood of plant life."

Pure extracted liquid chlorophyll is available and can be used in cases of the above internal and external conditions. Use only chlorophyll that is extracted from alfalfa or other plants; avoid the chemically manufactured variety. The standard dosage for internal use is one tablespoon chlorophyll in ½ cup of water, twice daily. However, to achieve the maximum benefits of taking chlorophyll internally, the many green plants, grasses, and algae that contain abundant raw chlorophyll are preferred because each offers it own additional properties.

The chlorophyll-rich foods discussed below appear as remedies throughout this text. From a planetary perspective, this is due to the cooling, calming, and generally peaceful quality they engender in an environment filled with aggression, hostility, noise, and other *yang* excesses. On the personal level, some people take these foods to mask the effects of an unwholesome diet, lack of exercise, and other stressful life patterns. This way of using green foods brings only marginal results. Poor diet and negative habits must also be stopped for a full healing effect.

Micro-Algae

Certain algae, especially the micro-algae spirulina, chlorella, and wild blue-green (*Aphanizomenon flos-aquae*), contain more chlorophyll than any other foods, and their chlorophyll content can be more than double depending on their growing conditions. These aquatic plants are the most accepted and best-known micro-algae at this time. Spiral-shaped and emerald to blue-green in color, their size is measured in microns (millionths of a meter).

These primitive organisms were among the first life forms. In blue-green algae such as spirulina, we find three and one-half billion years of life on this planet encoded in their nucleic acids (RNA/DNA). At the same time, all micro-algae supply that fresh burst of primal essence that manifested when life was in its birthing stages. At a moment in history when the survival of the human species is in jeopardy, many people have begun instinctively to turn to these original life forms for nutritional support.

Micro-algae exist on the edge between the plant and animal kingdoms, and offer some unique nutritional advantages. In their dried state—the usual commercial form of these products—we find, in addition to chlorophyll, the highest sources of protein, beta-carotene, and nucleic acids of any animal or plant food. Their very large store of nucleic acids (RNA and DNA) is known to benefit cellular renewal and to reverse aging. Too much nucleic acid, however, can raise the uric acid level in the body, causing calcium depletion, kidney stones, and gout. Such problems haven't generally arisen because standard dosages of micro-algae contain safe amounts of nucleic acid.

Since spirulina and chlorella are often grown in a controlled medium, their mineralization and other dynamic features can be altered toward the maximum values for human nutrition. For example, when minerals are added to the waters in which these micro-algae grow, they exhibit a higher mineral content.

The green and blue-green micro-algae all contain abundant chlorophyll and therefore can be used in the applications given earlier for chlorophyll. In fact, the majority of rejuvenating and cleansing benefits claimed by the various producers of these foods result from their chlorophyll content. Since they all contain ample protein, beta-carotene, omega-3 and/or GLA fatty acids, and nucleic acid, it is understandable that these micro-algae will share some common healing properties. In the sections which follow, the unique properties and best uses of each type of micro-alga will be given. Once specific properties are identified, it is then clear that certain algae will be better suited to specific imbalances and certain types of individuals. All micro-alga distributors refute this idea, quite possibly because such descriptions can limit sales. Most makers of health products, including the alga producers, claim their products are good for virtually everyone.

However, we have found some distinct properties of algae that define and, in a few cases, limit their usage. These properties are derived from a combination of nutritional data, East Asian perspectives, and observations of many users, the majority of them satisfied. Nevertheless, the negative experiences, which undoubtedly are a small minority, still need to be heard. We include one such account a little later.

The medical use of algae is not yet approved in the United States by the Food and Drug Administration, but the many benefits attributed to them by doctors in Japan and elsewhere clearly reflect their intrinsic and unique nutritional power.[14] In recent years, researchers have increasingly studied micro-algae because they contain anti-fungal and anti-bacterial biochemicals not found in other plant or animal species.

In a press release in late 1989 to *The New York Times,* the National Cancer Institute announced that a group of scientists had found sulfolipid extracts from a blue-green marine alga to be active against the AIDS virus. (Spirulina contains approximately 4 milligrams sulfolipids per 10-gram sample; wild blue-green *[Aphanizomenon]* is also thought to contain these compounds.) When we contacted the research team, one of the researchers told us, "It is unlikely that ingestion of the crude alga will bring about any specific therapeutic benefit. The sulfolipids are broken down rapidly by the digestive system into their component parts. One of the difficult tasks ahead will be the formulation of the sulfolipids in a manner which allow them to reach their target."[15]

Spirulina

In general, the blue-green micro-alga spirulina is nurturing, tonifying, and useful for overcoming deficiencies, but at the same time offers cleansing action because of its rich chlorophyll content. Its use by those with weakness and poor assimilation is explained by the fact that its nutrients are easy to digest and absorb.* For example, much of its protein is in the form of biliprotein, which has been predigested by the algae. A good portion of its carbohydrate is also broken down into rhamnose, and a small but important part is glycogen. These supply enduring energy soon after ingestion.

The special form of protein in spirulina benefits those with problems resulting from excessive animal protein, which does not assimilate well and further burdens the body with waste products. Thus, people who have eaten too many animal products and refined foods—typically those who are overweight, diabetic, hypoglycemic, cancerous, arthritic, or suffering from similar degenerations—often benefit from the relatively pure quality of the protein in spirulina. Of course, spirulina protein is in the context of massive amounts of beta-carotene, chlorophyll, fatty acid GLA, and other nutrients.

By eating only 10–15 grams daily of protein in this form, the body normally becomes satisfied and animal protein is craved less. In addition, the severe liver damage resulting from malnutrition, alcoholism, or the consumption of nutrient-destroying food or drugs can be treated effectively by this type of nutrition. Spirulina also protects the kidneys against injury that occurs from taking strong prescription medication.[18]

Properties: Slightly salty flavor; cooling; increases *yin* fluids; is highly nutritive (nourishes the body); detoxifies the kidneys and liver; builds and enriches the blood; cleanses the arteries; enhances intestinal flora; and inhibits the growth of fungi, bacteria, and yeasts.

Used in the treatment of: Anemia, hepatitis, gastritis and other inflammations, diabetes, hypoglycemia, obesity, overeating, malnourishment, poor skin tone, and most chronic skin outbreaks; offers ample immune-strengthening nutrients such as beta-carotene, chlorophyll, and gamma linolenic acid (GLA). It is contraindicated for those with signs of *coldness* accompanied by water retention or other forms of *dampness* (mucus, yeasts, cysts, etc.) in the lower abdomen.

Important to note in the area of prevention, spirulina is richly supplied with the blue pigment phycocyanin, a biliprotein which has been shown to inhibit cancer-colony formation.[19] Predominant blue pigmentation in food is rare. The blue color tends to promote astringency, a drawing together. The chemical reality of spirulina's blue color is demonstrated by its effect in the brain. Here phycocyanin helps draw together amino acids for neurotransmitter formation, which increases mental capacity.[20]

---

*The protein digestibility of spirulina is rated at 85%, versus about 20% for beef.[16, 17]

The unsaturated fatty acid gamma linolenic acid (GLA) and its associated prostaglandin PGE$_1$ have been researched extensively in recent years, notably in the area of immunity. Most people are deficient in GLA, but the wealth of GLA applications (listed earlier in the *Oils and Fats* chapter) is economically obtained by using spirulina, one of the richest sources.

The cell wall of spirulina has a special nature. It is composed entirely of mucopolysaccharides (MPs). These are complex sugars interlaced with amino acids, simple sugars, and in some instances, protein. Thus MPs contain only completely digestible nutrients instead of the indigestible cellulose wall typical of other micro-algae, plants, and seeds.

MPs are credited with strengthening body tissues, especially the connective tissues, while making them more elastic and resilient. They also are strongly anti-inflammatory.[21] All these attributes are most important for those who are very active physically and for older people as well. Because of the high incidence of heart disease in the West, MPs are sometimes used to reinforce the tissues of the heart and guard against artery deterioration. They further protect the vascular system by lowering blood fat.[22]

Chlorella

Chlorella is another well-known algal food of high nutritional value somewhat comparable to that of spirulina, but containing a little less protein, just a fraction of the beta-carotene, and more than twice the nucleic acid and chlorophyll. It is generally more expensive than spirulina because of the processing required to improve the digestibility of a tough outer cell wall.

Once thought of as a liability that inhibited assimilation, the cell wall has been found to be valuable. It binds with heavy metals, pesticides, and such carcinogens as PCBs (polychlorobiphenyls) and carries these toxins safely out of the body. Another feature of the cell wall is a substructure that contains complex polysaccharides. These substances, which function differently than the mucopolysaccharides of blue-green algae, stimulate interferon production as well as other anti-tumor and immune-enhancing activity.[23-26] The cell wall also contains compounds related to those found in bacteria that fortify immunity and protect against mutation.[27] The law of similars ("like cures like") offers another approach to understanding the immune-strengthening quality of chlorella: an organism with a tough outer cell wall may well possess the basic properties which strengthen our own cellular structure against invading organisms and toxins.

The minute size of chlorella (6 microns) requires centrifuge-type harvesting, which further adds to its cost. This technical requirement can put the cultivation of chlorella out of reach of individuals and small communities. Nonetheless, because of its abundance of nucleic acid and chlorophyll, the cost of these two nutrients in chlorella is comparable to their cost in other green micro-algae. For example, one buys more spirulina than chlorella to obtain equal amounts of chlorophyll and nucleic acid.

Many people use chlorella for a nutrient factor isolated in the 1950s and not available in other green foods: "Chlorella Growth Factor" (CGF). CGF is related to the special nature of chlorella's nucleic acid.

The nucleic acid in the human body (RNA/DNA) is responsible for directing cellular renewal, growth, and repair. The amount of nucleic acid in the body decreases with age; in fact, insufficient nucleic acid causes premature aging as well as weakened immunity. Nucleic acid is depleted by lack of exercise, stress, pollution, and poor diet. Replenishing RNA/DNA is therefore important to every aspect of bodily health and longevity. Since chlorella has a true nucleus, it is a more evolved organism than the other common green micro-algae and therefore may offer superior-quality RNA/DNA. This particular aspect of its RNA/DNA, measured by the CGF, strengthens immunity by improving the activity of T- and B-cells, which defend against viruses and other invading microorganisms, and macrophages, which destroy cancer and cellular debris in general.[28-31]

The major uses of chlorella are similar to those of spirulina, although there are significant differences. Chlorella may be considered the least cooling, most tonifying, and most gently cleansing of the micro-algae. It is the safest to use for *deficiencies*. CGF makes chlorella most useful for improving growth patterns in children, maintaining health in old age, healing injuries, and initiating growth where it has been stunted from disease or degeneration, including Alzheimer's disease, sciatica, palsy, seizures, multiple sclerosis, nervousness, and other nerve disorders. (These imbalances, as they manifest in Americans, often fall under the *wind damp* category in Chinese medicine.)

Chlorella Growth Factor promotes normal growth but does not stimulate the growth of disease processes such as tumors. Because its chlorophyll content is one of the highest of any food, chlorella is useful for the many conditions which benefit from chlorophyll's purification, renewal, and anti-inflammatory properties. Treatment of viruses and fungi which sap energy, such as candida-overgrowth, Epstein-Barr virus, chronic fatigue immune deficiency syndrome (CFIDS), and AIDS, is advanced by the immune-enhancing qualities of CGF as well as the antiviral effect of chlorophyll. All blood sugar imbalances—diabetes, hypoglycemia, manic depression—are greatly helped because much of chlorella's protein, like that of spirulina, is predigested and ready to work to smooth out blood sugar fluctuations.

Chlorella contains a greater quantity of fatty acids than either spirulina or wild blue-green. About 20% of these fatty acids are the artery-cleansing, omega-3, alpha-linolenic variety; perhaps this is one reason chlorella has been shown to be so effective in reducing cholesterol in the body and preventing atherosclerosis.[32, 33]

Chlorella does not contain the biliprotein phycocyanin found in blue-green algae such as spirulina and wild blue-green; therefore it does not have this anti-cancer dimension. Those who benefit from the immune-strengthening value of CGF and also want phycocyanin can simply add a blue-green alga. Any two or more micro-algae combine well, especially if both are needed. In general, other uses of chlorella seem to parallel those of other green foods. Because most chlorella on the market has more than 23% of its caloric content as fat, this micro-alga is generally not useful in the treatment of obesity.

Wild Blue-Green

A third micro-alga, *Aphanizomenon flos-aquae,* which we call "wild blue-green," grows wild in Klamath Lake in Oregon and is processed by various low-temperature drying methods that preserve cellular integrity. By comparison, most commercial micro-algae are cultivated, and dried with at least some use of heat. Wild blue-green is currently sold under various trade names, frequently as a mail-order product, and its proponents claim it contains optimum nutrition as a result of its pristine habitat and heatless processing. The fact that this alga is wild is itself one recommendation for its use, since everyone regularly needs at least some amount of wild food in the diet.

Wild blue-green has by far the most extreme properties of the commonly available micro-algae, and one needs to take precautions when using it. Like many strong substances, it has remarkable healing value when applied correctly. Even this alga's growth pattern exhibits an extreme nature. Under certain not-well-understood conditions—perhaps as a result of increased light and heat in late summer—wild blue-green can transform into an exceptionally toxic plant, so poisonous that toxicologists rate it "very fast death factor (VFDF)," since ingestion causes death in animals within five minutes.[34, 35] Most of the research citing the toxin in wild blue-green involves samples from lakes in the northeastern United States. William T. Barry, Northwest algal expert, limnologist, and professor at Gonzaga University in Spokane, Washington, claims that he has never found wild blue-green in its toxic state in Klamath Lake.[36] The companies that harvest there make the same claim and purport to monitor the product closely. As an assurance of the safety of wild blue-green in its normal, non-toxic state, several studies show that the products currently coming from Klamath Lake are completely safe.[37]

But what if the alga becomes toxic only rarely, and in amounts that would be hard to detect during processing? Research from the 1950s and -60s suggests that toxic blooms of wild blue-green did occur in the lake.[38] According to Barry, even this remote possibility is "covered," as the freeze-drying process apparently denatures the toxin. Knowing this poisonous aspect of wild blue-green, we gain respect for its powerful nature; also, as its toxic potential is exposed, individuals who want to harvest their own fresh wild blue-green will be warned.

Interestingly, native peoples have used naturally occurring blue-green algae (spirulina) in Latin America and Africa for hundreds, if not thousands, of years, but there is no record of Native Americans using wild blue-green *(Aphanizomenon)*. The fact that wild blue-green can transform into a toxin may be one explanation. Another may be its bitter flavor.

It is the bitter flavor that enters and influences the "heart-mind" system, according to traditional Chinese medicine. Many of the strongest herbal nervines such as valerian root are intensely bitter.

Because bitter substances can focus the mind, certain bitter foods including wild blue-green and peyote have been used to improve concentration during meditation and prayer. (Peyote is the much stronger of the two, often causing vomiting and hallucination, while wild blue-green offers a mental "buzz and blissed-out feeling,"[39] in the words of Viktoras Kulvinskas, author of *Survival into the 21st Century*.) Overcoming depression or a sluggish physical/mental condition with a mental stimulant such as wild blue-green is an excellent application of food-as-medicine. Gaining spiritual insight with reliance on any substance, however, can be counter-productive because it becomes more difficult to focus the mind without the substance. Perhaps this is one reason the sweet flavor (from whole foods and unrefined sweeteners) was emphasized in the earliest Vedic and Buddhist scriptures of India. Sugars gently activate the mind and require the aspirant to learn mental discipline to gain spiritual awareness; in general, the use of foods that strongly affect consciousness is discouraged in the original teachings of these "middle path" practices.

Properties and Uses: Wild blue-green is bitter, cooling, drying, mildly diuretic, a neurostimulant, an anti-depressant, and a relaxant; it also reduces *dampness* and overcomes liver stagnancy. Therefore, wild blue-green is excellent for the overweight, robust, *excessive* person, or those with *dampness* and/or *heat;* the depressed, flabby, modern person who has grown up with an excess of meats, eggs, dairy, and rich, greasy, refined, chemical-laden foods does exceedingly well in general with wild blue-green. Of course, those who are not as unbalanced also flourish with this micro-alga, as long as they have at least some signs of *excess*.

Because wild blue-green stimulates the opening of neural pathways, it has great value in treating cocaine, amphetamine, and other neuro-stimulant addictions. It also shows promise in the treatment of Alzheimer's disease. Those who have dulled their nervous system with too much salty food, including excesses of soy sauce and miso, usually benefit from wild blue-green. Moderate to large doses of wild blue-green have been therapeutically useful for cancer, arthritis, multiple sclerosis, candida overgrowth, and similar degenerations; it dries the *dampness* that supports these conditions and simultaneously acts as a mood elevator, although it must be taken in moderate amounts by those in frail conditions. In general, wild blue-green should be used cautiously by the person with a *cold* constitution if weakness, thinness, *dryness,* and/or "spaciness" are also part of the diagnostic picture.

Slim's Wild Blue-Green Adventure

A person whom we shall call "Slim" has a *dry,* thin, mentally unfocused, sensitive, and *cold* constitution. He had benefited from taking spirulina, and upon hearing that wild blue-green was more powerful, decided to try it. After three days of taking ¼ gram once or twice a day, he felt less focused and colder. He consulted with me about this, and I told him that someone with his constitution does not do well with too much bitter flavor, because bitter foods in general reduce weight, are drying and cooling, and can make the highly sensitive person lose his or her mental focus. Slim communicated this information to the president and a top salesman of the wild blue-green company. Each thought their product could not have such an effect. Slim was then encouraged by the salesman to take wild blue-green for at least a month, because "he had obviously been experiencing only a temporary healing reaction." Not wanting to miss out on the possibility of gaining more robust health, Slim decided to give the product another try for one month.

Taking the same quarter-gram dosage as before, he soon began feeling weak and cold. The next symptom was apathy and unproductivity; he would gaze out into space for hours. (Ayurveda confirms this experience—the *vata,* spacey individual becomes much more so with the consumption of bitter foods.) After three weeks Slim felt still colder, even though it was warm weather, and he lost weight rapidly from his already-meager frame. He also noticed an absence of sexual desire and the beginning of an aching sensation in the lower back. In the final week, he felt "wasted" and incapable of doing his work, and developed a sort of asthmatic wheezing. The thought and taste of wild blue-green was nauseating.

All symptoms gradually lifted when Slim stopped taking the micro-alga. However, it took about five months to regain his former mental concentration and physical strength, and even after this length of time, he still experienced occasional wheezing.

Slim's experience demonstrates that wild blue-green, like many strong substances, is not a panacea. Ingestion by the wrong person can be devastating. It is simply a question of the effect of too much bitter flavor on a *cold* and *deficient* person. On the other hand, in the *excessive* and overly robust individual, wild blue-green can liberate energy (bitter foods supply energy by burning up fat), support mental focus and alertness, strengthen reproductive ability, and be generally beneficial. This does not mean that everyone who benefits from wild blue-green will continue to do so indefinitely. It is best to regularly check its effect. One sign of overuse is a cold and inflexible personality, and another is weakness and lack of mental focus. However, for many people, wild blue-green continually provides balance; one must simply pay attention.

We estimate that only about 5% of the American population will have negative results from taking wild blue-green. Another 20% will have mixed results or short-term benefits. This *deficient, cold,* and/or "ungrounded" quarter of the population will normally do better with chlorella or spirulina, although for some, all micro-algae may be contraindicated. At the other end of the diagnostic spectrum, 25% of the population with *excessive* signs are the ideal candidates for wild blue-green as described earlier, and even though they will improve with other micro-algae, the benefits will not equal those derived from wild blue-green. Thus, the estimated 25% of the population who receive mixed or negative results from wild blue-green is balanced by another 25% who will experience exceptional results. The middle 50% is not so clearly defined, but in general it seems most people in this category have major health issues that would benefit from any of the micro-algae. By weighing the characteristics of each alga carefully, an optimal choice can be made.

Dunaliella

Recently, another micro-alga, the golden *Dunaliella salinas,* has been found to be nutritionally valuable. Although low in chlorophyll and not as high in protein and certain other nutrients as the micro-algae discussed earlier, it offers exceptional amounts of vitamin A in the form of beta-carotene. Its protein level of 18%, although high compared to most vegetable foods, is moderate in light of the 60% levels of other micro-algae; therefore, dunaliella may be better for individuals who have conditions resulting from excess protein with vitamin A/beta-carotene deficiency. It is often combined with spirulina or other micro-algae in the treatment of cancer and skin diseases. (See "Vitamin A and Beta-Carotene" later in this chapter for dosage.)

Micro-Algae Dosage

When the exceptional amounts of chlorophyll, protein, or other nutrients in micro-algae are sought for treating disease conditions, correct dosage can run a wide range, so the amount needs to be adapted according to varying needs. For dietary supplementation, prevention of disease, and immune enhancement, nearly all micro-algae come with directions for a single recommended dosage. However, the optimum dosage level depends on several factors. Each micro-alga has unique properties and advantages, so we suggest that individuals develop a personal dosage based on their own levels of activity, weight, and health. It is best to start with the minimum dosage and increase it according to your needs. An ideal dosage level results in more energy and fewer cravings.

Digestive upset or a mild frontal headache from micro-algae usually indicates a beneficial healing reaction, although in some cases too much is being taken. In either case, take less for a few weeks (try $\frac{1}{5}$ to $\frac{1}{10}$ the standard dosage). When the dosage is then increased to a moderate level and there is still no reaction, it indicates that the upset or headache was caused by the release of a layer of toxins in the body, that is now complete. The more unbalanced or toxic the person, the less micro-algae should be taken in the beginning. For renewing the liver and similar major projects, plan on taking micro-algae for at least one year. As a general rule, take these and all other supplements a maximum of six days a week. Micro-algae can be taken between meals when there is an energy need, at the beginning of meals, or to replace a missed meal.

There have been some complaints, based on evidence from colonic irrigations, about the incomplete intestinal absorption of micro-algae tablets. Micro-algae are hydrophilic (water-loving). To be digested, the dehydrated and compressed tablets need to be broken down by chewing, and then reconstituted by drinking ample fluid afterwards. The fluid can be soup at mealtime, but if water is drunk, it should be taken at least one half-hour before meals to avoid diluting digestive juices. Those with an aversion to chewing up dry tablets can soak them in water an hour or more before ingestion, or use powders or granules mixed with liquids or moist foods.

Spirulina Dosage: Spirulina is available in powder, capsules, and tablets, and is sometimes found as liquid extracts or flakes. For purposes of prevention, most people benefit from a "standard" 10-gram dosage: one heaping teaspoon of powder or 5 grams of tablets, twice a day. Double this amount (20 grams/day) is normally an effective upper dosage range for imbalances such as diabetes, hypoglycemia, cataracts, and anemia. More than this, however, is not toxic. Athletes and others with large energy requirements sometimes take 20 grams two or three times a day. (See "Choosing Micro-Algae and Cereal Grass" later in this chapter for other uses and dosages.) Pregnancy and lactation require at least 20% more protein than normal. Dosages for children are given in Chapter 21.

Finding the best way to take spirulina powder so that the flavor and texture are acceptable is important. For some people, it takes a week or two to learn to appreciate the flavor. The powder mixes easily with moist food or liquids and is often incorporated into soups, sauces, and dressings. To combine spirulina with water, juice, a warm grain beverage or root tea, put in a blender for just a second at low speed to keep from foaming; if a blender is unavailable, a little lemon juice added to the powder makes mixing with liquid easier. Avoid putting a spoon containing spirulina powder into liquids—the powder will stick to the spoon. Simply add the powder slowly to the liquid while stirring.

Spirulina Dosage Options

Measures For Using Powder			Milligrams For Tablet/Capsule Usage
1 rounded teaspoon	=	3 grams	= 3,000 mg.
1 heaping teaspoon	=	5 grams	= 5,000 mg.
1 tablespoon	=	7.5 grams	= 7,500 mg.
1 rounded tablespoon	=	10 grams	= 10,000 mg.

Chlorella and Wild Blue-Green Dosages: These micro-algae are used similarly to spirulina, although generally in smaller amounts. Since chlorella has a high concentration of chlorophyll and nucleic acids (RNA/DNA), the daily dosage level for prevention is two to three grams. Six to twelve grams per day is commonly needed during stressful conditions or disease processes. Chlorella is normally available in tablets or packets containing a measured amount of granules.

As a result of wild-crafting, low-temperature processing, its massive chlorophyll content, and bitter principle, wild blue-green is very active; one to two grams constitute a "standard" daily dosage. Three to ten grams per day is an effective dosage during disease or stress. It is usually best to divide this dosage into three equal portions to be taken three times daily. Wild blue-green is most often available in capsules or granules. One teaspoon of granules equals 1.5 grams; one table-spoon equals 4.5 grams. Because of its strong cleansing action, this alga should not be taken during pregnancy unless the body has been accustomed to it for at least one year prior to conception.

Outstanding Nutrients in Spirulina, Chlorella, and Wild Blue-Green Compared with Other Sources				
100-gram samples				
	Spirulina	**Chlorella**	**Wild Blue-Green**	**Other Highest Sources**
Protein*	68%	55%	60%	Brewer's Yeast 45%
Vitamin A	250,000 I.U.	55,000 I.U.	70,000 I.U.	Carrots 28,000 I.U.
(from carotene)				Cereal Grass 10,000–50,000 I.U.
				Dunaliella 8,300,000 I.U.
Iron	58 mg.	133 mg.	130 mg.	Beef Liver 6.5 mg.
Chlorophyll*	.7–1.1%	2–3%	3–6%	Alfalfa .2%
				Cereal Grass .2–.54%
DNA/RNA*	4.5%	13%	N/A	Sardines .8%

*Percentage of total weight
Note: The micro-algae, alfalfa, wheat grass, and brewer's yeast are dry measures.

Wheat and Barley Grass

Cereal grasses are another group of high-chlorophyll foods. Commercially, these usually appear as either wheat or barley grass (greens), and are also available in powders and tablets. It is easy to grow wheat grass at home.

The major therapeutic properties of wheat and barley grass are nearly identical, although barley grass may digest a little more easily. People with allergies to wheat or other cereals are almost never allergic to them in their grass stage. In the dried form, these grasses rank just behind the micro-algae in chlorophyll and vitamin A. Their protein levels are 20%—about the same as many meats—but of course their amino acid/protein profile is quite different. Most cereal grasses also contain trace amounts of vitamin B_{12} and many other nutrients. Wheat grass can pick up more than ninety minerals out of the estimated possible 102 found in rich soil.

In addition to high nutrient content, cereal grasses offer unique digestive enzymes not available in such concentration in other foods. The hundreds of enzymes they contain help resolve indigestible and toxic substances in food. Also present is the anti-oxidant enzyme superoxide dismutase (SOD)* and the special fraction P4D1.[40, 41] Both of these substances slow cellular deterioration and mutation and are therefore useful in the treatment of degenerative disease and in the reversal of aging.

According to various experiments, P4D1 works by stimulating the renewal of RNA/DNA. In one test it successfully activated the renewal of cellular DNA that was severely damaged by X-rays.[41] P4D1 also has exceptional anti-inflammatory properties, even more powerful than those of steroids such as cortisone.[41] This explains in part the remarkable healing action we have witnessed in cases of arthritis and inflammatory conditions in general. And unlike steroids and other "pain-killer" drugs, P4D1 exhibits no side effects or toxicity.

SOD is the enzyme in healthy cells which protects them from the highly destructive "free radicals" formed when radiation, bad air, chemical-laden food, and other toxins damage the body. SOD is either greatly lacking or completely absent in cells that are cancerous.

The carbohydrate structure of cereal grass has special value. Like that in certain micro-algae, it contains large quantities of mucopolysaccharides (MPs). These MPs, similar in activity to those discussed earlier in spirulina, also have the ability to strengthen all body tissues—including those of the heart and arteries—lower blood fat, and reduce inflammations.

Thus, the cereal grasses contain anti-inflammatory properties in at least three biologic dimensions: chlorophyll, P4D1, and mucopolysaccharides.

There is some question about the value of slowly-grown, dried cereal grasses compared with the fresh variety. At least one major cereal grass company in the United States plants wheat in the fall or early spring, so that it undergoes cool temperatures and several months of slow growth. It is then carefully dried. By comparison, fresh wheat grass grown in a warm climate or indoors for the customary seven days may contain as little as 25% of the chlorophyll, vitamin A, and other nutrients found in the cold-weather crop. Nevertheless, homegrown cereal grasses are valuable because their fresh state preserves certain enzymes that can be lost in the drying process. Such fresh juices are more cooling than juices from dried grass powders and therefore are especially helpful for the robust person with *heat* or *excess* signs such as yellow tongue coating, aversion to heat, strong radial pulse, loud voice, reddish complexion, and an extroverted or forceful manner.

---

*SOD is abundant in all chlorophyll-rich foods as well as in sprouts. Cereal grass is an especially high source.

Wheat Grass Cultivation

To grow wheat grass indoors, spread wheat berries on one inch of fertile soil, ideally mixed 50% with peat moss (from a garden supply store). The soil can be in a tray or box. Cover seeds with ½ inch of soil and moisten daily just enough for the grass to grow. When the grass reaches about five inches in height, it is cut off and its essential fluid extracted in a wheat grass juicer, or it can be chewed very thoroughly. (The pulp residue from chewing can be discarded.) Once cut, the wheat grass is allowed to regrow for two more harvests.

Properties and Uses: Compared with spirulina and chlorella, cereal grass is more cooling and more quickly cleansing of toxins in the body; but it is less cooling and cleansing than wild blue-green. Its strong digestive properties help those with liver excesses, slow digestion, and gastro-intestinal inflammation.

Specific medicinal uses[42] of wheat and other cereal grasses have traditionally included the treatment of arthritis, bruises,* burns,* cancer, constipation, emphysema, gangrene,* poison oak rash,* rheumatism, and wounds.*

For these external conditions (*), apply locally: 1) cereal grass juice; 2) a cloth soaked in the juice; or 3) a poultice of crushed grass pulp. External healing is hastened when the cereal grass is also taken internally.

Additional, more recent applications[43] include the treatment of hypertension, cholesterol excess, anemia, hepatitis, obesity, diabetes, peptic ulcer, hypoglycemia, fatigue, hemorrhoids, prostate difficulties, premenstrual syndrome (PMS), muscle debility, and toxicity from lead, mercury, and other heavy metals.

Deficient, passive people who tend toward weakness or *coldness* should use cereal grasses carefully and in smaller amounts. The micro-algae chlorella or spirulina may be wiser choices in these cases.

Dosage: Cereal grass juice is very concentrated; even one ounce has therapeutic value, and not more than two ounces are to be taken at one time. (More than two ounces is not toxic, but does not generally increase effectiveness.) It should be thoroughly insalivated before swallowing. Powders from dehydrated juices are available and are likewise very concentrated; one rounded teaspoon of juice powder is mixed with ½ cup of water. Whole leaf grass is also available in tablets or powders, and these may be taken in larger amounts than the dried juice powders—up to ten grams of tablets or a heaping tablespoon of powder. For prevention, gradual renewal, added nutrients, and to counter the effects of toxins in food and the environment, use wheat or other cereal grasses once a day; for disease conditions, two or three times daily.

Scheduling, Reactions, and Seasonal Attunement: To overcome the tendency to overeat, or to purge candida yeasts, take grass juice, tablets, or powder mixed with water at the beginning of meals. (The powders and tablets are better than fresh juices for treating excessive candida-type yeasts in the digestive tract.) Otherwise, if the grasses are needed for prevention, as a supplement, or for disease conditions, they are ideally taken one hour or more before meals, on an empty stomach. When they are used *only* as a nutritional supplement, another option is to take them at the end of a meal.

Some people may experience a mild reaction to cereal grass involving diarrhea, headache, or other discomforts. These reactions will normally occur no more than a few times, and indicate detoxification. If they continue, then too much is being taken, or the cereal grass is not appropriate.

The season to emphasize highly cleansing chlorophyll food is the springtime, when purification and rejuvenation cycles are at their height.

Choosing Micro-Algae and Cereal Grass

Very often, people have difficulty deciding which chlorophyll-rich food is best. Overlapping qualities in these foods do exist. Even the same product will vary depending on how it is grown, harvested, and processed. Nevertheless, the basic properties of each of these foods usually remain intact. If indicated, a combination of more than one micro-alga and cereal grass can be taken in a program tailored to individual needs.

General Guidelines

The suggestions which follow apply to all uses of cereal grass and micro-algae, including those not mentioned specifically in this section. For example, if using these green foods during fasting, one has choices based on whether there are signs of *excess* or *deficiency*, *heat*, *cold*, or *dampness;* choices can be further clarified with insights from the next section, "Considerations and Specific Uses."

Spirulina and chlorella are cooling and cleansing; wild blue-green and cereal grass are even more so. Therefore, the robust and **excessive** person (red complexion, strong pulse and voice, thick tongue coating, energetic nature) will benefit from any of these four, but the best balance is provided by cereal grass and/or wild blue-green.

In the **deficient** person (pale or sallow complexion, weakness, frailty, introverted nature, little or no tongue coating), spirulina and chlorella are generally helpful, while wild blue-green and cereal grass should be taken cautiously.

The person with a **cold** constitution (feels cold often, pale complexion, has an aversion to the cold) will do best with chlorella or small doses of spirulina, because chlorella (followed closely by spirulina) is less cooling than other micro-algae or cereal grasses. The person with *cold* signs accompanied by lower abdominal edema, mucus, cysts, tumors, or similar *damp* conditions in this region of the body should avoid spirulina, although spirulina is often beneficial for these conditions when *coldness* is not a factor. People who have a *cold* constitution—especially when accompanied by dryness, thinness, *deficiency*, or lack of groundedness (spaciness)—should avoid wild blue-green, and use cereal grass sparingly.

The person with **heat** signs (feels hot often, deep red tongue, yellow tongue coating, has an aversion to heat) and inflammatory conditions including arthritis, ulcers, hepatitis, gastritis, pancreatitis, or canker sores can be treated most efficiently with wheat- or barley-grass products because of their P4D1 fraction and chlorophyll. A little less effective but very useful are any of the green micro-algae. Spirulina and chlorella are especially good remedies for the *deficient* person with inflammation and other *heat* signs.

For cancer, AIDS, Epstein-Barr syndrome, multiple sclerosis, rheumatoid arthritis, tumors, candida overgrowth, excessive mucus, edema, and other conditions associated with **dampness**, wild blue-green is generally the most useful. Individuals who are not particularly *excessive* will benefit from a moderate dosage of 1.5–2 grams. The upper dosage ranges of cereal grass, chlorella (excellent for disorders with immune malfunction), spirulina, and dunaliella are also beneficial additions (often spirulina and dunaliella are used together). One may choose the one or two most appropriate of these green foods based on their properties.

For the robust person who has a *dampness*-related disease accompanied by clear signs of *excess*, 10 grams daily or more of wild blue-green is a therapeutic dosage. Also recommended: cereal grass 2–3 times a day; the other micro-algae can be added if indicated.

In cases of frailty or severe weakness, chlorella or spirulina is the best choice. In addition to these, 1 gram of wild blue-green once or twice daily lifts the heavy mentality and depression that accompany *damp*, weak conditions.

Considerations and Specific Uses

Economy: Those who need substantial amounts of dietary GLA fatty acid, beta-carotene, and easily digested protein can choose spirulina as the most economical source. The economy of spirulina is due to its simple harvesting and processing. The processing of chlorella and wild blue-green is more complex—these micro-algae seem destined to remain dietary supplements, whereas spirulina has potential as a principal food and protein source.

When considering other nutrients, cost comparisons differ. Depending on the particular crop of wild blue-green and spirulina, chlorella will usually be the most economical source of chlorophyll. Additionally, some properties and nutritional factors cannot be compared because they exist in only one type of micro-alga. For example, CGF is found only in chlorella, and phycocyanin is unique to blue-green algae. And the cost of any one micro-algae from different sources can vary widely. Spirulina prices differ most—by as much as 300%. Tablets and capsules are always more expensive.

Vitamin/mineral supplement: Wild blue-green and wheat and barley grasses grown on rich soil during a cold season have the most balanced vitamin/mineral contents. Spirulina and chlorella have varying nutrient concentrations, depending on their cultivation; in most cases these too offer an excellent array of vitamins and minerals.

Exercise supplement: Those who do strenuous physical exercise need superior fluid metabolism to keep their sinews and joints flexible and free of inflammation.

Spirulina provides these *(yin)* fluids better than the other micro-algae or cereal grasses. However, if inflammations persist in spite of spirulina use, then a wise addition is cereal grass, with its specific anti-inflammatory properties discussed earlier. In fact, cereal grass can be recommended as a protection against inflammation during most endurance sports contests and work-outs, where extreme body heat is generated.

The unique macro-nutrients of spirulina—its particular forms of protein, carbohydrates, and fatty acids—are abundantly available in the 15- to 20-gram dosage range. For example, the protein from 20 grams of spirulina may be equivalent to several ounces of meat because of the superior assimilability of spirulina and its relative lack of toxic metabolic by-products. Other attributes of spirulina: its predigested protein provides building material soon after ingestion, without the energy-draining side effects of meat protein; its mucopolysaccharides relax and strengthen connective tissue while reducing the possibility of inflammation; its simple carbohydrates yield immediate yet sustained energy; its GLA fatty acids improve hormonal balance; and its protein-bonded vitamins and minerals, as found in all whole foods, assimilate better than the synthetic variety. Spirulina can generally be considered an appropriate food for those who exercise vigorously, as evidenced by the many world-class athletes who use it.

The chlorophyll of cereal grass and all green micro-algae is helpful for detoxifying the liver, kidneys, and blood of impurities that result from strenuous physical exertion.

The proteins, carbohydrates, and several other nutrients in spirulina are also available from chlorella and wild blue-green in much the same form, but in smaller amounts in their normal dosage range—these micro-algae are seldom used in 15-gram doses the way spirulina is. Nevertheless, there are other reasons that athletes benefit from chlorella and wild blue-green. Chlorella Growth Factor promotes growth and repair of tissues of all kinds, including nerve tissue. The cerebral stimulus from wild blue-green can liberate surprising amounts of stored physical energy; it also improves mental concentration in the robust individual, an essential factor in competitive sports.

Depression: Wild blue-green excels for lifting bad moods; spirulina, chlorella, and cereal grass are also useful.

Anemia: All cereal grasses and green micro-algae discussed in this section are good blood tonics, but spirulina and chlorella are best for building up blood deficiency caused by weak digestive absorption and poor spleen-pancreas function, because these micro-algae are less cooling and cleansing than wild blue-green and wheat or barley grass. (See "Blood Deficiency" in Chapter 31.)

Malnutrition: Chlorella and especially spirulina have long records of use for emaciation and malnutrition in people of all ages. They also treat childhood malabsorption syndrome, when digestion in children all but ceases. To treat this and malnutrition in general, either of these micro-algae can become a major feature of the diet.

Aging and poor immunity: Premature aging and immune system breakdown come about most rapidly from free-radical damage. Superb protection against such damage is offered by the fraction P4D1 and the anti-oxidant combination of beta-carotene and superoxide dismutase (SOD), all found within a rich matrix of other nutrients in cereal grass. In addition to protection, P4D1 activates renewal of damaged nucleic acids (RNA/DNA). The great quantity of digestive enzymes in cereal grass improves digestive absorption so that more immune-strengthening, anti-aging nutrients can be utilized.

Similarly, the nucleic acids and beta-carotene in micro-algae are effective for retarding aging and fortifying immunity. Although cereal grass provides the best single protection, adding micro-algae has even greater effectiveness. As discussed earlier, those who are *deficient* and/or *cold* will usually do better taking spirulina or chlorella and using cereal grass carefully.

Weight loss: A central factor in weight loss is the fatty acid GLA, of which spirulina is the richest source. Next best for weight loss are wild blue-green and cereal grass. Chlorella helps regulate body weight in general in persons with weak digestive energy (poor absorption, lack of appetite, loose stools), but is usually not an effective weight loss remedy for those with a dietary history rich in meat, dairy, and eggs.

Hypoglycemia and diabetes: All three green micro-algae—spirulina, chlorella, and wild blue-green—are ideal for controlling hypoglycemia because they contain a sufficient quantity of predigested carbohydrates to supply energy that endures. Also, the predigested protein in these calms blood sugar turbulence in both hypo- and hyperglycemia (diabetes). To simply control sugar cravings, as little as $\frac{1}{2}$ gram of any of these micro-algae, taken at the time of craving, is often an effective remedy. Spirulina is the best choice when larger amounts of protein are needed for rebuilding the sugar-regulating function of the adrenals, liver, and pancreas, because its standard dosage provides sufficient protein for this purpose. Since diabetes usually entails a lack of natural GLA fatty acid synthesis in the body,[44] spirulina has been particularly useful here.[45]

Liver renewal: General liver rejuvenation can be assisted by choosing micro-algae or wheat grass according to the "General Guidelines" section above. For complete renewal in every case, plan on taking the appropriate green food(s) for at least one year. (See *Wood Element*, Chapter 24, for suggestions on liver renewal and a discussion of liver syndromes.)

Other specific liver patterns: A fiery or excessive liver signified by *heat* signs such as red eyes, flushed face, and a tendency toward anger is best overcome by using substantial amounts of wheat grass or wild blue-green. Dunaliella is also a helpful addition because of its cooling, detoxifying nature.

When there is severe liver damage from long-term use of alcohol or drugs, easily digested protein is indicated, and any of the green micro-algae fulfill this need. In these cases of liver excess and liver damage, wild blue-green and chlorella are best taken in the 10-gram/day range, much higher than their normal dosage.

Spirulina dosage for these conditions is about 20 grams/day.

Liver stagnancy with signs such as spasm, swellings (especially of the throat), pain, and depression can benefit from the standard dosage of any of the micro-algae or wheat grass.

Greens in the Diet

Remember that *every* green food has helpful amounts of chlorophyll and can be used for building blood, cleansing, and controlling the growth of unwanted microorganisms. The high-oxalate greens such as spinach, beet greens, and chard, however, must be taken in limited quantities by those with mineral deficiencies or loose stools because of the laxative and calcium-depleting effect of their substantial oxalic acid content. Appropriate chlorophyll-rich foods, chosen mostly from the common green vegetables, can healthfully occupy 15–20% of the diet of modern people. This relatively high percentage is recommended especially for those living in very polluted areas. While this intense period, which begins a new era in our history, offers certain advantages, the many toxic effects of the environment and common diet need to be countered with the green color of renewal.

Vitamin A and Beta-Carotene

All chlorophyll (green) plants have certain pigments known as carotenes. Chlorophyll and carotene, in fact, work synergistically in several ways. One vital relationship occurs when chlorophyll activates enzymes which produce vitamins E and K, and help convert carotene into vitamin A. For this reason, green sources of carotene convert more than twice as much of their carotene into vitamin A as do yellow foods. This increased action catalyzed by chlorophyll is helpful for those who are deficient in vitamin A, but it is not always essential since the carotene not converted has other functions.

"Beta" carotene makes up the majority of carotene in plants, and from a plethora of current studies is thought to be especially beneficial in treating cancer, tumors, and other diseases related to weakened immunity. While vitamin A and beta-carotene appear almost interchangeably in the discussions that follow, it is helpful to keep in mind that beta carotene is only one source of vitamin A and at the same time has additional nutrient features, particularly in the area of immune enhancement.

Causes of the Widespread Vitamin A Deficit

One of the most widely recognized nutritional deficiencies of recent times is of vitamin A. Not only are too few A-rich green and yellow vegetables consumed, but liver, the one good source of vitamin A in the animal kingdom, is often neglected. Beef liver contains 44,000 I.U. of vitamin A per 3½-ounce serving. However, it may be fortunate when liver is not eaten, not only for reasons of compassion, but because commercially raised animals are all too likely to be saturated with chemicals, hormones, and drugs, and these accumulate in their livers.

Lack of food in the diet containing vitamin A is an obvious reason for its deficiency, but its multiple functions provide another. Vitamin A plays many key roles in the metabolic processes of the liver. This organ is overworked in most people because of the consumption of rich, greasy, toxin-laden, highly processed food, and from overeating in general. With such a diet, one can hardly know how much vitamin A is sufficient; some nutritionists now advise five or ten times the Recommended Dietary Allowance.

When people on an excessive diet show vitamin A deficiency, clearly the first course of action is to see if the deficiency resolves through simple moderation. Many vegetarians who eat too much fat in the form of nuts, seeds, and oils—and ingest excess protein from grains and legumes—also show vitamin A deficiency patterns such as flaky scalp, dry skin, and premature aging (from insufficient RNA—see below).

Once an excessive diet is moderated, then vitamin A can help re-establish proper liver function. An advantage of using the beta-carotene (of vegetables) as a source of vitamin A is its non-toxic property. Any excess of beta-carotene is stored in the body until needed, whereas vitamin A from animal products (retinol) is toxic in large doses. Research with cancers indicates that beta-carotene has an anti-tumor effect which is far superior to retinol.[46]

Major Properties of Vitamin A

- Essential for the correct metabolism of protein by the body.
- Greatly enhances production of RNA, which transmits to each cell vital information on function and renewal.
- Protects the body at the level of the skin, tissue, and cell surfaces: protects mucous membranes of the mouth, nose, throat, and lungs, reducing susceptibility to infections; neutralizes the effects of air pollution on these areas; softens skin and increases its resistance to disease; fortifies the flow of protective *qi* energy; on the cellular level, strengthens cell walls to inhibit penetration by viruses.
- Helps build and repair bones, teeth, hair, nails, skin, and the mucous membranes of the lungs and in the digestive and reproductive tracts. Helps form rich blood, maintains good vision, and protects against night blindness.
- Activates the thymus gland and immune system.

Specific Actions Attributed to Beta-Carotene Foods

More than twenty-five years of worldwide research indicates that people who consume foods with more than average amounts of beta-carotene have a lower incidence of cancer of the lungs, stomach, colon, bladder, uterus, ovaries, and skin. The National Research Council also supports the use of vitamin A/beta-carotene foods in cancer prevention;[47] in one nineteen-year study reported in a British medical journal, *The Lancet,* there was a seven-fold decrease in cancer incidences among heavy smokers who also had comparatively high beta-carotene intake.[48]

According to Charles Simone, M.D., author of *Cancer and Nutrition* (McGraw-Hill, 1983), beta-carotene is the "most potent free-radical neutralizer or scavenger known today . . . [it] blocks the process by which a normal cell can turn malignant."

Note: Only foods rich in beta-carotene appear to prevent cancer; isolated beta-carotene in supplements has not been proven effective.[49,50]

Food Sources of Vitamin A from Carotene

in International Units
100-gram (3½-ounce) Samples*

Dunaliella	8,300,000	Green onions	5,000
Spirulina	250,000	Watercress	4,900
Wild blue-green	70,000	Winter squash	4,200
Wheat/Barley grass	66,000	Collard	3,300
Chlorella	55,000	Swiss chard	3,300
Carrot	28,000	Chinese cabbage	3,000
Sweet potato	26,000	Apricot	2,700
Kale	8,900	Romaine lettuce	2,600
Parsley	8,500	Persimmon	1,800
Spinach	8,100	Cantaloupe	1,800
Turnip green	7,600	Peach	400
Beet green	6,100		

*Note: only the dunaliella, spirulina, wild blue-green, chlorella, and wheat/barley grass samples are dried.

Signs of Vitamin A Deficiency

Deficiency often appears as rough, dry, prematurely aged and wrinkled skin; skin diseases in general; loss of sense of smell; allergies; dandruff; night blindness; eye inflammation; and dryness of the mucous membranes of the mouth and of the respiratory and reproductive systems.

Dosage: The Recommended Dietary Allowance of vitamin A is 4,000–5,000 I.U. daily for adults and 1,500–4,000 for children. Those who are pregnant, lactating, or undergoing a disease process usually have greater requirements. More vitamin A is needed in the cooler seasons and also by those who use their eyes extensively for reading or other focused work.

To heal the causes of deficiency, very often vitamin A/beta-carotene foods need to be emphasized for a year or more. The effect in the body of vitamin A from food is much more potent than from synthetic supplements, so for deficiencies one may start with what is considered a relatively small amount—perhaps several times the RDA, or about 15,000–25,000 I.U. daily.

Food choices can be based on other properties. For example, a person with constipation should choose more yellow foods rather than blue-green. (Yellow food stimulates peristalsis, whereas blue cools and astringes.) Someone with inflammations would do better with the chlorophyll-rich blue or green foods. The taste of the food will help guide the quantity needed, since the sense of taste will usually tell a person when enough has been eaten. If wheat grass or micro-alga tablets are used, chewing them well will increase their absorption as well as give a clue to optimal dosage level.

Good results can normally be seen from adequate beta-carotene intake, not only for disease conditions but for bolstering wellness and increasing the attributes of vitality and longevity. Middle-aged people who have lustrous, wrinkle-free skin have invariably had beta-carotene-rich diets for many years, often during their growing years.

It is good to remember that the highest vitamin A/beta-carotene sources, the micro-algae, are ingested in relatively small amounts. For example, typical servings of spirulina range from a teaspoon (three grams) to a tablespoon (7.5 grams) or heaping tablespoon (ten grams), yielding 7,500, 18,750, and 25,000 I.U. of vitamin A, respectively. A 3½-ounce portion of kale provides 8,300 I.U., while the same amount of carrots offers 28,000 I.U. Thus, good amounts of vitamin A are available from typical servings of either vegetables or micro-algae.

To obtain the highest therapeutic levels of vitamin A/beta-carotene, dunaliella might be the best choice. One 300-milligram tablet (¹⁄₁₀ teaspoon of powder) provides over 25,000 I.U.; a teaspoonful supplies 250,000 I.U. This level of intake is not considered dangerous when beta-carotene is in a whole food such as micro-algae, but massive amounts, unless required for therapeutic purposes, may eventually create imbalance. This is true of any nutrient or food, even though it may be a completely non-toxic substance. A good indication of too much beta-carotene intake is a yellowing of the skin (carotenemia).

Commercial forms of pure beta-carotene are nearly always synthetic. Long-term results from the whole-food sources will be better.

There can be a wide variance in the beta-carotene content of different samples of the same food. In various 3½-ounce samples, carrots may fluctuate between 100 and 20,000 I.U., and one Hawaiian grower of spirulina purportedly obtains more than 500,000 I.U. per sample—more than double the average. Because of the vast differences in soils and chemicals used in farming, nutrients in land-grown food vary more than the micro-algae. Knowing the sources of food and choosing for quality ensures more nutrients.

There are some conditions in which beta-carotene and other carotenoids do not convert well into vitamin A in the body. Among these are diabetes mellitus and hypothyroidism. In these cases, the vitamin A of animal products (retinol) becomes a useful substitute. This does not mean that beta-carotene should be neglected altogether, since it is possible that many of its immune functions derive from the portion that does not convert to vitamin A.[46]

Survival Simplified

In anticipation of a crisis that would result in disruption of the food supply, many individuals have put aside stores of freeze-dried survival rations containing their favorite foods. There is a degree of wisdom in having a secure food supply, since this affects the stability of one's emotions in ways that are not always conscious.

However, there is a simpler alternative to commercially preserved food supplies. Non-perishables such as grains, legumes, seaweeds, and salt can be kept in sufficient quantity to last a year or more if carefully stored. In any event, this is certainly the most economical and convenient way to purchase these items.

Grains and legumes and their products can be prepared with endless variety. In addition, for fresh high-nutrient food, all seeds (grains, beans, peas, and lentils) can be sprouted, and the grasses from wheat, rye, barley, or oats will supply nourishing greens. In a crisis involving radiation or a plague, these foods are excellent immunity-builders, and the cereal grasses, seaweeds, and salty foods detoxify radiation. Seeds, of course, can be re-planted each year, so they represent a renewable food supply.

Medical statistics show that during World War II, people in Norway experienced the best health of their lives. Heart disease, cancer, and schizophrenia incidences suddenly dropped forty percent. They ate more of their traditional foods—whole grains, beans, vegetables, and fresh fish—but little of the meat, margarine (hydrogenated oils), refined sugar, or processed foods that had become a major part of their pre-war diets.[1, 2] Ideally, this present generation will discover health and vitality through choice rather than crisis.

Enjoyment of Food

The way you eat is an expression of who you are, regardless of the quality of the food. The enjoyment of good food and company creates such an inner joy that it's possible to taste the sweetest of nectar in even the simplest of food. Without this joy, and with no blessing offered, the most wholesome, delicious food can seem tasteless and leave the soul hungry. People who eat only for the taste or according to a diet or nutritional value often develop cravings for something they aren't getting. They bring turmoil into their lives and homes in their constant search, and they eat to satisfy a misplaced hunger.

Overeating and Aging

Overeating, a popular pastime in the wealthy nations, is thought to be the major cause of premature aging (see also "Aging" in Chapter 28). Fifty years of research have shown that when a nourishing diet is eaten sparingly, aging is retarded; the maximum life span and immunity are extended in all animal species so far tested, from protozoa to worms, insects, fish, and rodents as well as humans.[1, 2] In fact, consumption of too much rich and denatured food is responsible for most of our civilized diseases, such as obesity, cancer, and diabetes. Overeating by vegetarians also occurs regularly, and while it may not always result in weight gain, it invariably causes weakness, digestive upset, and accelerated aging.

On an emotional level, overeating results from excessive and undifferentiated desire, which also leads one to choose an unnecessarily great variety of foods. Each food has a unique flavor which the appetite control center of the hypothalamus recognizes. Before it feels satisfied, the hypothalamus seeks a certain amount of every flavor it has sampled. Thus it is very difficult not to overeat a meal of many ingredients.

Another cause of an unusually huge appetite is parasites. Symptoms and cures are listed under "Parasites" in Chapter 7 and Appendix A.

Refined foods may also contribute to overeating, according to a scientific study reported by the U.S. Agricultural Research Service (March 1, 1999). An explanation is that one is biologically conditioned over millions of years of human evolution to consume whole foods; excessive eating may represent an instinctive craving to obtain nutrients that are lost during refining. Common foods depleted in nutrients include "white" refined: sugar, pasta, bread, pastries, and rice; refined oils, and reduced-fat dairy.

Habitual overeating, especially of meat and strong flavors, inflames the lining of the stomach. According to Chinese medicine, excess *heat* in the stomach is itself a cause of overeating, but even when this *heat*-overeating cycle is broken, one still must change underlying habits, which may have become imbedded in the body's cells and organs over many years.

Achieving a Balanced Appetite

1. Overcome excess desires which manifest in elaborate, complex meals. At the same time, begin eating simply.
2. If overeating is habitual, consume raw vegetables and fruit regularly to cool a fiery stomach. Celery is especially good. When it is difficult to stop eating, eat celery to help end the meal. Also try eating more meals of whole fruit or vegetables or their juices. However, bitter vegetables such as celery, lettuce, and raw plant food worsen the condition of overeaters with a thin, *dry,* nervous, or *deficient* constitution. These individuals would wisely choose to eat cooked vegetables or fruit. Especially helpful for reducing stomach inflammation in all overeaters are cooked cabbage and an herbal tea of slippery elm bark.
3. In general, more liquid needs to be in the diet of overeaters, for example, soups and stews. When there is thirst between meals, herbal and other beverages including water can be taken. In addition, concentrated chlorophyll products such as wheat grass, spirulina and other micro-algae, and dark leafy greens also cool the stomach. (See *Green Food Products, C*hapter 16, for help in choosing the most appropriate chlorophyll foods.)
4. Reduce consumption of foods which may inflame the stomach: meats, fried or oily food, nuts, seeds, and very salty or warming flavors (garlic and other members of the onion family, and cinnamon, ginger, cumin, fennel, caraway, hot peppers, etc.).
5. Never eat yourself full. A helpful rule is offered in the teachings of the ancient Essenes, who lived long and vigorous lives: Stop eating when two-thirds full.[3]
6. Breathe deeply and chew thoroughly. Both of these practices encourage patience and help reduce desire.

The Art of Chewing

Eating begins with the simple art of chewing. Chew well to polarize the food with your system and in order to make smooth digestion possible.

If under pressure at meals, simply chew, and let the chewing relax you. Then you can be grateful and enjoy the whole spectrum of tastes and aromas that make up the meal.

Carbohydrate digestion begins in the mouth. Thorough chewing turns grains and other complex carbohydrates into satisfying sugars and makes oils, proteins, and minerals available for maximum absorption. Whole vegetal foods, especially whole grains, must be mixed with saliva and chewed until liquid to release their full nutritional value. Without adequate chewing you will feel heavy and dull, develop gas, and be undernourished. Meats, fats, sweets, and processed foods satisfy the immediate desire for taste, but soon dull the taste buds. The more they are chewed, the worse they taste. The more whole carbohydrate foods are chewed, the sweeter they become. Dry bread, common dry "rice cakes" found in most food stores, and whole grains without sauce encourage one to chew. Because digestion becomes so efficient, the body begins to feel wonderfully light.

To get started in the correct habit of chewing, try counting the chewing of each bite thirty to fifty times at the beginning of each meal. It helps to put down your fork/spoon/chopsticks between bites.

American nutritionist Horace Fletcher (1849–1919) became famous for Fletcherism, the art of thorough mastication. Ancient Japanese and Chinese traditions also teach the benefits of chewing well. Most modern people must re-learn this forgotten art in order to make a successful transition to whole foods.

Other Concerns About Eating and Nourishment

- Do not be so rigid or self-righteous about your diet as to annoy anyone. A bad relationship is more poisonous than one of Grandma's sugar cookies. If you desire such a treat, it is better to have it than stuff yourself with rice to suppress the desire. This causes mental anguish and arrogance.
- Set aside a special time and place for meals in a clean environment, surrounded with pleasant sounds, aromas, colors, and conversation. Avoid emotionally charged subjects and confused, scattered talk or thoughts. Avoid eating while tired, too hot or too cold, worried, angry, standing, watching TV, reading, or before bathing. These activities make the food hard to digest. Relax and get comfortable. Perhaps undertake self-reflection about your condition. Eating is a time to receive offerings in the form of food to nurture and revitalize your body. Nurture your thought as well. Consider your manners insofar as they represent your intention toward others. Give attention to the unique qualities of each food and the work involved in bringing it to you.
- Relax after eating, but do not fall asleep or into a stupor. Relaxation helps you digest your food and sleep well at night.
- Give thanks before and after eating.
- Choose the majority of your foods from local growers. (This helps not only your health but your local economy and also the environment by using fewer resources for shipping and refrigeration.) Eat according to your health and constitutional needs.
- Liquids and food should not be too hot or too cold. This is especially important for infants and children. Heat debilitates the stomach and creates acidity. Cold paralyzes it.
- Drinking with meals dilutes the digestive juices. However, a small amount of warm water—four ounces or less—is acceptable. In general, drink water or herbal teas ten to twenty minutes before meals and at least half an hour after fruit meals, two hours after a meal rich in starches and plant proteins such as grains and legumes, and four hours after a meal containing meat, eggs, or dairy products.

Meal Schedules:
The Nature of One, Two, or Three Daily Meals

In order to arrive at a health-promoting eating schedule, one may want to take into account important physiological factors.

The night and early morning hours before approximately five A.M. are passive times of the day when the digestive organs need to rest. The liver in particular needs to complete numerous subtle metabolic functions unhampered by the early stages of digestive activity. One of these functions is blood purification, which is interrupted and altered when late meals are eaten. According to the "Chinese clock," the most active time for the liver is between one and three A.M.

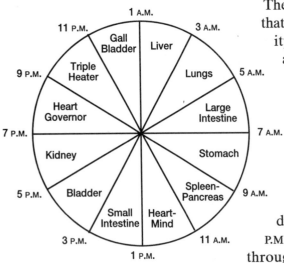

The Chinese clock is an ancient observation that the body's internal organs have peak activity during two-hour intervals. This theory also suggests that an organ's minimum activity is twelve hours away from its peak interval. For example, the peak activity of the stomach is from seven to nine A.M., and its minimum activity is twelve hours later, from seven to nine P.M.

The further away from peak liver activity the meal is taken, the more completely the liver can perform its several hundred functions. If the last meal is eaten at six P.M., seven hours are available for food to go through preliminary digestive processes. Since grains and legumes stay in the stomach for up to three hours, the remaining three hours or so in the small intestine for assimilation is none too long; the products of assimilation must then be processed by the liver. Thus, many Far-Eastern spiritual practitioners eat one meal a day before noon. In this way there will be at least twelve hours before the liver has its greatest activity.

The types of food eaten on a single meal plan can vary greatly since there are almost twenty-four hours to complete digestion. Some kinds of foods that present difficulty because of their long digestive time can actually be beneficial to people with a single meal schedule. For example, the peanut greatly slows the metabolic rate; this effect poses a problem for those eating multiple meals. However, peanuts are traditionally sought after by those eating once a day. Foods such as the potato which build the *yin* fluids are valued since the body contracts and easily dehydrates during its day-long fast; dark leafy greens are also emphasized, since these also help maintain the body's fluids.

When the single meal is eaten within an hour of noon, it falls during the heart-mind time interval. At this time the intuitions are heightened, and choices for *what is eaten* and *how much* are clearer—an especially important consideration when there is only one opportunity each day for choosing foods.

Serious Chinese Zen monks and their American counterparts still maintain a single-meal dietary practice. They are sufficiently energized (by this and their other practices) that their only "sleep" is from midnight until three A.M., during which time they sit in meditation. Three A.M. is the beginning of the lungs' two-hour cycle, the ideal time to arise and do breathing exercises. Many yogis and meditators will naturally arise between three and five A.M., a time of day when the *prana* (*qi* and breath) vitality is heightened. Furthermore, because the body is not burdened by digestion, the entire eight-hour time period between three A.M. and the single meal at eleven A.M. can be an exceptional time of day for profound spiritual experience.

This example of one daily meal—and the way it complements a lifestyle centered upon self-awareness—is important, since it sets the groundwork for understanding more common eating patterns. It illustrates two central ideas: one, that eating late at night can cause the liver and its subtle metabolic processes to work less efficiently; and two, that with less food one generally has more energy, greater clarity, and a need for far less sleep. However, the daily single meal is not recommended for those without strong discipline, since they may eat two or three meals' worth of food at the single meal. Otherwise, it is a good practice for nearly everyone one day of the week—a day to rest the digestive organs with one simple meal. Blood-sugar problems that may arise will be discussed later.

Two Meals Per Day

The two-meal daily schedule is optimum for most people who have adjusted to a grain-and-vegetable diet. In the morning, there should be an hour or two after rising before eating so that the body and internal organs can gradually adjust from dormancy to a state of more active energy. In any case, wait until hungry before eating. Often hunger will not occur until several hours into the morning.

According to biological rhythms portrayed by the Chinese clock, the hours between seven and nine A.M. are the optimal time to eat, since they are the most active time for the stomach, although nine to eleven A.M.—the interval when pancreatic activity is emphasized—is also a good time, if this is when hunger signals. This meal must be moist enough to help with morning dehydration, and must also have sufficient calories, protein, and carbohydrates to support one in the warmest and most active part of the day, the afternoon.

The first meal should be larger than the second, and should be prepared with more water. For example, if cereal creams (such as rice cream) are eaten, they are normally prepared with several times more water than the whole unmilled grain. And if unmilled grains are included, they too can be cooked with extra water. In general, the first meal of the two-meal schedule can contain lightly cooked or raw items. An exception is made for persons with signs of *coldness* or *deficiency*. They should have at most only minor amounts of raw or lightly cooked foods.

The second meal can be in the mid-afternoon or later, preferably before sunset or seven P.M., whichever comes first. With sunset the body receives the signal to begin more internal metabolic and hormonal processes, and the stomach is considered an exterior organ (compared with the liver or pancreas). Seven P.M. also initiates the weakest period of time for the stomach. We have seen the best therapeutic results from eating the last meal earlier in the afternoon, around three or four P.M. This allows a good nine hours before the time of heightened activity of the liver. As the second meal is moved later in the day, which is necessary for many working people, its quantity should become less. When later meals are eaten, it is best to stay up for at least four hours afterward.

The last meal should be smaller in quantity, since the inactive part of the day is approaching. It should also contain more cooked food because of the night's cool and internal qualities. Therefore the last meal naturally includes inner-directing food: root vegetables and concentrated proteins such as lentils or tempeh can be emphasized. These are general tendencies, and do not mean that the first meal cannot contain proteins and root vegetables.

Three-Meal Schedule

The three-meal-per-day plan is perhaps most practical for the greatest number of people. When one has grown up with the rhythm of three meals, it is best to stay with this rhythm until the body signals it is time for a change. This normally occurs when the pancreas, liver, adrenals, and other organs are sufficiently healed so that blood-sugar levels are stabilized. Once stability is reached, one will usually be hungry only two times a day.

The three-meal plan reflects most people's low blood-sugar conditions, and also clearly delineates the three periods of the day. Optimally, the first meal is taken during the stomach interval between seven and nine A.M., but of course not until hunger is felt. Like the first meal of the two-meal plan, it is ideally warm and prepared with ample water, but it does not need the variety of raw or lightly cooked items since it only takes one through the cooler time of day. (A raw, cleansing option is described later.) This should be a simple meal. A typical example is mild miso-ginger soup and one grain such as oatmeal or sweet rice cream.

The second meal, usually at noon or shortly thereafter, can be the largest meal of the day. It requires more variety, and for those who are neither *cold* nor *deficient*, it is the best time to eat cooling food (such as salad) since it must balance the hottest and most active part of the day. The afternoon is when blood-sugar levels dip to their lowest point.

The last meal should be the smallest; it is cooked and ideally contains a concentrated protein such as legumes, nuts, seeds, dairy, or if needed for *deficiency*, other animal products. It is eaten at least four hours after the second meal and preferably before seven P.M.

The Morning Elixir

Upon awakening, one is often thirsty but not hungry. Because of dehydration during sleep, and the fact that sleep is an internal process, one will often desire expansive liquids to satisfy dryness and bring the energy up and out of its dormant phase. When the body is stiff and the mind unclear after rising, it means that the liver has not completed its necessary blood purification. This condition reflects either habitual or recent overeating, consumption of too many animal products, intoxicants, or poor-quality food, improper food combining, and/or late eating.

Even healthy people, however, are usually a little thirsty after sleep. When one awakens with high energy and a clear mind, then only thirst needs to be satisfied. This can be done with just a small amount of herbal tea or water. If there is a groggy condition, more cleansing fluids can be drunk in order to purify the system at this time. Typical beverages—which we call "elixirs" because of their refreshing and detoxifying qualities—are listed in the following chart according to their cleansing nature. They are best at least slightly warmed in order to add an expansive quality, and in no case should they be served cooler than room temperature.

If one tends toward *coldness* or weakness, then it is safest to stay near the top of the list. As *excessive* signs (thick tongue coating, reddish complexion, strong voice, forceful pulse, and robust body and personality) become more prominent, a person benefits more from the more strongly cleansing elixirs. If *damp* conditions exist such as obesity, edema, candida yeast overgrowth, and carbuncles, then bitter

	Elixir	**Examples**
less cleansing	warming teas	ginger, fenugreek, cinnamon, star anise, fennel, spearmint
	vegetable broth	cabbage, parsley
	micro-alga drink	spirulina or chlorella
	water	plain or with squeezed lemon
	vegetable juice	carrot, celery
	fruit juice	apple, prune, grape, orange
	barley/wheat-grass juice	freshly extracted, or from commercial wheat- or barley-grass powders
	wild micro-alga drink	freeze-dried wild blue-green micro-alga (*Aphanizomenon*)
	root teas	burdock, dandelion, chicory (usually with roasted barley in coffee substitutes)
more cleansing	flower teas	chamomile, red clover blossoms, orange blossoms

plants such as burdock, dandelion, chicory, chamomile, wild blue-green micro-alga, and cereal grasses are beneficial.

The Purifying Morning Meal

The morning is an important time for cleansing since it is the time that one has been without food longest. In addition to the morning elixir, those who need a gradual cleansing program for any reason—especially if moving away from an extremely rich diet—may choose to eat primarily purifying foods for the first meal. One would normally choose only vegetables or fruits for a purifying meal. People who generally do best with these foods are robust, strong, and have signs of *excess* and/or *heat*. When a tendency exists toward candida overgrowth, weak digestion with loose stools, or low blood sugar, fruit is *not* recommended.

If fruit or vegetables are eaten in the earlier, cooler part of the day, they usually create better balance when they are at least slightly cooked. If the first meal is eaten close to the afternoon, then the cooling value of eating some of the food raw should be considered. Nevertheless, individuals with pronounced *excess* and *heat* signs often benefit from raw food at any time. In deciding between cooked or raw food, one should always first consider personal health signs before temperature fluctuations of the day.

Local Food

As a person becomes more balanced, food that grows well in the native locale becomes more appealing, and eating according to the daily, seasonal, and climatic influences takes on greater importance. Local plant and animal foods are generated from similar soil, water, and air, and share the same climatic conditions. Thus they are uniquely adapted to support the life of their area's inhabitants. For this reason, some people maintain that it is best to eat 100% of the diet from one's own region (loosely defining "region" as within a 300- to 500-mile radius encompassing all areas with similar environmental patterns). We feel an ideal percentage may be around 90%. Since many soils are deficient in some nutrients, there is a likelihood of gaining the deficient nutrients by sampling food from other areas. Also, when a small portion of the diet originates from another area of the planet, a link is created to that area, insofar as food partakes of numerous qualities indigenous to where it is grown.

Between-Meal Snacks For Low Blood Sugar

Adjusting to any new meal schedule may take time, and perhaps the biggest obstacle comes from low blood sugar. When the blood sugar level falls, a person can easily become depressed and weak. (See *Blood Sugar Imbalances,* Chapter 29.) Even though it is not a good practice to eat between meals, it is necessary in some cases when three meals a day are insufficient. The best choices of between-meal snacks include complex carbohydrates and proteins. Sometimes these are the same food; rice cakes, for instance, have good percentages of both. Starchy veg-

Meal Scheduling Summary

Number of Daily Meals

	Three Meals per Day	Two Meals per Day	One Meal per Day
Type of Person Recommended For:	Those who work hard physically, or have low blood sugar (crave sweets), or are beginning a transition to a grain- and vegetable-based diet.	Those who have adjusted to a grain-and-vegetable diet; this plan helps develop good physical and/or mental qualities.	Those who have firm discipline. This plan can support advanced development of mind and spirit.

Optimum Meal Times

First Meal	7–9 A.M.	7–11 A.M.	11 A.M.–1 P.M.
Second Meal	11 A.M.–1 P.M.	3–6 P.M.	
Third Meal	4–7 P.M.		

Meal Size and Special Features

First Meal	A) Simple and of moderate size, prepared with ample water and cooked, or B) a cleansing meal of vegetables or fruit for those who need purification.	Larger, more varied, containing some lightly cooked or raw food.	Moderate in size with sufficient variety; prepared with ample water and containing some raw or lightly cooked items. Dark, leafy greens are helpful.
Second Meal	Largest in size and greatest variety, containing some lightly cooked or raw food.	Smaller, simpler, and cooked. Contains the most protein; root vegetables are emphasized.	
Third Meal	Smallest size and cooked; may contain the most protein; root vegetables are emphasized.		

etables, especially carrots, quickly raise blood sugar levels. Micro-algae and bee pollen also are used successfully for this purpose. The easiest choice for a snack, of course, is the concentrated sweeteners and fruits, since they satisfy quickly—but they may cause even lower blood sugar later. Fruit and sweeteners vary greatly in their ability to stabilize blood sugar (see *Sweeteners,* Chapter 11). The previous chart summarizes the suggestions for the three meal schedules.

For All Meal Plans

A) The Morning Elixir: Soon after rising, quench thirst with water, herbal tea, vegetable broths, green drinks (wheat/barley grass or spirulina drinks), or vegetable or fruit juice. These drinks should be at least slightly warm.

B) Interval between rising and first meal: Wait one to two hours or more before first meal; eat only when hungry—this applies to all meals.

C) Very weak or sick people should eat according to condition and hunger. See *Excess and Deficiency,* Chapter 6.

Food Combinations

The Importance of Food Combining

Too much elaborate food encourages nearly everyone—even people who normally live moderately—to overindulge. The consequence is digestive fermentation, contaminated blood, and a confused mind. Common digestive disturbances from poor food combining include decreased nutrient assimilation, intestinal gas, and abdominal pain and swelling. If such eating practices continue over time, degenerative conditions can ensue.

Food combining and most other successful nutritional guidelines follow a central physiological principle: Proper and complete assimilation of food is a result of the action of digestive enzymes. Different types of food (even foods within the same group, such as two different grains) require their own unique enzymes.

When many different ingredients are eaten at the same meal, the body becomes confused and is not able to manufacture all of the necessary enzymes simultaneously. At this point digestion still takes place, but partially through bacterial action, which always causes fermentation and the associated problems mentioned earlier.

When the protein in any food is digested enzymatically, the result is that amino acids are made available to repair and maintain the body. Bacterial digestion also makes amino acids available, but creates additional poisonous by-products such as ptomaines and leucomaines. Similarly, bacterial fermentation of starch results in toxic products—alcohols, acetic acid, lactic acid, and carbon dioxide. The healthful digestion of starch by enzymes yields only simple sugars. Digestive fermentation is not to be confused with more healthful, controlled fermentations such as those used in sourdough products, sauerkraut, miso, tempeh, etc.

Some people tolerate certain food combinations that others do not. During a time of illness or crisis, it may be imperative to adhere to stricter than usual rules of food combining. In any case, when a grain- and vegetable-based diet is followed without good results, it is usually due to improper food combining.

Three food-combining plans are offered here. Plan A is only for those with normal digestion and without serious health conditions; Plan B, the most effective program for digestive excellence, is needed most by persons with poor digestion and/or major health problems; Plan C, a one-pot meal, can include more or less restrictive combinations, depending on the person's digestive strength. It is well-suited to individuals deficient in *yin* fluids.

The food-combining principles of Plan B reflect the eating patterns of our earliest ancestors, when a food was eaten either alone or combined with only one or two other foods. Such primitive eating patterns were practiced for tens of thousands of years and are the foundation of our digestive capacities. For those in a weakened or stressed condition, it is most beneficial and natural to revert to such a simple dietary plan.

Eating simply when in good health is also a way to preserve vitality. A meal of few foods does not mean a paucity of nutrients, since each meal can contain foods different from those of the last meal.

Some of the healthiest people eat simply, as do many children, who are more closely in touch with their instincts. Instincts become stronger during sickness—thus the tendency for ailing people to know what they need (often the simplest fare). Most people will do best when, after exploring their tolerances, they choose suitable parts from each of the following plans.

The rules of Plan A recognize that many people need to eat foods in a certain order and combination for satisfactory digestion.

Plan A: Food Combining for Better Digestion

Fundamental Rule: Simpler meals digest better.

Rule 1. Place highest-protein foods at the beginning of the meal.

The highest-protein foods have priority because they require copious stomach acids, whereas the starches and other foods, by comparison, use very little. Generally, the foods with the highest protein are legumes, nuts, seeds, and animal products. When protein-rich foods are eaten after starches and other food, stomach acids will not be sufficient for their digestion.

Rule 2. The salty foods should be eaten before foods of other flavors.

A small amount of soup can be eaten first if it contains salty high-protein and enzyme-rich products like miso or soy sauce, which activate and encourage digestion. Otherwise, soup dilutes the initial digestive juices needed for protein breakdown and should be saved for the end of the meal. Salty foods go before other flavors since salt has a strongly descending (*yin*) aspect and gravitates to the bottom of the stomach, stimulating gastric juices for the digestion of all other food. When a salty product such as pickles or salt plum is eaten at the end of the meal in small quantity, it can help resolve the gastric chaos resulting from overeating or combining too many foods.

When the stomach is distressed, traditional Chinese medicine teaches that its normally descending energy tends to "ascend," with signs of belching, vomiting, or heartburn; salt can help to reverse this condition, although too much salt can worsen it. The best use of salt is in combination with food near the beginning of a meal; its application as an after-dinner digestive aid is a special use. Legumes are best eaten before grains, not only because of their higher protein content but because they are generally prepared with more salt to aid in their palatability and digestion.

Rule 3. Proteins, fats, and starches combine best with green and non-starchy vegetables.

Green vegetables are the food best eaten at the same time as proteins or starches; however, it is not customary for people with normal digestion to isolate proteins from starches and eat them first, combined only with green and non-starchy vegetables. While such isolation can still be helpful, the minimal intention of Plan A is that when protein, starches, and greens are in the same meal, protein food is emphasized at the beginning of the meal and eaten with generous amounts of green vegetables to aid its digestion. The relationship between greens and protein digestion is discussed in the chapter on protein and vitamin B_{12}.

The relationship of protein foods to starches should also be considered, because the interdigestibility of protein and starch is influenced by the proportion of each. A concentrated protein digests much more easily if it is consumed in relatively small amounts. For example, many people digest a bean and grain meal better if the ratio of beans to grains is at most one-to-two, although ratios as low as one-to-seven are often advisable. (Plan B, described later, is for those who must not combine protein and starch.)

In any meal, protein foods are difficult to digest completely. Excess protein, particularly that of animal origin, is the major dietary source of indigestion and sickness in the West and other areas of the world where it is consumed. The problem with protein in the form of animal products is that it nearly always contains substantial saturated fat. These and most other fats and oils greatly slow the digestion of protein. The situation is made even worse when animal products already rich in fat are fried in cooking oils. The key to using fats and oils (e.g. butter, cream, cooking and salad oils) is to minimize their consumption, especially in the protein-rich meal.

Starches, like proteins, fats, and oils, combine well with green and low-starch vegetables, and less well with other starches, since each type of starch requires a slightly different digestive environment. Ideally, a single starch per meal is preferable, although most healthy people can tolerate two grains, or one grain and another starch in vegetable form. For example, the nutrition and digestibility of a meal which already contains rye bread and beets—two starches—would not necessarily be improved if the bread included another grain such as wheat, since the less-efficient digestion of both grains would tend to offset the added nutrients of the wheat. This is especially true in persons with subnormal digestion.

Rule 4. Fruit and sweetened foods should be eaten alone, or in small amounts at the end of a meal.

Because of their relatively simple carbohydrate structure, fruits and concentrated sweeteners pose a special problem when combined with other foods. When eaten in a meal, they digest first and tend to monopolize all the digestive functions; the other foods wait, and ferment. Fruits and sweeteners mix most poorly with starches and proteins; their combination with green vegetables is not necessarily objectionable. Lettuce and celery, for example, are commonly thought by many food-combining experts to aid the digestion of fruit and simple sugars. In a meal of proteins or starches, we recommend that the fruit or dessert be eaten at the end of the meal, preceded by a large green lettuce salad. This order is due to the expansive and ascending nature of the sweet flavor. In fact, the green salad would be a much better way to end a starch or protein meal.

Ideally fruit, either raw or cooked, and products made with sweeteners are eaten by themselves as refreshing snacks or energizing small meals. Consider an oatmeal-raisin-almond cookie made with amasake sweetener. This combination of starch, fruit, protein, and concentrated sweetener, as good as it may taste, offers a strong challenge to any digestive system, even if not eaten after a meal of several other ingredients.

Plan A: Recommended Order of Eating

I   **Protein**
miso soup*
beans, nuts
cheese, eggs
fish, meat

II   **Starch**
rice
bread
potato
winter squash

III   **Salad**
raw vegetables
sprouts

IV   **Dessert**
fruit
dishes sweetened with
fruit, dried fruit,
and/or concentrated
sweeteners such as
molasses and maple syrup

eaten with
Green and **Non-Starchy**
Vegetables (cooked or raw)
kale
cabbage
broccoli
turnip greens
mushroom
radish

The above four phases of Plan A are not a recommendation that all four categories should appear in a balanced meal. In almost every case, the fewer the types of food in a meal, the better the digestion.

*Soup is eaten first if it is a salty enzyme-rich soup made with miso or soy sauce. A light vegetable soup is eaten at the end of a meal.

Notes: 1) Further examples of protein, starch, and green and non-starchy foods appear later in this chapter. 2) The recipe section contains a large variety of vegetarian dishes, ranging from the very simple to the relatively complex. The more complex recipes are intended for people who have good digestion, and especially for those in transition from a complex diet, who still desire strong flavors in foods. Even then, these recipes are for occasional use only.

Plan B: Food Combining for Best Digestion

Plan B—with some features of Plan A but more restrictive—is the ultimate plan for the person with sensitive or otherwise poor digestion. It is also the best plan for anyone in times of sickness.

Individuals in good health, of course, might wisely choose to follow Plan B to boost their vitality. It is also an effective plan when greater focus and clarity are desired. Some people find it a helpful practice to follow Plan B at least one day per week.

Plan B has two basic rules: 1) Eat protein and starchy foods in separate meals; each combines best with green and non-starchy vegetables; 2) fruits are eaten alone. However, several exceptions to these rules make Plan B quite flexible.

Plan B Food Combining: Exceptions

Special Combinations for High-Fat Proteins, Fats, and Oils

The protein foods highest in fats—the "high-fat proteins"—include cheese, milk, yogurt, kefir, nuts, and oil-bearing seeds. These also combine best with green and non-starchy vegetables although they have an additional feature: they combine fairly well with sour (acidic) fruits. Thus almonds and sour apples; whole sesame butter and lemon sauce; yogurt and strawberries; and cottage cheese and grapefruit are all acceptable combinations of high-fat proteins with acid fruits.

Even though acid retards the digestion of protein, it does this no more than the abundance of fat in a high-fat protein food. Moreover, acids actually help in the digestion of fats, and if combined with protein before it is eaten, also help break down protein chains. On the other hand, taking acids at the time of protein ingestion inhibits the secretion of stomach acids, which are needed for complete protein digestion. By marinating proteins such as meats and beans in vinegar or other acids, however, the acids combine with and dismantle protein chains before they enter the stomach, and very little acid, if any, is in a free state to inhibit gastric acid during digestion. This is particularly true of meats that are cooked after marination (described in the *Protein and Vitamin B$_{12}$* chapter).

In this chapter, we will call "fats" and "oils" those foods that derive nearly all of their caloric energy from their fatty acid content. These are to be distinguished from the high-fat proteins above because fats and oils contain comparatively little protein. Examples include lard, butter, olives, avocados, cream, sour cream, and oils (e.g., flax, sesame, olive, coconut, *ghee* [clarified butter]). Fats and oils, however, unlike proteins and high-fat proteins, do not greatly retard the digestion of starches. Thus bread with butter, rice and olives, potato with avocado, and cream or fresh flax oil on oatmeal make fairly good combinations. The digestion of fats and oils, similar to all protein foods, is greatly aided by consuming them with green vegetables. In starchy meals, therefore, they digest best when accompanied by abundant leafy greens.

Fats and oils also combine with acid fruits. One often sees this combination in lemon and oil salad dressings.

Regardless how well they are combined with other foods, any excess of fatty/oily food in the body wreaks havoc on the liver.

Drink Milk Alone

According to the Old Testament, milk is not to be consumed with meat. In nature, mammals take milk by itself; even when weaning, they will not take milk at the same time other foods are being eaten. Milk that is consumed along with another food tends to curdle around it, insulating it from digestion. Curdled (fermented) milk products such as cheese, yogurt, and buttermilk do not cause this problem, and like the other proteins, combine very well with green vegetables.

Fruit Exceptions

Melons are eaten alone since they digest very rapidly; any other food they are eaten with slows their digestion, causing fermentation.

Lemons, limes, and tomatoes are acid fruits that also combine with green and low-starch vegetables. This is very useful information for making salads, especially of the high-protein variety, since we already know that acid fruit combines with high-fat protein. For example, a high-protein salad can include greens and a high-fat protein (nuts, seeds, avocado, or yogurt), combined with lemon, lime, and/or tomato.

Celery and lettuce, as noted, are two vegetables that can be eaten with fruit in general and even enhance the digestion of fruit and simple sugars. From the perspective of traditional Chinese medicine, lettuce and celery have the ability to dry *damp* conditions, including the fermentation in the digestive tract which regularly occurs when sweet foods are eaten. (Lettuce and celery are discussed further in "Balancing Sweet Foods and Maintaining Calcium," page 227.)

Drinking fruit juice between meals can upset digestion unless two hours have passed since a starch meal or four hours after a meal containing concentrated proteins. Those who need the cleansing, cooling qualities of most fruit—individuals who are overheated, toxic, and show signs of *excess* from a dietary history of too much meat and other rich food—may do well with one meal of the day, usually the first, consisting entirely of fruit. This is an especially good idea for anyone if fruit and fruit juices are being combined poorly with foods such as grains and vegetables or are being eaten soon afterward; it is much better to have one completely fruit or fruit-juice meal. Please refer to "Fruit" in the recipe section for warming/cooling and other properties of common fruits.

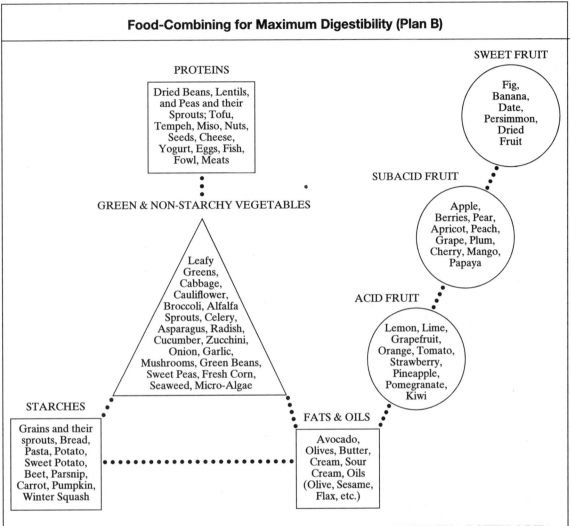

Food-Combining for Maximum Digestibility (Plan B)

PROTEINS

Dried Beans, Lentils, and Peas and their Sprouts; Tofu, Tempeh, Miso, Nuts, Seeds, Cheese, Yogurt, Eggs, Fish, Fowl, Meats

SWEET FRUIT

Fig, Banana, Date, Persimmon, Dried Fruit

GREEN & NON-STARCHY VEGETABLES

SUBACID FRUIT

Apple, Berries, Pear, Apricot, Peach, Grape, Plum, Cherry, Mango, Papaya

Leafy Greens, Cabbage, Cauliflower, Broccoli, Alfalfa Sprouts, Celery, Asparagus, Radish, Cucumber, Zucchini, Onion, Garlic, Mushrooms, Green Beans, Sweet Peas, Fresh Corn, Seaweed, Micro-Algae

ACID FRUIT

Lemon, Lime, Grapefruit, Orange, Tomato, Strawberry, Pineapple, Pomegranate, Kiwi

STARCHES

Grains and their sprouts, Bread, Pasta, Potato, Sweet Potato, Beet, Parsnip, Carrot, Pumpkin, Winter Squash

FATS & OILS

Avocado, Olives, Butter, Cream, Sour Cream, Oils (Olive, Sesame, Flax, etc.)

FOODS THAT CAN BE COMBINED AT A MEAL ARE *DIRECTLY* CONNECTED BY A DOTTED LINE.*

Restrictions and Special Combinations:
- At most take either one protein or one starch per meal.
- Take melons alone.
- Take milk alone.
- Lemon, lime, and tomato (which are acid fruits) combine well with green and non-starchy vegetables.
- Lettuce and celery (which are green vegetables) combine well with all fruits.
- Nuts, oil-rich seeds, cheese, yogurt, kefir, and other fermented dairy foods (which are high-fat proteins) combine well with acid fruits.

*Examples: Either proteins or starches combine well with green and non-starchy vegetables, but not at the same meal (no dotted line between starches and proteins); likewise, sweet and acid fruits do not combine well with each other.

Plan B Examples

Protein Meals
- sesame-seed yogurt on steamed kale and alfalfa sprouts
- almond-lemon sauce on broccoli
- lentil-hijiki seaweed soup and sauerkraut
- hatcho (soy only) miso-seaweed mushroom soup
- sprouted mung bean-lettuce-parsley salad
- tofu, cabbage, fresh sweet pea stew
- tempeh-radish-spirulina sauce over watercress
- sliced orange sections in yogurt
- grated goat cheese on endive-tomato salad

Starch Meals
- buckwheat groats and cabbage-mushroom soup
- sweet potato with avocado butter and parsley garnish
- shredded beet, beet green, and radish sprout salad
- rice-nori seaweed rolls
- carrots, sweet corn, and green beans topped with fresh flax oil
- sprouted wheat bread
- quinoa cereal with brussels sprouts and cauliflower
- winter squash and turnip greens
- potato and sour cream
- avocado and sprout sandwich
- oatmeal-dulse cereal with butter

Leafy Green and Low-Starch Vegetables
This group combines most widely of all, and encourages the digestion of proteins and starches (see examples in protein and starch meals). Each member of this group also combines well with all other members, although mix three or four at most for better digestion. Meals of only leafy green and low-starch vegetables are usually either salads or cooked vegetable dishes, and examples are obvious and plentiful. Relatively high protein sources are available in this group: fresh sweet corn, fresh peas, and green beans; also seaweeds and micro-algae such as spirulina and chlorella. Eating only from this group is highly cleansing; the fruits are even more so.

Fruit Meals
- stewed dried apricots and raisins
- apple-pear juice
- cantaloupe
- tomato-lettuce salad
- diced apples and celery
- crushed pineapple with almonds
- huckleberries
- fresh figs
- bananas and peaches

In the following chart Plan B is summarized and is listed alongside Plan A for comparison.

Food Combining Plans A and B

Food Group	Examples	Plan A: Combining For Better Digestion	Plan B: Combining For Maximum Digestibility
Proteins	Legumes (beans, lentils, peas), bean sprouts, tofu, tempeh, miso, soy soy sauce; all meats, fish, eggs	Combine best with green and non-starchy vegetables. Protein foods are best eaten before starches and fats. At most two proteins per meal.	All proteins combine only with green and non-starchy vegetables; an exception is that high-fat proteins also combine with acid fruit. One protein food only per meal.
High-Fat Proteins	Nuts, oil-bearing seeds, dairy products		
Fats and Oils	Avocado, butter, cream, sour cream, oils (olive, sesame, flax, ghee, etc.)	Combine best with green and non-starchy vegetables. Combine fairly well with starches and acid fruit. Eat in small amounts.	Combine only with green and non-starchy vegetables, starches, and acid fruit. One fat or oil only per meal.
Starches	All grains and cereals including bread, pasta, and sprouted grains; potato, sweet potato, beet, carrot, parsnip, winter squash, pumpkin	Combine best with green and non-starchy vegetables, and are best eaten after protein foods. At most two starches per meal.	Combine only with green and non-starchy vegetables and fats and oils. One starchy food only at a meal.

Green and Non-Starchy Vegetables—The Hub of Food Combining

Leafy Green Vegetables	Chard, kale, spinach, parsley, watercress, lettuce, cabbage, bok choy; turnip, mustard, collard and beet greens; sprouts of alfalfa, cabbage, radish, and mustard; seaweed and micro-algae (spirulina, wild blue-green, chlorella); wheat and barley grass	Combine with all other foods.	Combine with all other vegetables, proteins, starches, fats, oils, and three acid fruits—lemon, lime, and tomato.
Non-Starchy Vegetables	Cucumber, broccoli, cauliflower, celery, turnip, radish, onion, green bean, sweet corn, sweet pea, zucchini, leek, garlic, eggplant, bell pepper, mushroom, asparagus, summer squash, okra	Combine with all other foods.	Combine the same as leafy green vegetables above.

Food Combining Plans A and B (continued)

Food Group	Examples	Plan A: Combining For Better Digestion	Plan B: Combining For Maximum Digestibility
Fruit			
Sweet:	Banana, fresh fig, raisin, all dried fruit, date, persimmon	Preferably eaten alone, although can be eaten at end of meal, ideally preceded by a green salad.* Fruit combines with other fruit according to rules of Plan B.	Eat as a meal by itself. Exceptions: all fruits combine with lettuce and celery, and acid fruits combine with fats, oils, and high-fat protein. All fruit combines with all other fruit except sweet and acid fruits do not mix, and melons are best eaten alone. Combine only two or three fruits at once.
Subacid:	Apple, berries, apricot, peach, grape, plum, pear, cherry, mango, papaya, nectarine		
Acid:	Orange, lemon, lime, grapefruit, pineapple, currant, pomegranate, tomato, sour apple, strawberry, kiwi		
Melons:	Watermelon, cantaloupe, casaba, etc.		
Concentrated Sweeteners			
	Honey, maple syrup, rice syrup, barley malt, amasake (rice-koji ferment), dried unrefined cane juice, fruit syrups and juices, and the herbs stevia and licorice	Sweetened products such as herbal teas with honey and desserts are eaten alone for best digestion. If combined with a meal, they are taken at the end in small amounts, ideally preceded by a green salad.*	Eat alone (e.g., amasake drink)—not with any other foods except herbal teas or water.

*The greens recommended for this salad are lettuce and/or celery.

Plan C: The One-Pot Meal

Traditions in India and China use foods of multiple ingredients for healing when they are prepared correctly.

In Plan C, as in Plan A, one may combine a number of foods at a single meal. But instead of focusing on the order of foods eaten, it calls for cooking all ingredients for a meal in a single pot with ample water. Typical examples of one-pot meals are soups, stews, and congees (see "Congees" in recipe section). One-pot meals in East Asia may include ingredients such as grains, vegetables, legumes, seeds, herbs, and/or meat. The way this plan works to minimize digestive problems resulting from combining ingredients is explained by Robert Svoboda in *Prakruti, Your Ayurvedic Constitution* (Geocom, 1989): In a one-pot meal, ". . . the

various foods have settled their differences in the pot, fought out whatever needed to be fought out, and come to some conclusion, which you then consume."
This plan differs from foods cooked with little or no water in that a slowly cooked
watery medium allows the chemicals of all ingredients to interact more completely.
In a sense, the foods are being pre-digested in the pot.

Plan C is good for those who are weak or chronically ill. If digestion is also
poor, C meals should be simpler, but need not be as strict as Plan B because of
the harmonizing effect that occurs when foods slowly cook together in ample
water. The watery nature of these meals recommends them to those with deficient
yin fluids syndrome as well as those who cannot chew their food thoroughly.

The Art of Presentation

An essential aspect of food-combining is its overall appearance—the way the
food is mixed with other food in terms of texture, size, color, and arrangement.
Food that is impatiently prepared without a sense of care and nourishment will
look and taste that way, and will have a poor effect on the health of those who
eat it.

Awareness of presentation transforms the meal, helping one to eat less yet
gain greater nourishment; the meal will be more appreciated and therefore eaten
more consciously, which translates physically into improved assimilation. Intuitions are heightened and better choices made regarding the order, combinations,
and amounts of the foods to be eaten.

When accomplished as an art at the highest level, food presentation is elegant
in its simplicity. There are no absolute rules in this art, and the following are
specific suggestions to stimulate your creativity.

- Prepare food simply but with appeal to the eyes, and with enough variety to
  awaken the appetite and nourish the body.
- Present only a few dishes at a meal and serve something different at the next
  meal.
- Present each dish so that it stands by itself yet helps balance the meal.
- Create a contrast with color, shape, and texture, and include all five flavors in
  the right amounts (see *Therapeutic Use of the Five Flavors,* Chapter 23).
- Serve light foods with heavy ones, sweet foods with sour ones. Balance a soft
  dish with a crunchy one. Enliven a bland dish with a bright color.

It must be remembered that food combining and presentation are but two
important dimensions of meal planning. Choosing foods which balance specific
conditions and unique constitutions is also of vital importance. For example, people who are *deficient, cold,* or suffering from candida overgrowth may not do well
with cooling fruits.

Allergies and Food Combining

The study of allergies has become one way of understanding nearly every health problem. Common allergic reactions to foods and other substances range from frequent colds, hay fever, sore throats, and mucus problems to skin diseases, fatigue, depression, insomnia, headache, and digestive disturbances.

Looked at in the most basic terms, an allergic reaction to food is simply a message from the body that a particular food is not appropriate. Reactions to denatured, refined, and imbalanced foods are actually helpful, since we then know that these foods are damaging our health, and can choose to avoid them. However, allergic reactions may also commonly occur from supposedly wholesome items such as whole wheat, corn, soy, and a number of other unprocessed foods, raising the question of why such products cannot be tolerated.

What we have discovered is that people with allergic reactions to certain foods are not always allergic to those foods, but are reacting to poor food combinations.

In the case of whole wheat, for instance, people seldom simply combine it with leafy greens and/or low-starch vegetables alone. Most often, it is in the form of bread—in a sandwich with such proteins as cheese, meat, or peanut butter. In the morning it is eaten as toast with eggs and bacon. Vegetarians will often use nut or seed butters on bread, or serve it with legumes.

To discover one's food sensitivities, first apply Plan B, the simplest food combining, to the diet. At this point, most allergies cease. If this is the case, then one may expand a little, and find which *combinations* of foods can be tolerated. On the other hand, if allergies continue while strictly following Plan B, then one should begin eliminating suspected foods, starting with those which are craved most (these are usually the ones producing the allergic reaction). Keep a daily record of what is eaten and any changes in reactions. Once the allergen is identified, it may or may not have to be eliminated.

Allergies and the Sproutable Foods

For allergies to wheat and similar foods that do not clear up under Plan B, another option is available—sprouting. When wheat (or any other seed) is sprouted, it seldom produces an allergic reaction. Sprouted wheat can be made into breads (see recipes) or cooked as a cereal dish; it can even be eaten raw in warmer climates or seasons, and is especially good for those with a *hot* internal climate. Sprouting may be tried with other potentially allergenic foods such as soybeans, lentils, grains, and many varieties of seeds. In most preparations of whole grains or legumes, we have suggested in the recipe section that they be presoaked for several hours. Soaking removes phytic acid* and also initiates the process of sprouting.

---

*Phytic acid in grains and legumes interferes with the assimilation of their minerals, especially zinc.

Depending on how far a seed is allowed to sprout, it develops from a protein or starch to a leafy green or low-starch vegetable. For the purpose of food combining, most grain sprouts are still listed as starches and legume sprouts as proteins since the normal sprouting time does not completely transform their character beyond their original food groups. However, sprouting converts much of their starch into simple sugars, and their protein into free amino acids; meanwhile, free fatty acids have been created from the fats. Enzymes and vitamins are increased, as well as a variety of mineral bonds on the amino acids (forms of chelation).

For these reasons, the sprouting of grains, legumes, and other seeds makes them much more digestible. Soaking grains and legumes before cooking may be sufficient to relieve allergies, but further sprouting may also be necessary. The method for sprouting can be found under "Sprouts" in the recipe section. Finally, it is important to recognize the cooling, cleansing nature of sprouts; they clearly benefit the fiery, robust individual, but when eaten in excess they can weaken digestion and worsen the condition of those who are *deficient* and *cold*. The cooling and cleansing qualities of sprouts may be reduced by lightly cooking them.

The Four-Day and Six-Week Plans

The majority of allergies by far are to foods that cannot be sprouted, dairy and egg allergies being the most prevalent. When allergies to these items persist in spite of simple food combining, they should of course be avoided. In the case of these and all allergens, however, temporary avoidance may be all that is required. Many allergy sufferers find they are no longer sensitive to a food if it appears in their diet no more than once every four days. Others find that allergies to a particular food clear up when they totally abstain from it for six weeks.

Physical and Mental Sources of Allergy

In the last few decades, more and more people have reported hypersensitivity to nearly every imaginable substance. Allergic reactions extend beyond food to animal hair, dust, water, sunlight, etc. On a psychological level, these physical aggravations may be related to feelings of isolation, separation, even arrogance—an inability to accept the world as it is. Physiologically, they represent poor immunity and a major malfunction in the antigen-deactivating capacity of the liver. (An interesting East/West correspondence is that arrogance is also associated with a malfunctioning liver, according to ancient Chinese physiology.)

Perhaps the most important remedy for allergies is to work toward fewer feelings of separation and self-importance. Then, if one consistently follows a simple, high-quality diet, the liver will gradually be rebuilt and its ability to neutralize allergenic substances restored. To hasten the process, any chlorophyll-rich foods such as micro-algae and cereal grasses may be emphasized. These are helpful for clearing allergies because of their immune-enhancing, anti-inflammatory properties as well as their abundant supply of omega-3 and/or GLA fatty acids (as discussed in the *Green Food Products* chapter).

Candida overgrowth is also implicated in extensive allergies. To determine whether candida treatments are appropriate, please refer to "Candida Overgrowth Symptoms," page 72.

Fasting and Purification

Fasting and purification can be an uplifting experience that enhances health and attitude, depending on why and how it is done. One may fast by eating nothing, eating a single food, or by eliminating one or more foods from the diet. The fast can last a day to several days, or for several weeks. Almost all modern affluent people need to fast from a lifelong daily schedule of three meals supplemented with between-meal snacks. Virtually every religious and healing tradition recommends fasting for therapeutic or spiritual advantages.[1]

Many of our primitive ancestors fasted. In the spring of the year when winter supplies ran low, they typically fasted one or more weeks on little more than water and spring greens. Contemporary fasting usually involves abundant fruit and vegetable juices. However, excessive fasting on juices can seriously impair the metabolic rate and digestive strength ("spleen-pancreas digestive fire" in Chinese healing), cool and weaken the body, and sometimes result in abnormal weight gain after the fast. To avoid these adverse reactions, the type of fast should be matched to the individual.

Cleansing and Building

The word "fast" itself indicates an important feature of a fast. It signifies a speeding-up of the cleansing and renewal process by slowing down the normal digestive routine. "Cleansing" is a relative term. It generally means the purging of toxins and residues we have accumulated by using too many building foods (those rich in fats and proteins which build tissue most rapidly). While it is best to alternate cleansing and building, in most cases people eat far more building foods than cleansing ones. For this reason the cleansing foods and methods of a fast are the usual remedies for most diseases of excess. A common assumption is that quicker cleansing is better, and most people interested in quick results want to use very rapid cleansing methods such as fruit and vegetable juices. Although the quicker methods can be valuable therapeutically, we have found that the slower, milder fasts with selected whole foods foster a consciousness of patience and a faith in the wisdom of living with gentler cycles. Such fasts can bring remarkable healing to those who lead stressful lives.

The cycles of cleansing and building can be separated: by overeating rich, building foods and then abruptly fasting, one experiences two distinct phases. Cleansing and building by the principles in this book integrates the two cycles. The majority of one's diet should be foods with some of both properties. Vegetables are considered cleansing yet are also mildly building since they contain significant amounts of protein, starch, minerals, and fats—the materials with which we are built and maintained. On the other hand, grains, beans, nuts, and seeds are building foods but contain sulfur, fiber, and other cleansing qualities. Even so, building and cleansing activities in the body are rarely at the same level at a given time. For example, in the winter months building will predominate, and at warmer times, cleansing will inevitably prevail.

Once a person is stabilized on a middle-path dietary regime, the extreme cleanses become less attractive than they may once have been. After limiting the intake of heavily building foods for a while, a certain degree of balance is automatically achieved, and the most appropriate fasts occur during the times we simply eat only a grain, or a few vegetables or fruit for a day or so.

Fasting and the Acid- and Mucus-Forming Foods

Because of the types of foods many of us have ingested during the greater part of our lives, certain food groups work better in a fast than others, depending on the food residues that need to be eliminated. These residues are most often from the acid-forming, high-fat, and/or mucus-forming categories. Examples are meats, fish, poultry, eggs, most dairy,* most grains and legumes,** refined sugars, drugs, and chemicals.*** When the body is too acidic as a result of these foods, disease and infections proliferate. This is especially the case in arthritic and rheumatic conditions.

The body should be slightly alkaline in order to build an alkaline reserve for acid-forming conditions such as stress, lack of exercise, or poor dietary habits. The most alkaline-producing foods are the fruits, vegetables, sprouts, cereal grasses, and herbs. (See "Cleansing and Building Foods" chart later in this chapter.) The acid and alkaline balance can also be changed dramatically by simple practices, including soaking mildly acid-forming foods such as whole grains and legumes before cooking them (as recommended uniformly in this book's recipes). This starts the sprouting process, which is alkalizing. Another highly alkaline-forming process is to chew thoroughly such complex carbohydrates as grains, vegetables, and legumes in order to mix them with saliva, a very alkaline fluid. The correct ratio of acid and alkaline foods in the diet is difficult to know, since the balance is altered

---

*Most dairy is acid-forming. Milk is approximately neutral in acid/alkaline but high in mucus-forming attributes such as fat.

**Millet and roasted buckwheat are slightly alkalizing. Soy and lima beans are extremely alkalizing.

***Many but not all drugs and chemicals are acid-forming.

by chewing, food preparation, exercise and lifestyle, and even our level of positive thinking. However, those who are prone to infections, viruses, excess mucus problems, and other generally toxic acidic conditions need to increase exercise, become more conscious, and have a lighter, more alkalizing diet.

The quality of coating on the mucous membranes of the body is important; animal products can build a heavy mucus that obstructs the breathing, sinuses, urinary tract, and general digestion. Many complex carbohydrates (grains, beans, lentils, seeds) promote mucus also, although it is generally beneficial instead of obstructive if moderate amounts of food are chewed well and other healthful, non-mucus-forming habits are practiced, such as not eating late at night. Even though grains are generally somewhat mucus- and acid-forming, they can still be very helpful as fasting foods for those without mucus problems if these and other suggestions given later are followed.

Many people maintain the idea that the intake during a fast should consist of only water or, at most, juices. However, we have found fasting on vegetables, fruit, or grains to be very successful. It is an experiment in moderation that minimizes the possibility of a post-fast binge. Technically slower than more intense fasts, it is safer and less stressful for those coming from a very rich dietary background.

The final factor to consider is the generally tonifying and building qualities of grains compared with the eliminative nature of vegetables and fruits. If one has signs of *heat* (feels too hot, dislikes heat, drinks copious amounts of cool beverages, red complexion) or *excess* (robust person, strong voice, forceful pulse, thick tongue coating), then it is wiser to use raw vegetables, fruits, or their juices for fasting. Those who have symptoms of *coldness* (chills, pallor, aversion to the cold and an unusual attraction to warmth) would do better with a fast of cooked vegetables or grains, perhaps with the addition of warming herb teas suggested later in this chapter. Those with pronounced signs of *deficiency* (weak, thin—more than 12 pounds underweight, pale, little or no tongue coating) should not fast. Those with only slight *deficiency* signs can benefit from short fasts of grain, with chlorella or spirulina micro-algae as an optional supplement. To help make food choices, check the therapeutic properties in "Grains," "Vegetables," and "Fruit" in the recipe section.

On a liquid fast, hunger occurs on the second or third day and then disappears. When hunger later reappears, it is a sign that the body has fasted long enough. Because of the accumulation of excess acids, fats, mucus, poisons, infections, drugs, and heavy metals that the modern person carries, we recommend no more than a seven-day fast on fluids or a fourteen-day fast on specific solid foods if it is not supervised by someone with experience, since the discharge of toxins could be more than the organs of elimination can handle. Shorter one-day or even half-day fasts can be very helpful if they are done weekly.

Five Fasts

I. Raw Fruit, Vegetable, or Liquid Fast

For those making a transition to primarily whole vegetarian foods from a background of abundant animal products, and who do not have signs of *coldness* or *deficiency*, try a salad fast of either raw vegetables or raw fruit such as carrots, cabbage, apples, etc. Herbal teas, water, or juices can be drunk according to thirst. The individual with candida overgrowth must avoid fruit and fruit juice.

Note: Most fruits and vegetables do not combine well at the same meal—exceptions are celery and lettuce, which can be eaten with fruit—see *Food Combinations* chapter.

For the strong person with signs of *excess* try one or more of these:

A. Fruit juices; vegetable juices; and/or barley- or wheat-grass drinks made from cereal grass powders or freshly pressed grasses. Common vegetable juices include carrot, beet, celery, cabbage, parsley, and other greens. Carrot is one of the safest juices to use. Smaller amounts of other vegetables are often juiced with carrots for variety and for the benefit of their specific properties. The cleansing, healing traits of fruit, vegetable, and cereal grass juices in a fast act more quickly than water alone.

B. Herbal tea formulas such as 1) Two parts burdock root *(Arctium lappa)* and 1 part red clover blossoms *(Trifolium pratense):* for impure blood, skin diseases, arthritis, and excess weight; 2) Two parts dandelion root *(Taraxacum officinalis)*, 1 part fennel seed *(Foeniculum vulgare)*, 1 part flax seed *(Linum usitatissimum)*, 1 part fenugreek seed *(Trigonella foenumgraecum),* and ½ part licorice root *(Glycyrrhiza glabra):* for excessive mucus, weak lungs, gastro-intestinal inflammations, liver excesses, hunger in the first few days of the fast, and quicker cleansing; or choose other herbs according to specific needs.

C. Pure water or water with a squeeze of lemon.

The total daily consumption of juices, teas, and/or water on a liquid fast will ideally fall between six and eight glasses, although more can be taken if thirsty. Most people do well when one-half to two-thirds of the total fluid consumed comes from fruit, vegetable, and grass juices, and the remainder from teas and water. Fluids should be room temperature when drunk, not cold. Juices can be diluted by half with water to slow down the fast.

II. Steamed-Vegetable Fast

If you have overeaten consistently, consuming excess sweets, nuts, beans, grains, dairy, or eggs, and your condition is a little on the *cool* and *deficient* side, then consider a fast of lightly steamed vegetables of your choice. Take at most three different vegetables at a time, although one or two is preferable. Drink water or herbal teas according to thirst.

III. Whole-Grain Fast

The person who wants to improve mental focus and whose constitution ranges from fairly balanced to slightly *deficient* and thin, or *cold,* will normally benefit from a whole-grain fast for at least three days. Chew each bite thirty to fifty times. Rice and various other whole grains may be used. Millet is recommended for its alkaline, detoxifying nature. Wheat and other grain sprouts are also alkaline, and less cooling when steamed. Take water or a grain beverage if thirsty between meals. Warming herb teas such as cinnamon bark and dried ginger root can be used by those with *cold* signs. Ideal breads to use in a fast include traditional, naturally leavened (sourdough) bread of unrefined grain and Essene-style bread of sprouted grain. The grain fast in the form of bread and water for one or two days a week has recently been recommended to the world through several children who experienced the apparition of "Our Lady of Medjugorje" at Medjugorje, Yugoslavia.[2] (The messages for spiritual renewal given to children at Medjugorje are similar to ones given at Lourdes, France, and Fátima, Portugal, in the earlier part of this century.)

A mung bean and rice fast, commonly used by yogis, is referred to as "the food of the gods" because of its balancing effect on every facet of the body and mind. Mung beans are more valuable than other legumes for fasting because of their ability to purge toxins from the body. Cooking them with a little seaweed enhances their detoxifying nature. Various grains can be substituted. The results are improved when mung beans and the grain are eaten at separate meals, with the beans, perhaps as a soup, at the last meal of the day. The cooling effect of mung beans can be reduced for the *cold* person by adding warming spices in the last 20 minutes of cooking. Try black peppercorn, fennel, cumin, and/or dried ginger.

IV. Micro-Algae Fast

This is a good fast for those with blood sugar imbalances and attendant sugar cravings, and for those who find fasting difficult. Micro-algae are often combined with a vegetable or fruit juice, herb tea, or other liquid fast. When micro-algae are taken with a cooked grain or vegetable fast, the combination becomes the safest fast for people who tend to be slightly weak or thin. It is also ideal for people who must maintain a busy schedule while fasting. One seldom experiences hunger or other difficulty. Use micro-algae mixed into liquid two or three times a day. Each time, take approximately 5 grams of spirulina, 1½ grams chlorella, or ¾ gram wild blue-green *(Aphanizomenon flos-aquae).* At the start of the fast halve this dosage for three days unless you are already in the habit of using micro-algae. Refer to the *Green Food Products* chapter to find out which one (or more) micro-alga is most appropriate for you.

V. Absolute Fast

The oxygen charge from this fast on air is best for individuals who have such *damp* excesses as water retention, candida overgrowth, too much body weight, abundant mucus, or sluggishness. Absolute fasting is not appropriate for the thin or over-*heated* person. Without preparation and close supervision, it is not safe for most people to extend this fast beyond a day and a half (36 hours). Such a fast general-ly accomplishes in this time what other fasts take several days to do. Eat or drink nothing for 36 hours: begin at 6 or 7 one evening; end early the second morning.

Absolute fasting is the most profound fast with the fewest distractions: one drops every aspect of solid and liquid nourishment and is sustained with the breath of life. Thus it is the fast which best encourages concentration on the ultimate and absolute nature of reality.

Native Americans would customarily fast on air for four days (96 hours) and end it by drinking 3–4 quarts of an herbal tea (peppermint works well) followed by regurgitation and a sweat lodge. Regurgitation removes toxins in the stomach, and sweating helps excrete poisons that have accumulated in the lymphatic system near the skin. Over the years we have witnessed dozens of people successfully follow this four-day prayer fast in an isolated tepee on ceremonial grounds in northern California. Each day of the fast a different lesson is brought by a spiritual teacher, who also monitors the condition of the faster.

An ancient Middle Eastern ritual included a forty-day absolute fast undertak-en by the most evolved members of the highly disciplined Essene desert commu-nities. Other Essenes also fasted for forty days, but on moist fruit (twenty days), fruit juice (ten to seventeen days), and water (three to ten days).[3] A life of prayer, ritual, and pure vegetarian food prepared all members well for fasting. The Essene sect is thought to have been founded by the prophet Elijah.[4] Members were not-ed for longevity and often lived 120 years. Moses and Jesus Christ were also recorded as completing forty-day absolute fasts.[5]

For Good Fasting

A. Use pure water and foods. Freshly pressed juices are preferable although unrefined, organic, bottled juices may be used.

B. Chew food very well. This includes "chewing" liquids—mixing them with saliva—before swallowing.

C. The quantity of liquid or food can be somewhat determined by your intuition, which is remarkably heightened while fasting. Nevertheless, in fasts on whole fruits, vegetables, or grains, never eat to the point of feeling full. Try eating no more than twice daily unless very hungry.

D. Get sufficient mental and physical rest, and keep warm. When feeling cold, add freshly ground black peppercorn to ingredients in a whole-food fast, or drink teas of warming herbs such as black peppercorn, dried ginger, cinnamon bark, fennel, fenugreek, and/or rosemary.

E. Daily enemas are traditional with fasts. They are often useful for those with slow digestion, although they are not as important for those fasting on grains, veg-etables, or fruit as for those on tea, water, or juices. Headaches that occur during fast-ing can be caused by stagnant intestines. In this case enemas are a speedy remedy.

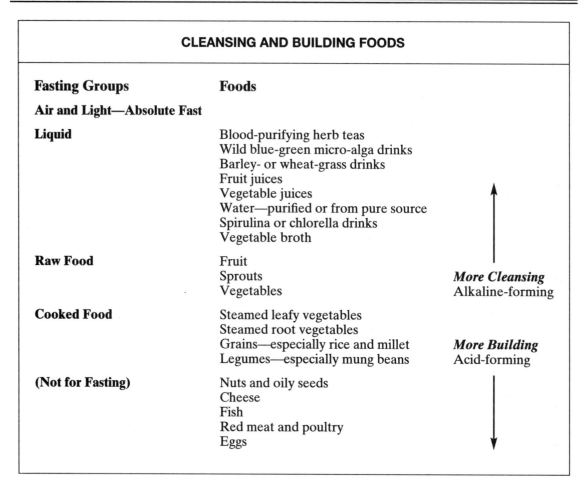

CLEANSING AND BUILDING FOODS

Fasting Groups	Foods	
Air and Light—Absolute Fast		
Liquid	Blood-purifying herb teas	
	Wild blue-green micro-alga drinks	
	Barley- or wheat-grass drinks	
	Fruit juices	
	Vegetable juices	
	Water—purified or from pure source	
	Spirulina or chlorella drinks	
	Vegetable broth	
Raw Food	Fruit	
	Sprouts	*More Cleansing*
	Vegetables	Alkaline-forming
Cooked Food	Steamed leafy vegetables	
	Steamed root vegetables	
	Grains—especially rice and millet	*More Building*
	Legumes—especially mung beans	Acid-forming
(Not for Fasting)	Nuts and oily seeds	
	Cheese	
	Fish	
	Red meat and poultry	
	Eggs	

For enemas, one may use pure water; or for better results use teas of chamomile, yarrow, or catnip made with water that does not contain chlorine or fluoride. Other helpful processes which assist in cleansing are dry-brush treatments, baths, and saunas; walks and moderate exercise; sun and air baths. Avoid heavy labor, though light work is possible for most people. Those fasting on liquids or air should avoid driving or using equipment that requires normal reflexes, since response time is slower during these fasts.

F. Complete a series of small fasts before attempting a long one.

G. Start and break the fast gradually by taking one-third of the length of the fast on each end of the fast (one day for a three-day fast) to add foods from other fasting groups at levels closely below that used on the fast. (See the "Cleansing and Building" chart.) For example, in preparation for and in breaking a vegetable or fruit juice fast, one may choose any other liquids, raw vegetables, sprouts, and cooked vegetables. When starting and breaking a raw-vegetable fast, one can include raw and cooked vegetables, sprouts, and a small amount of grain. A grain fast can be prepared for and ended with such typical vegetarian fare as grains, vegetables, legumes, a few almonds, and perhaps an animal product such as yogurt.

When breaking this and all fasts, the most important rule is to not overeat. The success of a fast depends on how well it is broken, for the desire to binge can be overwhelming. If one immediately puts all the excesses back in that came out during the fast, any benefit is doubtful.

Reasons for Fasting

- To overcome emotional attachments to food.
- To cure physical and mental stagnancy, which manifests as poor appetite, apathy, fatigue, mental depression, and many other chronic ailments.
- For purification of the body before a change of diet to better one's health.
- As a seasonal cleansing: The foods eaten during summer and winter are more extreme. Some people find it beneficial to fast soon after the end of these seasons to make the transition smoother into the more moderate seasons of spring and autumn. Spring fasting, for example, rids the body of the heavy, fatty, and salty foods of winter and prepares it for the activity of summer. Autumn fasting eliminates the residues from excess sweet and cooling foods of the summer and prepares one for the storage season of the winter. An appropriate healing action to take in the autumn is the selected whole-grain or vegetable fast. High in fiber, this fast is particularly beneficial for the colon (see *Metal Element* chapter).
- For spiritual reasons: To strengthen one's spiritual practice, prayer, or meditation; prior to and during times of ritual—for example, a wedding or an equinox ceremony; for special holy days.
- To enhance one's mental awareness, sleep, and dreams.

When Not To Fast

- In cold weather, an extended fast can be harmful.
- During serious physical or mental degenerations, unless advised by a knowledgeable doctor or other qualified health practitioner.
- If one is starving or deprived of proper nutrition.
- During pregnancy or lactation. It is more beneficial to nourish one's body during these times with a health-building diet.

Appropriate fasting has been found to cure virtually every disorder involving excess as well as to increase lifespan, but one should exercise caution on the longer fasts. Regardless of the fasting procedures, the vitally important factors are the attitude and learning during the fast, including the conviction to make what was learned a part of daily life.

Food for Spiritual Practices and Retreats

Fasting or at least dietary restraint has been used in every culture to support spiritual practices. Because spiritual disciplines clarify the mind and energize the body, fasting and all food choices are made much simpler.

A special opportunity for transformation is a retreat or similar function centered on the unfolding of an individual's spiritual nature. The food at such an event should not be overly emphasized; however, there are preparations and types of food that can benefit the entire process. The following suggestions are modeled after several East Asian traditions that can be applied to any primarily vegetarian retreat.

Perhaps the "three *gunas*" of ancient East Indian philosophy are the most important guidelines to use when relating food to consciousness. The Tamasic *guna* includes dark personality traits, irritability, and emotional states that lead to degenerative conditions. Tamasic foods supporting these conditions are of poor quality, overly cooked, strongly processed, and/or partly spoiled. Meats are Tamasic if they are cured or come from sluggish animals that are fed unnatural substances such as drugs and hormones. In general, Tamasic foods depress one's spirit.

The Rajasic *guna* is characterized by those who are aggressive and worldly. Their energy derives from stimulating foods and not from spiritual awareness. Rajasic food must be of reasonable quality and freshly prepared. It is rich-tasting and well cooked with ample flavors and spices. However, Rajasic food is not extreme; overly spicy and heavily cooked food is Tamasic. Rajasic meats come from freshly caught fish and wild game.

The Sattvic *guna* addresses the needs of those participating in spiritual and scholarly activity. The foods of this category specifically affect the consciousness in an uplifting way. Such foods create equilibrium; they neither drive the energy of the body nor overly influence the mind. One who partakes of Sattvic foods can more easily be motivated from internal guidance because such foods promote a peaceful mentality. Sattvic foods are freshly prepared, moderately cooked, and are not heavily spiced or salted. Sattvic foods include freshly drawn milk, fruit, grains, vegetables, legumes, nuts, and seeds. Preparation is important. For example, neither commercially processed milk nor pre-cooked canned food are considered Sattvic. See Summary, Chapter 52, for discussions on Sattva.

A retreat which incorporates prolonged meditations and other lengthy spiritual practices has additional dietary requirements. One's body becomes more contracted and produces greater internal warmth. It is necessary to take in the right amount of liquids and cooling foods to maintain a balance yet keep from losing focus. Digestive absorption is greatly enhanced during sessions of meditation and prayer, and so very simple food at this time will be the most satisfying. Even though strict food-combining rules *per se* are rarely followed by most spiritual adepts, such individuals often follow similar principles in their fasting and simple meal plans. For example, meals during Chinese *zuo ch'an* meditation sessions typically include grains served with mostly above-ground green vegetables cooked in broth with a minimum of roots and beans.

When beans are desired at a retreat, two of the most useful are soybean products in the form of tofu and tempeh, and mung bean sprouts. These supply ample *(yin)* fluids to the body and are cooling. All grains are valuable—barley and millet especially moisten and cool the body; wheat also cools while it calms and fortifies the spirit and strengthens the heart and mind. It therefore supports mental focus and spiritual awareness. An excellent form of wheat is cooked wheat sprouts. Fruit is best eaten in the morning or afternoon as a meal by itself. Milk is also ideally taken by itself, although other dairy such as yogurt or cheese combines well at a meal with citrus.

Cooked food is used almost exclusively in traditional monasteries and by nearly all recognized meditation masters. Even the ancient Essenes, who lived in hot, arid regions, lightly cooked their wheat sprouts with solar heat. Although more nutrients are available from raw food, it may be that fewer of these nutrients are absorbed compared with lightly cooked food. According to Chinese medicine, cooked food strengthens the digestive absorption and transport of nutrients. To the spiritual seeker this means that cooked food supplies better nutrition to the nervous system and hormonal/glandular centers. Without this nourishment, one's consciousness can become more easily unbalanced; the person will be less peaceful and therefore find greater difficulty in focusing on one's True Nature (God). It may be because of these principles that Gautama Buddha, in the *Shurangama Sutra*, recommends cooked food in order to avoid aggravations. Of course, these ideas do not mean that raw food should never be eaten. Fresh uncooked food has vitally important therapeutic value for the excessive individuals who need it. Most people with heavy meat and processed-food backgrounds are in this category. Thus, a little raw food or at least very lightly cooked food at retreats in America and Europe will create balance for the majority of participants.

Further considerations include cutting down or eliminating such strong ingredients as salt, oil, and harsh spices. Avoid heavily cooked foods as well as foods with a highly pungent taste (onions, chives, garlic, leek, and shallots), for they can cause excessive desire and the consequent loss of concentration (see "onion family" in recipe section). Food is best taken only once or twice a day. However, one may wish to have broth or herbal teas at other times. If you like, maintain silence during meals.

Food for Children

A child can be reared as a vegetarian as long as the parents are knowledgeable and conscientious. There is no room for junk food, excessive sweets, or random food selection. A child's growth requires adequate calories and protein for energy to build strong internal organs and to keep the body healthy and developing properly.

Teaching Good Eating Habits

- Many of the earliest habits of a nursing infant are instilled during breast-feeding. If the mother is peaceful and eats wholesome foods, the child will not only receive nourishing milk, but experience the harmonious quality of the mother and her diet. It is said in Chinese folk medicine that when an angry mother's milk is placed in the sunlight, it dries with a purple color; normal milk dries white.

- The first solid food given will determine what a nursing infant will desire later on. If you give your baby primarily food with sweeteners, oil, or salt, it will always crave very sweet, oily, or salty food.

- After weaning a child, continue to provide yourself with a good diet and your children will sense this; it will be easier for them to accept your guidance toward whole, nutritious food.

- Listen to your children's needs and let them change their own eating patterns. Allow them to select foods from outside sources when they are older, and help them to reflect on how different foods affect their behavior—what foods make them sick or feel well.

- A nourishing, harmonious environment is often the most important factor in a child's diet. The family is stabilized by sharing at least one meal of the day together, at a regular time. Blessing the food, holding hands in a circle or enjoying a choice of pre-dinner songs will add a great deal of meaning to a child's life, as well as help form a good attitude toward food. Never air grievances or have angry or disagreeable discussions at mealtime.

- Even when they are babies, encourage children to chew well or at least hold the food in their mouths until it is thoroughly mixed with saliva. Chew together and make it enjoyable.

- Parents who urge their children to eat too much or too fast, or when they are excited or tired, may be creating finicky eaters. Be flexible, and let children rest or play until they are hungry, or let them miss an occasional meal. Toddlers have small stomachs. It's best to give them small meals and nutritious snacks if necessary.

- Sometimes food is too coarse, soggy, or just plain boring. Make an attempt to make food more interesting and delicious. Do not force children to eat because you think it is healthy. It is normal for children to lose their appetites for a few days at a time.

- To stimulate their creativity and interest in food, let your children help you cook (stirring, modeling dough into fun shapes, etc.). Make the main meal the most interesting and important.

- Dish up small servings and let your children ask for more, or let them help themselves.

- Do not bribe your child with a dessert as a reward for eating the meal or for other good behavior. If you withhold dessert as punishment, you will instill in a child the notion that dessert is the most special, yet forbidden food. Linking sweet rewards to good behavior teaches children to identify food—especially sweets—with emotional nourishment rather than biological development, resulting in eating disorders of many kinds.

- Give a small amount of new food to a child at first. If he or she protests, make no fuss, and give them less next time. (Don't be surprised when one day your child likes it.)
- Ask friends and family not to give your child sweets or "junk food," but more nutritious snacks or desserts.
- When children change their eating patterns, it could be a normal stage of development, or the first sign of illness. It is best to give them simple food and let them rest until it passes, or to seek advice.

Food for Babies

With the advent of the career-oriented mother who is often absent from her newborn infant, it is of utmost importance for the health of her child that excellent nutrition not be neglected. Making poor nutritional choices for an infant will usually mean health problems throughout life, not to mention the additional costs and time involved in caring for an unhealthy child. A career mother may be making a wise and even financially sound choice to invest six months' to a year's time away from work to be close to her newborn. Here is one recommended method of feeding and weaning an infant:

During the first six months, the ideal diet of an infant is nearly all mother's milk. Starting at about six months, puréed vegetables and other foods are accepted, and milk consumption may naturally and gradually decrease to 50% of the diet at the age of one year. Between one year and eighteen months, milk is still of great value but may decrease to around 25% of the diet, depending on the baby. At eighteen months the first molar usually appears, signaling that the pancreatic enzymes are being manufactured more efficiently. Over the next six months babies will usually desire less milk, and may wean themselves.

This two-year schedule is only a general one, and the process will vary depending on the individual child's rate of development. In some cases babies will wean themselves after six or eight months, or not willingly want to be weaned at all. There are also many instances among modern people in which the mother is not able to give milk, or the baby is not able to accept what is given. In the latter case, very often an adjustment in the mother's diet will make milk more acceptable. She can eat fewer combinations of food at meals (see *Food Combinations* chapter) and avoid refined, processed foods.

A Chinese herbal remedy to improve an infant's ability to digest milk is sprouted barley, prepared according to the method for sprouts given later in this chapter. Rice sprouts may be substituted but take longer to sprout and are a little less effective. (Whole barley must be used—pearled barley will not sprout.) Another remedy is a grain tea of roasted rice: roast one part rice in a skillet until dark brown; add three parts water; simmer for 20 minutes, and then pour off the tea and give several ounces of it to the infant once or twice daily.

When Mother's Milk Is Not Available

If mother's milk is not available, or for some reason cannot be accepted by the baby, here are four other options:

1. Another mother's milk (wet nurse).
2. Goat's milk, preferably from organically raised goats.
3. Highest quality milk replacement formula.
4. Unhomogenized cow's milk, preferably from organically raised cows.

Each of these four choices will usually need to be supplemented—number 1 the least, and 2, 3, and 4 progressively more so. Choices for supplementation depend on the age of the infant, and include soy products, sprouts, seed, nut, and sprout milks, and animal products, which are discussed a little later. Milk choices also can supplement each other. For example, if the milk of a wet nurse is insufficient in quantity, goat's milk can be used to make up the difference. In the event that animal milks are used, especially cow's milk, their usefulness is noticeably increased by adding chlorophyll foods such as cooked green vegetables to the diet. This combination is explained in the *Calcium* chapter. (Vegetables should be juiced for the youngest infants.)

We are not suggesting that many foods need to be mixed at the same feeding time, but that they be included in the diet at different times. Milk, for example, is best taken by itself. Digestion in children, and babies in particular, is highly responsive and sensitive. Many of the "fits" and colics of infants are a result of poor food combinations. Healthy children of all ages generally prefer simple meals.

Raw and Pasteurized Milks

A Sattvic food in Ayurveda, fresh cow's milk is said to help one develop awareness. According to teachers of this ancient healing art, milk is for those with strong digestion who need to gain weight. Furthermore, to be useful in the body it must be of high quality—ideally freshly drawn from well-treated cows, not homogenized, and taken in moderate amounts. Milk can be difficult for anyone to digest, and especially for infants because of their immature digestive organs. Thus in Ayurvedic prescriptions it is frequently boiled and flavored with a pinch of warming spice such as cardamom, ginger, turmeric, or nutmeg to improve its digestibility. For most infants, simmering an onion in milk has a similar, though milder, effect—it cuts down on mucus generation and enhances assimilation.

From a nutritional perspective, raw cow's milk is superior to pasteurized milk in terms of its beneficial enzymes, but must be certified free of harmful microorganisms. If there is any uncertainty, sterilizing the milk with a quick boil will not only destroy bacteria but even eliminate certain dangerous microbes that survive pasteurization. If it is done quickly then cooled, a minimum of nutrients is lost.

Human milk contains four times more whey protein than cow's milk, and half the amount of casein protein. Whey protein is water-soluble and very easy to digest, whereas casein is not soluble and is thus harder to break down. This may be part of the reason that, in many areas of the world, cow's milk—even very clean milk—is always brought to a quick boil, then cooled.

Bringing milk to a boil breaks down protein chains completely, makes them easier to assimilate, and causes fewer allergic reactions. This milk is safer for all infants and more acceptable for children with weakened digestion. Pasteurization takes place at a temperature below boiling and so it only partially dismantles the protein structure. Such an intermediate breakdown makes milk even more difficult to digest.[1] So if pasteurized milk is used, it is important to finish the protein breakdown with a quick boil.

In contrast, raw goat's milk is already in a very digestible form for most of those with weak digestion, and is not improved by heating. Nevertheless, bringing it to a boil is recommended if for some reason it is not clean. Goats are usually healthy, and any contamination would most likely be introduced after milking.

Homogenized Milk

During the years of the Korean conflict, medical personnel were shocked to discover that autopsies of some young American soldiers revealed arterial deposits and deterioration, a condition previously thought to exist only in the elderly.[2] More recently, children as young as three years of age are exhibiting varying degrees of fatty deposits in their arteries. Some researchers now feel that homogenized milk may play a role in this vascular degeneration.[3]

Homogenization allows the enzyme xanthine oxidase in the milk cream to enter the bloodstream instead of being excreted, as would normally occur. When this enzyme enters the heart and arteries, it damages the membranes, creating scar tissue. Cholesterol accumulates on the scars and gradually clogs the arteries.[3]

An Ayurvedic insight is that homogenization makes the fat in milk nearly indigestible; when consumed, toxic residues *(ama)* form in the body.[4]

Dairy Quality

One of the most vital issues to consider about milk is its quality. Modern animal milk generally has 400% more pesticides than an equivalent sample of grains or vegetables. Human milk, especially that of carnivores, contains considerably more pesticide residue than the milk of other animals.

In addition to pesticides that animals ingest on sprayed plants and feed, livestock raised for meat, eggs, or dairy frequently receive rations of hormones to stimulate growth and production, along with antibiotics to protect against disease. After their milk is tested, many mothers are told by doctors that they must eat fewer animal products in order for their milk to fall to safe levels of heavy metals, steroids, pesticides, and antibiotics.[5]

Animal versus Human Milk

When milk animals are raised without drugs or antibiotics, on unsprayed feed and forage, and children have no allergic or mucous response, then animal milk can be a beneficial dietary supplement. If it is used as the sole food source for infants, we have some reservations, since its higher protein value is designed to create the faster-growing skeleton and body and slower mental development of an animal (a calf will quadruple in weight during the first six months, whereas an infant's weight will only double). Mother's milk, with four to five times the linoleic acid,* encourages faster nervous-system and brain development.

Cow's Milk

Compared with human milk, cow's milk is deficient in lactose and vitamins B_1, C, E, and A. It has three times the minerals in far different proportions. For example, phosphorus and calcium are equally represented in cow's milk, whereas the ratio in mother's milk is two-and-a-half times as much calcium as phosphorus. Also, the type of lactose in cow's milk, called alpha-lactose, does not produce the necessary *Bacillus bifidus* flora in babies' intestines. Mother's milk, which has beta-lactose, encourages *Bacillus bifidus* to grow.

These and many other differences do not mean that cow's milk cannot be used to some benefit, but it clearly cannot be a complete substitute for mother's milk. It should be only a supplemental part of an infant's diet. According to several East Asian traditions, cow's milk is considered a tonic for weakness and *deficiency*, and is thought to be healthful for those who tend toward thinness and *dryness*. For these and most other purposes, however, goat's milk is usually superior.

Goat's Milk

Even though goat's and cow's milk have some similar nutritional features, goat's milk differs in many basic qualities including taste, mineral content, and chemistry in general.

Goats are very clean animals and, given the opportunity, enjoy browsing on a variety of bushes, herbs, and barks that are rich in minerals and other nutrients usually lacking in the bodies of modern people. For example, goat's milk is one of the best fluorine sources, nearly ten times higher than cow's milk. Dietary fluorine helps build immunity, protect teeth, and strengthen bones; fluorine, however, is lost in pasteurization. Chemical sodium fluoride in the water supply does not have the same healing properties.

Goat's milk has been a remedy for people in weakened and convalescent conditions in many traditional cultures. It has specific uses in the treatment of ema-

---

*The essential fatty acid linoleic acid, and a fatty acid generated from it, gamma-linolenic acid, are both well supplied in human milk and are necessary for correct nerve-tissue development.

ciation, malnutrition, anemia, stomach ulcers, nervous exhaustion, and loss of energy; goat's milk also enriches the intestinal flora and can be beneficial in cases of constipation. Its astringent property can treat diarrhea as well. It is often used to tonify both the young and the old, and has been generally recognized as a wholesome baby food.

Not every infant can tolerate goat's milk, although most do well with it, even most of those who are allergic to cow's milk or do not tolerate mother's milk. Occasionally goat's milk is easier to digest than mother's milk if the mother is emotionally upset, chemically toxic, or imbalanced in other ways. One very important advantage of goat's milk over cow's milk is its soft curd and smaller fat globules, which make it far more digestible; in most other respects as well, goat's milk offers more healthful results. There are numerous examples of rubicund and robust vegetarian infants and children whose diet is supplemented with goat's milk and its products. Because of the nature of its fat structure, goat's milk is already homogenized in its natural state; however, it is often pasteurized commercially. For maximum benefit and flavor, it should be fresh. Drinking it just after milking, before it cools, is recommended for those who most require its therapeutic values.

Mother's Milk

Although goat's milk can usually supplement an infant's diet when mother's milk is not available or accepted, human milk has special factors not found in animal milks or in milk replacement formulas. Many studies indicate that infants who receive adequate mother's milk are less prone to infant death, have better immunity, and generally suffer fewer diseases throughout life.[6, 7]

If mothers do decide to work during the first months after giving birth, their milk can be expressed in the morning by hand or with a breast pump (available through most pharmacies), and should be kept cool for use later in the day. If the mother must be away for several days, she can withdraw extra milk daily and freeze it in a closed container, since it would spoil after a day or so at temperatures above freezing. Even though it has been demonstrated that extracting mother's milk and then feeding it in a bottle has less value than when it is suckled directly from the mother,[8] it is obvious that mother's milk from a bottle is far better than bottled animal milk or milk substitutes.

Fermented Dairy Products

The enzyme rennin is secreted in the stomach by most children from birth to age seven (girls) or eight (boys). This enzyme coagulates milk and helps in the digestion process. Without rennin secretion, many people are allergic to milk. However, soured milk products including buttermilk, kefir, yogurt, and cottage cheese are already predigested by the bacterial action of the souring process and are digested much better by the great majority of people who lack rennin. In addition, other properties of milk are transformed by the souring: lactose is converted to lactic acid, and casein is partially broken down. Many individuals, especially from cultures where dairy is not common, have lactose intolerance, but they sometimes can digest fermented milk (although there may also be unknown factors of intolerance present). If dairy is to be used at all by older children and adults, we nearly always recommend the fermented and soured, raw milk products. Those people with a heritage from areas of the world such as northern Europe, where milk has been a major dietary feature for many generations, will generally tolerate dairy better.

Dairy Summary

- For infant nutrition, mother's milk is nearly always superior to animal milks and formulas.
- Children and infants may benefit from animal milk or its products if they are not overused. Avoid low-fat dairy; full-fat dairy aids utilization of fat-soluble vitamins A and D—for bone development and maintenance.
- Milk does not combine well with other foods at the same meal. It is best taken alone, and should not be drunk cold.
- Chlorophyll foods such as green vegetables increase the usefulness of dairy products.
- Raw milk from organically fed animals is greatly preferred; bringing raw cow's milk to a boil quickly, then cooling it, makes it more assimilable, less reactive and safer for infants, and more acceptable for children with weak, sensitive digestion. Its digestibility is also enhanced by adding a pinch of spice (ginger, turmeric, cardamom, etc.) or, for infants, simmering an onion in it.
- Commercially pasteurized milk should also be brought to a boil. Avoid homogenized milk.
- Children with an intolerance to milk digest fermented or soured milk products more easily, as does everyone over seven years of age.
- Milk of goat origin is usually more healthful than cow's milk.
- A child should avoid dairy foods if they cause allergies or mucus problems.

Food Groups and Proportions

Milk intake generally begins to decrease after about six months of age. At this time, and until the age of eighteen months, the most acceptable foods in addition to milk are those that are low in complex carbohydrates. These include:

1. Sprouts of grains, legumes, and other seeds (their carbohydrate is turned to sugar)
2. Milks made from sprouts, seeds, and nuts—prepare according to directions given below in "Cereal or Milk from Sprouts" and in the recipe section in "Grain and Seed Milks."
3. Vegetable juices, particularly carrot juice (its complex carbohydrate is in the pulp), low-starch vegetables, and small amounts of all sea vegetables
4. Soy preparations including tempeh, natto, and soy milk
5. Fruits, avocados, and to a minor extent, fruit juices

For infants under eighteen months, solid-food items such as vegetables, sprouts, soy foods, and fruits are best cooked, puréed and, if desired, diluted with water. Tofu and tempeh should be cooked very well by simmering. Overuse of fruit, especially citrus fruits, and all raw fruit and vegetable juices, can weaken digestion. Regular use of raw juices is most appropriate during clear signs of *excess* (red face, screaming, thick tongue coating).

Sometimes unsprouted cereals and other high-starch foods are craved. These can be prepared according to the directions which follow. The suggestion to pre-chew these foods is especially helpful for babies under eighteen months.

After the age of about eighteen months (with the appearance of the first molar), non-sprouted cereals, legumes, and starchy vegetables can be introduced to the diet gradually. It is important that the grains and legumes be pre-soaked before cooking, to at least initiate the sprouting process and thus eliminate phytic acid, which depletes valuable minerals in infants. The following preparations are most appropriate for babies who follow the gradual weaning pattern described earlier and are about eighteen months or older. Of course, they are also suitable for babies who wean at a different rate or desire such foods earlier.

Preparation of Baby Food During and After Weaning

Suggested Proportions in the Diet
         40–60% grains and cereal preparations
         20–40% vegetables
          5–10% legumes (beans, peas, lentils, fermented soy products), dairy,
                   and/or other animal products
          5–10% fruit
         A small amount of sea vegetables, nuts, and seeds

Vegetables, legumes, seeds, and seaweeds should be cooked until very soft, and then mashed or chewed by an adult until creamy or liquid. As children get older and learn to chew, food can be cooked and mashed less.

Recipes for Cereal or Milk

Grain Cereal	*Grain/Seed/Sea Vegetable Cereal*	
⅓ each: brown rice	90%	whole oat groats or
sweet brown rice		brown rice
oat groats, millet,	5%	sesame seeds or almonds
kamut, or quinoa	5%	wakame

Presoak all ingredients in either recipe for 6 or more hours, and discard soak water. In the recipe with wakame, soak the wakame separately, cut into ¼ by 1-inch pieces, and use its soak water to enrich other dishes. Add 6–7 cups water for each cup of grain. Bring ingredients almost to a boil. Lower heat and simmer, covered, 2–3 hours, or leave on very low heat overnight. Mash into a cream or milky liquid.

Milk from Cereal: Squeeze milky liquid through a cheesecloth. (Do not discard cereal residue.) Add water if necessary.

Variation: Occasionally add rice syrup or barley malt.

Cereal or Milk from Sprouts: Blend or purée wheat, lentil, mung, or barley sprouts in a little water for a baby meal. For milk, blend sprouts with water or rejuvelac (water in which wheat sprouts have soaked—described in recipe section), then strain or squeeze through cheesecloth or a nylon sprout bag. Another method for making sprout milk is to juice the sprouts and add water or rejuvelac for the desired consistency. Sprouts are high in vitamins, minerals, and enzymes and support fast growth in babies and children in general. Use sprouts more often in the spring and summer and less in the fall and winter, and also less for children and infants who are weak, pale, and passive *(deficient)*. Alfalfa sprouts in particular are too cooling and cleansing for the frail child. See "Sprouts" in the recipe section for directions on making sprouts.

Animal Product Quality

Numerous studies during the last twenty years indicate that vegetable foods in general contain far fewer pesticide/herbicide residues than dairy products (as discussed earlier), and less than one-tenth the amount found in red meats, fish, and fowl;[9, 10] also, foods of plant origin contain virtually none of the hormones, antibiotics, and other drugs that saturate our commercial animal products.

Children are in a very dynamic growth process, and it should be a priority to feed them the cleanest foods possible to build the biologic foundation for the rest of their lives. Even if relatively pure animal products are found, the residues such as excess mucus or uric acid resulting from their digestion can be a problem. Therefore, whole foods from the plant kingdom should comprise the bulk of a child's diet.

The Vegetarian Child

All necessary nutrients—protein, fats, calories, minerals, vitamins, enzymes, etc.— are abundantly available in a purely vegetarian diet with the possible exception of vitamin B_{12} (see *Protein and Vitamin B_{12}* chapter). As a prevention against B_{12} deficiency, give vegetarian children one fifty-microgram B_{12} tablet a week.

There are a number of common foods in children's diets that limit nutrient assimilation, listed later in the section "Foods to Use with Caution." Besides poor foods, several other factors require special attention in the diets of children:

A child's digestive system is quite immature until age two and therefore does not assimilate protein or carbohydrates as efficiently as that of an adult.

Secondly, children—infants in particular—seldom chew the essential vegetarian foods such as grains, legumes, and vegetables well enough for optimal assimilation.

Finally, most children in the highly developed nations of the West have an ancestral background rich in animal products, and therefore may find it biologically difficult to adapt to a completely vegetarian diet at a time when tremendous nutritional assets are needed to fuel their rapid growth and development. Nevertheless, most children will thrive on a primarily vegetarian diet of quality wholesome foods if these foods are prepared correctly (e.g., puréed for very young children.)

For the three reasons above, nearly all vegetarian children require *some* animal products after weaning, in order to flourish. Regular use of goat's milk and its products, or other high-quality dairy products, is usually all that is needed from the realm of animal foods for completely supporting a vegetarian child's development. When dairy is not tolerated, especially nutritious plant and animal products may be necessary if deficiencies arise.

Food for Preventing and Treating Deficiencies

If your children show *deficiencies,* if they are pale, weak, and frail, inactive and not growing, changing their diet may help. If a *deficient* child is being breast-fed, then the mother should improve her nutrition or other factors in her life, to increase her general health.

Deficiency in children is often related to a lack of *ojas,* an essence of the body described by Ayurveda. *Ojas* at the beginning of life provides immunity, strength, and the development of intellect. Since the *ojas* of the mother is absorbed by the unborn young in the last two months of pregnancy, premature babies are often *ojas*-deficient. The best source of *ojas* after birth is the milk of the mother. Clarified butter *(ghee)* and almonds also enhance this essence. Building *ojas* is a gradual process. As an aid for children who lack good immunity and strength, combine approximately one teaspoon of clarified butter and/or a few ounces of almond milk with their food several times a week. (See clarified butter and almond milk in index to locate recipes.) When the *ojas* is improved, other tonic foods are better utilized by the body.

Taken in small amounts, fish and naturally raised fowl and other meats can be a helpful tonic against *deficiency.* However, for reasons given throughout this chapter, children may be better off if primary needs can be met by dairy, plant, and microorganism-rich sources.

The vegetal foods listed below assist in the treatment of general *deficiency* associated with an inadequate diet in children (and others). Of course, many other approaches are possible. One of the main uses of these foods is to diminish the need for animal products by all children, not just those who are *deficient.*

None of the following foods should be a sole source of nutrition for infants or children. They are intended to be part of a balanced diet. If used for deficiency, moderate, regularly given amounts work best. Further information on these products is found in the *Protein and Vitamin B$_{12}$* chapter and the recipe section.

Soy

Soybean products are commonly used in the West for infant malnutrition, usually in the forms of poor quality soymilk and infant formulas. The soybean, however, is a good source of protein and calcium, and it is one of the few significant common plant sources of the essential fatty acid alpha-linolenic acid. This lipid, when metabolized into DHA, is a vital component in the structural development of the brain and must be adequately supplied during the first years of life (further discussion of these fatty acids appears in the *Oils and Fats* chapter). The soybean is cooling and must be used in conjunction with other foods; otherwise it may weaken the kidney/adrenal function and thereby limit proper growth. Soybeans are also strongly alkaline, and may be difficult to digest.

The soybean becomes less cooling and more digestible in fermented forms such as tempeh, miso, and natto—a soy product similar to tempeh that is becoming more widely available. Miso has valuable enzymes in addition to the other soybean nutrients, but because of its high salt content must be used in very small amounts for children. Some of the most common soy products—soymilk, infant soy formula, soy protein concentrates—are not whole foods, have denatured proteins, are de-mineralizing, and therefore are not healthful foods for children. Tofu is quite cooling to the kidney-adrenals and should be used sparingly.

Micro-Algae

University and government studies in Mexico show spirulina to be helpful in infant malnutrition. Likewise, the Chinese have successfully administered spirulina for *deficiency*, and spirulina in conjunction with fish has been used to correct the most severe cases of childhood malnutrition for more than fifty years through the efforts of Dr. John McMillin, whose work is described in the *Oils and Fats* chapter.

Perhaps the most outstanding of spirulina's nutritional features for curing deficiency is its exceptionally high level of the fatty acid GLA. It also contains substantial omega-3 alpha-linolenic acid. GLA is important for growth and development, and is found most abundantly in mother's milk; spirulina is the next-highest whole-food source. We sometimes recommend spirulina for people who were never breast-fed, in order to foster the hormonal and mental development that may never have occurred because of lack of proper nutrition in infancy.

Chlorella micro-algae is also useful for deficiencies and infant malnutrition. It contains many of the same nutrients as spirulina but is better for the extremely weak and frail child because it is a little less cooling and cleansing.

Wild blue-green *(Aphanizomenon flos-aquae)* is a bitter and highly cleansing micro-algae and as such is not advisable in cases of *deficiency*. For the nutritional values of micro-algae, see the *Green Food Products* chapter.

Micro-Algae and Soy Dosage: Under one year of age, babies can use ½ teaspoon (1.25 grams) of spirulina or ¼ teaspoon (0.6 grams) chlorella up to twice a day; ⅛ teaspoon of light miso once a day; and ½ ounce of tempeh or natto once a day. These amounts can be doubled by the time the child reaches eighteen months of age. In severe *deficiency*, the amounts of these foods can be increased by taking them more often rather than in larger doses. A child over seven would use a maximum of one tablespoon (7.5 grams) of spirulina or 1½ teaspoon (4 grams) chlorella per day, one teaspoon of miso and three ounces tempeh or natto per day.

Tempeh and natto must be cooked—preferably simmered in a covered pot for 20 minutes. For infants, they are then puréed and mixed with any food or liquid. For best assimilation, mix miso and micro-algae first with a little warm water, and then combine this solution with other foods or drinks. Use these and all supplements at most six days a week.

Amaranth and Quinoa

The dried, powdered sprouts of amaranth are now being used in Mexico in baby food. Both amaranth and quinoa grains have more calcium and protein than milk (see discussion of amaranth and quinoa under "Grains" in recipe section). They combine with other grains such as wheat to form higher amino-acid protein profiles than meats. Amaranth and quinoa supply a high level of balanced nutrition when used in cereal or grain milk recipes. Their sprouts are valuable, but they cannot always be counted on to sprout; their germination rate depends on the variety and age of the seed. These grains have a slightly bitter flavor, making them inappropriate for *deficiency* when taken alone. However, the bitterness diminishes with sprouting. When sprouting is not possible, we recommend they always be combined with another sweet cereal such as rice, oats, sweet rice, or barley. If the combination cereal is still too bitter for the child to accept, a little rice syrup can be added.

*   *   *

Certain practices are vitally important for overcoming *deficiencies*. For example, a *deficient* mother will often improve in health simply by chewing her food more thoroughly. Also, food given to a baby can be pre-chewed by the mother, which is a necessity when giving food that is not well-mashed. Chewing for the baby can greatly increase assimilation of nutrients.

Royal Jelly and Other Animal Products

If vegetarian nutrition and proper feeding methods fail to correct *deficiencies* in children, one may try animal products, perhaps first the goat and other dairy products mentioned earlier. However, when these cannot be used, sometimes other animal foods can help.

Royal jelly, the food that transforms a common worker bee into a queen bee, allowing her to live twenty times longer, is thought to contain the highest complete nutrition of any food. It promotes growth and development, and is commonly used for both infant and general malnutrition. It is available commercially in a number of forms, and can be given daily to infants in approximately 50-milligram doses to benefit nearly every sort of *deficiency*. Children's dosage is 75 mg. for each fifty pounds of body weight. Some royal jelly preparations contain ginseng, which is usually too strong for children and should be avoided.

An idea based on ancient practice is still in use by nutritionists and others who are aware of its value. It is a way to extract the nutritional essence of an animal without giving the difficult-to-digest flesh to a baby or child. Using bones from an organically raised animal (poultry is preferred), break the bones and cook them just below boiling for eighteen hours. Add water as necessary. Root vegetables may be added. Slightly acid vegetables such as carrots, celery, squash, and beets help to extract minerals and other nutrients from the bones and their marrows into the broth. A tablespoon of apple cider vinegar or lemon juice will do the same. When cooked, remove the bones and use this broth alone, or as a liquid base for other foods.

The advantage of this animal-product soup is its unique nutrition from the marrow, which is known in China to promote growth and development. Such a broth from broken bones and vegetables is called "longevity soup." Historical precedents for this practice exist in most other traditional cultures as well, including Native America, where children were given bones to suck out the marrow. People who are vegetarian for ethical reasons may see this as not directly involved in taking animal life, since bones can be obtained that would otherwise be discarded. A word of caution: Avoid animals raised where lead has deposited from auto exhausts or other sources over the years, since lead collects in the bones and marrow of animals. Today more than ever it is important to know about the sources of the food you give your children.

One of the vital nutrients in marrow is the omega-3 fatty acid DHA, which is required for the development of the brain, eyes, and other organs in infants. We know from the *Oils and Fats* chapter that modern mothers and their infants often lack adequate omega-3s. Oils from certain fish and flax seed are the most commonly used sources of these fatty acids. In the 1940s children received the first "vitamin supplement"—just 10 drops or so of cod liver oil. Today this oil is often given to weak infants and children who contract frequent colds, flus, and other infectious diseases. It also treats extended colic as well as irritations in the digestive system and in all other body tissues. Its preformed omega-3 fatty acids, vitamins A and D, and other nutrients not only help build nerve, brain, and bone tissues, but strengthen all cells and their immunity. It has been considered an essential supplement for premature and formula-fed babies.

Lactating mothers can also take it for their deficient infants. For pronounced deficiencies during pregnancy and early infancy, fish oil is thought to be more helpful than omega-3 plant oils, which may not contribute enough DHA. Likewise, infants may not form sufficient DHA from vegetable omega-3 sources for a number of months, so cod liver oil and other fish oils are considered more effective. For best results use fish oils from clean ocean areas. *Cod liver oil daily dosage:* Babies: approximately 8 drops orally from a medicine dropper or in their formula; dosage can increase to 12 drops for premature birth, not receiving mother's milk, or poor immunity. Pregnant and lactating women: 1 to 2 teaspoons; children are given less according to weight. Emulsified oils taste better and are one-third cod liver oil, so the dosage of these is triple the above.

The Chinese regard such developmental problems as failure to grow or incomplete closure of the skull bones as an indication of *jing* insufficiency. A number of the foods recommended in this section for overcoming *deficiency* may be used to restore *jing*. These and others, along with an explanation of the *jing* concept, appear in the *Water Element* chapter. In serious *jing* deficiency, appropriate choices of any of the *jing*-enhancing foods can form a nutritional base for the powerful *jing* tonics that treat pronounced maldevelopment in children. (See "deer antler" and "tortoise shell," page 365.)

Because of the strong nature of flesh foods (including meat, eggs, chicken, and fish), they are best considered medicinal condiments for children rather than main fare. Their use is most appropriate in the cooler seasons, when weakened conditions are more prevalent. Mincing to the size appropriate for the child and cooking these foods in soups or stews makes their effects milder and generally more beneficial (this applies to people of all ages). If ingredients in a soup are cut too large for a child, the whole soup can be blended after it is cooked. Other ways to make the effects of animal foods less extreme are discussed at the end of the chapter *Protein and Vitamin B$_{12}$*. If any of the meat products do help a child's *deficiencies*, they can be used intermittently or else discontinued when the *deficiency* is resolved, in order to avoid the build-up of toxic by-products.

Foods to Use with Caution

- Flours (especially wheat) promote infant mucus and allergies. Avoid them for the first two years. Children over two with reactions to wheat can sometimes tolerate kamut or spelt pastas and breads; these ancient grains and products made from them are well-accepted by most children, and are increasingly available in stores carrying whole foods.

- Raw onions and garlic are too stimulating for regular use by children, but make good medicine for colds. Garlic is helpful in ridding children of worms if taken daily for a week. To give garlic in a form children can accept, slice it thin and place it between thin slices of apple—an apple-garlic sandwich. (The apple will disguise the acrid flavor.) Most children also tolerate minced garlic mixed into a thin miso-water paste or into honey. Garlic pills or capsules can be used for children who are old enough to swallow them. When the mother eats garlic (or any herb) the essential qualities usually come through the milk, so caution is advised while nursing.

- Use no salt under ten months of age. Then begin with one grain, and increase slowly. There is sufficient natural salt for children in grains, vegetables, and small amounts of sea vegetables. Excess salt is too hard on their kidneys and also tends to inhibit growth.

- Avoid common refined and rancid cooking oils as well as margarine, shortening, and the many commercial "treats" made with hydrogenated oils. All of these fats and oils block fat metabolism, resulting in greater likelihood of incomplete nervous system development, emotional instability, and degenerative diseases later in life.

- Too much raw food can weaken children, especially infants and toddlers, by reducing their digestive strength. Being susceptible to parasites, children can also have their digestion and general health undermined by parasitic infestations as a result of eating raw vegetables. Lettuce, radishes, carrots, and potatoes, for example, frequently harbor parasites. (Removal of parasites from salad vegetables is discussed on page 572.) When a child has *deficiency* signs (thinness, low energy, pale complexion, weak voice, introversion), feels cold, or has loose stools, uncooked food should be restricted. During phases of *excess* (aggression, loud voice—possible screaming or yelling, thick tongue coating) and/or *heat* (red face, wants cold fluids and few clothes), a child usually needs to eat more salad, fruit, and raw or lightly cooked sprouts. Juices from vegetables, sprouts, or barley-grass concentrates are also helpful.
- Avoid refined sweeteners such as fructose and white sugar.
- Chocolate contains a caffeine-like substance (theobromine) and oxalic acid, which can inhibit calcium absorption; as a confection, it nearly always is combined with mucus-forming refined sugar and processed milk.
- Raw honey sometimes contains small amounts of the toxin botulin. When the quantity of this toxin is low, it is easily denatured in the mature digestive tract. However, the underdeveloped digestive systems of most infants do not have this ability, and botulin in raw honey has been known to cause infant death (this acute food poisoning is called "botulism"). Botulin may not be completely destroyed even in cooked honey, and since it is also not always specified whether commercial honey is raw or cooked, it is safest to avoid giving any honey to children who are less than eighteen months of age.
- Fruit: use primarily when children are fully vital. Too much fruit can encourage colds, runny noses, ear problems, and general weakness. It is best taken cooked in cold weather, especially for the weak or frail child.
- Always dilute fruit juices, and serve them warm or at room temperature. Juice is more concentrated and weakening than whole fruit.
- Infants who bottle-feed on sweet juices, milk, and/or carrot juice several hours daily are at risk of losing their front teeth to decay.[11]
- Buckwheat is overly drying and stimulating for most children and can cause hyperactivity and nervousness when eaten regularly.
- Sautéed, fried, or heavily pressure-cooked foods can be too concentrated for children. Cooking without oil is generally more appropriate.
- Limit or avoid strong spices and condiments.

A child's digestive system is delicate and can change dramatically with ingestion of strongly polarized foods. Many traumas and obstructions of later life are a result of extreme experiences in childhood. We have noticed that unfortunate health and traumatic conditions are usually accompanied by nutritional extremes. Children are easily influenced. If they are given excesses of very expansive, dispersive foods, they become scattered and weak very quickly (e.g., strong spices, refined sugars, too much tropical fruit). Fortunately, they revert to normal nearly as quickly. The same applies to an excess of highly concentrated foods (meats, eggs, salt, etc.). When children grow up swinging between nutritional extremes, it is more difficult for them to root out that tendency later on. However, as mentioned before, small amounts of animal products to supplement *deficiencies* is not extreme.

Food and Behavior

People who think that food has little effect on behavior need only observe the difference in children who begin to eat a balanced whole-food diet. The effect on adults is similar but takes longer because of inertia and the stored toxins that first must be released. One hyperactive child we knew was consistently chaotic and quite rude for several years. His mother decided to feed him primarily unrefined vegetarian foods, and after three weeks, his behavior changed dramatically. He became courteous, happy, and a pleasure to be around.

The child who eats an excess of poor-quality red meats is usually aggressive and/or emotionally stressed because of at least one factor—most common meats are high in the fatty acid arachidonate, which forms hormone-like prostaglandins of the E_2 series in the body (discussed in the *Oils and Fats* chapter). An excess of these promotes mental and physical inflammation, and thus aggression. As aggression-based internal stress accumulates, intoxicants become more attractive later in life for their (temporary) relaxing value.

When refined sugar is dominant in the diet, moodiness is commonplace as a result of sugar imbalances in the blood and brain.

Positive results have been obtained just by eliminating processed sugars, other refined foods, and foods which contain chemical ingredients and preservatives. Such dietary improvements have been spreading during the last decade in many areas of the United States and Canada, often at the request of the local school administration. (See note 14, page 695, for discussion on Attention Deficit Hyperactivity Disorder—ADHD.)

Certainly not all childhood behavior problems can be solved by simple dietary changes. Children, like adults, sometimes refuse to eat wholesome food. In other cases, dietary changes are too extreme. There may be too many natural sweets and fruit juices, too many salty foods and nut butters, or food may be ill-prepared.

Some problems with children's behavior may be constitutional problems resistant to quick dietary healing. Very often, however, the seemingly incorrigible child simply craves another kind of nurture besides a good diet—the influence of parents who live in emotional balance.

Suggestions for Conception and Pregnancy

Many of the imbalances that people exhibit throughout life originate in prenatal deficiencies, which often reflect the diet and overall vitality of the parents during conception and pregnancy.[12] Since it takes months to make deep improvements in health, we advise both men and women to strengthen themselves well before conceiving children.

Taoist Prohibitions at the Time of Conception[13]

Taoism is a 2,600-year-old philosophical/religious system of China; its practices are intended to bring one into harmony with the *Tao* or unsurpassed "Way." The following prohibitions have been developed through careful observation of the vitality of children over thousands of years. Some of the suggestions are commonly known and accepted in the West, while others concerning the weather and celibacy may seem peculiar. Whether they become widely accepted will depend on the experience of Westerners using them.

A child will be much healthier if sex is avoided throughout the pregnancy. This is not only a Taoist claim but also a recommendation of Tibetan and Indian Yogic traditions. This suggestion is often poorly received by people in the West. However, it is a most important recommendation in cultures which have closely observed its effect. This author concurs with this prohibition and has witnessed remarkable differences in the emotional integrity and awareness of children whose parents chose celibacy during pregnancy, compared to their siblings who developed when the parents were not celibate. The impact on the fetus of hormonal and other physiological changes resulting from sexual activity is a ripe area for future scientific investigation. Because complete celibacy is considered to be out of the question for most married people, perhaps this prohibition can at least serve as a recommendation for moderation in sexual activity during pregnancy.

Neither partner should be under the influence of any intoxicants nor in the habit of using intoxicants.

Do not conceive during strong winds or storms.

Do not conceive if either partner is weak or sick.

If conception is difficult, it may help to avoid sexual activity, which will allow the body to strengthen; frequent and uncontrolled sex can be weakening to the reproductive system, resulting in less fertility.

During Pregnancy

- Pregnant women should eat according to their intuitions, since they are heightened at this time. Usually it is best to include a wide variety of nutritious foods. Vegetarians may be drawn to dairy, eggs, fish, or other animal products during pregnancy. This is particularly the case with recent vegetarians. It often takes a dozen or more years to completely acclimate to a primarily vegetarian diet when one has a heritage of centuries of animal food over-consumption.
- Do not dramatically alter the diet, since the toxins released in major changes will affect the fetus. The following dietary suggestions, however, are safe to follow.
- Avoid all intoxicants and strong substances, including cigarettes, alcohol, marijuana, coffee, unnecessary medicines, etc.

- Bitter herbs should be avoided unless prescribed for a medical purpose; seaweeds should be restricted in pregnancy except for treating signs of *heat* and *excess* (robust character, loud voice, red face/eyes, dark yellow, scanty urine, thick yellow tongue coating, forceful pulse).
- Replace refined foods with whole, fresh food; for example, use whole-grain breads instead of white bread, mineral-rich sweeteners such as rice or barley malt, honey or molasses instead of refined sugar or synthetic sweeteners, and fresh vegetables instead of canned.
- Eat sufficient green vegetables. These contain nutrients needed in greater quantities during pregnancy: omega-3 fatty acids (necessary for fetal brain development), folic acid (works with vitamin B_{12} to build blood and promote fetal growth), and magnesium (essential for calcium uptake). The safest of the highly concentrated chlorophyll foods during pregnancy is wheat- or barley-grass (see *Green Food Products* chapter for dosage). Green vegetables are likewise important during nursing and are a Japanese folk remedy to increase milk supply.
- Avoid "mega-doses" of vitamins and other nutrients without a specific medical reason. Most prenatal supplements contain safe nutrient levels and are helpful if the diet is not of high quality. Strict vegetarians (vegans) should take a vitamin B_{12} supplement.
- Maintain a daily awareness practice such as quiet contemplation, meditation, and/or prayer.
- Get regular moderate exercise, outdoors if possible, in sunlight and fresh air.

The Child Within

Understanding the nature of life, why and how individuals come into being, and the purpose behind procreation are fundamental questions that are not often satisfactorily dealt with, even by parents. When we are able to accept the mystery of life equally with our logical, explainable reality, we begin to enter the world of the child and can begin to grow with our children.

Children come literally from our insides and will continually relate to those deep places within us where we sorely need awareness. The surprising and sometimes shocking actions of children are most often just those areas of our subconscious we have refused to face. It can be a "shock" to experience emotional and physical expressions from which we have shielded ourselves so completely.

Healing and Bonding

In every instance, we have observed that people who have chronic problems with their offspring have not worked on themselves. When parents heal themselves by making deep attitudinal changes, and support these with appropriate actions in their lives, invariably the children will also start clearing their own negative behavior. Because of the depth of bonding in a family, it is not always necessary to communicate directly about such kinds of healing. It is often simply felt, even thousands of miles away.

When are the effects of a parent's transformation felt most strongly by children? When there is truly meaningful change—when at least the most rigid outer layer of resistance, including stagnant mental conditioning, begins to melt. This is marked by the purging of physical toxins that have supported a stale mentality. Sometimes this process takes months or years, since often we *say* we are changing before actually making the level of commitment necessary for a deeply penetrating transformation. For instance, many people will start a new diet, stop intoxicants, and still find a way to maintain a poor attitude. When we really are renewed, we feel it both in spirit and throughout the body.

We have had equal success in recommending that children initiate change in order to help their parents; all other close or "bonded" relationships, including husband/wife and even close friends, also work in this same way.

Our family relationships are the ones that present us with the experiences and lessons we need to work on extensively. Many modern families choose to break up rather than persevere in solving problems that arise. Those who succeed in creating a balanced family in this time of great social transformation acquire limitless patience and learn to work with compassionate understanding.

The ultimate food for children is life with parents with these qualities.

Part III

The Five Element and Organ Systems

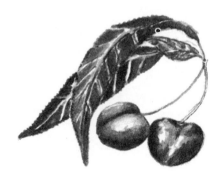

Five Element Correspondences

Five Elements	Wood	Fire	Earth	Metal	Water
HUMAN BODY					
Yin Solid Organ	Liver	Heart-Mind	Spleen-Pancreas	Lungs	Kidneys
Yang Hollow Organ	Gallbladder	Small Intestine	Stomach	Large Intestine	Urinary Bladder
Sense Organ Sense	Eyes/ Sight	Tongue/ Speech	Mouth/ Taste	Nose/ Smell	Ears/ Hearing
Tissue	Tendons and sinews	Blood vessels	Muscles and flesh	Skin and hair	Bones
Emotion	Anger and impatience	Joy	Worry and anxiety	Grief and melancholy	Fear and fright
Voice Sound	Shouting	Laughing	Singing	Weeping	Groaning
Fluid Emitted	Tears	Sweat	Saliva	Mucus	Urine
Paramita*	Patience	Wisdom and concentration	Giving	Vigor	Keeping moral precepts
NATURE					
Season	Spring	Summer	Late Summer	Autumn	Winter
Environmental Influence	Wind	Heat	Dampness	Dryness	Cold
Development	Birth	Growth	Transformation	Harvest	Storing
Color	Green	Red	Yellow	White	Black/dark
Taste	Sour	Bitter	Sweet	Pungent	Salty
Orientation	East	South	Middle	West	North
Grain	Wheat, oats	Corn, amaranth	Millet, barley	Rice	Beans

Paramita in Sanskrit means "to go across," often in the sense of crossing a sea of pain and suffering. Here the *paramitas* are ways to correct imbalances in the Elements. For example, in the Wood Element, anger is overcome with patience; in Earth, weakness in the spleen-pancreas and stomach can be helped by giving. The *paramita* of "keeping moral precepts" means to hold the five traditional precepts of avoiding killing, lying, stealing, sexual misconduct, and intoxicants. A good moral foundation supports a strong biologic foundation, and we will discuss in the *Water Element* chapter how the kidney-adrenal function is the root and foundation of the body.

Five Elements:
Seasonal Attunement and the
Organs in Harmony and Disease

he Five Elements system of the ancient Chinese serves as an aid for understanding the limitless correspondences that pervade every facet of life. In
the Six Divisions and Six Influences we discovered simple yet effective patterns that describe the constitution and condition of an individual. The Five Elements take another diagnostic step toward unification of the person, including
the internal organs, emotions, body parts, and environment, linking these with
five dynamic categories that empower and control one another by means of "Creation" and "Control" cycles.

The Five Element system was developed by Chinese sages who saw reality in
terms of the most direct (and easily overlooked) relationships. For example, they
noted that kidney imbalance is related to fear and bone disorders. How accurate
is this system? Several thousand years later the associations originally set forth
are still enlightening to those who apply them. Their accuracy has been verified by
countless successful practitioners of Chinese medicine.

The traditional medicine of China does not stop with the one-word descriptions listed under each of the Five Elements. Rather than being a rigorous system in itself, the Five Elements function as a faint shadow of the entire body of
Chinese medical philosophy and practice, acting as reminders of certain principles. Thus, for in-depth clinical applications, the words in a Five Elements chart
must be interpreted and fit into the elegant and precise texture of Chinese physiology. In dietary healing, however, one needs only a working knowledge of the
basic and most important features of this physiological schema. In the Five Element
chapters that follow we offer the basics of Chinese physiology, and each Five Element discussion is preceded by a description of seasonal correspondences.

Seasonal Attunement

The ancient Chinese believed that the seasons have a profound cyclical effect on
human growth and well-being—that we are influenced by climatic changes and
should live in harmony with them. For example, as summer *(yang)* draws to a
close we may be aware that fall and winter *(yin)* are just around the corner, and so
our body and mind, day by day, make gradual adjustments. If one lives in a climate with cold winters, it is necessary that the blood be thicker as the weather
grows cold; consciously preparing for this change can help make the winter a time
of beauty and comfort instead of a time to dread. This process is undertaken in part
by knowing how to choose and prepare food according to the seasons.

Harmony with the seasons is second nature to the balanced person. Unfortunately, most of us have blunted our instinctual awareness; only through practices that bring us close to the cycles of Nature do we begin to hear the voice of our own nature clearly. Gradually the practices become internalized, and more complete trust in our intuition is possible. The earliest classics of the East (and West) suggest we follow our spiritual guidance (*yang*—heaven's domain) and at the same time accord with Nature (*yin*—earth):

> The principle of the interaction of the four seasons and of *yin* and *yang* is the foundation of everything in creation. Thus sages nurture their *yang* in the spring and summer and *yin* in the fall and winter in order to follow the rule of rules; therefore, unified with everything in creation, sages maintain themselves continuously at the Gate of Life.—*Inner Classic*

One misunderstanding often arises regarding the use of flavors for seasonal attunement. The flavor associated with each Element affects the organ in that Element in specific, therapeutic ways, but it is not used for general attunement to the associated season.* The key to understanding this lies in the difference between specific and general uses. For example, the bitter flavor's cooling, contracting, *yin* properties are of special value in treating over*heated* conditions of various organ systems, particularly those of the heart, so bitter is assigned to the Fire Element. To generally attune to summer, however, one must become more *yang* and expansive, like the summer itself, by using hot spices. Fortunately, these cause cooling through sweating, by pushing *yang* to its extreme. (Recall that *yin* and *yang* at their extremes transform readily into each other.)

If one is attuned to the summer by being hot on the body's surface so that the sensation of hot weather is not overbearing, and by being able to sweat when necessary, the bitter flavor will be required only occasionally for cooling, if at all. Therefore, in the following Five Element chapters, a distinction is made between the use of flavors for seasonal attunement and their use in therapy.

The Organs in Harmony and Disease

After seasonal considerations, the discussions in the Five Element chapters turn to the basic language and diagnostic methods used in the Chinese physiology of the organs; the remedies for the most widely encountered syndromes of each organ system are also given. The Five Element relationships are thus put into a workable perspective; we see that related areas have to respond when changes occur in any area. For example, if the functioning of the liver can be improved, then the other categories listed under Wood will also improve. The person undoubtedly will be more patient and less angry, vision may improve, tendons and ligaments may become stronger and more flexible, a gall bladder problem may vanish, and so on. Conversely, by developing patience and strengthening ligaments and tendons,

---

*The salty flavor is an exception and is discussed in the *Water Element* chapter.

the liver will benefit. It is obvious that such simple, easily observed connections between our symptoms and internal organs are an invaluable aid in diagnosis. Prevention is emphasized, since the Five Elements and other evaluation methods in this book will usually indicate subtle imbalances long before a medical crisis occurs.

Creation and Control Cycles

Not only are the correspondences within each Element important, but the Elements influence one another, as mentioned earlier. The method of influence is described in elaborate detail by Chinese physiology. A shorthand way of remembering and using these influences is the Five Element Creation and Control Cycles.

Below is an introduction to these cycles as explained in the *Nei Ching*, which we refer to as the *Inner Classic*.

Creation Cycle
Wood burns to make
Fire whose ashes decompose into
Earth where are born and mined
Metals which enrich
Water which nourishes trees (Wood).

Control Cycle
Wood is cut by Metal.
Fire is extinguished by Water.
Earth is penetrated by Wood.
Metal is melted by Fire.
Water is channeled and
contained by Earth.

The Creation Cycle: Observe from the preceding charts how the organs correspond to the various Elements. For example, the heart is associated with Fire, the liver with Wood, etc. The Creation Cycle shows how one organ, sometimes called the "mother," "creates" or "feeds" the following organ, its son, through a strengthening flow of energy. Example: The heart strengthens its son, the spleen-pancreas; the spleen-pancreas strengthens its son, the lungs. If one organ becomes deficient, it may draw excessively from the preceding organ (its mother) and deplete it, and at the same time it will not have the ability to strengthen the next organ, its son. Thus, one of the best ways to strengthen the heart (Fire) is to first improve its mother, the liver (Wood).

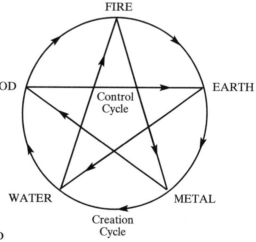

Creation and Control Cycles

Likewise, a weakness from one season will be expressed in the following season. Example: Diarrhea in late summer can lead to bronchitis in the fall. This is due to the correspondence of late summer to the Earth Element, which is also the domain of the spleen-pancreas and stomach. The fall is the season in which the Metal Element and lungs are emphasized.

The Control (Destruction) Cycle: This cycle represents the process by which Elements "check and balance" one another. When the balancing is normal and healthful, it can be called the Control Cycle. If it is not, a Control Cycle can become a Destruction Cycle. This occurs when an organ becomes hyperactive or excessive in some way and then, instead of beneficially controlling the next organ in the Control Cycle, attacks it. See the Control Cycle in the preceding chart.

Control Cycle example: Balanced kidneys protect the heart, since the *yin* fluid of the kidneys is distributed throughout the body and protects the heart from inflammation.

Destruction Cycle example: Kidneys that cause excessive fluid retention weaken the heart (Water can put out Fire). This relationship is confirmed by modern medical science, and now many who have heart and circulatory problems such as hypertension are given diuretics to shed excess water.

In the Creation and Control Cycles we see the dynamics inherent in the Five Elements and their organ systems—they are not solitary, fixed entities but interrelated flows of energy and substances, all in a state of transformation. The flows among the organs described in Chinese physiology include *qi* energy, fluids, nutrients, emotions, and many other factors, all working in an orderly and harmonious fashion when health is present.

> The sages follow the laws of Nature and therefore their bodies are free from strange diseases. They do not lose any of their natural functions and their spirit of life is never exhausted.
>
> —*Inner Classic*

Thus, Chinese physiology, in conjunction with Five Element theory, presents the entire person—bodily functions, tissues, and organs as well as mental and emotional aspects—as correspondences that influence one another. This orderly system suggests a perfection in the inter-connection of all things, and thereby enhances our sense of unity. Such a vision of reality inspires hope and engenders clarity in what may otherwise seem a random and chaotic universe.

Therapeutic Use of the Five Flavors

The flavor of food is sometimes difficult to describe, yet it provides insight into the therapeutic dimensions and actions of the food. The Five-Element associations listed earlier are valuable, but for purposes of dietary healing, we must also know the flavors in terms of their thermal nature (warming/cooling value), their many remedial actions (moistening, drying, astringent, purgative, antibiotic, dispersing, tonifying, etc.), where their energy is directed in the body, and how they are used therapeutically in various organ systems, not just the organs they relate to in the Five Elements. The bitter flavor of dandelion, for example, reduces both *heat* and *damp* conditions in general, particularly in those areas affected by the liver, spleen-pancreas, lungs, and heart. Dandelion and other bitter foods also tend to direct energy inward and toward the lower part of the body.

The system of flavors we will use has been developed by traditional Chinese healers. Occasionally in this system a food is assigned a flavor that does not correspond with the taste. This occurs because flavors are designated in part to reflect the properties of the food, and thus some assigned flavors may differ from the acknowledged taste.

A number of foods have two or more flavors to take into consideration, such as vinegar, which is both bitter and sour. Such a food is used therapeutically only if both flavors are needed.

Two flavors—pungent and sweet—are considered *yang,* tend to be warming, and direct energy outward and higher in the body. The remaining three flavors— sour, bitter, and salty—are *yin* and cooling, and conduct energy lower and inward.

In addition, according to Chinese physiology as well as the Five Elements theory, the flavors "enter" (are most closely associated with) the internal organs in this way:

- the sour flavor enters the liver and gall bladder;
- the bitter flavor enters the heart and small intestine;
- the sweet flavor enters the spleen-pancreas and stomach;
- the pungent flavor enters the lungs and large intestine;
- the salty flavor enters the kidneys and bladder.

In the diet of a healthy person the flavors should be balanced, with the sweet flavor predominating, because the Earth Element and its associated flavor—sweetness—are considered the most central aspect of the body and its nourishment. Such balancing is quite simple. It means that each day the sweet flavor—the primary flavor of most carbohydrates such as grains, vegetables, legumes, nuts, seeds, and fruit—should be accompanied by small amounts of bitter, salty, pungent, and sour foods. Very often these primarily sweet carbohydrates will contain sufficient secondary flavors themselves; otherwise, condiments can be used. When health is poor and during acute disease conditions, it is usually helpful to change just two flavors, emphasizing one obviously important flavor and restricting a contraindicated one.

The flavors not only create balance but also bring a person into harmony with seasonal influences. Invariably, the question arises how to balance flavors that attune to the seasons but contradict individual needs. The answer is first to balance the individual, then to work for seasonal attunement as much as possible without violating the individual's internal climate. For example, a person with edema cannot ordinarily tolerate salt, and so even though more salt is normally used in the winter, those with edema should not increase salt. Instead, they can emphasize the bitter flavor, which is drying and also helps attune the individual to the colder season.

The quantity of flavors is important. If a flavor is generally helpful for an organ function, too much of that flavor has an opposite and weakening effect. This is often seen in the use of the sweet flavor, which benefits the spleen-pancreas and digestive function. However, when too much is taken, the result is weakening of digestive absorption, mucus accumulation, and blood sugar imbalances such as diabetes.

Pungent (including acrid, spicy, hot, and aromatic flavors)

Properties: A *yang* flavor; expansive, dispersive; when the pungent flavor has a warming energy (see examples below), it stimulates circulation of energy and blood, tending to move energy upwards and outwards to the periphery of the body.

Uses of the Pungent Flavor: Stimulates digestion, disperses mucus caused by highly mucus-forming foods such as dairy products and meats, and offers protection against mucus conditions such as the common cold. The diaphoretic pungents such as mint, cayenne, elder flower, scallion, garlic, and chamomile are used to induce sweating during a common cold or other *exterior* condition. They can also lighten the effects of grains, legumes, nuts, and seeds, all of which have moderate mucus-forming properties; they disperse stagnant blood and increase *qi* energy as well. Some of the extremely pungent flavors such as garlic, mugwort, and cayenne destroy or expel parasites. In the West, pungency is consumed most often in the form of alcoholic beverages. Unfortunately, though these substances have some beneficial short-term effect, they ultimately cause necrosis, especially brain-cell death.

Organ Functions:
1. The pungent flavor enters and clears the lungs of mucus conditions (do not use warming pungents [see examples below] if there are *heat* conditions anywhere in the body).
2. It improves digestive activity, which is ruled by the spleen-pancreas, and expels gas from the intestines.
3. According to the *Inner Classic,* pungent flavor "moistens the kidneys," which affect fluids in the entire body. One result of this is an increase of saliva and sweat from the action of certain pungents such as ginger. The hot pungent herbs also tend to be good for *cold,* contracted conditions of the kidneys, warming and relaxing them.
4. The pungent flavor stimulates blood circulation and is cardiotonic.
5. It helps clear obstructions and improve sluggish liver function.

Seasonal attunement: The pungent flavor (in alliance with the full sweet flavor) attunes a person to the spring. Those pungent flavors that are also hot provide the interior environment of, and attune the body to, summer; these include cayenne, black pepper, hot green and red peppers, and fresh ginger. One may also use certain hot pungent flavors—most notably dried ginger and cinnamon—for overcoming signs of *coldness,* since these herbs are deeply warming for a relatively long span of time. Cayenne and other peppers are also warming, but are so extreme that they change to a cooling effect after thirty minutes or so.

Individuals Most Benefited: Those who are sluggish, dull, lethargic, or excessively heavy benefit from the pungent flavor (as well as from the bitter flavor). Those inclined to *damp*/mucous conditions of the Metal Element organs (lungs and colon) can add pungent flavors for prevention and treatment. The person with *cold* signs improves with the use of warming pungents.

Certain pungent flavors can be beneficial for *dry,* thin individuals or those who tend toward *wind* conditions of nervous, restless activity. Such flavors are found in the seed pungents which relax the nervous system and improve digestion: fennel, dill, caraway, anise, coriander, and cumin. The pungent roots ginger, onion (cooked), and horseradish, along with black peppercorn, act as stimulants and also help promote general stability and smooth circulation of energy. However, not all pungent flavors are appropriate for the *dry* or unstable person (see below).

Cautions: Some pungent flavors worsen the condition of the *dry, windy,* nervous, or thin person. These include sage, raw onion, and *all* hot peppers, especially cayenne. According to the *Inner Classic,* "In *qi* diseases, avoid too much pungent food." This applies in times of deficient *qi* including weakness, or stagnant *qi* of the sort involved in obstructions and constrictions. Also avoid the many warming pungents when *heat* signs exist. Those who are overweight from overeating should choose cooling pungents.

Examples: Warming pungents: spearmint, rosemary, scallion, garlic and all onion family members, cinnamon bark and branch, cloves, fresh and dried ginger root, black pepper, all hot peppers, cayenne, fennel, anise, dill, mustard greens, horseradish, basil, and nutmeg. Cooling pungents: peppermint, marjoram, elder flowers, white pepper, and radish and its leaves. Neutral pungents: taro, turnip, and kohlrabi.

The pungency of some foods is diminished by cooking. The loss of pungency in moderate simmering is easily noticeable in many common vegetables including turnip, cabbage, the onion family, and horseradish. With mild steaming some pungency is preserved, but for full effect, eat the heat-sensitive pungents raw or pickled. Pungent leafy herbs such as the mints should be steeped, although most barks and roots such as ginger and cinnamon need to be simmered.

Salty

Properties: A *yin*, cooling effect; tends to move energy downward and inward; has "centering," earthy qualities; moistens *dryness;* softens hardened lumps and stiffness; improves digestion; detoxifies the body; and can purge the bowels and promote emesis.

Uses of the Salty Flavor: The salty flavor may be increased in the diet to soften lumps, for example, hardened lymph nodes, cataracts, and other knottings of the muscles and glands. Salt is used internally for constipation, abdominal swelling and pain, and externally for impure blood conditions with *heat* signs, such as most skin discharges, sore throat (in a hot water gargle), and pyorrhea (brush teeth with fine salt). Salt counteracts toxins in the body, is an appetant (increases appetite), and is greatly overused, especially in the form of common table salt, which is poor quality. (See the chapter on salt for additional insight into its nature and uses.)

Organ Functions: The salty flavor, associated with the Water Element, "enters" the kidneys and is also considered a "proper" flavor for the spleen-pancreas, where it strengthens the digestive function. Salt also fortifies a weak heart-mind and improves mental concentration.

Seasonal Attunement: The descending, cooling nature of the salty flavor attunes one to the colder seasons and climates, and should be used progressively more throughout fall and winter.

Individuals Most Benefited: Foods with a salty flavor moisten and calm the thin, *dry,* nervous person.

Cautions: Salt must be greatly restricted by those with *damp,* overweight, lethargic, or edemic conditions, and also by those with high blood pressure. Seaweeds, which are salty, are an exception to these restrictions, because their iodine and trace minerals speed up metabolism. Although salt is *yin* by nature, too much salt has the opposite effect, according to Ayurvedic tradition, and should be used very sparingly by aggressive people. Those with blood toxicity need to monitor their use of the salty flavor as well. "Do not eat much salt in blood diseases."—*Inner Classic*

Examples: Salt, seaweed (kelp, kombu, bladderwrack, dulse, etc.); barley and millet have some salty quality although they are primarily sweet. Products made with substantial amounts of salt include soy sauce, miso, pickles, umeboshi (salt plum), and gomasio (sesame salt).

Sour

Properties: A *yin,* cooling quality; causes contraction and has a gathering, absorbent, astringent effect, to prevent or reverse abnormal leakage of fluids and energy, and to dry and firm up tissues.

Uses of the Sour Flavor: Used in the treatment of urinary dripping, excessive perspiration, hemorrhage, diarrhea, and weak, sagging tissues including flaccid skin, hemorrhoids, and uterine prolapse. The sour flavor derives from a great variety of acids, some of the most common being citric acid, tannic acid, and ascorbic acid (vitamin C). The most sour flavors such as found in black and green teas and blackberry leaves can be classified as "astringent." However, not all remedies that stop bleeding, diarrhea, and other "loose" problems are sour or astringent in taste, and specific remedies for such conditions are given in later chapters.

Organ Functions: The sour flavor is most active in the liver, where it counteracts the effects of rich, greasy food, functioning as a solvent and breaking down fats and protein. Sourness helps in digestion to dissolve minerals for improved assimilation, and can help strengthen weakened lungs. Sour-tasting food is also the "proper food" for the "heart-mind" (the Chinese concept of the union of heart and mind), as it plays a role in organizing scattered mental patterns.

Seasonal Attunement: Sour food draws one into harmony with the fall, the time of gathering (harvesting) and the beginning of the period of contraction, with the onset of cooler weather.

Individuals Most Benefited: Sour flavors collect and hold together the dispersed, capriciously changing personality. Sour foods do not occur frequently enough in the modern diet.

Cautions: Those with *dampness,* heaviness of mind or body, constipation, and constrictions should use the sour flavor sparingly. "In diseases of the sinews (tendons and ligaments), do not eat much sour food."—*Inner Classic*

Examples: Most sour foods also have other prominent flavors, as seen below.

Sour	**Sour and Sweet**
hawthorne berry	aduki bean
lemon	apple
lime	blackberry
pickles	cheese
rose hip	grape
sauerkraut	huckleberry
sour apple (crab apple)	mango
sour plum	olive
	raspberry
Sour and Bitter	sourdough bread
vinegar	tangerine
	tomato
Sour and Pungent	yogurt
leek	

Bitter

Properties: A *yin,* cooling effect; causes contraction and encourages the energy of the body to descend. Reduces the *excessive* person (robust, extroverted, with thick tongue coating, loud voice, reddish complexion, etc.). Bitterness is antipyretic, lowering fever; it will also dry fluids and drain *dampness.* Certain bitter foods and herbs have a purgative effect and induce bowel movement.

Uses of the Bitter Flavor: Helpful for inflammations, infections, and overly moist, *damp* conditions specified below. Also used for constipation. Perhaps the most underused and least appreciated of the flavors.

Organ Functions: The bitter flavor is closely identified with the Fire Element and heart, where it clears *heat* and cleans arteries of *damp* mucoid deposits of cholesterol and fats, in general tending to lower blood pressure. (Celery is a specific food for this purpose.) The bitter flavor also clears stagnancy and cools *heat* in the liver (normally caused by overconsumption of rich foods).

Bitter foods and herbs drain various *damp*-associated conditions in the forms of candida yeast overgrowth, parasites, mucus, swellings, skin eruptions, abscesses, growths, tumors, cysts, obesity, and all moist accumulations including edema in the regions governed by the spleen-pancreas (the intestines and the flesh of the body). Bitter also increases intestinal muscle contractions.

The kidneys and lungs are said to be tonified and vitalized by bitter flavors. Bitter is superb for removing mucous/*heat* conditions in the lungs, signified by yellow phlegm discharges. Even though bitter is the flavor that enters the heart, according to the *Inner Classic,* it is the "proper" flavor for the lungs.

Seasonal Attunement: One progressively increases the use of the bitter flavor throughout the fall and winter, in order to contract and channel energy lower into the body for the colder season. *Heat* symptoms that arise during any season can be neutralized by the bitter flavor.

Individuals Most Benefited: Slow, overweight, lethargic, watery *(damp)* individuals; also overheated, aggressive persons are cooled by the bitter flavor.

Cautions: Persons who are *deficient, cold,* weak, thin, nervous, and *dry* should limit bitter food intake. And "those with bone diseases should not eat much bitter food."—*Inner Classic*

Examples: For a strong bitter flavor as an aid in major imbalances, try the commonly available bitter herbs such as dandelion leaf or root, burdock leaf or root, yarrow, chamomile, hops, valerian, chaparral, echinacea, and pau d'arco. Their various properties should be researched before use. To make bitter herbs and foods more palatable, they can be cooked with a little licorice root, stevia leaf, or other sweetener. Following are some common bitter foods, the majority of which exhibit other flavors as well:

Bitter
alfalfa
bitter melon
romaine lettuce
rye

Bitter and Pungent
citrus peel (also sweet)
radish leaf
scallion
turnip (also sweet)
white pepper

Bitter and Sweet
amaranth
asparagus
celery
lettuce
papaya
quinoa

Bitter and Sour
vinegar

Sweet

Properties: A *yang* flavor, regularly subdivided into full sweet (more tonifying and strengthening) and empty sweet (more cleansing and cooling—the flavor that occurs in most fruits). The sweet flavor, especially when found in warming food, helps energy expand upward and outward in the body. It is a harmonizing flavor with a slowing, relaxing effect. Sweet foods build the *yin* of the body—the tissues and fluids—and therefore tonify the thin and *dry* person; such foods also act to strengthen weakness and *deficiency* in general.

Uses of the Sweet Flavor: Especially in the form of complex carbohydrates, sweet food is the center of most traditional diets; it energizes yet relaxes the body, nerves, and brain. Sweetness is used to reduce the harsh taste of bitter foods and to retard acute disease symptoms. Sweet foods, in the form of complex carbohydrates such as grains, vegetables, and legumes, if not cooling varieties, are suitable for treating the *cold* or *deficient* person. Most dairy and animal products are considered sweet, and these may be necessary for extreme *deficiencies*. More information on the sweet flavor appears in the *Sweetners* chapter.

Organ Functions: The sweet flavor "enters" and strengthens the spleen-pancreas and is said to be an appropriate food for the liver, since it soothes aggressive liver emotions such as anger and impatience. It is traditionally used to calm acute liver attacks. Sweet food also moistens *dry* conditions of the lungs, and slows an overactive heart and mind.

Seasonal Attunement: The sweet flavor is appropriate in every season, and especially desirable for harmony at the time of the equinoxes and solstices, as well as during late summer, the juncture between summer and fall.

Warming and/or ascending sweet foods attune one to the upsurges of spring, as do warming pungent foods. Examples of warming sweet foods that acclimate one to springtime include spearmint (also pungent), sweet rice, sweet potato, mochi, amasake, rice syrup, molasses, sunflower seed, pinenut, walnut, and cherry. Sweet-flavored foods with an ascending direction and thermally neutral effect are cabbage, carrot, shiitake mushroom, fig, yam, and peas. Since not many fresh fruits and vegetables are available in most temperate climates in the spring, these can be stored dried, canned, or taken as juice. Some of them also keep well in a root cellar. As with all therapeutic substances, their other properties should always be taken into account.

Individuals Most Benefited: The *dry, cold,* nervous, thin, weak, or scattered person needs whole sweet foods in greater quantity; the aggressive person benefits from the retarding effect of the sweet flavor. When the sweet flavor is used in the form of grains, then wheat, rice, and oats often benefit both these individuals.

Cautions: The sluggish, overweight individual, or those with other *damp* signs, including mucous conditions, should take very sweet foods sparingly and even whole-food carbohydrates moderately. Chewing carbohydrates well makes them much less mucus-forming and therefore has a lighter, less *damp* impact on digestion.

According to the Chinese healing arts, too much sweet food damages the kidneys and spleen-pancreas, weakens the bones, and causes head-hair loss. The *Inner Classic* warns not to eat much sweet food when diseases of the flesh are present (including obesity, tumors, and edema).

Examples: All of the grains number among the most important sweet foods, although rye, quinoa, and amaranth also are quite bitter. All legumes (beans, peas, lentils) and most meats and dairy products are considered sweet. Below is a sampling of foods from other categories that have a sweet flavor:

Fruits	Vegetables	Nuts & Seeds
apple	beet	almond
apricot	button mushroom	chestnut
cherry	cabbage (p)	coconut
date	carrot	sesame seed and oil
fig	celery (b)	sunflower seed
grape (s)	chard	walnut
grapefruit (s)	cucumber	
olive (s)	eggplant	**Sweeteners**
papaya (b)	kuzu	amasake
peach (s)	lettuce (b)	barley malt
pear (ss)	potato	honey*
strawberry (s)	shiitake mushroom	molasses
tomato (s)	spearmint (p)	rice syrup
	squash	whole sugar
	sweet potato	(unrefined cane juice
	yam	powder)

b = also bitter; p = also pungent; s = also sour; ss = also slightly sour

*Although sweet to the taste, raw honey has a pungent, drying effect on the body after digestion. It dries up *damp,* overweight, and mucous conditions, but is not useful for those with a *dry, deficient,* thin, nervous, or over*heated* constitution. Honey that has been heated in processing or cooking has the moistening effect of other concentrated sweeteners (effective in overcoming *dryness* and aggravating to *damp*/mucous conditions).

Wood Element

Spring

Spring is a new beginning—the time of year to "rise early with the sun" and take "brisk walks," which as the *Inner Classic* reminds us, are *yang* activities, reflecting the ascending and active nature of spring. One cannot help but notice plant life pushing upwards after winter's slumber. The sight of the green color of tender young plants nourishes the soul through the eyes, so the appetite for food decreases and the body naturally cleanses itself, not only of food residues, but of excessive desire and the accompanying emotions of dissatisfaction, impatience, and anger as well. The metaphorical membrane over the eyes and mind disappears, and vision becomes clearer. Things are seen in new ways.

This is a time for contacting your true nature and giving attention to self-awareness and self-expression. The *Inner Classic* defines the vital relationships which describe springtime:

> The supernatural forces of spring create wind in Heaven and wood upon the Earth. Within the body they create the liver and the tendons; they create the green color . . . and give the voice the ability to make a shouting sound . . . they create the eyes, the sour flavor, and the emotion anger.

Spring Foods

This is the season to attend to the liver and gall bladder. In spring we naturally eat less, or even fast, to cleanse the body of the fats and heavy foods of winter. The diet should be the lightest of the year and contain foods which emphasize the *yang*, ascending, and expansive qualities of spring—young plants, fresh greens, sprouts, and immature wheat or other cereal grasses. Salty foods such as soy sauce, miso, and sodium-rich meats all have a strong component of sinking energy and are best limited during springtime. Too many heavy foods clog the liver, resulting in spring fits and fevers.

The expansive, rising quality of sweet and pungent-flavored foods is recommended by the classics* as a means of creating a personal spring within. For this effect, one can use a little concentrated sweetener with pungent herbs, such as honey/mint tea. The pungent cooking herbs—basil, fennel, marjoram, rosemary, caraway, dill, bay leaf—are desirable at this time. Most of the complex carbohydrates such as grains, legumes, and seeds have a primarily sweet flavor which increases with sprouting. Young beets, carrots, and other sweet starchy vegetables, thinned from the spring garden, provide a refreshing sweet flavor. Certain intensely pungent flavors are traditionally employed in the spring by Western folk healers as medicine: a week-long daily dose of raw onions and garlic acts as a vermifuge to rid the body of parasites. A traditional Japanese parasiticide is the sweet-pungent combination of mochi and mugwort—pounded sweet rice with mugwort.

Renewal and Raw Food

Food preparation becomes simpler in the spring. Raw and sprouted foods can be emphasized. In Ayurveda, these foods are termed *vatic,* meaning "wind-like." According to Ayurvedic thought, they encourage quickness, rapid movement, and

---

*Recommended by Li Shih-chen, the remarkable 16th-century herbalist who compiled the most extensive Chinese *materia medica,* the *Pentsao.*

outward activity in general. They are also cleansing and cooling.

Spring, the first season of the year, represents youth. Raw foods are thought to bring about renewal by reminding the body of the earlier, more youthful stages of human development, a time before the use of fire when man was extremely active physically, generating abundant heat; thus early peoples found balance in the cooling effect of raw foods. All the stages of our evolution are still encoded within us; going back through the layers of our evolution to more primal biological states is necessary if renewal is to be complete.

Raw food consumption should increase with signs of *heat* in the individual, in warmer climates, and during times of greater physical activity. Most people do well taking at least a little raw food daily, with greater amounts in the spring and summer diets. Nevertheless, there are limitations; as discussed in the *Earth Element* chapter, uncooked foods taken in excess can weaken digestion and trigger excessive cleansing reactions, and should not be used at all if there is bowel inflammation. Raw foods must be used cautiously in individuals with signs of weakness and *deficiency.*

Spring Cooking

Most people living in temperate climates, including most of the United States and Europe, need to cook the majority of their food to maintain climatic and digestive balance. In the spring, food is best cooked for a shorter time but at higher temperatures; in this way the food is not as thoroughly cooked, especially the inner part. If oil is used in spring cooking, a quick high-temperature sauté method is appropriate. When cooking with water, light steaming or minimal simmering is ideal.

The Liver in Harmony and Disease

This Wood-Element organ is perhaps the most congested of all organs in the modern person. Too much fat, chemicals, intoxicants, and denatured food all disrupt the hundreds of intricate biochemical processes of the liver. Traditional Chinese physiology tells us that the healthy liver establishes a smooth and soothing flow of energy through the whole person, in both body and mind. When the liver is harmonious, there is never stress or tension. People with vital livers are calm; they also have unerring judgment and can be naturally effective as leaders and decision-makers. When obstructed, stagnant, or overheated, the energy flow in the liver and throughout the body is hampered, resulting in myriad physical and emotional problems.

Symptoms of Liver Imbalance

Emotional: One of the first signs of liver disharmony is emotional difficulty related to anger: impatience, frustration, resentment, violence, belligerence, rudeness, edginess, arrogance, stubbornness, aggression, and an impulsive and/or explosive personality. When these emotions are repressed without an opportunity for transformation, they cause depression. Mood swings as well as emotional excesses in general are liver-related.

Physical: Numerous signs exist, ranging from the superficial and subtle to the deeper and obvious. In order to recognize the signs and the imbalances they represent, we now look at the most prevalent liver syndromes and the dietary principles for resolving them.

Common Syndromes of the Liver

Liver Stagnation. Many liver conditions involve *excess* of one kind or another. The most frequent kind occurs when too much food is eaten—especially rich, greasy food—and the liver becomes swollen and sluggish in its attempt to circulate *qi* energy smoothly through the body. The *qi* then stagnates in the liver and is not properly distributed.

Since it is *qi* that guides the flow of fluids and nourishment, swelling occurs in certain areas of the body when the liver is swollen and its *qi* is stagnant. (Swelling is a sign of excess.) The most common locations of swelling are near the liver/gall bladder acupuncture meridians or other liver-related regions. The thyroid gland, for example, governs how fast fats are burned by the body, and it is often thought in Western physiology to be related to the liver. When the liver is stagnant, a lump may be felt in the throat, even though one cannot physically be found; when a goiter exists (an enlarged thyroid, visible as a swelling at the front of the neck), this is also a sign of a congested liver. The chest or abdomen may also become distended, or the breasts enlarged. Swellings or lumps can occur in the neck, groin, sides of the body, and the lateral portion of the thighs. In addition, accumulations such as tumors and cancerous growths are liver-related, although the mass itself is considered a form of pathogenic *dampness* which generally indicates spleen-pancreas imbalance.

The Liver Rules the Tendons and Eyes. When *qi* energy and fluid flows in the body are deficient, then the tendons are not "moistened" and can easily tear, become inflamed, or cause unusual contraction or weakness in their related muscles. A common result of these conditions is an inflexible and rigid body.

Likewise, the eyes become inflamed, swollen, or pulled out of focus by the muscles that control them. Since the liver acupuncture meridian passes through and thereby influences the tissues surrounding the eyes, the eyes are directly affected by the liver in many ways. Cataracts, glaucoma, inflamed, red or dry eyes, night blindness, excessive tearing, near- or far-sightedness, and other visual abnormalities basically mirror the condition of the liver.

Many writers and therapists who teach vision correction suggest a dietary method that has proved beneficial for most Westerners at least partly because of its remedial effect on the liver. It includes primarily vegetarian food, with an emphasis on fresh raw vegetables and sprouts. One is advised to undereat and to take the last meal of the day in the afternoon. As discussed earlier in this text, eating moderate amounts of food and avoiding late meals allow the liver and gall bladder ample time to prepare for regeneration during their four-hour cycle of peak energy defined by the Chinese Clock—from 11:00 P.M. to 3:00 A.M.

From our perspective, the *qi* energy of raw food does stimulate the energy flow of a stagnant liver. In fact, the B vitamin known as folic acid is considered by some researchers as the quintessential nutrient in the correction of myopia.[1] This vitamin is also the most heat-sensitive and so is available only in raw food; it is found in abundance in green leafy vegetables and all sprouts. (All specific dietary suggestions are summarized later in this chapter.)

The Liver Stores and Purifies the Blood. The liver is said to be in charge of the storage of the blood, allowing more blood into circulation during periods of greater activity. While in storage, the blood is processed and purified. However, if the liver is stagnant, then blood purification may be inadequate, leading to the release of toxins through the skin. Impure blood is a cause of acne, eczema, carbuncles, boils, acidosis, and allergies; in addition, toxic blood feeds all degenerative conditions, including cancer and arthritis.

If the storage of blood malfunctions, the menses may be overabundant, irregular, scant, or lacking entirely. These last three can occur as a result of insufficient liver blood. Other signs of such a **liver blood deficiency** syndrome may include anemia, general bodily dryness, tendon/ligament/muscle spasms or numbness (blood lubricates and nourishes the tissues), pale fingernail beds and face, and spots in the visual field. In many problems with the liver, its blood and *yin* fluids in general are low and need to be enriched. The spleen-pancreas and kidneys also cause problems with the blood, its production, and the flow of menstrual blood. (These concepts will be developed in later chapters.)

Liver Heat. Longstanding liver stagnancy wears down the system. Taxed with excess, an expanded liver continually struggles toward balance, and thus generates *heat*. In fact, most *heat* signs in people with a rich diet are related to liver excess. Liver *heat* symptoms are fueled by the overconsumption of intoxicants, fats, meats, cheese, and eggs. Even though these concentrated foods are not all warming, *heat* develops as they block the normal functioning of the liver, and this blocking/stagnating effect occurs most often when these foods predominate in the diet. Liver *heat* exhibits general *heat* signs (aversion to heat, red tongue with yellow coating, constipation, great desire for cold fluids), as well as those that are specific to the liver: inflamed eyes, anger, headaches (especially migraine), dizziness, and/or high blood pressure.

In order to reduce stagnancy or heat, the kidneys—"mother of the liver"—must produce extra *yin* fluids, which in this case act as a coolant and decongestant. If the liver never rests from a state of congestion, neither do the kidneys rest, and eventually the kidney *yin* function weakens. A **liver *yin* deficiency** syndrome and the resulting minor *heat* signs develop as the *yin* of the liver diminishes and the kidneys strain to increase *yin* fluid production. Signs of such *"deficiency heat"* include any of the general *deficient yin* symptoms: fresh red tongue and cheeks, small but frequent thirst, hot palms and soles, and insomnia; when lack of *yin* specifically affects the liver, additional symptoms may include irritability, dry eyes, nervousness, and depression.

Sometimes *(excess) heat* and *deficiency heat* coexist in the liver, with signs of *heat* appearing in one area of the body, and *deficiency heat* appearing elsewhere. If this occurs, one needs to use not only cooling foods but also those which support the capacity of the kidneys to produce *yin* fluids.

The Effect of Excess on the Family of Organs

Liver excess profoundly affects not only the blood but the spleen-pancreas and stomach functions by invading these digestive organs through the Five Element Control Cycle (Earth is penetrated by Wood), thereby causing ulcers, abdominal inflammations, diabetes, gas, and indigestion in general. Since the spleen-pancreas directly influences the intestines, inflammatory conditions such as colitis and enteritis can also frequently be traced to liver overload in stress-filled, overfed people.

Finally, most cases of heart disease are related to liver stagnation, which inhibits the natural energetic flow of the Five Element Creative Cycle from the liver to the heart (Wood feeds Fire). It is no surprise that nearly everyone with heart deficiencies can be seen to follow the pattern of liver stagnation. Over time, this contributes to the great variety of vascular diseases that plague modern people.

One of the most efficient ways of improving the condition of the liver is to give its excess a place to go, and the obvious place is where it naturally flows—to its son, the heart. From the Five Element perspective, an excessive and "greedy" liver not only steals from its mother, the kidneys, but, as we have just seen, also refuses to give sufficient energy to its own son, the heart. Therefore, by strengthening the heart and encouraging it to receive energy, the liver is encouraged to release its excess, which in turn relieves the stress placed on the kidneys. The emotional pattern that often occurs in such an exchange takes the form of resentment and repressed emotions of a stagnant liver being transformed to the joy and compassion of the newly open and focused heart. Methods for improving the heart appear in the *Fire Element* chapter.

Since the liver is implicated in so many diverse illnesses, it is helpful to have concepts that explain and unify its effects. *"Wind,"* the climate of the Wood Element, is one such concept.

Wind and the Nature of Liver Disharmony

Wind, a *yang* climatic force associated with the liver and Wood Element, is described in the Chinese classics as the external environmental influence that enters the body most often in combination with the other climates. Thus one frequently speaks of *wind* combined with *heat, cold, damp,* or *dry* conditions. An example is the common cold, which is usually characterized as a blend of either *wind* and *heat* or *wind* and *cold.* This does not mean that climate is the only factor. The common cold is precipitated by contact with a virus, which proliferates when a person's protective *qi* (immunity) is weakened by one or more of many possible causes, including overexposure to wind and other adverse climates. The remedy for such typically mild conditions involves the sweating process described in the *Interior/Exterior* chapter.

Deeper, *interior wind* conditions affecting the liver can also enter the body from exposure to wind, but most deep "liver *wind*" imbalances are patterns of chaotic change in the body merely symbolized by the wind, and originate from liver stagnancy and *heat:* "*Heat* gives rise to *wind*" is how traditional Chinese medicine expresses this relationship.

A typical American pattern is *heat*-driven high blood pressure from an excess of fatty, cholesterol-rich animal products. As *heat* rises, a turbulent condition *(wind)* can easily develop in the blood vessels of the brain (dizziness), often resulting in their rupture (stroke). Cleansing the arteries and reducing this kind of high blood pressure is not a difficult task when the correct diet is followed. (See "Cleansing the Heart and Arteries" in Chapter 10.)

The general signs of *wind* conditions in the body parallel the wind-like qualities of change and fluctuation: moving pains, convulsions, tremors, cramps, seizures, strokes, emotional turmoil, nervousness, uncertainty, spasms, itching, dizziness. However, conditions of *wind* which damage certain organs and systems may result in stasis: rigidity, paralysis (occurs frequently after a stroke and its accompanying dizziness), coma, and numbness. In these cases one may envision wind extreme enough to damage the system, much as a strong enough wind can break the mast of a sailboat. (This is one example of the ancient teaching that extreme *yang* transforms to *yin* and vice versa.)

Wind symptoms can arise in any season, but are more prevalent in the spring. One may notice a similarity between the instability of *wind* and the nervous, irritable, unstable signs of the *yin*-deficient person. Recalling that *yin* is the principle that nurtures, stabilizes, cools, and calms, it is clear that sufficient *yin* fluids stabilize the liver and inhibit the generation of *yang* influences such as wind and *heat.* Thus, a shortage of *yin* fluids contributes to both *wind* and the *heat* that frequently causes it.

Gall Bladder Renewal

When the liver is consistently stagnant, sediment often settles out of the bile and forms accumulations that resemble stones, sand, or mud in the gall bladder. Since the gall bladder acts as a reservoir for bile, it becomes less efficient when clogged with sediment, and acute problems result when stones become lodged in the bile duct leading from the gall bladder to the duodenum.

Symptoms of Sediment in the Gall Bladder: indigestion, flatulence, periodic pain below the right front side of the rib cage, tension in the back of the shoulders near the neck, bitter taste in the mouth, chest pain. Most chronically ill people need gall bladder cleansing before recovery is complete; this includes individuals who regularly experience stress.

Gradual Gall Bladder Cleanse: During this process, avoid foods richest in saturated fats and cholesterol—heavy meats, dairy, and eggs. Also avoid peanuts and eat other nuts and seeds sparingly, if at all. Eat primarily unrefined grains, vegetables, fruits, and legumes. Such a diet gradually clears the gall bladder. Pears, parsnips, seaweeds, lemons, limes, and the spice turmeric hasten gallstone removal, and can be emphasized in the diet during the entire cleanse. Radish also removes deposits and stones from the gall bladder. For 21 days, eat just one or two radishes a day between meals; in addition, drink three cups of cleavers (*Galium aparine*) tea, or five cups of chamomile *(Anthemis nobilis)* tea each day. Finally, pour five teaspoons of fresh, cold-pressed flax oil over food at one meal of the day, or use half this amount at two daily meals. The dosage can vary proportionally according to weight (a 160-pound person needs about five teaspoons). Flax oil should be taken six days a week for two months. This diet and its specific stone-dissolving foods and herbs are usually sufficient to remove all sediment.

The "Gall Bladder Flush" described below may be taken if the gradual method is inconvenient. Tests performed by a physician can confirm the presence of gallstones. In cases of very large stones which cannot be flushed through the bile duct, the gradual method above is appropriate.

Gall Bladder Flush: One can often quickly purge the gall bladder of stones and other sediment with a one-day ritual commonly called the "Gall Bladder Flush." There are many variations on this, but one of the simplest and most effective is the following:

Beginning in the morning and throughout the day, eat only apples, preferably organic, as many as desired, but at least four or five. Apples of the green variety seem most effective, although all apples will help soften the stones. Water, herbal teas, and/or apple juice may also be taken. At bed-time, warm up two-thirds of a cup of virgin olive oil to body temperature and mix in one-third of a cup of fresh lemon juice. Slowly sip the entire mixture, and then immediately go to bed, lying on the right side, with the right leg drawn up. In the morning all stones should pass in the stool. This flush should be done with the guidance of an experienced health practitioner. This remedy has undoubtedly made gall-bladder operations unnecessary in thousands of likely candidates. An added benefit is that gall-bladder cleansing clears residues of excess from the liver as well.

A mild variation of the Gall Bladder Flush: For five consecutive days, ingest on an empty stomach two tablespoons of olive oil followed by two tablespoons of lemon juice.

The Source of Disharmony

Getting to the root of liver imbalance is a matter of understanding the fundamental cause of all disease. Too many desires—whether for sex, fame, power, security, money, or rich-tasting foods—can stimulate a person to eat excessively. Even in cases where not much is eaten, desire can blind proper judgment, so that inappropriate actions and diet may be chosen.

Most importantly, regardless of diet, emotions themselves when driven by the desire-complex of greed, anger, and resentment greatly damage liver function. Unresolved emotional issues are stored physically as residues of excess in the liver, while emotional clarification unlocks and releases these residues. Therefore, as the diet improves, it is necessary to liberate emotional obstructions. Any of various awareness methods can help; practices which cut through emotional obstructions, discussed in the *Interior/Exterior: Building Immunity* chapter, also apply here. If the awareness work is neglected, an emotional cripple can find a way to pervert even a sound diet so that it supports his or her current disturbances.

Summary of Common Liver Syndromes

Since various liver imbalances can develop from the same set of circumstances, the following syndromes are often found simultaneously, to different degrees, in one individual.

Note: The physical signs do not correspond on a one-to-one basis with the emotional signs on the same line.

I. Stagnant Liver. Characterized by obstructed *qi* energy flow.

Physical Signs	Emotional Signs
nervous system disorders	emotional repression
allergies	anger
lumps, swellings, scrofula, mastitis	frustration
distended abdomen, chest, or breasts	resentment
chronic indigestion	impatience
menstrual problems	edginess
stress, neck and back tension	depression
fatigue	moodiness
rigid, inflexible body	impulsiveness
eye problems	emotional attachments
impure blood, skin disorders	poor judgment
finger- or toenail problems	difficulty in making decisions
slow rising in morning	mental rigidity
muscular pain	negativity
tendon problems	
wiry, tight radial pulse	

• The tongue varies with the degree of stagnancy from a normal, light-red color to a dark hue, often tinged with blue, green, or violet.

Dietary Suggestions for Stagnant Liver Syndrome (see "Dietary Principles" below): A (avoidance of a liver-stagnating diet), B (pungent and raw anti-stagnancy foods), C (harmonizers), D (bitter and sour liver-excess reducers), E (detoxifying and cooling foods), and H (liver-rejuvenators). Note: Cooling and raw foods must be used with care by those with signs of *coldness* and/or *deficiency*.

Summary of Common Liver Syndromes (continued)

II. Liver Heat. Characterized by *heat* signs.

Physical Signs	**Emotional Signs**
red face	frequent impatience and anger
red, dry eyes	irritability
red tongue	explosive personality
splitting headaches	shouting
insomnia	willfulness
menopausal disorders	arrogance
low backache, weak legs	rudeness
high blood pressure	aggression
indigestion; constipation	violence
fast pulse and other *heat* signs	

Dietary Suggestions for Liver Heat (see "Dietary Principles" below): A (avoidance of a liver-stagnating diet); part 2) of B (raw anti-stagnancy foods); C (harmonizers), D (bitter and sour liver-excess reducers), E (detoxifying and cooling foods), and H (liver-rejuvenators).

III. Deficient Liver Yin and Blood.

Physical Signs   **Emotional Signs**

Deficient liver *yin* signs:

- dizziness
- dry eyes and weak vision
- night blindness
- ringing in the ears
- menopausal discomfort
- dry, brittle nails
- general deficient *yin* signs:
  - fresh red cheeks and tongue
  - hot palms and soles
  - night sweats and afternoon fevers
  - frequent but small thirst

Emotional Signs:
- depression
- nervous tension
- irritability

Deficient liver blood signs: (same as above)

- weak tendons and sinews
- muscle spasms and palpitations
- spots in visual field
- dry eyes and unclear vision
- pale fingernail beds
- ringing in the ears
- irregular menses
- scanty or absent menstruation
- general deficient blood signs:
  - numbness, dizziness,
  - pale tongue and face, dry skin,
  - insomnia and memory loss

Summary of Common Liver Syndromes (continued)

Dietary Suggestions for Deficient Liver *Yin* and Blood (see "Dietary Principles" below): A (avoidance of a liver-stagnating diet), C (harmonizers), F (liver *yin* and blood nurturers—use applicable remedies for deficiencies of the *yin* or blood of the liver), and H (liver-rejuvenators).

IV. Liver Wind. Characterized by instability and rapid movement. Usually combines with *heat, cold, damp,* or *dryness.* Can be caused by liver stagnancy, *heat,* or insufficient *yin* fluids.

Physical Signs	**Emotional Signs**
pain that comes and goes, or moves	manic-depression
spasms, cramps	nervousness
dizziness, vertigo	fits
tremors, palsy, twitching	unstable personality
pulsating headache	"the perpetual traveler"
ringing in ears	agitation
paralysis	emotional turmoil
dryness in upper body	inability to keep commitments
	uneasiness

Dietary Suggestions for Liver Wind (see "Dietary Principles" below): A (avoidance of a liver-stagnating diet); part 2) of B (raw anti-stagnancy foods); E (detoxifying and cooling foods), G (*wind* reducers), and H (liver-rejuvenators). Note: Cooling and raw foods must be used with care by those with signs of *coldness* and/or *deficiency.*

Dietary Principles for Healing the Liver

A. Dietary strategies to relieve a stagnant, swollen liver are essential since nearly all liver imbalances, including liver-related *heat,* blood and *yin* deficiencies, and *wind,* originate with stagnancy. The first remedy in every case (except malnutrition) is to eat less. One should also eliminate or greatly reduce certain foods which obstruct and/or damage the liver. These include foods high in saturated fats (lard, mammal meats, cream, cheese, and eggs—see *Oils and Fats* chapter), hydrogenated and poor-quality fats (such as shortening, margarine, refined and rancid oils), excesses of nuts and seeds, chemicals in food and water, prescription drugs (consult your physician before discontinuing), all intoxicants, and highly processed, refined foods.

B. 1) Foods which stimulate the liver out of stagnancy include moderately pungent foods, spices, and herbs: watercress, all the members of the onion family, mustard greens, turmeric, basil, bay leaf, cardamom, marjoram, cumin, fennel, dill, ginger, black pepper, horseradish, rosemary, various mints, lemon balm (*Melissa officinalis*), angelica root (*Angelica archangelica*), and prickly ash bark (*Xanthoxylum americanum*). Too much extremely pungent food, however, such as fiery hot peppers, can damage those with liver stagnation, and especially those with *heat* signs. Some anti-stagnancy foods are not pungent, or only mildly so: beets, taro root, sweet rice, amasake, strawberry, peach, cherry, chestnut, pine nut, and vegetables of the *Brassica* genus—cabbage, turnip root, kohlrabi, cauliflower, broccoli, and brussels sprouts.

Alcoholic beverages are pungent and temporarily combat liver stagnancy, but ultimately cause cell destruction and should be avoided.

2) Raw foods—sprouted grains, beans, and seeds, fresh vegetables and fruits—also stimulate liver energy flow.

C. Foods which harmonize the liver to a smooth flow of emotional/physical energy are necessary. Many of these foods are sweet in nature. As mentioned earlier in regard to springtime foods, the grains, vegetables, legumes, and other complex carbohydrates are ideal sweet foods for long-term liver harmony. During times of depression or other acute symptoms of liver imbalance, the concentrated sweeteners are often craved. Honey, used sparingly, is especially helpful since it has a detoxifying nature. Mixed with apple cider vinegar, it has an even stronger effect (see "Bitter and sour foods" below). Other minimally processed sweeteners, valuable during the initial stages of detoxification, are stevia powder, unrefined cane-juice granules, whole sugar cane, and licorice root. Barley malt, date sugar, molasses, and rice syrup are warming and stimulate *qi* energy flow. They are useful for treating stagnancy except where there is *heat* or *heat*-generated *wind*.

D. Bitter and sour foods reduce excesses of the liver. Perhaps the most powerful common remedy for quickly removing liver stagnation and the accompanying depression and indigestion is vinegar. Choose unrefined apple-cider, brown-rice, rice-wine, or other quality vinegars. The flavor of vinegar is both bitter and sour, and has detoxifying and highly activating properties. Its effect is improved by mixing it with honey—one teaspoon of each per cup of water. Vinegar should not be relied on indefinitely; the basic diet must be improved instead. Since vinegar is warming, it can worsen the condition of those with *heat* signs; instead, substitute lemon, lime, or grapefruit, which are also bitter/sour but cooling and more gradually acting.

Other bitter foods are rye, romaine lettuce, asparagus, amaranth, quinoa, alfalfa, radish leaves, and citrus peel. The many bitter herbs, particularly dandelion root *(Taraxacum officinalis)*, bupleurum *(Bupleurum falcatum;* Mandarin: *chai hu)*, chaparral *(Larrea divaricata)*, milk thistle seeds *(Silybum marianum)*, Oregon grape root *(Mahonia repens)*, and chamomile flowers *(Anthemis nobilis)*, offer excellent liver-cleansing effects. Licorice root *(Glycyrrhiza glabra)* can be used with bitter herbs to mask and mollify their harsh flavor.

Note: The above bitter-flavored examples must be used sparingly by the frail, generally *deficient* person. Bupleurum is more effective and less depleting in *deficiencies* when taken in the Chinese anti-stagnancy formula "Bupleurum Sedative Pills," listed on page 432. One reason for this formula's effects is its peony root *(Paeonia lactiflora;* Mandarin: *bai shao),* which has both bitter and sour flavors, and is one of the only herbs to treat each of the major syndromes of the liver.

Peony, a blood and *yin* tonic, reduces liver stagnancy gently and harmoniously—in a fashion symbolized by the soft, delicate quality of the peony flower itself; peony root also enhances the effects of any of the strongly bitter, aromatic herbs (including those above), while simultaneously making them less drying to the body's *yin* and blood. One may choose, for example, to mix equal parts of dandelion and peony roots with one-third part each of licorice root and turmeric. This formula combines the above principles of using pungent, sweet, sour, and bitter flavors with a blood and *yin* preserver such as peony root (other blood/*yin* tonics listed in "F" below may be taken instead of peony). An even milder-acting formula for reducing liver stagnancy or *heat* in the overly sensitive or frail person is two parts peony to one of licorice. The common herbs lemon balm, peppermint, and chamomile also are mild, and more effective than generally acknowledged, but lack the tonic action of peony.

E. Foods for detoxifying and cooling the liver: mung beans and their sprouts, celery, seaweeds (kelp is very helpful in liver stagnancy), lettuce, cucumber, watercress, tofu, millet, plum, chlorophyll-rich foods (see "H" below), mushrooms,† rhubarb root *(Rheum palmatum)* or stem,† radish,† and daikon radish.†

These last four (†) are especially effective in reducing toxicity resulting from overconsumption of meat. Rhubarb root and stem are the strongest of these remedies and also have laxative properties.

F. Foods for building liver *yin* and blood. Insufficient *yin* of the liver—causing *"deficiency heat"*—requires foods which tonify the *yin* fluids in general; of the above foods in "E," mung beans, mung sprouts, chlorophyll-rich foods, cucumber, tofu, and millet are appropriate, while seaweed, watercress, and plum improve water metabolism. Fresh cold-pressed flax oil and extracted oils of borage, evening primrose, or black currant seeds significantly improve the *yin* status of the liver. Taking sufficient liquids in general is helpful. The blood tonics below marked "*" also build the liver *yin*. Improving the kidney *yin* function is always beneficial in cases of liver *yin* deficiency; aloe vera gel is among the best kidney *yin* herbal tonics for building liver *yin* (see "Kidney *Yin* Deficiency," page 357).

When liver blood (an aspect of the *yin* that needs to be addressed separately) is deficient, it can be built up with general blood tonics such as spirulina and other chlorophyll-rich foods, dark grapes, blackberries, huckleberries, raspberries, and blackstrap molasses; in severe cases, gelatin* or organic animal liver* is useful. Helpful herbs include *dang gui* root *(Angelica sinensis),* prepared rehmannia root *(Rehmannia glutinosa),** peony root,* and yellow dock root *(Rumex crispus).* The three Chinese herbs—*dang gui,* rehmannia, and peony—can be used singly but are even more effective taken together (in equal parts). The combination is particularly beneficial for the *cold,* frail, or *deficient* person. To build the blood in general, see "Blood Deficiency," page 387.

G. Foods and spices which reduce liver *wind* symptoms: celery (c), basil (w), sage (n), fennel (w), dried or fresh ginger (w), anise (w), oats (w), black soybean (n), black sesame seed (n), kuzu (c), pine nut (w), coconut (n), fresh cold-pressed flax oil (n), and shrimp (w); common wind-quelling herbs include chamomile *(Anthemis nobilis)* (n), peony root (c), lobelia *(Lobelia inflata)* (n), scullcap *(Scutellaria laterifolia)* (n), valerian *(Valeriana officinalis)* (w). These foods and herbs are generally effective against *wind;* however, when *wind* occurs in combination with *heat* (including *deficient yin*-induced *heat*), then cooling foods such as those in "E" above can be added while avoiding the warming (w) remedies. Conversely, avoid the cooling remedies (c) in *wind* conditions marked with *coldness.* Neutral remedies (n) may be used in either case.

Foods that especially worsen *wind* conditions are eggs, crab meat, and buckwheat.

H. Foods which accelerate liver rejuvenation: the chlorophyll-rich foods, including cereal grasses and their products (such as wheat- or barley-grass juice powders), and also the micro-algae—spirulina, wild blue-green *(Aphanizomenon),* and chlorella. These foods are very useful in most cases of liver *excess,* stagnancy, *heat,* and *wind;* limitations on their use are discussed in the *Green Food Products* chapter. Cereal grass and micro-algae products which are processed at low temperatures are preferable because certain nutrients, particularly their omega-3 and gamma-linolenic fatty acids, are better preserved. Other green foods are also beneficial: parsley, kale, watercress, alfalfa, and collard greens, for example.

When the liver is depleted as a result of severe malnutrition from an exceptionally deficient diet or alcoholism, there are several proven remedies: a) the fresh milk of goats, cows, or sheep; b) spirulina in conjunction with fish gruel; c) a soup or congee containing liver from such organically raised livestock as sheep, beef, or chicken (if there exist *heat* signs such as often accompany alcoholism, avoid chicken liver because of its warming nature). These remedies are particularly applicable when the person has unmistakable signs of *deficiency* including a weak pulse, pallor, lassitude, weak voice and respiration, and a withdrawn personality.

*   *   *

In some people, liver malfunction may be related to the absence of mother's milk as an infant; those who were not breast-fed are more likely to develop immune deficiencies, allergies, and other liver-related disorders.[2, 3, 4] The liberal use of spirulina and other chlorophyll foods supplies the liver with immune-enhancing essential fatty acids—particularly the omega-3 and gamma-linolenic acid (GLA) variety—that it may have been lacking since birth. Introducing these foods into the diet of those with essential-fatty-acid deficiency, regardless of the person's age, encourages more complete liver function.

An Alcohol- and Drug-Abused Liver

An exceptional case of liver renewal is that of Phillip Raphael, a musician with an eighteen-year history of heroin addiction followed by twelve years of alcoholism and other drug dependencies. After these thirty years of substance abuse and poor health, he fell gravely ill. Two doctors diagnosed him as dying from liver failure with no hope of survival, whereupon he made a firm resolve to live. The following plan represents the main features of his cleansing program, various parts of which he followed for one to three years. (All parts of the plan were followed for at least one year.)

1. A diet of wheat grass, wheat-grass juice, spirulina, and fresh vegetable juices, including up to one quart of carrot juice daily; he also took fruit juices, to a lesser extent. He regularly ate small amounts of brown rice, his only cooked food.

2. Fasts on fruit, vegetable, and wheat-grass juices, for seven to ten days each month.

3. An herbal formula consisting of *qi*-stimulating herbs (fennel, anise, and cayenne), harmonizing and demulcent herbs (licorice and fenugreek), and a highly cleansing bitter herb (chaparral).

4. Weekly colonic irrigation and/or enema.

5. Periodic liver/gall bladder flushes (as described earlier in this chapter).

From the beginning of the cleansing process, Raphael felt his life returning. Over the next few years, he gradually introduced other foods: a variety of sprouts, raw vegetables, tofu, tempeh, and more brown rice. After a year on more solid foods, we suggested that he increase his consumption of cooked foods by adding lightly steamed vegetables. Immediately he noticed easier digestion and better assimilation. Cooked food seemed to accelerate the healing process, especially that of his colon. He had more bodily warmth and mental focus.

Other important factors in his recovery: correct food-combining, avoiding between-meal snacks, and a small final meal of the day.

Such an extreme and lengthy cleansing process is not recommended unless it is absolutely necessary; in this case, Raphael almost died during certain phases of the process. The first five years of his recovery were characterized by cleansing, and his body gradually returned to normal functioning. During the next several years, he established a higher level of wellness and has felt the subtle rhythm of his cells being restored. (Possessing an unusually strong constitution and signs of *excess* and *heat* during most of the recovery process, he benefited from a cleansing diet of mostly uncooked food. *Deficient* and *cold* people would benefit more from cooked foods.)

This example is offered to demonstrate the virtue of a number of points made earlier for liver renewal: foods which are *qi*-stimulating, cooling, harmonizing, cleansing, and rich in chlorophyll. In cases of general *excess*, fasting and colon cleansing are often useful.

Fire Element

Summer

To unify with summer, a *yang* season, the *Inner Classic* suggests we express the *yang* principle—expansion, growth, lightness, outward activity, brightness, and creativity. The following suggestions for lifestyle and diet reflect this principle.

Summer is a period of luxurious growth. To be in harmony with the atmosphere of summer, awaken early in the morning and reach to the sun for nourishment to flourish as the gardens do. Work, play, travel, be joyful, and grow into selfless service. The bounty of the outside world enters and enlivens us.

Summer Food and Preparation

Use plenty of brightly colored summer fruits and vegetables, and enjoy creating beautiful meals—make a dazzling display with the colors of the food, and design a floral arrangement for the table. Cook lightly and regularly add a little spicy, pungent, or even fiery flavor. When sautéing, use high heat for a very short time, and steam or simmer foods as quickly as possible. Use little salt and more water.

Summer offers abundant variety, and the diet should reflect this. Minerals and oils are sweated out of the body, and their loss can cause weakness if they are not replaced by a varied diet. To be more comfortable, drink hot liquids and take warm showers to induce sudden sweating and to cool the body. Summer heat combined with too much cold food weakens the digestive organs. Coldness causes contraction; it holds in sweat and heat, and interferes with digestion. Iced drinks and ice cream actually contract the stomach and stop digestion. (They are best avoided.)

On the hottest days, create a cool atmosphere (picnics, patio meals, etc.) and serve more cooling fresh foods such as salads, sprouts (especially mung, soy, and alfalfa), fruit, cucumber, tofu, and flower and leaf teas including chrysanthemum, mint, and chamomile. Common fruits which cool summer heat best are apples, watermelon, lemons, and limes. Mung bean soup or tea is another specific remedy. Also, the dispersing hot-flavored spices are considered appropriate in the warmest weather. At first their effect is to increase warmth, but ultimately they bring body heat out to the surface to be dispersed. With heat on the surface, one's body mirrors the summer climate and therefore will be less affected by it. Red and green hot peppers, cayenne red pepper, fresh (not dried) ginger, horseradish, and black pepper are all ideal for this purpose. However, if too many dispersing foods are taken, then weakness and loss of *yang* will result, and the ability to stay warm and vital in the cooler seasons is lost.

At the other extreme, heavy foods on hot days cause sluggishness. Such foods include meats, eggs, and excesses of nuts, seeds, and grains. Eating less and lightly on hot, bright days is a natural, healthful practice, a pattern easily forgotten when we neither pay attention nor change according to our internal rhythms.

When conditions of *heat* become lodged in the *interior* of the body due to a hot climate, poor diet, or other factors, the symptoms and cures are the same as those discussed under *"heat"* in the Six Divisions. *Summer heat*, the condition that arises from overexposure to high temperatures, is also summarized at the end of the *Six Divisions* chapters (page 101). According to the *Inner Classic,* the following are the major Fire Element correspondences:

> The supernatural forces of Summer create heat in the Heavens and fire on Earth; they create the heart and the pulse within the body . . . the red color, the tongue, and the ability to express laughter . . . they create the bitter flavor, and the emotions of happiness and joy.

The Heart in Harmony and Disease

The Fire Element rules the heart and small intestine. In Chinese healing tradition, the heart includes not only the organ itself but also the concept—shared by Western people—of the heart as a mental/emotional center, reflected in our phrases: "Have a heart!", "Put your heart into it!", or "Learn by heart." Dean Ornish, M.D., heart specialist at the University of California at San Francisco, has developed from his experience a similar awareness: "I think the mind is where heart disease begins for many people."[5] The Romanized word for heart in China is *xin,* which is often translated as "heart-mind." Thus, according to the Chinese medical definition, the heart not only regulates blood circulation but also controls consciousness, spirit, sleep, memory, and houses the mind. In this way the heart, together with the liver, is related to the nervous system and brain. The advantage of using this expanded definition is that it accords with reality—the heart acupuncture meridian affects both the physical heart and the mind. It is well-known that emotions affect the actual functioning of the heart, seen in the speed and strength of the pulses. We will refer to the various aspects of this expanded "heart-mind" definition as appropriate.

The heart in harmony: Those with healthy hearts are genuinely friendly. They are also humble, not out of convention but because they actually feel small in comparison to the wonders they perceive with their open hearts and aware minds. Clarity is a central attribute of those with a harmonious heart-mind. They seem to see effortlessly through problems to arrive at brilliant solutions.

General Symptoms of a Heart-Mind Imbalance

- Scattered and confused mind
- Excess or no laughter
- A ruddy or very pale face
- Speech problems (stuttering, excess verbiage, confused speech)
- Depression
- Mental illness
- Loss of memory
- Poor circulation
- Weak spirit
- Aversion to heat

Heart disease, simply on the physical level, is the largest health problem in the United States. If we include failings of the heart's mental aspect, these statistics are tremendously increased. Furthermore, chronic degenerative conditions such as cancer, arthritis, and insanity, which often arise from a lack of mental clarity, make strengthening the heart-mind system a treatment priority in East Asian medicine for these and other degenerative conditions.

Numerous nutritional studies indicate that heart and nervous system problems are related to calcium metabolism. Coffee, alcohol, tobacco, refined salt, sugar, refined flour, aluminum, pesticides, marijuana, and other intoxicants all interfere with calcium absorption. Equally damaging is excess protein in the diet. Cultures with high-protein diets have elevated levels of heart disease and osteoporosis. More information about improving calcium utilization is in the *Calcium* chapter.

The physical aspect which we recognize as heart disease is well-defined; by comparison, the mental aspects are less readily identified. The Chinese use the concept of *shen* to describe the spirit that resides in the heart and is responsible for the quality of one's consciousness.

In contrast to the widespread *excesses* of the liver, most heart problems involve *deficiency*. Very often, when treating heart imbalance in Chinese medicine, the heart itself is not directly treated. The heart relies on other organs for its nourishment and energy, so the great majority of heart problems are caused by and treated through the imbalances in other organ systems. The most prevalent heart disharmonies are summarized below.

Common Syndromes of the Heart-Mind

Deficiencies of the *yin* and the blood of the heart. Both the *yin* and blood have similar effects on the spirit *(shen)*. A *yang* principle, the spirit needs the *yin* and blood for stability; otherwise it "escapes" from the heart, causing incessant wandering of the mind. In more extreme cases an unstable spirit brings on insomnia, memory loss, irregular or racing heartbeat, excessive dreaming, irrational behavior, or insanity. (Spirit-stabilizing remedies are listed later.) To distinguish between *yin* and blood deficiencies, the person with a lack of *yin* tends to have minor heat signs: a fresh-red tongue and cheeks, fast and thin pulse, hot palms and soles, and an abrupt or nervous manner. Deficient blood signs: pale tongue, face, and nail beds; thin pulse and sluggishness.

Hypertension and hyperthyroidism are often thought to be caused in part by insufficient *yin*. The cooling value of the *yin* also protects the heart from inflammation. Very often a lack of *yin* occurs because of an excessive liver that consumes too much of the body's *yin*. Another cause may be deficient kidneys, as the kidneys are the root source of both *yin* and *yang*. To enrich the *yin*, it is important to first reduce any possible liver excess (pages 319–329). Next, warming substances which deplete the *yin* should be avoided: coffee, alcohol, tobacco, and others listed under "Kidney *Yin* Deficiency" (page 358). The remedies which tonify kidney *yin* work well for improving heart *yin;* especially valuable are fresh wheat germ, wheat berries (in food or as wheat-berry tea), and mung beans. In addition to the herbs for kidney *yin* deficiency, one may add lily bulb *(Lilium*-related species; Mandarin: *bai he)* and/or raw rehmannia root *(Rehmannia glutinosa*; Mandarin: *sheng di huang).* As discussed in the *Metal Element* chapter, tiger lily and other lily bulbs may be used interchangeably.

Deficient blood most often results from a weak spleen-pancreas and/or kidneys (both of these organs play a role in the manufacture of the blood). A basic plan to fortify the blood is given in "Blood Deficiency," pages 387 and 388. Three herbs which specifically enrich the blood and transport it to the heart include *dang gui* root *(Angelica sinensis),* processed rehmannia root *(Rehmannia glutinosa*; Mandarin: *shu di huang),* and red sage root *(Salvia miltorrhiza*; Mandarin: *dan shen).* Each herb may be taken alone. *Dang gui* in combination with processed rehmannia, a warming remedy, is especially effective for conditions with signs of *coldness.* Red sage root, a bitter herb, is more useful when there is a tendency to develop *dampness* or mucus excesses in the body.

In the last 100 years, the tense, hyperactive aspects of personality have predominated, and the *yin* aspects—the receptive, relaxed, feminine, and the earth itself—have been damaged. In response, a number of idiomatic expressions of the language have spontaneously emerged which seem to reflect, even encourage, the *yin* processes in the body. Beginning in indigenous music circles, and now among the general populace, the term "cool" that appears in phrases like "keep your cool" has come to mean calm, collected, and relaxed, and this is exactly how the *yin* fluids affect the functioning of the mind and spirit.

Deficiencies of the *qi* energy and *yang* of the heart. Both of these weaknesses bring about a disturbed spirit with signs of heart imbalance such as palpitations, irregular and weak pulses, pale tongue, and lethargy. A lack of *yang* (the warming principle) will also have signs of *coldness.* Typically, the *qi* energy of the heart is greatly lacking in modern people, or not smoothly distributed. The *qi* directs the flow of fluids and blood through the heart, so weak *qi* flow also causes the symptoms of *yin* and blood deficiency mentioned above.

Diseases described by modern medicine that often correspond to the signs of heart *qi* and *yang* deficiency are: hardening and thickening of the arteries of the heart, severe chest pains, nervous disorders, general body weakness, and depression.

The *yang* of the heart is furnished to a large extent by the kidneys, so deficient heart *yang* is related to deficient kidney *yang.* The *qi* of the heart is derived from the lungs and spleen-pancreas, so weakness in these organs always causes a deficiency of heart *qi.* Such problems can also be part of a liver stagnation pattern, which thwarts smooth distribution of *qi* to the heart.

A more fundamental reason for poor *qi* flow exists than the organ imbalances already outlined—a poor spirit. In Chinese medicine the spirit is said to rule the *qi,* so that the quality of one's spirit influences the smoothness and power of *qi* flow.

A strong *qi* flow is often observed in yogis and t'ai chi adepts who can alter their heartbeat and other vital functions to a remarkable degree because their practices empower the spirit. In t'ai chi, for example, "the guiding principle is to follow the spirit."

> Controlling the spirit facilitates the movement of *qi*.
>
> —*Inner Classic*

In summary, treatment for deficient heart *qi* should consider the possibilities of deficient spleen-pancreas *qi* (page 341), deficient lung *qi* (page 351) and stagnant liver *qi* (page 319). Improving the spirit *(shen)* can be essential for vitalizing heart *qi*. (See "Healing the Heart" later in this chapter for suggestions on tonifying the spirit.)

Stagnant heart blood. This condition often arises when too little heart *qi* or *yang* energy is available to move the blood. Stabbing pains, purple face or tongue, lassitude, palpitations, and shortness of breath are typical symptoms. Mucus may also be a cause of obstructed blood; if this is the case, then the coating on the tongue will typically be thick and greasy. In cases of mucus, one considers the source—improperly digested food and/or an excess of mucus-forming foods. Since mucus is a *damp* substance, one should avoid dietary factors which contribute to *dampness* (page 344). Stagnant heart blood patterns frequently occur in cases of coronary artery disease, heart inflammation, and angina.

Stagnant blood in general and as it applies to the heart is outlined in "Stagnant Blood," pages 392–395. *Dang gui* and red sage root, recommended above for deficient heart blood, are excellent anti-stagnancy remedies.

Cold or hot mucus-foam. These substances are a light type of "mucus." When they "invade" the heart, they disorganize the spirit/consciousness *(shen)*. Mental illness is often associated with the clouding of the spirit by "an invisible mucoid foam." Such mucus patterns may also cause thick tongue coating, abnormal behavior, and sometimes drooling.

In hot mucus cases, the foam obstructs the nervous system, bringing on disorders such as encephalitis, *wind*-induced apoplexy, and epilepsy. These conditions are accompanied by *heat* and *yang* signs in general: yellow tongue coating, fast pulse, and sudden, forceful, or violent movement. Cold mucus is heavier, more condensed and symptomatic of *yin* behavior—passivity, self-obsession, lack of good sense, a slow, stuck manner, and talking to oneself; the pulse is also slow and the tongue coating white.

Most cases of mucus improve if strongly mucus-forming foods are reduced: milk and dairy products, ice cream, eggs, meats, sugar, peanuts, and refined foods such as white flour. In hot mucus cases, one must avoid warming substances such as cigarettes, coffee, alcohol, and red meats. For cold mucus, one needs more warming foods and spices and especially must avoid the cooler mucus-generating foods—dairy, eggs, and refined flours. Also beware of habits that contribute to excessive mucus, such as eating complicated meals, failing to chew food thoroughly, and drinking cold liquids with meals. (For both hot and cold mucus-foam, see "Dietary Factors Which Contribute to Dampness" on page 344.)

Healing the Heart

As discussed above, the *qi, yang,* blood, and fluid deficiencies of the heart are cured when the kidneys, spleen-pancreas, lungs, and/or liver are restored to balance. In addition, consuming fewer mucus-forming foods cuts mucus problems off at their source, but it is not uncommon for fat and mucoid deposits to remain in the heart and arteries. How these deposits influence heart syndromes and disease patterns depends on the individual. When indicated, the methods given in the *Oils and Fats* chapter for rejuvenating the vascular system form a foundation for heart syndrome treatments and other refinements in this chapter.

In addition to balancing the heart through the other organs and vascular cleansing methods, there are specific spirit-clarifying methods. One such method is the use of speech, which is said to issue forth from the heart. The condition of the heart is reflected in the awareness of one's spoken words. Conversely, by improving our awareness of our speech, we strengthen the heart; the scattered mind and its spirit can be collected and organized through mindful speech patterns. Examples of these and other traditional spirit-focusing practices are prayer, meditation, devotional singing, mantras (chanting), affirmations, and silent contemplation on uplifting images.

For such practices to be beneficial, they need to be done attentively rather than mechanically. Establishing a strong, calm, and clear mind promotes more efficient healing of all organ systems. Having such a mind has other therapeutic benefits as well—it enables one to better withstand pain.

> When the heart is serene, pain seems negligible.
>
> —*Inner Classic*

At the beginning of any course of treatment, it is wise to first calm the mind and balance the spirit. For instance, some schools of acupuncture/acupressure start treatments on the area of the upper back at the heart-associated acupuncture point (Bl 15). This point is well known for calming the heart and spirit. Such treatment accords with the *Inner Classic* on this subject: "All proper needling [and healing] first treats the spirit." At most traditional healing events, a prayer is customarily offered first to heighten spiritual awareness. Grace before meals also has this effect.

Calming and Focusing the Mind

We of the "information age" tend to have mental hyperactivity. Energy from excessive thought and worry races through the head while the heart is impoverished. In severe cases, the *yang* aspects of the heart—*heat, qi* energy, and spirit—flood upward into the head. An excess of these qualities can cause fever, headache, irritability, insomnia, and mental disturbances. In general, the dietary cure for this condition involves improving the *yin* of the heart, so that spirit is held in the heart by a protective barrier of *yin* essences; similarly, *heat* and *qi* are also restrained.

When spirit becomes sufficiently concentrated in the heart, superficial thinking stops and integrated thought begins. One becomes fully present, and rather than thinking about "reality," thought *becomes* reality. Ultimately thought is experienced as the creation of reality, and the person feels happy (the associated emotion of a healthy heart) with living so directly and simply. Obviously, there are limitless gradations of consciousness on the way to unity. In generally accepted terms, mental health is present when a person is functional, rational, and has no "mental disease." One may easily find, however, by using basic awareness practices and a little dietary discipline that mental wellness extends indefinitely beyond this neutral stage.

Dietary suggestions for calming and focusing the mind: A simple diet with occasional light fasting goes a long way toward creating deep, peaceful thinking. In addition, one should avoid food habits which scatter the mind or overheat the body and thus deplete the *yin* fluids. Too many ingredients in meals, very spicy or rich foods, refined sugar, alcohol, coffee, late-night eating, and large evening meals can cause insomnia as well as a profusion of mental chatter during the day. The following substances reduce nervousness, treat insomnia, and improve mental focus by quieting the spirit and helping it stay centered in the heart.

- Oyster shell: excellent for building the *yin* of the heart. Also lowers floating *yang* as described above. Can be eaten in the form of "oyster-shell calcium," which is available at stores that sell nutritional supplements.
- Grain: whole wheat, brown rice, and oats gently but profoundly calm the mind.
- Mushrooms: nearly every form of these fungi have cerebral effects. *Poria cocos,* one of the most common Chinese "herbs," is used to settle the nerves and improve fluid balance. The *ling zhi* mushroom of China (*reishi* in Japan), becoming widely available in the West as an immune tonic, directly nurtures the heart, soothes the spirit, and calms the mind.
- Silicon foods: oatstraw tea, barley gruel, oat groat tea, cucumber, celery, lettuce, and celery/lettuce juice. Silicon foods improve calcium metabolism and strengthen nerve and heart tissue.
- Fruit: mulberries and lemons calm the mind (mulberries have the stronger effect of the two). Schisandra berries *(Schisandra chinensis;* Mandarin: *wu wei zi)* calm the spirit and are prescribed in Chinese herbology for insomnia and to aid memory recall and concentration. Their astringent nature lends them to treating frequent urination, nocturnal emissions, diarrhea, and excessive sweating.
- Seeds: jujube seeds *(Ziziphus jujuba/spinosa;* Mandarin: *suan zoa ren)* are a widely used Chinese herbal remedy for calming the spirit; they are thought to directly nourish the heart. Chia seed also has sedative action.
- Spices: dill and basil can be used in both food and teas for their calming effect.
- Herbs: regular use of chamomile *(Anthemis nobilis),* catnip *(Nepeta cataria),* scullcap *(Scutellaria laterifolia),* or valerian *(Valeriana officinalis)* is helpful for

the nervous person or insomniac, until the diet is improved to the extent that herbs are unnecessary. Taking rose hips with these herbs supplies vitamin C for soothing the nerves.
- Animal products: quality cow and goat milk and clarified butter *(ghee)* nourish the spirit of the heart in those who can tolerate these foods. For insomnia, the best way to take milk is the classic folk remedy prescription—drinking it warm before bed.

The Calming Effect of Whole Foods

From the Five Element correspondences, we know that the bitter flavor of any food "enters" and affects the heart. There it has multiple actions: cleansing the physical heart and associated arteries of deposits; sedating and lowering the *yang* qualities in the head and concentrating them in the heart (bitterness has a descending, centering property); cooling an overheated heart; and toning up a stagnant liver, thereby making more energy available for the heart via the Creation Cycle. The bitter aspect of grains such as wheat and rice is in their germ and bran; these, however, are removed in processing refined wheat flour and white rice. Also, the essential fatty acids in the grain germ and the B vitamins which reside primarily in the germ and bran have a definite healing and sustaining effect on the nerves.

Magnesium in foods is healing to the heart but is virtually lost in the milling of grains and the refining of most other foods. Magnesium allows calcium to function properly in the tissues of the heart and nerves; it also restrains the "anxiety peptide," a complex of amino acids in the brain which appears to contribute to anxiety.[6] Green foods are rich in magnesium because this mineral is positioned at the center of every chlorophyll molecule; interestingly, green in color healing is said to bring peace and harmony.

In recent years, the amino acid L-tryptophan has been taken widely as a supplement to calm the mind, promote sound sleep, and relieve depression. These healing effects are due to serotonin, a neurotransmitter in the brain which requires L-tryptophan for its formation. Eosinophilia-myalgia syndrome, a painful blood disorder possibly resulting from faulty L-tryptophan synthesis, was discovered in 1989 among hundreds of people taking it in supplement form.[7] A safer way to get L-tryptophan is in food, where it has been produced by nature, in the context of all the cofactors necessary for its proper functioning, as has been the case since the dawn of time. Most foods contain L-tryptophan, but the other amino acids in a high-protein diet compete with its use in the formation of serotonin. Research has demonstrated that a high-carbohydrate diet maximizes the presence of L-tryptophan in the brain. People who eat a carbohydrate-based diet of quality whole foods invariably are calm, rarely depressed, and able to sleep soundly.

Mental Depression. Melancholy, despair, and other aspects of mental depression are now more common than ever; in fact, according to Martin Seligman, professor of psychology at the University of Pennsylvania and author of *Learned Optimism* (1990), people born after World War II have almost ten times the depression rate of their parents and grandparents. Women are also twice as likely to suffer from depression as men. Certainly everyone's delicate, feminine, *yin* quality is easily damaged by excessive competition and stress; in most women, however, *yin* predominates and is more externally accessible; therefore women in general (and sensitive men) especially need to protect themselves from various forms of external harshness.

Mental depression is experienced in the mind but usually rooted in a stagnant liver. The remedies given earlier in the *Wood Element* chapter for clearing such stagnancy are appropriate. At the same time, foods used in both the East and the West for lifting depression can be taken as short-term remedies while the liver is being renewed. These foods also work well for treating the minor depression that nearly everyone experiences occasionally. They are: brown rice, cucumber, apples, cabbage, fresh wheat germ, kuzu root, wild blue-green micro-algae *(Aphanizomenon flos-aquae),* and apple cider vinegar. Including one of these foods in each meal is usually adequate. Wild blue-green and vinegar act more specifically than the other foods. *Dosage:* 1 teaspoon vinegar in a little water, while experiencing depression, up to three times daily; 1.5 grams wild blue-green one to three times daily. Severe chronic depression often accompanies other, deeper imbalances, and expert diagnosis should be sought.

Earth Element

Late Summer: The Interchange of All Seasons

Late summer, a short and relatively unrecognized "season," is approximately the last month of summer and the middle of the Chinese year.* It is the point of transition from *yang* to *yin,* between the expansive growth phases of spring and summer and the inward, cooler, more mysterious fall and winter seasons. A pleasant, tranquil, and flourishing season, it is as if time stops here and activity becomes effortless, dreamlike. Unity, harmony, and the middle way are summoned between the extremes.

To attune with late summer, one may listen to its subtle currents, as if living at the instant where the pendulum reverses its swing. Find the rhythms and cycles that make life simple and harmonious. Rigid or discordant mental/physical conditions can be transformed through centering practices that take one beyond all

---

*The Chinese year begins in February, with the exact day varying slightly each year.

conditions—for example, meditation with a Zen practice of breathing as an infant, into the abdomen, our physical center.

> The Earth Element, represented by the spleen-pancreas, regulates the "center," that which is constant, from where it harmonizes the effects of the four seasons.
>
> —*Inner Classic*

The Interchanges of the Seasons

The Earth Element has a strong influence over the fifteen days surrounding each of the two equinoxes and two solstices (7½ days before and after).* These are neutral buffers between the seasons, which change at the equinoxes and solstices. These interchange periods represent pivotal pauses in the light patterns we experience from the sun, the center of our solar systeem.

Late Summer and the Interchanges: Food and its Preparation

To attune with these seasons, choose some foods for each meal that are harmonizing and represent the center—mildly sweet foods, yellow or golden foods, round foods, and/or foods known to harmonize the center—millet, corn, carrots, cabbage, garbanzo beans, soybeans, squash, potatoes, string beans, yams, tofu, sweet potatoes, sweet rice, rice, amaranth, peas, chestnuts, filberts, apricots, and cantaloupe.

Food should be prepared simply, with a minimum of seasonings and a mild taste. Avoid complicated dishes and combinations of foods. Moderation should also guide other aspects of food preparation, including cooking time, methods and temperature, and the use of water and cooking oil. Of course, one may follow these practices to help sustain balance and middle-path experiences at any time.

The seasonal interchanges are traditional times of purification in many cultures. A short—perhaps three-day—single-grain fast during the fall and winter interchanges, and a vegetable or fruit fast on the cusps of spring and summer, bring one to the "center" during seasonal transitions.

The major Earth Element relationships defined by the *Inner Classic* are the following:

> The mysterious forces of the Earth create moisture in the Heaven and fertile soil upon the earth; they create the flesh within the body and the stomach [and spleen-pancreas]. They create the yellow color . . . and give the voice the ability to sing . . . they create the mouth [and sense of taste], the sweet flavor, and the emotions of anxiety and worry.

---

*The fifteen days surrounding the equinoxes and solstices amount to sixty days. The addition of the late summer month, running concurrently with the last month of summer, gives the Earth Element dominion over the same number of days as the other elements.

The Spleen-Pancreas in Harmony and Disease

The Earth Element's related organs, the spleen-pancreas* and stomach, are primarily responsible for the digestion and distribution of food and nutrients. The *qi* energy and other essences extracted from digestion are used by the body to create *wei qi* energy (immunity), vitality, warmth, and formation of the tissues and mental functions.

Those with a balanced spleen-pancreas are generally hard-working, practical, and responsible. They like to nurture themselves and others and are strong, active, and stable. They have endurance and good appetites and digestion; their limbs have strength; they tend to be orderly and careful, and often excel at some creative activity. They have fertile imaginations.

Those with general signs of spleen-pancreas imbalance are characterized by chronic tiredness, physical and mental stagnation, and compulsive, "stuck" behavior that prevents them from creatively developing their personalities. They typically have weak digestion, often accompanied by nausea, poor appetite, dull sense of taste, abdominal bloating, hard lumps in the abdomen, and loose stools. Blood-sugar imbalances may be part of the picture. When they have weight problems, they tend to be overweight without overeating, or thin and unable to gain weight. They tend to have sallow complexions and are often sloppy in appearance, live in disorder, and accumulate useless possessions.

Specific Syndromes of the Spleen-Pancreas

Deficient *qi* energy of the spleen-pancreas is common among poorly nourished people, including those who are malnourished due to a diet of refined, highly processed foods. The spleen-pancreas rules the extraction of *qi* energy and other nourishment from food in the digestive tract; most intestinal remedies in traditional Chinese medicine are directed toward the spleen-pancreas. To understand this relationship between the spleen-pancreas and intestines, consider the actual function of the pancreas: to secrete pancreatic enzymes into the small intestine. The health of the pancreas determines the quantity and strength of these enzymes, which in turn largely determine how well nutrients are absorbed through the small intestine.

---

*"Spleen" is a misnomer of early translators; when the term "spleen-pancreas" is used, it refers solely to the pancreas and its constellation of activities in both Chinese and modern physiology. The hyphenation of "spleen" to "pancreas" is used here for the sake of continuity with the many texts that have retained the term "spleen" from the first translations.

The blood-storage function of the spleen of modern physiology is part of the liver function of Chinese medicine; thus the spleen can be thought of as a separate lobe of the liver. The Chinese traditionally considered the liver to be on both sides of the body.

Symptoms of weak spleen-pancreas *qi:* loose stools, general weakness, fatigue, pale tongue with a thin white coating, weak pulse, and any of the other general signs of spleen-pancreas imbalance listed above. Imbalances commonly caused by weak spleen-pancreas *qi* include food sensitivities, nervous indigestion, anemia, chronic diarrhea or dysentery, ulcers, and pain in the upper abdomen.

Those with spleen-pancreas *qi* deficiency are predisposed to additional problems. The *qi* of the spleen-pancreas, often called the "middle *qi,*" animates the periphery of the body. The strength of the arms and legs depends on this *qi,* and weak limbs signify a deficiency of it. Another function of middle *qi* is to hold the internal organs in place; prolapses such as hemorrhoids and prolapsed uterus, kidneys, stomach, or intestines are usually a result of insufficient middle *qi.*

Dietary suggestions for deficient spleen-pancreas *qi:* The dietary treatment for this *qi* deficiency involves foods that are either warming (denoted by "†" below) or at least neutral in thermal nature. Foods with cooling properties weaken the digestion. Likewise, food that is cold in temperature extinguishes the "digestive fire"; in fact, just the process of warming up cold food absorbs a fair amount of the body's digestive energy.

Foods which correct *deficiency*, including most complex carbohydrates and certain animal products, are also recommended. Such foods are basically sweet and/or pungent; well-cooked rice is one of the best gradually acting spleen-pancreas tonics (see "congee" in recipe section); oats,† spelt,† sweet rice,† and pounded sweet rice (mochi)† also are excellent. Other beneficial foods:

1. The carbohydrate-rich vegetables: winter squash,† carrot, rutabaga, parsnip,† turnip, garbanzo beans, black beans,† peas, sweet potato,† yam, pumpkin;
2. The pungent vegetables and spices: onion,† leek,† black pepper,† ginger,† cinnamon,† fennel,† garlic,† nutmeg;†
3. Small amounts of certain sweeteners and cooked fruits: rice syrup,† barley malt,† molasses;† cherry† and date.†
4. If the *deficiency* is severe, small amounts of animal products prepared in a soup or congee may be helpful: mackerel, tuna, halibut, anchovy,† beef,† beef liver or kidney,† chicken,† turkey,† or lamb.† Butter† is the only recommended dairy product.

Food must be chewed well and taken in easily digestible form. Small, frequent meals are necessary at the beginning of the healing process, and all food should be at least moderately well-cooked. A weak spleen-pancreas indicates neglect or ignorance of the Earth Element at the level of food; properly preparing food with nurturing care imparts healing essence.

Deficient digestive fire. If a spleen-pancreas *qi* energy deficiency is allowed to worsen, it can degenerate into what is called "deficiency of digestive fire." Whenever fire—the *yang*, warming principle—is lacking, such an imbalance has all the symptoms of *qi* deficiency, but deficient digestive fire also shows signs of *cold* digestion that clearly distinguish it. These include watery stools (rather than loose), possibly containing undigested food. Further signs of *coldness* are: aversion to cold weather; cold hands and feet; clear urine; and pallor; also, the tongue is pale, swollen, and wet, with teeth indentations in the sides.

To balance this lack of fire, follow the deficient spleen-pancreas *qi* recommendations—with the exception of sweet rice, which is contraindicated in digestive fire deficiency. In addition, emphasize more warming herbs and foods such as those marked "†" in the "Dietary suggestions" above. When using ginger, the dried form (available as an herb) is better than fresh ginger for improving digestive fire.

Foods to restrict in deficient *qi* or fire of the spleen-pancreas: excessive raw vegetables, fruit (especially citrus), sprouts, and cereal grasses; cooling foods such as tomato, spinach, chard, tofu, millet, amaranth, seaweeds, wild blue-green microalgae, and salt; too many very sweet foods, liquids, and dairy products; and vinegar. Care must be taken not to push the liver to a state of excess. Large meals and rich foods are avoided; nuts, seeds, and oils are eaten in small amounts to nullify the Destructive Cycle activity of an excessive liver on the spleen-pancreas. Liver excess is perhaps the major cause of spleen-pancreas weakness.

Dampness, Mucus, and Microbes

The amount and quality of *dampness* present in the digestive tract and throughout the body are further measures of the health of the spleen-pancreas and therefore of digestion in general. The concept of *dampness* unifies many separate mucous, bacterial, viral, and yeast imbalances in the body under a few simple dietary treatments.

Dampness, a *yin* disorder, includes any overly wet or moist condition in the body. It can come from the environment, or it can be due to poor diet or internal organ weakness. *Damp* excesses in the digestive tract, lungs, bladder, sexual organs, and elsewhere most often appear as: 1) various types of mucoid deposits or moist accumulations such as edema, cysts, tumors, and cancers; or 2) an overgrowth of yeasts, viruses, putrefactive bacteria, amoebas, and/or parasites. These two groups are related to each other, since nearly every chronic mucous condition appears in the context of a proliferation of microorganisms.[8-14]

Symptoms of dampness: Dampness can invade the joints and acupuncture channels. Movement becomes difficult, numbness may appear, and if there is pain, it is fixed in one place. Any part or all of the body can be affected by *damp* swelling or edema. *Dampness* in the form of mucus also affects the heart and lungs, and is the cause of the most common problems in these organs. (Symptoms are described in the *Fire* and *Metal Element* chapters.) When *dampness* affects the spleen-pancreas—the intestines and digestion in general—symptoms may include feelings of heaviness, particularly in the head, lack of appetite, bloated abdomen, and watery stools; the coating on the tongue is thick and possibly dirty or greasy. In many cases, the cause of digestive *dampness* is the deficient *qi* or fire patterns discussed earlier. *Damp* diseases in general have a sluggish, stagnant quality and often take a long time to cure.

Dampness and Degenerative Disease

Many chronic illnesses involve *dampness*. Fully two-thirds of the typical diet in the United States consists of animal products, which promote any of the various types of *dampness* mentioned earlier. In addition, *dampness* often combines with *heat, wind* and/or *cold,* so these other factors must be taken into account when formulating a dietary plan. Cancer, multiple sclerosis, AIDS, chronic fatigue syndrome, rheumatoid arthritis, and other apparently virus- or microorganism-related degenerations usually involve pathogenic *dampness* in conjunction with various other contributing factors.

These kinds of conditions, true to the nature of deeply situated *dampness,* are not easily resolved by either traditional healing methods or modern medicine. Each case needs to be diagnosed and treated individually. However, there do seem to be common threads running through such imbalances: most of these conditions begin with yeast excesses in the digestive tract, and most respond to a diet that is not *dampness*-inducing, i.e., which is low in fats and mucus-forming food and high in whole, unprocessed vegetal foods. Nearly all such afflicted individuals improve if foods are added that decrease *dampness* in general. In addition, specific herbal, acupuncture, exercise, awareness, and other therapies can be custom-tailored to each individual.

Exercise is essential. Just as a damp cloth does not mold if it is hung out in circulating air, appropriate exercise oxygenates the body. (Oxygenation methods are discussed in the *Interior/Exterior: Building Immunity* chapter.) The beneficial effect of exercise on the *damp* condition of obesity is well-known. Listed next are the dietary factors to avoid in *dampness,* followed by those which are recommended; these suggestions form a dietary foundation for healing the multitude of imbalances in which *dampness* is a central feature.

Dietary Factors Which Contribute to Dampness

• Too much raw, cold, sweet, or mucus-forming food.

The digestive "fire" of the spleen-pancreas is extinguished by an excess of raw food, including too many raw fruits, vegetables, sprouts, and juices, which cause a thin, watery mucus or *dampness*. A similar effect occurs from too much cold food—normally, food should be room temperature or warmer. The appropriate amount of raw food in the diet depends on the strength and condition of the individual, the climate, and the person's level of activity. Robust and over*heated* people usually benefit from an increased intake of raw foods; warm climate and greater physical activity also increase one's ability to tolerate raw food in the diet.

Signs of excess raw-food consumption include weakness, coldness, and watery stools. Many vegetarian raw-food zealots have severely damaged their health by not knowing when to introduce some cooked food. At the same time, it must be emphasized that numerous disease conditions involving general *excess* (robust, extroverted nature, reddish complexion, thick tongue coating, forceful pulses) have been overcome with the cleansing action and therapeutic use of raw food.

Intake of highly sweet and other mucus-forming foods needs to be limited; these include meats, eggs, dairy products, fats such as lard and butter (avoid hydrogenated fats such as margarine altogether), oils, oily foods such as nuts and seeds (especially peanuts), and foods containing concentrated sweeteners. Simple sugars from sweeteners and fruits, taken in excess, also encourage the growth of infections and yeasts. Those who are afflicted with *dampness* related to *Candida albicans* yeasts should follow the candida dietary plan (page 73), which is more specific than this plan.

A small amount of mucus, however, is necessary in the digestive tract and along all mucous membranes. Moderate amounts of complex carbohydrates (grains, vegetables, legumes) in the diet supply a light and beneficial coating, although large amounts create excessive deposits. Overconsumption of dairy, eggs, or meat causes the thickest, stickiest mucous conditions. Other contributors include:

- Food that is refined or highly processed, rotten, stale, parasite-infested, or chemically treated.
- Too many ingredients in a meal (poor food combining).
- Late-night eating.
- Overeating.

Products with several *damp*-causing properties seem to have much worse effects than the mere sum of their properties. Ice cream, for instance, is very sweet, cold, highly mucus-producing, and often full of chemical additives; furthermore, its concentrated sweeteners and often added sweet fruits do not combine well with dairy, a high-fat protein. In the author's healing practice, regular consumption of ice cream contributes to abdominal lumps, cysts, tumors, and other *damp* conditions in general. Ice cream substitutes, even those made of high-quality ingredients, are very sweet and cold, and therefore support *damp* excesses and should be avoided by susceptible individuals.

Foods Which Dry Dampness: Rye, amaranth, corn, aduki beans, celery, lettuce, pumpkin, scallion, alfalfa, turnip, kohlrabi, white pepper, raw honey; all bitter herbs such as chaparral *(Larrea divaricata),* chamomile *(Anthemis nobilis),* and pau d'arco *(Tabevulia);* and the micro-algae dunaliella and wild blue-green *(Aphanizomenon).* Raw goat's milk is the one dairy product that will not usually contribute to *damp* conditions in the body.

Exterior Dampness. *Damp* conditions are not only diet-related. Overexposure to dampness in the environment will worsen internal *damp* conditions. "Damp environment" applies not only to weather but to other damp situations like sitting too long on cold, damp ground.

Waste and the Earth Element

The Earth Element represents the *yin,* nurturing, and receptive qualities of life. From this perspective, rampant hypoglycemia, cancer, constipation, and other afflictions related to faulty nurture begin to be transformed to health with a general respect for the Earth, for the food it offers, and for the human body, created from the material of the Earth. Those who respect the bounties of the Earth do not waste food or anything useful. By consuming only what is needed, they minimize the toxins and the depletion of the soil involved in industrial agriculture and food production. Respect and awareness for one's own body also influences one to stop the consumption of denatured, refined foods, and compassion limits the eating of meat in quantities beyond what is medicinally necessary.

To halt the destruction of the feminine, *yin* quality in general, it is helpful to see the entire process of how we live on the Earth as equivalent to what we receive from it in health and security. It is surprising how many environmentalists find no fault with eating glazed, greasy, white-flour doughnuts, while dedicated at the same time to cleaning up the streams and land. Our own bloodstreams and internal physical terrain must be cleaned as well to effect a total and unified change, one that brings a conscious merger of the individual spirit with the soul of the Earth.

Metal Element

Autumn

Fall is the season of harvest, a time to pull inward and gather together on all levels, a time to store up fuel, food, and warm clothing, a time to study and plan for the approaching stillness of winter. Everything in nature contracts and moves its essence inward and downward. Leaves and fruit fall, seeds dry, the sap of trees goes into the roots. The earth's grasses start to lose their deep green color, turning lighter and drier.

> The forces of Autumn create dryness in Heaven and metal on Earth; they create the lung organ and the skin upon the body . . . and the nose, and the white color, and the pungent flavor . . . the emotion grief, and the ability to make a weeping sound.
>
> —*Inner Classic*

Autumn Foods

To prepare food which reflects the qualities of autumn, we must be aware of its abundant yet contracting nature. This awareness can be heightened by choices for more astringent as well as heartier flavors and foods. In addition, cooking methods should involve more focused preparation to supply the greater energy required by a cooler season.

The essence of food is received through the sense of smell, which is related to the Metal Element and lungs. The appetite is stimulated by the warm fragrance of baked and sautéed food—concentrated foods and roots thicken the blood for cooler weather.

The fall is the time to organize the open and perhaps scattered patterns of the previous warmer seasons. To stimulate this activity in the body, to focus mentally, and to begin the process of contraction, add more sour flavored foods. These include sourdough bread, sauerkraut, olives, pickles, leeks, aduki beans, salt plums, rose hip tea, vinegar, cheese, yogurt, lemons, limes, grapefruit, and the sour varieties of apples, plums, and grapes. Be cautious with extremely sour foods, because small amounts have a strong effect.

In general, cook with less water, and at lower heat, for longer periods of time. This internalizes one's focus. Likewise, the bitter and salty flavors move energy strongly inward and downward; ideally, they are gradually introduced as the fall progresses into winter. Salty and bitter-flavored foods are discussed further in the following *Water Element* chapter.

Dryness

When dry climates prevail, it is important to know how to offset their effects. When a person has a *dry* condition, it usually is related to the lungs, and could have been caused by imbalances in the diet, excessive activity, adverse climate, and/or organ malfunction. The major symptoms of *dryness* in the body are thirst, dryness of the skin, nose, lips, and throat, and itchiness; those who are chronically *dry* also tend to have a thin body type.

To counter dry weather and treat conditions of *dryness* in the body in any season, foods which moisten can be emphasized: soybean products, including tofu, tempeh, and soy milk; spinach, barley, millet, pear, apple, persimmon, loquat, seaweeds, black and white fungus, almond, pinenut, peanut, sesame seed, honey (cooked), barley malt, rice syrup, milk and dairy products, eggs, clam, crab, oyster, mussel, herring, and pork. Using a little salt in cooking also moistens *dryness*.

Dairy and other animal products are more appropriate for those whose *dryness* is accompanied by weakness, frailty, and other signs of *deficiency*. The *dry* person's condition is frequently a result of inadequate *yin* fluids in the body, and therefore many of the remedies for nourishing the *yin* also treat *dryness*. Those with *dryness* should use bitter, aromatic, and/or warming foods with caution. These foods, which include many spices and herbs, dry the body.

The Lungs in Harmony and Disease

The lungs receive the *qi* vital force of the air and mix it with the *qi* extracted from food. This combination of *qi* and associated nutrients is then distributed throughout the body and is of particular importance in protecting the surfaces of the body (including the mucous membranes and interior surfaces of the lungs) from viruses, bacteria, and other invading pathogens. The strength of the lungs depends on their *qi.*

In health, lung *qi* energy is characterized by its ability to consolidate, gather together, maintain strength, and unify against disease at every level, including cellular immunity. The personality of those with strong lungs is influenced by this *qi:* they seem unified, hold onto their direction, create order, and are effective at what they do. How well we "hold on" and "let go" can be expressed in terms of emotional attachment. The colon is the *yang* organ paired with the lungs, and its obvious function is releasing what is no longer needed. In Chinese healing traditions, this release is on emotional and psychic levels as well as physical.

Attachments as an Indicator of Lung Vitality

Those with healthy lungs tend to hold onto their principles and keep their commitments, but when it comes time to let go of an object or relationship, they sense this and do it without emotional repression, feeling the associated grief and sadness, but soon resolving it. In comparison, those with weak lungs may experience loss with confusion and attempt to stifle their sadness, never completely letting go. At the same time, they can be disorderly and either lose their possessions easily or else hold onto them with unreasonable attachment.

Resolving Grief and Sadness

Grief is the emotion associated with the lungs and colon. Grief that is expressed and resolved strengthens the internal basis of health, but repressed grief causes long-term contraction in the lungs, which interferes with their function of dispersing nutrients and *qi;* ultimately, the lungs become congested with undistributed matter. Virtually everyone with lung and colon problems, regardless of the source of the problem, has unresolved sadness that needs to be cleared. Understanding the inward nature of this emotion offers a clue to working with it.

The contracting force of grief, if used constructively, clears repression: it encourages us to look within, to identify unresolved sorrows, and to transform them by simply being mindful of them. Sharing such feelings with others can also help dissipate them. By focusing internally, one heals those areas where deep illness may otherwise develop. Turbid emotions and thoughts can be cleansed by long, deep breathing. The expansive quality of pungent foods, the flavor that first "enters" the lungs, can assist in clearing grief.

The Physical Indications of Lung Vitality

Before assessing lung vitality, it is useful to consider three additional relationships:
1. The lungs are said to "open" to the nose; this means that the sinuses, bronchials, air passageways, and the nose itself are all influenced by the lungs.
2. The health of the skin, including the mucous membranes and their inherent immunity, reflect lung health.
3. The amount and quality of mucus relate to the lungs.

The individual with healthy lungs maintains a light, moist, protective coating on all mucous membranes; in conjunction with well-nourished and energized skin, this wards off extreme weather influences as well as viruses and other pathogens. Such a person is protected against infectious diseases like colds and flus and has good immunity in general.

In contrast, both dryness and excessive mucus in the membranes, sinus problems, nasal congestion, lung and bronchial conditions, frequent colds, and susceptibility to contagions all indicate lung imbalance.

Because the *qi* and nutrients directed by balanced lungs nourish the periphery of the body, the person with strong lungs has soft, lustrous skin and glossy hair. Skin that is dry, dull, or rough is a sign of lung imbalance.

Causes of Common Lung Disorders

In addition to unresolved grief, many problems of the lungs (and colon) are due to a sedentary lifestyle. Insufficient activity encourages poor respiration and elimination. Lung and colon problems are also aggravated by a faulty diet: overeating; not eating roughage; consuming too much meat, dairy, and other congesting foods; using drugs, cigarettes, and processed foods. Poor eating habits cause mucus to be deposited in the lungs, which blocks their proper functioning. Colds, allergies, sinus problems, bronchitis, and asthma are among the problems that may result. Furthermore, toxins build up in the lungs and colon and create tension, exhaustion, hair and skin problems, and pale complexion. The following syndromes illustrate more precisely how these various conditions manifest in the lungs, and thus shed light on their cure. (Colon and intestinal/digestive problems in general are addressed in the *Earth Element* and *Diseases and Their Dietary Treatment* chapters.)

Common Syndromes of the Lungs

The first lung syndrome, the onset of conditions such as the common cold and flu, has been described earlier as an *exterior* invasion of the lungs by *wind* (see pages 68 and 321). If such *exterior* conditions are not cleared up, they can develop into *heat* in the lungs.

Heat **congesting the lungs** will usually have *exterior* symptoms such as fevers accompanied by chills, and a red tongue with a dry, yellow coating. In addition, there is a dry cough, shortness of breath, and a painful sore throat; there may also be thick, yellow-green sputum with pus, or even rank, bloody pus; and yellow nasal discharge. Treatment involves adding foods and herbs which cool the *heat* and transform sputum in the lungs.

Useful foods and herbs: watercress, cantaloupe, apple, persimmon, peach, pear, strawberry, citrus, seaweeds (e.g., agar, nori, kelp), mushroom, daikon radish, radish, carrot, pumpkin, kuzu, cabbage, bok choy, cauliflower, chard, papaya, and white fungus; herbs include horehound leaf and chickweed.

The majority of the diet should be in the form of soups. Soups and congees of millet, barley, or rice are cooling and soothing for lung *heat*. The most effective of the above foods are watercress and white fungus. White fungus *(bai mu er)* is available at many groceries and herb stores. Drinking freely of horehound *(Marrubium vulgare)* or chickweed *(Stellaria media)* tea is helpful.

Avoid: warming and/or congesting foods including coffee, alcohol, lamb, chicken, beef, warming fish (e.g., trout, salmon, anchovy), onion family members (especially garlic), cinnamon, ginger, fennel, and other warming foods and spices.

Phlegm in the lungs is most often brought about by weak digestion (weak spleen-pancreas *qi*) that causes mucus. It can also result from too much mucus-forming food. In either case, mucus accumulates in the lungs; symptoms include cough, shortness of breath, wheezing, or asthma accompanied by sticky phlegm. The tongue coating is greasy and white if the phlegm is cold; a greasy yellow coating indicates hot phlegm. Treatment includes foods that transform, reduce, or expel phlegm.

Useful foods, spices, and herbs: fennel(w), fenugreek(w), flaxseed(n), cayenne(w), watercress(c), garlic and other members of the onion family(w), horseradish(w), turnip(n), fresh ginger(w), radish(c), daikon radish(c), mushroom(n), cereal grass(c) and seaweeds(c); herbs include nettles(c), coltsfoot(n), elecampane root(w), and mullein leaf(c). Items with a cooling thermal nature are denoted "c," warming "w," and neutral "n."

The general diet should consist of foods that digest easily and do not add any further mucus burden. These are vegetables, fruits, and sprouts; small amounts of legumes, grains, and almonds can usually be tolerated. It is best to eat simple, small meals. The above cooling remedies are useful for treating hot phlegm; the warming remedies treat cold phlegm; neutral remedies can be used for hot or cold phlegm. The herbs, spices, and seeds combine well to make teas. For hot phlegm, for example, one might choose mullein leaf *(Verbascum thaspus),* coltsfoot *(Tussilago farfara),* nettles *(Urtica urens),* and flaxseed; for cold phlegm, elecampane *(Inula helinium),* fresh ginger, and fenugreek.

Avoid: all dairy foods, mammal meats, peanuts, tofu, tempeh, miso, soy sauce, soy milk and other soy products, amasake and all other sweeteners except stevia leaf.

Deficient *yin* of the lungs occurs when there is a chronic lack of *yin* to cool and nourish the lungs. Such a condition is most often a result of a chronic lung infection, inflammation, or other long-term lung disease which drains the *yin* of the body. Insufficient *yin* of the lungs (or of any organ) suggests a deficiency of kidney *yin*, which enriches the *yin* of the entire body. Typical symptoms include dry, unproductive cough with little or no sputum (sometimes tinged with blood); periodic fever, frequent thirst, fresh-red cheeks and tongue, hot palms and soles, night sweats, thin and fast radial pulse. Treatment includes foods that tonify the lung *yin* as well as the kidney *yin*, the root of *yin* in the body.

Useful foods and herbs: Irish moss and other seaweeds, spirulina and chlorella micro-algae, orange, peach, pear, apple, watermelon, tomato, banana, string bean, soy milk, tofu, tempeh, sugar cane (and unrefined cane-juice powder), rice syrup, flaxseed, butter and other dairy products, egg, oyster, clam, and pork; herbs include marshmallow root, slippery elm bark, the bulbs of tiger lily and other lilies, rehmannia root (raw variety), and Solomon's seal root.

Deficient *yin* of the lungs requires consistent effort to cure completely. The basic diet should exclude all warming foods and spices such as those to avoid in "*heat* congesting the lungs," above. Too much bitter flavor in the diet is drying, and therefore also contraindicated; use very bitter herbs such as golden seal, dandelion, echinacea, and burdock cautiously if at all. If tolerated, dairy products and eggs should be of excellent quality and taken in small amounts.

Marshmallow root *(Althea officinalis)* is a valuable remedy in most cases of lung *yin* depletion and, in addition, is laxative; slippery elm *(Ulmus fulva)* has great nutritive value and can be recommended in cases of extreme wasting; Solomon's seal *(Polygonatum officinale)* is the most energizing of these *yin* tonics and is used traditionally in both China and the West. According to Michael Tierra in *Planetary Herbology*, most species of lily bulb *(Lilium*-related species) are edible except the "calla" lily—not a true lily. Lily bulb, a commonly available Chinese herb, has a sedative effect which makes it useful for cases of *yin* deficiency accompanied by nervousness or insomnia. Another common Chinese herb, raw rehmannia *(Rehmannia glutinosa)*, can also be used for *heat*-induced hemorrhages; for constipation and/or sore throat resulting from *yin* deficiency; and for canker and tongue sores. Avoid raw rehmannia in cases of *coldness* or weak digestion (spleen-pancreas *qi* deficiency) or in pregnancy accompanied by anemia.

Deficient *qi* of the lungs is a chronic, often debilitating lung pattern. Symptoms include weakness, fatigue, weak voice and limited speech, coughing, and shortness of breath. If the protective *qi* has also been weakened, there may be spontaneous sweating with any physical activity and poor immunity to contagions such as colds and flus. Deficient *qi* of the lungs can result from long-term lung diseases, particularly those with *heat* signs (including the minor *heat* signs of deficient lung *yin* discussed above). General lack of bodily *qi* can also cause this syndrome. The *qi* energy in the body is rooted in the kidney-adrenals, which in turn depend on the *qi* derived from food—a spleen-pancreas function.

The treatment is to supplement the *qi* energy of the lungs with foods and preparation methods that tonify the lung *qi* and improve the absorption of food *qi*.

Useful foods and herbs: rice, sweet rice, oats, carrot, mustard green, sweet potato, yam, potato, fresh ginger, garlic, molasses, rice syrup, barley malt, herring; herbs include elecampane root, spikenard root, and licorice root.

The diet should include primarily cooked food and restrict cooling or mucus-forming foods such as citrus fruits, salt, milk and other dairy products, cereal-grass products, spinach, chard, seaweeds, and micro-algae (chlorella is acceptable). Elecampane *(Inula helinium)*, spikenard *(Aralia racemosa, A. californica* and related species), and licorice *(Glycyrrhiza glabra* and related species) are effective separately or in combination. A typical formula combines licorice (½ part) with 1 part of either elecampane or spikenard.

Protecting the Lungs and Colon

Most people show signs of lung and colon weakness—their skin is not vital, they harbor old grief, hold unhealthy attachments to things and people, and tend to have mucus problems. Yet their condition is not outwardly serious and may not accurately fit into one of the syndromes discussed above.

In our experience, a good portion of people, when told that they have cancer, relate the news to their friends with statements like this: "But I've hardly been sick a day in my life, and I never even get a cold!" People in America who never get a cold are either exceptionally healthy or—more often—holding onto toxins that will contribute to serious diseases later. One or perhaps even two colds a year should not necessarily be considered an unhealthy sign, particularly if the level of toxins where the person lives and works is high. However, a mild lung and colon cleansing once a year, coupled with regular use of protective foods, may make colds and flus unnecessary. There will also be better distribution of *qi* energy and nutrients and fewer unhealthy emotional attachments. Most importantly, it will protect against the later development of more serious diseases.

Protective and Purifying Foods

Pungent foods: For both cleansing and protection, choose foods that specifically affect the lungs and colon. Pungent foods help disperse the stuck, mucus-laden energy of these organs. This traditional wisdom parallels more recent discoveries: Hispanics in the Los Angeles area who smoke have a surprisingly low incidence of respiratory problems, according to Dr. Irwin Ziment, a professor at the University of California School of Medicine at Los Angeles; based on this finding, he has prescribed chilies for lung-related problems for the last ten years.[15]

All pungent foods such as hot peppers and chilies can be used to protect the lungs, but at least some white pungents should be included because this color specifically affects the Metal Element. These include members of the onion family, especially garlic; also turnip, ginger, horseradish, cabbage,* radish,* daikon radish,* and white peppercorn.* Cooling foods denoted by "*" should be used if there are any *heat* or *deficient yin* signs (yellow mucus in small amounts, sensation of being too hot, red face, sore throat, hot palms and soles, night sweats, periodic fever); otherwise any of the foods are appropriate. Consuming all pungent foods raw maximizes their dispersing effect. They are still potent, however, when slightly cooked, and this is a better preparation method for those who are *deficient*.

Mucilaginous foods are important for mucous membrane renewal of the lungs and colon. These plants remove old, thick mucoid deposits and replace them with a clean, moist coating. Some of the best of these foods are seaweeds and certain herbs and seeds, for example kombu, marshmallow root, flaxseed, and fenugreek.

Dark green and golden-orange vegetables offer a protective effect because of their rich beta-carotene (provitamin A) content. As discussed in the *Green Food Products* chapter, beta-carotene protects the surfaces and mucous membranes of the body. This protection bolsters the peripheral immune activity of the *qi*. According to a variety of recent studies, beta-carotene foods appear to protect both the lungs and the colon against cancer.[16–19] Beta-carotene foods with particular protective value for these organs include carrot, winter squash, pumpkin, broccoli, parsley, kale, turnip and mustard greens, watercress, wheat or barley grass, common green, blue-green, and golden micro-algae, and the herbs yerba santa leaf, mullein leaf, and nettles.

The green members of this group are especially important, as their chlorophyll inhibits viruses and also helps the lungs discharge the residues from chemical fumes, coal dust, cigarette smoke, etc. (The herb yerba santa is a specific remedy for this purpose.) Green foods also improve the digestion of proteins and fats, which, when consumed excessively, are implicated in colon cancer.[16]

Fiber: To cleanse the lungs and colon, emphasize fiber foods. Sufficient fiber in the diet reduces the incidence of some cancers by more than 60%, and as a consequence the American Cancer Society now advocates 30% more fiber in the average diet. (The colon and lungs are the sites of the highest incidence of cancer in Americans.) Fiber is the indigestible portion of foods—the bran of grains, the pulp of fruits, and the cell walls of vegetables. There is essentially no edible fiber in animal products. While all fiber improves the functioning of the intestines, not all fiber is alike. Wheat bran has little effect on cholesterol, whereas pectin, a fiber in apples, cherries, carrots, and other produce, eliminates cholesterol from the digestive tract. The fiber in oats also has this capacity.

Research on colon health has shown fiber to be beneficial in curing and/or preventing appendicitis, colon cancer,* diverticulosis (pouches in the colon), constipation, and hemorrhoids.[20–26] Fiber encourages healthful bacterial growth in the colon, which aids in the assimilation of nutrients and the formation of cancer-resistant bowel acids. Fiber is also a source of pentose, an anti-cancer agent. Even though taking pure fiber can have therapeutic results in extreme cases, the most balanced approach is to eat a variety of different types of fiber in the form of whole vegetal foods. (All recipes in the recipe section are high in fiber.) For prevention, all fiber-rich foods are helpful; for an effective cleansing fast of a few days, choose the least mucus-forming fiber foods, vegetables and fruits.

Taking a variety of foods from the above groups in the daily diet acts to bolster immunity and lung/colon function in general. People with minor signs of lung and colon weakness and a rich dietary background also do well to fast for a few days each season on vegetables and fruits. These are best chosen from the pungent, white, golden-orange and green types, and can be supplemented with mucilaginous foods and herbs. Sample meals: broccoli-carrot-daikon-kelp soup; apples and pears (both are white foods except for the skins). For hunger between meals, try spirulina or barley-grass drinks, or flaxseed-marshmallow root tea.

---

*Research also indicates that dietary fiber may provide protection against cancers of the breast, stomach, ovary, endometrium, rectum, mouth, and pharynx.[24]

This general type of short fast does not have extreme effects; it is best suited to those who tend toward mucus problems, poor skin tone, have at least a moderate tongue coating, and are not frail or otherwise *deficient*. (See the *Fasting and Purification* chapter for other suggestions.) Again, specific lung and colon problems need to be addressed separately.

*   *   *

The Metal Element appears to be the weakest of the elements in modern people. By replacing the causes of common lung and colon disorders outlined earlier with wholesome, protective foods in conjunction with an active lifestyle, the lungs and colon are gradually renewed. Slow, steady progress, except in acute diseases of these organs, seems to work best. Sticky lung- and colon-related emotional attachments are not easily dislodged. When the dietary support for such attachments is suddenly removed by intense cleansing methods such as extreme fasting and repeated colonic irrigations, it may be all too easy to soon replace it with an even greater excess of heavy, mucus-promoting, attachment-supporting foods in the diet.

Water Element

Winter

Winter is the end of all the seasons. To unify with winter, one emphasizes the *yin* principle to become more receptive, introspective, and storage-oriented; one cools the surface of the body and warms the body's core. Cold and darkness drive one to seek inner warmth. It is a time to rest, to meditate deeply, refine the spiritual essence, and store physical energy—in the form of a little added weight—for the cold season. Even though the slow *yin* processes predominate, one must stay active enough to keep the spine and joints flexible.

> The forces of winter create cold in Heaven and water on Earth. They create the kidney organ and the bones within the body . . . the emotion fear, and the ability to make a groaning sound.
>
> —*Inner Classic*

Winter Food and Preparation

It is said that the kidneys "open to the ears," which means that hearing is related to the health of the kidneys, the organs most affected by wintertime. The ability to listen clearly is heightened in the cold, silent months. The sounds of cooking and voices from the kitchen stimulate the appetite. Warm hearty soups, whole grains, and roasted nuts sound good on cold days. Dried foods, small dark beans, seaweeds, and steamed winter greens fortify the kidneys in the winter. Cook foods longer, at lower temperatures and with less water.

Salty and Bitter: Flavors for the Cold Season

Both the salty and bitter foods are appropriate for winter, since they promote a sinking, centering quality which heightens the capacity for storage. Such foods also cool the exterior of the body and bring body heat deeper and lower; with a cooler surface, one notices the cold less. However, use salt with care; an excess tightens the Water organs (kidneys and bladder), causing coldness and overconsumption of water, which weakens these organs and affects the heart as well. Providing protection for the heart-mind in the winter is important and can be accomplished with the addition of a few bitter foods, since their flavor is said to "enter the heart."

Most common bitter foods are not wholly bitter, but combinations of bitter and other flavors. These foods include lettuce, watercress, endive, escarole, turnip, celery, asparagus, alfalfa, carrot top, rye, oats, quinoa, and amaranth. The bitter flavor is also part of the protective coating of some foods, e.g., citrus peels and the outermost leaves of cabbage (seldom on cabbage in stores). The strongest bitter qualities are in the herbal realm. Common examples are chicory root *(Cichorium intybus)*, burdock root *(Arctium lappa)*, horsetail *(Equisetum arvense)*, and chaparral *(Larrea divaricata)*. Roasted, ground chicory is available as a major ingredient in many coffee substitutes.

Salty foods include miso, soy sauce, seaweeds, salt, millet, barley, plus any food made salty by the addition of salt. Salt is overused in the typical diet, while the bitter flavor is under-represented. However, strong doses of bitter food are not needed except in the case of certain imbalances, but small, regular amounts in the winter nurture deep inner experiences and preserve joy in the heart.

After acclimating the body to winter with appropriate cooking methods and more salty and bitter foods, the *cold* person may still feel cold because of a lack of warming potential *(yang)* in the body. In this case, add more warming foods such as those listed later in this chapter under "Kidney *Yang* Deficiency." Subjecting the healthy body to a little cold nourishes the kidney-adrenal function, but excess cold weakens it.

The Kidneys in Harmony and Disease

The Water Element organs are the kidneys and the bladder. In Chinese physiology, these organs govern water metabolism and control the bladder. In addition, the kidneys are seen as the root and foundation of the body. They rule the lower part, including the sexual organs and their reproductive functions. They also provide energy and warmth. This concept of "kidneys" goes beyond that of Western physiology. To explain why these additional functions can reasonably be part of kidney function, adrenal gland activity is generally assigned to the Chinese concept of kidney. The adrenals contribute to the energy, warmth, sexuality, and other attributes of the body. The kidney-adrenal connection is clear since the adrenals are located directly on top of the kidneys and produce secretions that make kidney activities possible.

The kidneys, representing the roots of the body, are the foundation of all *yin* and *yang* qualities in the body. Thus, the kidney *yin* supports and affects the *yin* of the entire body; kidney *yang* acts as a foundation for all the *yang* of the body. Accordingly, traditional Chinese medicine describes the kidneys as the "palace of Fire and Water," and in any diagnosis involving the kidneys, one considers both their *yang* and *yin* aspects. For example, the person with healthy, vital kidneys is active yet calm, courageous but gentle, accomplishes a great deal without stress, and balances assertive action with nurture.

All problems with the kidneys show up in one or more specific areas of the body, its emotions, and its development patterns. Knowing these areas is invaluable in assessing kidney vitality.

General Symptoms of Kidney Imbalance

- all bone problems, especially those of the knees, lower back, and teeth
- hearing loss and ear infections and diseases
- head-hair problems—hair loss, split ends, premature graying
- any urinary, sexual, and reproductive imbalances
- poor growth and development of the mind and body; premature aging
- excessive fear and insecurity

The Water Element emotion is fear. Like the kidneys, fear is deeply rooted, and we are often not consciously aware of even major areas of fear and insecurity. A little healthy fear protects us and keeps us from foolhardiness. When excessive, however, fear fosters a general insecurity about life and also "injures" the kidneys. On the other hand, weak kidneys generate fearful feelings, which in turn block loving experiences. To explain this in terms of the Destruction Cycle: stressful, fear-ridden kidneys (Water Element) fail to remove excess water, which extinguishes the heart spirit (Fire Element) and its normal expressions of love and joy. Many people receive psychotherapy in an attempt to identify and dismantle deep insecurities. Often there is little success because the kidney-adrenal complex has not been renewed. By restoring the kidneys to any significant degree, one typically feels a tremendous elation as the dark cloud of fear lifts.

Common Syndromes of the Kidneys

The kidneys manifest imbalance primarily as deficiencies. The most prevalent types are insufficient *yang* and *yin;* also important is lack of *qi* energy. *Jing* essence deficiency is common among modern people, yet is seldom adequately dealt with.

Kidney *yin* deficiency indicates the kidneys are failing to supply adequate *yin* fluids. All areas of the body are affected, but particularly those organ systems which require *yin* most—the liver, heart, and lungs. Conversely, these organs draw from the kidney *yin* when deficient in their own, and can deplete it. Such a pattern is seen all too often in the West in cases of liver excess, which draws on the calming, cooling effect of *yin* fluids to balance its overheated, congested condition. In addition to the *heat*-reducing, sedative effect of kidney *yin,* its other attributes include the nurturing, moistening, supportive, stabilizing, and tissue-building qualities characteristic of the *yin* principle in general.

Symptoms of kidney yin deficiency include dizziness, ringing in the ears, dry throat, dry mouth, fever, low backache, weak legs, involuntary seminal emission, spontaneous sweating, thin, fast radial pulse, and distinctly red tongue. Signs of extreme deficiency of *yin* are emaciation and deep-red, shiny tongue.

Emotional and other characteristics: shortage of the *yin,* calming, receptive, grounding principle can manifest as agitation, irritation, nervousness, insecurity, and fear. The personality is not rooted or stable and may not be dependable; because of deep, often-unacknowledged insecurity, there is a tendency to move from one problem, place, or relationship to the next without ever getting down to the root issues.

Foods which nurture kidney yin: millet, barley, tofu, string bean, black bean, black soybean, mung bean and its sprouts, kidney bean and most other beans, kuzu root, watermelon and other melons, blackberry, mulberry, blueberry, huckleberry, water chestnut, wheat germ, potato, seaweeds, spirulina, chlorella, black sesame seed, sardine, crab, clam, eggs, pork, and cheese. Recommended herbs include marshmallow root *(Althea officinalis),* prepared rehmannia root *(Rehmannia glutinosa;* Mandarin: *shu di huang),* asparagus root *(Asparagus cochinchinensis;* Mandarin: *tian men dong),* aloe vera gel, and silver colloid.

Notes: Black sesame seeds are most appropriate for those with dry stools or constipation; it is an especially good remedy for older people with this condition as well as those with debilitating diseases marked by insufficient *yin. Yin* deficient debilitation often results from parasitic and microbial infections, in which case aloe gel and silver colloid are of exceptional benefit (see pages 437 and 661).

Asparagus root (not the stem) from common asparagus can be substituted for the Chinese asparagus root listed above. Both asparagus root and marshmallow root are especially helpful when deficient kidney *yin* depletes the lung *yin.* Prepared rehmannia root is the main herb in the Chinese "Rehmannia-Six" or "Six Flavor Tea Pills" formula, a six-herb combination found in all Chinese pharmacies as well as many other herb shops. It is perhaps the most widely used kidney *yin* tonic. This combination also contains herbs which strengthen the kidney and spleen *qi* energy. The herbs in this chapter, unless otherwise noted, are used according to the "Standard Herbal Preparation" given in the *Dietary Transition* chapter, page 110.

The animal products—particularly eggs, pork, and cheese—should be eaten in small amounts to avoid stimulating the liver into a *heat* or stagnant condition that drains the *yin* of the kidneys. For similar reasons, indulgence in emotions that provoke the liver should be avoided if possible: impatience, anger, stress, and emotional upset.

Because the kidney *yin* influences all the bodily *yin,* many of the above remedies can be seen to coincide with those given earlier in the *Six Divisions* chapter for "*deficient yin*" in general.

Avoid: Too much warming food such as coffee, alcohol, tobacco, lamb, cinnamon, cloves, ginger, and other hot spices. Also avoid overeating.

Kidney *yang* deficiency indicates that the warming, energizing, and controlling function of the kidneys is inadequate. The kidney *yang* is often compared to a fire that enkindles the spirit and animates all other life processes.

Typical symptoms: cold signs such as an aversion to cold, cold extremities, pale complexion, weak knees and lower back, mental lethargy and poor spirit, lack of sexual desire, irregular menses, clear vaginal discharge, sterility, frequent urination, clear urine, inability to urinate, edema, asthma, lack of will power and direction, and an enlarged, pale tongue. The person has a tendency to be inactive, indecisive, and unproductive.

The spleen-pancreas supplies the kidney *yang:* it makes possible efficient digestion and absorption of *yang* nutrition that enriches the kidney *yang.* Thus, many kidney *yang* deficiencies cannot be cured without an improvement in "digestive fire," as discussed in the *Earth Element* chapter. The kidney-adrenal function, when activated by its *yang* and *qi* attributes, "grasps" and absorbs the *qi* distributed by the lungs. If kidney *yang* or *qi* is lacking, a person may not be able to inhale deeply, or may develop "kidney-induced" asthma and/or shortness of breath.

Foods and spices which warm the kidney yang: cloves, fenugreek seeds, fennel seeds, anise seeds, black peppercorn, ginger (dried preferred), cinnamon bark, walnuts, black beans, onion family (garlic, onions, chives, scallions, leeks), quinoa, chicken, lamb, trout, and salmon.

Notes: Walnuts specifically improve the kidney *yang* and its capacity to "grasp the *qi*" and thus are a suitable remedy for chronic cough, wheezing, and other asthma symptoms caused by *cold* and deficient kidneys. Dosage: $\frac{1}{3}$ to 1 ounce daily. Caution: too many walnuts can cause "canker" mouth sores.

An effective vegetarian kidney *yang* formula: add several of the above warming spices and foods—dried ginger, onions, and fennel seeds, for example—to black bean-seaweed soup. When warming the kidney *yang,* it is a good practice to add a *yin* tonic such as seaweed to protect the *yin.*

Avoid: Cooling foods and fruits, raw foods, excessive salt; use seaweed cautiously.

Deficient kidney *qi* indicates that the kidneys lack sufficient energy to control the urine and semen. This can occur as a result of a congenital defect, sexual overindulgence, sexual activity at too early an age, or loss of control with aging.

Typical symptoms: low back pain, weak knees, pale tongue, weak, thin radial pulse, minor *cold* signs, frequent urination, incontinence, inability to urinate, dribbling urine, involuntary seminal emission, and other problems with urinary/seminal control.

Recommended foods and herbs: parsley, wheat berry, and sweet rice; herbs include rose hips, oyster shell, clam shell, schisandra fruit, raspberry and blackberry leaves, and gravel root.

Notes: Sweet rice is a mild-acting remedy—the major astringent property is in the roots of the sweet rice plant. Wheat berry has a little stronger action than sweet rice, but is not as effective as the other recommendations. It can be eaten as sourdough bread, cooked berries, or other unrefined forms of the grain; it can also be taken as an herbal tea. Crushed or whole oyster shell (*Ostrea gigas*; Mandarin: *mu li*) and clam shell (*Meritricix meritrix*; Mandarin: *hai ge ke*) are available from Chinese herb stores or can be gathered at clean ocean beach areas. In their whole form, these shells need to be crushed before decocting into a tea. Oyster-shell calcium supplements sold at nutritional outlets can also be taken. Rose hips (*Rosa*-related species), schisandra fruit (*Schisandra sinensis*; Mandarin: *wu wei zi*), gravel root (*Eupatorium purpureum*), and raspberry and blackberry leaves (*Rubus ideaus* and *Rubus villosus*) are taken as herbal teas. Parsley can be eaten fresh or infused as a tea.

Deficient kidney *qi* is related to deficient kidney *yang* (*yang* contains *qi*) but is not as deep an imbalance.

Damp-heat in the bladder (Bladder Infection) indicates that a *damp* condition in the bladder has combined with *heat*. This generally is seen in the form of an infection, and appears most frequently in women because of shorter, more easily infected urinary ducts; it also commonly affects those with arthritis, gout, and other overly acid conditions. Sexually transmitted diseases are very often characterized by *damp-heat* symptoms.

Symptoms: Frequent, burning or painful urination; the sensation of urine retention even after urination; possible fever, little appetite, great thirst, and cloudy, even blood-tinged urine.

Recommendations: Infections thrive in a *damp* environment caused by too many acid-forming foods: refined sugar and other concentrated sweeteners, too much meat, greasy, oily foods, and too much starch.

Bitter, cooling, and/or alkalizing foods clean out infections *(damp-heat),* so the majority of the diet should be vegetables and foods that remove *dampness* and *heat*. These would be cooling foods, usually with some bitterness. Overeating also increases *damp-heat,* so light eating on broths and herbal teas is recommended during the painful acute phase. Broth ingredients can be chosen from these foods: aduki beans (especially effective against *damp-heat*), lima beans, celery, carrots, winter squash, potatoes with skins, asparagus, mushrooms, and other vegetables that are not warming. Recommended fruit: lemon (diluted juice), cranberry (juice or tablets), and huckleberries. Beneficial herbal teas: uva ursi (*Arctostaphylos uva urse*), dandelion leaf (*Taraxacum officinalis*), plantain leaf (*Plantago major*), pipsissewa (*Chimaphila umbellata*), flax seed, and watermelon seed.

Notes: The most effective of the herbal remedies are uva ursi and pipsissewa, although prolonged use of uva ursi can be irritating to the urinary tract; pipsissewa is better for chronic bladder and kidney infections and long-term use. The leaves of the manzanita shrub *(Arctostaphylos manzanita)* of the American Pacific coastal region may be substituted for uva ursi, a close relative. Dandelion and plantain leaves also make good additions to broths; often thought of as common lawn weeds, each is nearly as effective as uva ursi for treating urinary infections. Most commercial cranberry juice is prepared with added sweeteners; it is best to find an unsweetened variety, or use tablets.

Chronic bladder and kidney infections suggest a kidney *yin* or *yang* deficiency. In cases of sexually transmitted diseases, the modified herpes program should be followed (see "Herpes," page 439).

Jing: The Source of Kidney Vitality

By improving the *qi*, *yin*, or *yang* of the kidneys, one also improves the *jing*, a deeper essence. The kidneys store *jing*, which determines one's vitality, resistance to disease, and longevity. *Jing* is also concentrated in the brain, ova, semen, and bone marrow. One is born with "congenital" *jing*, which influences individual constitution and development; the amount of congenital *jing* one receives corresponds to the health and constitution of the parents. This *jing* is irreplaceable and meant to serve one throughout life; once it is used up, life ceases. However, "acquired" *jing* can be obtained from food and can greatly magnify the activity of even small amounts of congenital *jing*. *Jing* is a more fundamental quality than *qi*, blood, or other substances in the body. A deficiency of *jing* does not have obvious *heat* or *cold* symptoms.

***Jing* deficiency** impairs growth and development and can cause birth defects in offspring, retarded physical and mental growth, slow or incomplete maturation, inadequate brain function, weak legs and bones, impotence and other reproductive problems, and early senility. One cannot have too much *jing*.

Other symptoms of *jing* deficiency include dizziness, loose teeth, loss of head hair, ringing in the ears, and weak, painful knees and lower back.

More important than adding *jing*-building remedies is preservation of congenital *jing* and the health of the kidneys by avoiding harmful habits:

Factors which Deplete Jing

1. Stress, fear, insecurity, and overwork.
2. a.) Too much semen loss in men greatly reduces *jing*, particularly when it occurs in old age.

    b.) Women bearing "too many" children, especially without rebuilding soon after each birth. "Too many" means more than their particular constitution can healthfully support.
3. Toxins in food and water; intoxicants such as alcohol, marijuana, cocaine, coffee, and tobacco; heavy metals such as mercury and lead; and aluminum (usually from cookware).

4. Excessive sweet-flavored food.

5. Too much dietary protein.

Nourishing the Jing

Everyone needs more vitality—there is no limit—and therefore everyone needs to nourish their *jing*. Without adequate *jing*, the foundation essence, nothing else functions properly in the body. Since all wholesome food contributes to acquired *jing*, the important question is, which foods work best to replenish this *jing* once it is depleted?

Before even the best *jing* tonics can act, they have to be digested, assimilated, and metabolized properly. Thus, one needs to first assess the health of the spleen-pancreas in terms of its digestive strength (*qi* and digestive fire). The liver assists in digestion, and because of its degenerate condition in most people, it usually needs renewal before *jing* can be efficiently bolstered. A basic relationship between the liver and kidneys is elucidated by the Chinese teaching that "the liver and kidneys are from the same source," which is why a number of kidney tonics also tonify the liver.

No one can say that any one food has all nutrients needed for optimum *jing* renewal; certainly a broad range of nutrients is needed from a variety of foods. However, Chinese tradition does specify foods that build *jing* rapidly when one is severely deficient. Other foods have *jing*-enhancing properties, but work more gradually.

Some people, depending on their constitution and condition, need specific foods to build their *jing*, while other foods are inappropriate. In the West, for example, many people in their sixties have considerable vitality. They have symptoms on the *excessive* side of the scale: their voices are strong, pulses forceful, complexions bright and reddish, they have outgoing personalities, and are generally robust. Yet their teeth and much of their hair fell out years earlier; they have little sexual drive, and chronic low backaches—all signs of *jing* deficiency.

Their *excessive* characteristics are usually fueled by a rich diet and hard work. As we shall soon see, certain rich meats, if eaten in small amounts, can strengthen the *jing;* however, large amounts are usually consumed by these people, along with stimulants such as coffee and refined sugar. Even though they realize substantial superficial energy from this lifestyle, stress and stimulants continually tax deep *jing* reserves. In addition, the kidneys barely keep up with such high energy demands, and are unable to store the deeper *jing* essence. Adding more meat, dairy, or other animal products as *jing* nourishment for people whose dietary problem originally resulted from these foods is a mistake. The robust person with signs of *excess* does best with vegetal-quality *jing* tonics and, if desired, small amounts of animal products so that the body does not react violently to a dramatic dietary change.

Finding Personal Jing Nourishment

Building *jing* with diet requires foods that promote the growth and development of the body and mind; such foods should also provide renewal, longevity, reproductive capacity, and protection from premature aging. The following foods have these qualities to varying degrees.

1. Micro-algae (chlorella, spirulina, wild blue-green), fish, liver, kidney, brain, bone and its marrow, human placenta, and cereal grass. These foods are rich in nucleic acids (RNA/DNA), which protect the body from degeneration. Nucleic acids contain the blueprint for cellular renewal and have been shown to initiate aging reversal.[27] The animal products among these foods are also rich in vitamin B_{12}. Western nutrition has shown B_{12} to influence the production of nucleic acids;[28] it is also the vitamin known to initiate growth and development.

Vitamin A, richly supplied in the above animal and vegetable foods, strengthens sexual development and reproduction, as well as protects against congenital birth defects[29]—all these properties are in the domain of *jing* activity. At the same time, most such foods contain ample omega-3 fatty acids, which are found in concentration in the body wherever there is *jing* storage—in the sperm, brain, liver, kidneys, bone marrow, and placenta. Omega-3s develop and maintain the nervous system, clean the arteries, and provide cellular integrity.

Notes: As discussed in the *Protein and Vitamin B_{12}* chapter, micro-algae are the best source of B_{12} of any food, according to certain tests. However, much of this B_{12} may be an ineffective analogue, and so one should take B_{12} supplements if no other sources of B_{12} besides micro-algae are in the diet. This is particularly true for the elderly, who have a greater need for the vitamin.

Cereal grass contains valuable amounts of nucleic acids, but nowhere near those of the micro-algae. It is included here because it contains the "P4D1" fraction discussed in the *Green Food Products* chapter, which is thought to repair damaged nucleic acid in the body. Cereal grass is also a source of omega-3 oils, and a rich source of provitamin A. One of the best nutritional reasons for using barley- or wheat-grass for *jing* stimulation is its "grass juice factor," its growth-promoting, reproduction-enhancing effect measured by researchers but not fully understood.[30–33]

"Chlorella Growth Factor" in chlorella is a similar phenomenon that promotes the vitality described by the concept of *jing*. (See page 233.)

The animal products mentioned above are considered strong tonics for growth and development in both the East and West. In China, human placenta *(Placenta hominis*; Mandarin: *zi he che)* is thought to be one of the best general tonics for wasting and debility. Chinese pharmacies carry it in a dried, powdered form; to use fresh placenta, wash it in water and cook in soups. It can be preserved for periodic use by slicing and freezing. Placenta is also used in such reproductive disorders as recurrent miscarriage, sterility, impotence, and insufficient lactation.[34] Placenta is a universal folk remedy for restoring vitality after childbirth, when *jing* deficiency is commonest in women of childbearing age. Placenta is said to be the only meat that comes from life rather than death.

When using kidney, liver, and other animal parts, it is important that they be from animals raised "organically." This especially applies to bone and marrow (see page 296 for "longevity" [marrow] soup recipe).

Chinese medicine considers the blood and *jing* to be closely related, and some *jing* tonics are also blood tonics, such as the B₁₂, micro-algae, wheat grass, liver, kidney, and placenta remedies given above. In a further blood/*jing* connection, Chinese medicine ascribes the health of the hair to both blood quality and vital, *jing*-rich kidneys.

2. Solomon's seal, almonds, milk, clarified butter *(ghee)*. *Jing* nutrition can include foods which build the bones and act as nutritive tonics. One such Western herbal tonic is Solomon's seal *(Polygonatum officinale;* Mandarin: *yu zhu).* Used extensively in the East, it plays a prominent role in a formula developed by Chinese mountain-dwelling Taoists, who reputedly use it to assist in learning levitation. Any such feat requires extraordinary vitality, which is measured in Chinese terms by *jing* and the degree of its conversion into other substances and energies of the body.

Almonds, milk, and clarified butter support *ojas,* a bodily essence described in Ayurveda which largely parallels the *jing* concept. Milk from any animal represents a close and subtle transformation of its blood. Babies typically get all of their *jing* nourishment from mother's milk during the first few months of life. All dairy, if it is of the highest quality and tolerated by the individual, supplements the *jing.* Clarified butter, when used as a cooking oil, improves the assimilation of nutrients, a most important factor in the formation of *jing.*

3. Nettles. A kidney tonic in the West, nettle leaves also thicken the head hair and enrich the blood, which further indicates their value in supplementing *jing.* Milarepa, an ancient sage of Tibet, fasted on nettles until his skin turned a light green hue. He eventually developed legendary psychic and physical powers. Nettles have been widely used in Europe to improve vitality. They can be eaten as a cooked green (light steaming removes the stinging property) or taken as an herb.

4. Royal jelly and bee pollen. These honey-bee products are thought to contain the most complete range of nutrients of any foods. Royal jelly is more concentrated in nutrients than bee pollen. They are both energy tonics and used in cases of general *deficiency.* Royal jelly promotes phenomenal physical growth, reproductive ability, and longevity in the queen bee. In humans it also strongly stimulates sexuality, and may help extend human life as well.[35] Bee pollen contains many of the same nutritional features as royal jelly, but in much smaller quantities, and is suitable for *jing* maintenance and mild cases of *jing* deficiency.

5. Dodder seeds *(Semen cuscutae;* Mandarin: *tu si zi),* prepared rehmannia root *(Rehmannia glutinosa;* Mandarin: *shu di huang),* deer antler *(Cornu cervi;* Mandarin: *lu rong),* tortoise shell *(Plastrum testudinis;* Mandarin: *gui ban),* chicken, and mussel. Dodder seeds and deer antler are potent Chinese *jing* tonics for those with serious depletion. Prepared rehmannia is a more gradually acting remedy, as are chicken and mussel.

6. As a foundation for the above and other substantial *jing* tonics, one should use foods which tonify and direct energy to the kidneys in general. The Five Element

prescription is beans and especially dark foods with the salty flavor, such as black beans cooked with a little seaweed and a pinch of unrefined sea salt. Among common foods, Chinese herbology recommends the following as generally beneficial for the kidneys: millet, wheat, black sesame seeds, black soybeans, chestnuts, mulberries, raspberries, strawberries, and walnuts.

Black or dark colors in clothing or food nourish the kidneys and conserve *jing*.

7. Ideal *jing* nourishment must also include spiritual practices, which can mobilize *jing,* infuse it with energy and spirit, and transform it into *qi* and *shen*.

As *jing* is spent in sexual activity (particularly in male emissions), the emphasis on celibacy by certain groups of spiritual seekers throughout history has served to preserve *jing* in both male and female participants. Persons with ample *jing,* however, may become agitated with sexual desire unless it is transformed into a spiritual essence. Celibate yogis, monks, nuns, and others accomplish the transformation by various means, including selfless service, devotional practices, and spiritual disciplines.

The most highly evolved spiritual masters of China and India were said to generate *sharira*—crystalline gems in their bodies—which were thought to be condensations of their *jing.* According to one theory, *sharira* indicate the degree of spiritual concentration. *Sharira* may be a highly unified substance that, when integrated into the living body, brings profound clairvoyance and attunement to spiritual guidance. Only the most evolved of modern masters have had one, or at most several, *sharira* appear in their ashes after cremation. (An exception is noted in reference 41 on page 697.) However, some of the most respected teachers in history had an abundance. Buddha, for example, was reportedly found to have 10,000 *sharira.* Because *sharira* seem to have miraculous properties, a certain reverence is customarily paid to them, much the same as the bones of saints in the West are treasured relics. (Bones harbor the marrow and therefore the particular quality of *jing* of the person.)

Choosing the Appropriate Jing Tonic

Those with *heat* signs (aversion to heat, great thirst, red tongue, yellow tongue coating, flushed face, and/or bloodshot eyes) or the minor *heat* signs of *deficient yin* (hot palms and soles, afternoon or tidal fevers, small but frequent thirst, night sweats, and/or fresh-red cheeks and tongue) should avoid or cautiously use warming *jing* remedies such as deer antler, chicken, liver and kidney from beef or lamb, walnuts, mussel, trout, salmon, and other warming fish. The most appropriate *jing* tonics for the person with signs of *deficient yin* are: prepared rehmannia, Solomon's seal, bone-marrow soup, placenta (especially if there are night sweats, debility, and emaciation), chlorella, spirulina, and black beans with seaweeds. These tonics, except for prepared rehmannia, are also beneficial for the person with *heat* signs. Additionally helpful for *heat* signs are wheat grass and wild blue-green micro-algae.

Those with signs of *excess* (robust, reddish complexion, forceful radial pulse, strong voice, and/or thick tongue coating) should choose from the following remedies: wheat- or barley-grass products, micro-algae (spirulina, chlorella, or wild blue-green), nettles, seaweed, pollen, almonds, Solomon's seal, bone-marrow soup, fish, and kidney. Dodder seeds, deer antler, and placenta are too tonifying to be recommended in cases of *excess*.

Those with signs of *deficiency* (frailty, pale or sallow complexion, weak radial pulse, introverted personality, and/or little or no tongue coating) can benefit most from dodder seeds (especially in cases of threatened miscarriage or a tendency to loose stools), prepared rehmannia, royal jelly, bee pollen, milk, clarified butter, placenta (especially if there is wasting and emaciation), and deer antler. However, cereal-grass products and wild blue-green micro-algae are best avoided.

Those with signs of *cold* (frequent feelings of coldness, aversion to the cold, pale complexion, and/or attraction to warm food and drinks) can benefit most from dodder seeds, clarified butter, deer antler, warming seafood (especially mussel; also salmon, anchovy, and trout), placenta, chicken, liver (particularly chicken or lamb), and kidney (especially lamb). Avoid cereal-grass products, wild blue-green, seaweeds, nettles, and Solomon's seal.

In children, severe *jing* deficiency manifests as stunted growth, mental retardation, learning disability, sluggish movement, skeletal weakness and deformities, and failure of the fontanel (skull bones) to close. For these conditions, deer antler is a specific remedy. Tortoise shell is preferred in cases of failure of the fontanel to close; it also treats stunted skeletal development.

Notes: If any type of meat is eaten as a *jing* tonic, one should follow the guidelines for preparation, dosage, quality, and moral awareness given at the end of *Protein and Vitamin B₁₂,* Chapter 9. The recommended herbs are frequently available in formulas which enhance their actions. Prepared rehmannia, for example, is sometimes difficult to digest and is often taken in the "Six Flavor Tea Pills" formula recommended earlier (page 357). These pills contain dioscorea, which strengthens digestion.

The Aging Process

Aging in America is commonly thought to be only a process of degeneration. Although aging usually involves physical decline, there are many people who maintain comparatively full physical and mental health throughout their later years. The main reason may be one's original constitution, yet it seems that certain practices contribute significantly to vitality in old age.

When people age gracefully, physical decline is more than compensated for by the development of wisdom. If we study the aged martial artists who can easily fend off younger, more muscular opponents, we see that their skills are not due to greater strength or speed but to the ability to "see" more clearly; a situation is "known" as or even before it happens.

Perhaps the most important factors for increasing vitality in old age are those practices which deepen spiritual awareness, along with an attitude that applies them consistently in daily life.

Dietary factors are also important for older people, since assimilation of nutrients decreases with age. Good nutrition, at all ages, is needed for building the vital essence *(jing)* of the kidneys. Without this essence, old age occurs rapidly.

Ayurveda describes aging as a process of increased *vata,* i.e., a tendency to become drier, thinner, more nervous and restless, with less appetite, more fear, and lighter sleep. Because of dryness, the likelihood of constipation increases. These symptoms of aging translate to *deficient yin* in Chinese medicine. Though less quickly than *yin, yang* warming, energizing, and controlling qualities also decrease: the older person tends to be more sensitive to the cold, has less physical energy, and sometimes has difficulty with urinary and bowel control.

All these aging processes, as suggested above, differ according to individuals. Ideally a person will experience the signs of aging mildly. The following plan, based on slowing the loss of *jing* and constitutional *yin* and *yang,* can contribute to graceful and dignified aging. As such, it serves to highlight important considerations during one's latter years.

Dietary Suggestions for Vitality in the Elderly

1. Avoid overeating. Overeating is the major cause of aging in wealthy countries (see page 251). Never eat to the point of being full. This recommendation is not only the first but the most important.

2. Do not eat late at night. Eat the last meal of each day as early as possible — it should be small in size and nourishing.

3. Avoid sudden, extreme diet changes. Gradual change is tolerated best.

4. Foods should be easily digestible. Cereal creams and purées may be necessary for those who cannot chew well.

5. Avoid weakening foods and restrict cooling foods. Examples of weakening foods: refined sugar and its products, intoxicants such as coffee and alcohol, too much salt, and highly processed foods. Examples of cooling foods are most raw vegetables, fruits and juices. Raw foods and fruit can be used to a greater extent if there are *heat* and *excess* symptoms.

Older people are often inclined to increase salt and sugar in their diets. One of many explanations is that both of these readily available substances moisten the body. Also, the sense of taste diminishes with age, and adding more salt and sugar makes food taste the way the person remembers it. An excess of salt, however, stimulates aging by increasing blood pressure, reducing mineral uptake from other foods, and depressing the spirit. A little honey or other high-quality sweetener moistens, strengthens, and harmonizes the body and mind, whereas too much sweetener—especially refined sugar—weakens all organ systems (see *Sweeteners* chapter). Instead of emphasizing these strong substances in the diet, the older person is wiser to use other moistening foods suggested below (number 9).

6. A high-protein diet of heavy meats weakens the bones of the older person and severely taxes the organs of digestion, respiration, and circulation. A younger

person digests meat more easily because of greater spleen-pancreas digestive energy. Those who need meat for conditions of weakness and *deficiency* should use it in small amounts; most digestible are the organ meats, fish, and marrow soup (one of the *jing* tonics mentioned above).

7. Organic minerals (organized by plant life) are the most fundamental nutrients. Marine animals whose diets are highest in the broad range of minerals found in seaweeds and other algae do not show obvious signs of cellular aging, and usually die from accidents. The cellular structure of adult whales is virtually identical to that of newborn whales.[36] By comparison, adult humans generally have massive cellular deterioration compared to infants. Some of the richest and most complete sources of organic minerals are seaweeds such as kelp, kombu, and wakame; wild blue-green micro-algae; and barley- or wheat-grass products. (Thin, frail, and *cold* people should avoid wild blue-green micro-algae and use cereal grasses cautiously.) Refined sugar, perhaps more than any other common food, devastates the mineral condition of the body.

8. Following the advice in number 3 above to make gradual changes, the majority of the diet can come from the carbohydrates such as whole grains, vegetables, legumes, nuts, seeds, seaweeds, and regional fruits. A variety of such fiber-rich carbohydrates cleans the heart and arteries and keeps the digestive tract functioning smoothly. If animal products, herbs, or other foods or nutrients are taken, complex carbohydrates make a good nutritional foundation.

Sprouts of grains, legumes, and seeds are an ideal way for older people to take these foods because sprouting breaks down fats, proteins, and starches into easily digestible forms. Nucleic acids (RNA and DNA) can increase tenfold in the sprouting process. Sprouts should be at least lightly cooked except for persons with *heat* or *excess* symptoms. Eating immature foods including sprouts, cereal-grass shoots (all barley- and wheat-grass products are made of young grass shoots), and young vegetables such as baby carrots adheres to the principle practiced in the ancient traditions of the Far East and the health clinics of Europe and America: immature foods keep a person young. Similarly, associating with young people and being physically, mentally, and socially active contribute to vitality throughout life.

9. Those who tend to be dry and thin should eat foods which improve *(yin)* moistening and fluid metabolism—millet, barley (soup), tofu, black soybeans, mung beans, seaweed (very effective), spirulina or chlorella micro-algae, wheat germ, and potatoes; also use seeds of black sesame or flax, especially if there is constipation from dryness. Walnuts also moisten the intestines and are a common remedy for constipation among the elderly in China. Bananas treat dryness-type constipation and, along with almonds, avocados, and coconut, are good for elderly people with a *vata* condition (who tend to be thin, dry, anxious, and nervous). Sardines, eggs, and other *yin*-building animal foods listed earlier may be necessary in extreme cases. Avoid prolonged use of very hot spices.

10. Include *jing*-nurturing foods. For best results, follow the guidelines in the previous section, "Choosing the Appropriate *Jing* Tonic." Some of these tonics are also

yin-building foods. Those who need animal products may choose those that specifically enrich *jing*. Unlike meats, the bee products royal jelly and pollen are especially good choices because they do not contribute harmful mucoid by-products of digestion. Although not a specific *jing* tonic, honey is one of the best sweeteners because it contains traces of the unique nutrients found in pollen and royal jelly, and also lubricates the intestines. Dairy products of high quality are beneficial during old age if they are tolerated (see guidelines in the *Protein* chapter). Because lactose intolerance increases with age, fermented dairy products are usually best: yogurt, buttermilk, soured milk, kefir, cottage cheese, etc. The robust older person and those with high-fat dietary backgrounds should use dairy cautiously.

11. Senility and other difficult aging problems can sometimes be helped by the *jing* tonics such as deer antler, dodder seeds, processed rehmannia, longevity soup, mussel, and chicken. Even when these foods do not effect a cure, they provide a good basis of nutritional enrichment for other remedies. One such remedy is *Ginkgo biloba* tree leaf, which has been shown in clinical studies to increase blood flow and neural transmission in the brain.[37, 38] An extract of the leaf of the ginkgo—the oldest living tree species—has reduced senile symptoms such as memory loss, vertigo, ringing in the ears, depression, and lack of vigilance.[39, 40] The micro-algae wild blue-green and chlorella have also been beneficial in certain cases of senility. Nutritional supplements, which are sometimes helpful—especially when the diet remains poor—are best taken with advice based on expert diagnosis.

12. Some degree of prostate enlargement occurs in 60% of men between the ages of forty to sixty; the percentage increases to nearly 90% by the age of seventy. This condition, known as benign prostatic hypertrophy (BPH) or hyperplasia, may result from imbalanced hormonal levels which create an overproduction of prostate cells. Symptoms include swelling, difficult and frequent urination, and dribbling urine. In Chinese medicine, prostate enlargement is usually seen as "damp heat in the lower burner," and kidney deficiency (see kidney syndromes listed in this chapter [pages 356–363], especially kidney *yang* and *qi* deficiencies).

Alcohol, stress, and elevated cholesterol levels may contribute greatly to BPH. BPH can be controlled by a balanced diet which lowers cholesterol levels (see pages 158–178), contains essential fatty acid rich oils, provides adequate minerals, especially zinc, and includes the above suggestions on aging. Avoid: alcohol, refined salt, excess salt (of any kind), shellfish, fried foods, excess fats, *dampness* promoting foods (see pages 344–345), non-organic foods (pesticides exacerbate BPH).

Studies indicate that an extract of *Pygeum africanum* is effective in treating prostatic hypertrophy.[42] The bark has been used in Europe for decades with no side-effects. Standard dosage of the extract is 100–200 mg. daily for several months. Saw palmetto herb is a rejuvenative tonic used for impotence and infertility. It is sweet, warming and is often combined in formulas with pygeum. Other herbs traditionally used in prostate formulas are chaparral, gravel root and *Hydrangea arborescens*. Lightly roasted pumpkin seeds may be eaten daily for their essential fatty acid and zinc content.

Part IV

Diseases and
Their Dietary Treatment

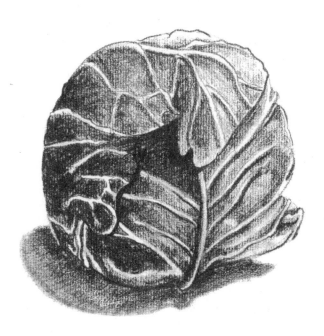

Blood Sugar Imbalances

Diabetes

Diabetes mellitus ("sugar diabetes") is a condition in which the body is unable to properly metabolize sugar. The most prominent symptoms of this imbalance are excessive thirst and frequent urination (other signs are given below); complications of diabetes frequently include blindness, heart disease, kidney failure, and circulation problems in the extremities. In sugar diabetes, the pancreas fails to produce either effective or sufficient insulin, a hormone which controls blood sugar levels. The result is hyperglycemia—excessive sugar in the blood stream.

Diabetes most often develops according to two basic patterns. In the juvenile-onset diabetes, the insulin-producing part of the pancreas is damaged and there is insulin insufficiency. Diabetes of this kind is difficult to cure. Even so, following a good diet with adequate starch and fiber can often make possible a reduction in insulin intake by about one-third, as well as reduce the incidence and severity of diabetic complications.[1-4]

In the more common kind of diabetes—adult-onset, which we will subsequently refer to as "diabetes"—enough insulin is produced, but its utilization in the cells of the body is simply blocked by the effects of a diet rich in fats.[5, 6] (Eating refined white sugar and other simple sugars also contributes to diabetes because in excess, these sugars convert to fat in the body.) When a low-fat diet based on complex carbohydrates such as unrefined grains, vegetables, and legumes is followed for several weeks, approximately 80% of diabetics can stop taking insulin and diabetic pills altogether, and the remaining 20% can reduce their intake.[7-9]

In both juvenile- and adult-onset diabetes, too much sugar enters the blood, the kidneys excrete it along with fluids, and urination becomes frequent and excessive. The drop in body fluids is often accompanied by thirst, inflammations, infections, thinness, red tongue, and similar signs (which match the *deficient yin* fluids syndrome of Chinese medicine).

The high-fat diet that often supports diabetes also causes liver stagnation, a condition of excess which imbalances the spleen-pancreas through the five Element Destruction Cycle, thereby making pancreatic secretions such as insulin less effective.

The obvious remedy is to consume less food, especially foods that stress the liver and weaken the spleen-pancreas. Thus one should limit greasy and fatty foods (meats, eggs, cheese, butter, excess oil, nuts, and seeds) and avoid denatured foods (refined, "white" flour and sugar, hydrogenated, synthetic fats such as margarine and shortening, intoxicants, and chemical ingredients) and very sweet, salty, and spicy foods. One should also avoid late-night eating and complex food combinations. Small, frequent meals (four or five daily) help to stimulate insulin production.

Nutritionists have identified chromium, zinc, and manganese as factors which control blood sugar levels. These minerals are removed in the refining process which produces white sugar, white flour, refined salt, and many other highly processed foods. In whole grains, these minerals reside in the bran. In China, where primarily refined grains are consumed, an innovative treatment for diabetes has arisen that is also a little-known American folk remedy[10]—adding wheat bran to the diet, which has been shown to lower blood sugar levels, quite possibly because of its concentration of the blood-sugar-controlling minerals.[11] Bran is also a rich source of silicon, a mineral thought by some nutritionists to improve pancreatic function.[12] (See *Calcium,* Chapter 15, for other silicon foods.)

In order to maximize mineral absorption, one can employ chlorophyll, a major catalyst of the vegetable kingdom which increases the utilization of all nutrients in humans,[13] therefore greatly enhancing the treatment of diabetes.[14, 15] Because chlorophyll catalyzes cell renewal,[13] it also makes the long-term outlook for diabetes brighter, as it can assist in rebuilding a damaged pancreas. Since diabetes often involves acidic blood,[16] general toxicity, and various inflammations, the alkalizing, detoxifying, and anti-inflammatory effect of chlorophyll is likewise useful. Even pure extracted liquid chlorophyll has been effective in treating diabetes,[17] although the high-chlorophyll foods—especially wheat or barley grass, spirulina, and chlorella—contain important additional minerals, enzymes, and other nutrients. To use chlorophyll products for diabetes, take the upper dosage range on a daily basis as described in *Green Foods Products,* Chapter 16.

The most basic practice for improving nutrient assimilation is proper chewing. Particularly with complex carbohydrates, whose digestion begins with saliva, thorough chewing is essential for their complete breakdown so that adequate minerals and other nutrients are absorbed. Feeling satisfied, the diabetic is less likely to overeat and more easily avoids the large meals which aggravate diabetes.

Deficiency Diabetes: Nearly all cases of diabetes are marked by one or more signs of *yin* deficiency. In this text, "deficiency diabetes" is further defined by signs of spleen-pancreas deficiency: poor appetite, fatigue, loose or watery stools, weak pulses, pallor, and introversion. These are not the typical diabetic symptoms observed in the wealthy countries, but they do occur. Individual differences in diabetic symptoms come about from the unique constitution and eating patterns of each diabetic person. In Third World countries, diabetes is not common, yet in the frail individual deficiency diabetes may arise from a denatured diet consisting mainly of white rice, refined sugar products, and a few fruits and vegetables. Mothers with diabetes occasionally have "deficiency diabetes" symptoms, because childbearing taxes the generative power of the spleen-pancreas. In fact, diabetes is much more common among mothers than other women. Women with three children, for example, are twice as likely to develop diabetes as women with no children; women with six children are at six times the risk.[18] Because of this factor, two out of three diabetics are women.

To overcome deficiency diabetes, all vegetables and fruits are cooked, and the spleen-pancreas-tonifying diet for overcoming weak *qi* is followed (page 342). The remaining dietary recommendations in this section, beginning with "Beneficial Oils," are also appropriate, and regular, small amounts of any of the animal products listed may be helpful during the initial phases of recovery. Quality cow dairy is particularly useful when general *deficiency* signs are present (frailty, thinness, weakness, and wasting). However, if there are loose stools or excess mucus, avoid cow dairy and, if available and tolerated, use raw goat dairy products instead. Of the recommended herbs, all are beneficial except dandelion root and leaf, which are too bitter and cleansing for deficiency diabetes.

Excess-Type Diabetes: A very different picture of diabetes often emerges in the robust person who has overindulged in a heavy meat-and-fat diet full of refined foods. This person may also have one or more symptoms of insufficient *yin*, but in addition is typically overweight and constipated, and shows general signs of *excess* such as a ruddy complexion, thick (possibly yellow) tongue coating, strong pulses, and an outward-oriented personality.

A diet abundant in cleansing foods such as raw vegetables and fruits should be followed for excess-type diabetes. Except for the banana, which has excellent detoxification properties, the fruits should be either acid or subacid, because the acidic, sour flavor lowers the blood sugar (examples are listed below). Lemons and grapefruit, in fact, reduce blood sugar levels so rapidly that one should be careful not to overuse insulin simultaneously. Appropriate animal products include moderate amounts of goat milk and/or goat yogurt; also useful in severe cases are broths or congees of clams, or of animal pancreas from beef, pork, lamb, or chicken. The other animal products listed in the chart below should be avoided in excess-type diabetes, except possibly in soups during the phase of transition from a very rich diet. Likewise, avoid all sweeteners in this kind of diabetes; the exceptions are stevia-leaf products and licorice-root powder or tea. Over time, synthetic sweeteners commonly used by diabetics lead to liver stagnancy.

Beneficial Oils

Because excessive and poor quality fats play such a prominent role in the typical diabetic etiology, small amounts of certain high-quality oils can hasten recovery. Cautious use of oil is urged in the early phases of the healing process because any excess taxes a liver in need of rejuvenation. We know from the *Oils and Fats* chapter that GLA oils regulate insulin and seem to protect against diabetic heart, eye, and kidney damage, and that these and the omega-3 oils help cleanse the heart and arteries. Another oil, the common linoleic fatty acid, has an insulin-sparing activity which enables insulin to be more effective.[19]

Fresh flax oil is one of the best sources of high-quality linoleic and omega-3 fatty acids. GLA fatty acids are available in evening primrose, borage, or black currant seed oils, and also in spirulina. (See *Oils and Fats* chapter, page 173 for GLA dosage, and page 165 for flax-oil dosage.) Note: Extracted omega-3-rich fish oils, concentrated in preformed EPA and DHA omega-3s, must be used sparingly by diabetics to avoid healing reactions; usually 1 gram/day is a safe dosage for the first month or so. Eating "omega-3 fish" does not generally cause reactions because their oils are eaten with minerals, amino acids, and various other nutrients in the fish which temper reactions and aid fatty-acid digestion.

Healing Considerations

Depending on the depth of the symptoms, most diabetics who decide to eat and live in harmony show significant improvement within at most a few months. Those on insulin can usually reduce their dosage *gradually* (under a doctor's supervision). As mentioned earlier, it is not uncommon for insulin to eventually become unnecessary.

Deficiency and excess-type diabetes are only two possibilities; very often there is a combination of these, with one type predominating. In addition, excess-type diabetes may change into the deficiency type. Other signs also need to be taken into account, especially if there is an extreme imbalance in the heart or other organ system(s). When a *deficient yin* or deficient kidney *yin* syndrome exists, add *yin*-nurturing food and herbal remedies (pages 65 and 357).

Eating a wide sampling of foods from the following list strengthens the pancreas, regulates blood sugar, and at the same time improves the fluid metabolism. (The individual properties of many of these foods are given in the recipe section and elsewhere in this book.) Diabetics should choose one or more of these foods daily as part of a primarily vegetarian diet of unrefined grains, vegetables, legumes, fruits,

---

Foods Commonly Used in the Treatment of Diabetes

Grains and Legumes
millet
rice
sweet rice
oats
fresh corn
whole wheat and its bran
tofu and soy products
mung bean
garbanzo bean

Chlorophyll Foods
wheat- or barley-grass
spirulina
chlorella
liquid chlorophyll

Vegetables and Fruits
string bean
carrot
radish
Jerusalem artichoke
turnip
asparagus
yam
spinach
avocado
pear
plum
lemon
grapefruit
lime
blueberry
huckleberry

Herbs
dandelion root and leaf
cedar berries
yarrow flowers
blueberry/huckleberry
  leaf

Sweeteners
licorice tea or powder
stevia powder or extract

Animal Products
clam, abalone
cow's milk, yogurt
pancreas of lamb, pork
  beef, or fowl
lamb kidney
chicken or goose
beef

herbs, and a limited amount of nuts and seeds.

Activity: Of equal importance to diet is vigorous exercise, which lowers blood sugar levels and thereby reduces the need for insulin. Exercise also improves the circulation, which tends to be poor in diabetics.

Hypoglycemia

Hypoglycemia, or low blood sugar, often develops from the same kind of dietary extremes that cause diabetes, but instead of a diabetic shortage of insulin, an excess is produced. In time, if insulin overproduction continues, the pancreas becomes overworked, and loses its ability to produce sufficient and/or effective insulin, the result being diabetes. This is why hypoglycemia often precedes the onset of diabetes.

To resolve a hypoglycemic condition, one must control insulin production. Avoiding denatured and refined foods is one answer, because these foods lack the minerals and other nutrients which control all metabolic activities, including insulin production. Refined flour or sugar, for example, is composed primarily of carbohydrates that deliver energy and warmth *(yang)*. The minerals that are refined away would have been incorporated into the blood, hormones, and various body fluids *(yin)* to cool, moisten, and subdue the burning of sugars into energy. The hypoglycemic body robs its own tissues of these needed minerals, thereby losing the deep controlling reserves that stabilize it during dietary extremes and stress in general. Thus, those with low blood sugar may notice major fluctuations in blood sugar levels according to what was eaten at the last meal.

The symptoms of hypoglycemia are many; the following is an incomplete but representative listing commonly found in medical texts dealing with blood sugar disorders. In the left column we have placed those disorders that are sometimes associated with a deficiency of *yin* in the body.

Symptoms of Hypoglycemia

insomnia	pale skin
sweating	headache
fast pulse	low blood pressure
hot flashes	craving for sweets
noise or light sensitivity	cool wet skin
ringing in ears	mental disturbances
temper tantrums	shortness of breath
dry or burning mouth	loss of appetite or constant hunger
worry, anxiety	blurred vision
dizziness	depression
restlessness	crying spells
lack of concentration	numbness, especially in mouth
hyperactivity	cold hands and feet

irritability	drowsiness
loss of sex drive	swollen feet
impotence	eye-ache
weakness in legs	distorted judgment
muscle pain or cramps	tightness in chest
fluttering feeling in chest	fatigue

High-protein diets have been (and sometimes still are) considered a cure for hypoglycemia, because protein digests slowly, supplies energy gradually, and does not trigger excess insulin production. But a high-protein diet causes other serious problems, as we have seen earlier in the *Protein and Vitamin B₁₂* and *Calcium* chapters. The high-protein foods that seem to work best over time are the chlorophyll-rich types recommended in diabetes—spirulina, chlorella, wild blue-green, and cereal-grass products. (See *Green Food Products,* Chapter 16, for guidelines.)

The principal dietary remedy for hypoglycemia is the complex carbohydrates in their whole forms. Grains, vegetables, and legumes, like animal proteins, take time to break down and metabolize, and also contain nutrients that regulate insulin production. The same dietary practices which successfully treat diabetes can be applied to hypoglycemia: thorough chewing, small frequent meals (six or seven a day), and simple food combining. A major difference in the diet itself can be the addition of a *little* more fatty food for hypoglycemics who are not overweight. Cheese, nuts, and seeds, in small quantities, make good snack foods; other fats such as butter and avocado can be used regularly. Small amounts of these kinds of foods offer a gradually acting, long-lasting energy and also have a generally retarding effect on hyperactivity.

Salt consumption must be curtailed because it reduces blood sugar. Seaweeds, however, which have a salty flavor, are useful because of their rich protein and mineral content.

Eat only whole fruits, not juices, which are too concentrated in simple sugars and lack the fiber and certain minerals of unpressed fruit. Overuse of even whole fruit, however, can precipitate extreme fluctuations in blood sugar, so their use should be limited. Citrus fruits tend to lower blood sugar quickly and should be avoided.

Wholesome concentrated sweeteners can be tolerated by most hypoglycemics if eaten occasionally and moderately. The best metabolize most slowly, are processed least, and thus contain the most complete nutrition. They include molasses, rice syrup, barley malt, and honey.

Of the foods listed earlier which are commonly used in the treatment of diabetes, all are useful for hypoglycemia with the exception of citrus fruits, plum, radish, turnip, spinach, sweet rice, yarrow flowers, and dandelion leaf (dandelion *root* is beneficial).

Hypoglycemic persons are not only mineral-deficient but also usually lack adequate essential fatty acids (EFAs); this often manifests in one or more of these signs: dry hair and skin, low body weight, poor glandular function (especially of the pancreas and adrenals), and liver/gall bladder-related imbalances (according to the liver function of Chinese medicine) such as irritability, depression, nervousness, pains and cramps. Adequate essential fatty acids are usually available in a diet based on unrefined vegetables, grains, legumes, and nuts and seeds. In the initial stages of healing hypoglycemia, however, it is helpful to add extra EFAs of exceptional quality such as those found in fresh, cold-pressed flax oil.

Deficient yin symptoms are as prevalent in hypoglycemia as they are in diabetes; similarly, add *yin*-nurturing foods and herbs when indicated.

The Hypoglycemic Personality

The hypoglycemic person usually has a long history of sugar abuse and is often drawn to sugar in an attempt to placate some deep, underlying emotional disharmony. Hypoglycemia, in turn, eventually causes its own set of problems. The brain needs adequate blood sugar at all times to function properly, so low blood sugar affects the mental processes. With insufficient sugar for the brain cells, the hypoglycemic person can develop foggy concepts or distorted moral senses;[20] in children, lack of blood sugar can lead to retardation and is often related to juvenile delinquency.[21] Alcoholism, based on overconsumption of sugar in the form of alcohol, nearly always has hypoglycemic symptoms.[22]

Low blood sugar is also prevalent in persons with disorders such as schizophrenia,* drug addiction, and obesity.[22] According to health educator Bernard Jensen, hypoglycemia symptoms occur in at least half the population of America.[23] Those smaller segments of the population most severely affected—some alcoholics and psychotics, for instance—have difficulty initiating change. Their successful recovery at first depends on the wisdom of those who treat them. Fortunately, there is an increasing realization by therapists that many addictions and mental disorders are linked to long-term faulty nutrition.

Clearly, one of the major factors in excessive sugar consumption is the level of meat consumption. We have discussed in previous chapters how too much meat in the diet causes sugar cravings as an attempt at establishing a protein/carbohydrate balance. We also know that excessive meat-eating generates prostaglandins that cause pain, inflammation, and depression, and that sugar and alcohol can temporarily reduce these burdens.

Overcoming such a hypoglycemic cycle often requires fresh insight and inspiration to change. Perhaps the most important issue in healing hypoglycemia and its dietary roots involves a moral awareness of how one lives on the Earth (refer to the earlier discussion: "Waste and the Earth Element," page 345).

---

*Schizophrenics are also frequently afflicted with celiac disease (gluten intolerance), to be discussed later.

The Stomach and Intestines

According to Chinese medical tradition, the stomach and spleen-pancreas work together as an organ pair. The stomach receives the food and continues the process of breaking it down that began in the mouth. The ancient Chinese described the stomach as extracting a "pure essence"* which is then sent to the spleen-pancreas to be manufactured into blood and *qi* energy.

The stomach conducts the semi-transformed food into the intestines for further assimilation, which is influenced by the strength of the spleen-pancreas. In contemporary terms, "spleen-pancreas strength" quite possibly translates as the quality and quantity of the pancreatic enzymes, which are secreted into the small intestine. Thus, for most problems of the small intestine, one can work with dietary principles that improve the spleen-pancreas.

When the stomach is unbalanced, it tends to become "overheated," in Chinese terminology, and is soothed by cooling drinks and moist foods. However, such foods can easily weaken the spleen-pancreas, a *yin* organ particularly sensitive to *dampness*, which generally benefits from warming, dry foods. To find a balance, the wisest dietary choices avoid overheating the stomach and thereby avoid the need for large quantities of water and cold drinks.

"Stomach Fire" and Heat-Induced Ulcers

Symptoms: "Stomach fire"† is a painful condition involving a burning sensation in the stomach, bleeding gums, excessive appetite, bad breath, and constipation. The tongue is unusually red and its coating thick and yellow. Stomach fire often causes inflammations such as ulcers of the stomach, duodenum, and mouth (canker sores), although inflammations also can occur from a *cold* stomach and other causes.

Dietary Suggestions for Stomach fire and Ulcers: Avoid fried foods, heated or poor-quality vegetable oils, red meats, coffee, hot spices (such as cinnamon, chili peppers, black pepper, and mustard), alcohol, excessive salt, vinegar, citrus fruit, plums, and chewing tobacco. To heal the inflamed lining of the stomach, use soothing, mucilaginous foods and preparations: waters, soups, or congees of oats, barley, or rice; honey-water, banana, avocado, tofu, and soy milk; milk, soured milk, or yogurt, all of goat origin; spinach, cucumber, cabbage, potato, and lettuce; chlorophyll-rich products such as cereal grass, micro-algae, and liquid chlorophyll;

---

*This essence may correspond in comparatively recent physiological knowledge to the small amounts of water, salts, sugars, and other nutrients which are absorbed through the gastric mucosa.[24]

†"Fire" in this context means excessive *heat* in the stomach. The term "digestive fire" is used elsewhere as a measure of *yang* energy available to support digestion.

378

and herbal teas of licorice root *(Glycyrrhiza glabra),* slippery elm *(Ulmus fulva),* marshmallow root *(Althea officinalis),* red raspberry leaf *(Rubus ideaus),* flax seed *(Linum usitatissimum),* or chamomile *(Anthemis nobilis).*

Raw cabbage juice, if taken on an empty stomach immediately after juicing, is more effective for healing ulcers than cooked cabbage. However, whole raw foods may cause irritations, so the remaining foods in the supporting diet—grains, vegetables, and sweet fruits—should be well-cooked, soft (even puréed when necessary), and easy to digest. The above remedies can be relied on exclusively during periods of severe inflammation; a typical selection might include rice-cabbage congee, goat milk, licorice-marshmallow-flax tea, and spirulina. After recovery from the acute phase has begun, one or more of the remedies can continue to be emphasized as part of the supporting diet.

Tongue Coating and Digestion

The coating on the tongue is an accurate reflection of the condition of the spleen-pancreas and digestive tract in general. By studying the tongue coating, the ancient Chinese arrived at the following guidelines, which are still widely used:

- A white coating, if thin, slightly moist, and evenly distributed, is normal; however, in disease this kind of coating may indicate *deficiency.* If a white coating appears very wet, it indicates *coldness, dampness,* deficient digestive fire, or other *yang* deficiency in the body; if dry, it signifies *heat* or lack of body fluid.
- A thick coating suggests a condition of *excess.*
- A yellow coating is a sign of *heat.*
- A black or gray coating is a sign of either extreme *heat* (coating is dry and tongue is red) or extreme *cold* (coating is wet and tongue is pale).
- A thick greasy-looking coating signifies an accumulation of mucus or other *damp* condition in the body.
- A "stripped" tongue—no coating and tongue looks shiny—indicates the *deficient yin* syndrome or weak digestion (deficient spleen-pancreas *qi*).
- A coating that appears to lie floating on the tongue surface denotes weak digestion (deficient spleen-pancreas *qi*). A normal coating appears rooted.

Colitis and Enteritis

These inflammations of the colon and small intestine can be generated by emotional repression and the related energy stagnation of the liver. Such inflammations are often tied to a dietary history of too much meat and a consequent excess of arachidonic acid in the body (see *Oils and Fats* chapter and "Liver Stagnation" in the *Wood Element* chapter). Typical symptoms of intestinal inflammation include abdominal pain and cramping, diarrhea, and rectal bleeding in severe cases. Because food is not being properly absorbed, there is often weight loss and weakness.

If *heat* signs exist such as a yellow tongue coating, the remedies for intestinal inflammation are the same as those for stomach fire, above. Of special usefulness are the chlorophyll products, including cereal grass, micro-algae, and liquid chlorophyll. However, other imbalances without *heat* signs may cause enterocolitis (inflammation of the small and large intestine), most often a lack of spleen-pancreas digestive fire or *qi* energy, or an excess of *dampness*. In these situations, one follows the recommendations given earlier for these imbalances (pages 342–344), and at the same time adheres to the stomach-fire diet. Although in this case exclude from that diet the most cooling remedies—lettuce, banana, soy products, spinach, cucumber, cereal grasses, micro-algae, marshmallow, and yogurt.

In intestinal inflammations of all types, chewing food well breaks it down better so that it is less irritating, stimulates proper pancreatic secretion, and provides well-insalivated complex carbohydrates which act like a healing salve on the intestinal coating. Raw food is not tolerated because it easily irritates delicate surfaces of inflamed intestines. Many of the symptoms of enteritis and colitis can be caused by dairy intolerances, which are sometimes merely intolerances to the poor quality of the dairy products used. (See "Dairy Recommendations," page 150.)

Of the herbal remedies applicable to stomach fire, flax seed requires special preparation in order to preserve its rich stores of linolenic acid, which counteracts the inflammatory influence of excessive arachidonic acid discussed earlier.

Warm-water flax seed extraction: Place one-quarter cup of flax seeds in one quart of warm, purified water for eight hours, then strain.

Flax seed tea is a highly effective European folk remedy for general gastrointestinal ulceration, inflammation, and bleeding (consult a physician in case of hemorrhage). It also makes a soothing enema for these conditions. Flax seed tea is still helpful when decocted by simmering in the usual manner, but less effective than the warm-water extract.

Two other useful remedies for all types of intestinal inflammation deserve mention: 1) several fresh figs daily (dried figs soaked in water may be substituted); and 2) one teaspoon of a strong decoction of black or green tea, taken four times daily (see "Tea" section, page 209).

Diverticulosis (herniation of the muscular coating of the colon) and Irritable Bowel Syndrome (spastic colon)

These common bowel syndromes each manifest symptoms of bloating, cramping, pain, and constipation followed by diarrhea. In disorders with muscular problems such as hernias and spasms, the liver is generally implicated.

Some medical advisers still prescribe a bland, low-residue (low fiber), refined-food diet of dairy, meat, white-flour products, and soft vegetables for these conditions. But anthropological investigations reveal that cultures with high-residue diets rarely have such gastrointestinal disorders,[25] supporting the theory that the soft, fiber-poor diet is the cause, and not the cure, for these ailments.

Studies in the last few decades show that unrefined, high-residue diets are helpful in these types of disorders.[26–28] From a mechanical standpoint alone, high-residue foods such as whole grains, vegetables, legumes, and sprouts pass much more smoothly through the intestines, making the possibility of spasms and hernias less likely. Also, these foods move other food residues along and keep the area around the site of hernias cleaner so that there is less likelihood of infection and inflammation. In addition to maintaining a high-residue diet, one must be cautious not to provoke the liver with intoxicants and foods containing excessive or poor-quality fats and oils. (See "Syndromes of the Liver" on pages 319–329 for further information on diagnosing and renewing the liver.)

Celiac Disease

This condition involves an inability to digest gluten, a protein found in the glutinous grains. Although not a commonly diagnosed condition, celiac disease may be more widespread than records indicate. The symptoms—diarrhea, abdominal pain, flatulence, weight loss, anemia, muscle cramps and spasms—are similar to other chronic intestinal disorders, and so may easily be misdiagnosed.

Gluten is the tough elastic protein in wheat, rye, and barley. Oats also contain substantial gluten, but for an unknown reason, do not cause problems in those with gluten intolerance.[29] In celiac disease, the gluten of the above cereals (except oats) is not digested, perhaps because of a lack of pancreatic enzymes. However, simple indigestion is not the only problem: during the disease process, the villi of the small intestine are destroyed, impairing the assimilation of nutrients from all foods. There are also many cases in which prior intestinal damage brings on celiac disease—this damage may be caused by mental stress, long-term use of laxatives, intestinal infections and/or parasites, excessive coffee-drinking, and protein deficiencies caused by anorexia or certain weight-loss regimes.

From the standpoint of Chinese medicine, the inability to digest any healthful food suggests a weakened spleen-pancreas severely lacking in energy and/or digestive fire. Certain of the aforementioned signs of celiac disease, namely diarrhea, abdominal pain, flatulence, weight loss, and anemia, are also signs of weak spleen-pancreas *qi* energy. Celiac patients with these symptoms need to follow the remedies for tonifying the spleen-pancreas: restrict cooling and highly mucus-forming foods (some celiacs do not improve unless both gluten and milk are withdrawn) and add more warming foods. (See "Deficient *Qi* Energy of the Spleen-Pancreas," page 342, for specific dietary suggestions.)

Often, persons with celiac disease are deficient in B vitamins and other nutrients supplied by whole grains. This need not be a problem—one can always choose from the non-glutinous varieties of grains such as rice, corn, millet, buckwheat, quinoa, and amaranth as well as oats. Sweet rice, a sticky grain not always tolerated by celiacs, is among the remedies for deficient spleen-pancreas qi (above) and deficient blood (below). Clearly, sweet rice-intolerant celiacs with these deficiencies should avoid sweet rice and use the other recommended remedies.

Because of nutrient malabsorption, the treatment of celiac disease must also address the likelihood of anemia and malnutrition, and can therefore include the blood-building remedies (see "Blood Deficiency," page 387). In order to restore the small intestines and the digestive system in general, the dietary approach should include recognition of possible liver stagnation (page 319) and the use of flax seed tea. Nettle leaf *(Urtica urens)* tea specifically encourages the renewal of intestinal villi, but it should not be taken while signs of *coldness* exist.

It appears that many schizophrenics have celiac disease.[30] They frequently manifest similar digestive symptoms, and carefully controlled studies show that schizophrenics generally improve faster on a gluten-free diet.[31, 32]

It is quite possible that among millions of people with sensitivities to wheat, a large number suffer from an inability to digest the gluten. Since celiac symptoms come and go, the condition may be prevalent in the general population, but to a minor and varying degree that depends on individuals' fluctuating eating patterns and emotional health. Those who suspect a gluten intolerance can try avoiding the glutinous grains and all their products for at least two months to see if symptoms are relieved. Celiacs who are severely afflicted can expect significant renewal to require one or more years of consistent effort.

Dysentery

This acute condition is marked by bacterial or amoebic contamination of the digestive tract. *Dampness* combines with *heat* in dysentery and there is burning liquid diarrhea, usually containing blood. The tongue is red with a yellow coating. For prevention, eat small meals when traveling—overeating makes the digestive system ripe for dysentery. Too much raw food in particular dampens the digestive fire and puts one at risk of picking up and becoming a breeding ground for the microorganisms that cause dysentery. If dysentery contamination is suspected in food, eating a clove of garlic before every meal provides excellent protection. Fresh lemon or lime juice taken on an empty stomach is also preventative.

The following remedies are taken three to five times daily.

- Remedies for dysentery: a) The beginning stages of bacterial dysentery and all stages of amoebic dysentery can usually be cured with raw garlic. b) Foods and herbs which treat acute symptoms of dysentery in general are: figs, soups of swiss chard, radish, eggplant, or yam; capsules or teas of golden seal *(Hydrastis canadensis),* nettle leaf *(Urtica urens),* or peppermint *(Mentha piperita).* A strong decoction of black or green tea is very useful (see "Tea," page 209). For treating chronic dysentery, either boiled tofu or a decoction of pomegranate rind is helpful. If *deficiency* signs, chills, undigested food in the stools, and a stripped tongue coating are present, add dried ginger-root tea. To maintain strength during dysentery, oat water can be taken, and a thin porridge of oats and tofu may be tolerated.

Diarrhea

This imbalance is a normal reaction by which the body clears out excessive or unwholesome food. Rancid, poisonous, or bacteria-contaminated foods are frequent causes of acute diarrhea. Chronic diarrhea, in most cases, is due to weakness in the digestive system, discussed earlier in the *Earth Element* chapter as deficient spleen-pancreas *qi* or fire, and as excessive *dampness.*

- General remedies for all types of diarrhea: rice or barley broth, blackberry juice, garlic (especially good for diarrhea from bacterial contamination), leek,* string bean, eggplant,* sunflower seed, umeboshi plum, crab apple,* olive,* aduki bean, sweet rice, button mushroom, and yam; carrot and buckwheat are beneficial in the treatment of chronic diarrhea.

    Diarrhea will often manifest with *heat* or *cold* signs, and different remedies may be called for accordingly.

- Specific remedies for "cold" diarrhea (watery stools, copious clear urine, chills, white, wet tongue coating): red, black, or cayenne pepper, cinnamon bark, Chinese or Korean ginseng, dried ginger, nutmeg, chestnut, chicken egg.

- Specific remedies for "hot" diarrhea (stools cause burning sensation in anus; yellow tongue coating, yellow urine, aversion to heat, desire for cold drinks): millet congee, tofu, mung bean, persimmon,* pineapple, and herb teas or capsules of raspberry leaves *(Rubus ideaus),* marjoram *(Origanum marjorana),* peppermint *(Mentha piperita),* or nettle leaf *(Urtica urens).*

The basic diet during diarrhea should be small meals that are well-chewed; especially helpful are gruels or congees of rice, barley, or oats, which can include other appropriate foods listed above. Take in ample fluids to counteract possible dehydration. Foods to avoid: honey, spinach, cow's milk, apricot, plum (umeboshi plum is beneficial), sesame seeds, oils, and any foods that are difficult to digest.

Constipation

Infrequent and/or difficult bowel movements are most often caused by one of two imbalances in the body:

1) Excess-type Constipation. This most common type of constipation results from an excessive liver with conditions of either *heat* or stagnancy. Liver *heat* dries up body fluids in general, and the stools become dry, hard, and difficult for the body to pass. Signs of *heat* affecting the intestines include a red dry tongue with a yellow coating.

Liver stagnancy inhibits correct *qi* energy flow, which in turn reduces peristalsis, the wavelike muscular contraction of the intestines. In stagnancy, the tongue

---

*These foods are considered "obstructive" and tend to retard the flows and movements in the body.

coating is thick while the tongue itself may vary from normal (light red) to dark red with a purple or blue-green hue.

The dietary guidelines for reducing liver excesses involve restriction of meats, fats, and other rich foods, and the addition of various cleansing, stimulating remedies (page 326). The herbal laxatives for cooling *heat* and increasing peristalsis include the bitter purgatives such as teas of barberry root *(Berberis vulgaris)*, rhubarb root *(Rheum palmatum)*, cascara sagrada bark *(Cascara sagrada),* and dandelion root *(Taraxacum officinalis)*—a very mild laxative. (Please refer to the chart at the end of this section for a summary of herbs and other suggested remedies for constipation.) These kinds of herbs are best combined with demulcent herbs, which protect the intestinal lining and replace its heavy mucous coating in cases of constipation with a lighter, cleaner mucilaginous coating. The demulcent herb licorice root has additional properties: it harmonizes any harsh aspect of bitter herbs and is itself mildly laxative as well. A typical herbal formula is a decoction of equal parts of a laxative herb such as cascara sagrada, a demulcent seed such as flax, and licorice root, taken in one-cup doses two to three times per day. Each of the four laxative herbs above is cooling, but rhubarb root is the best choice when strong *heat* signs are present. (Rhubarb is also a common Chinese remedy for appendicitis.) All of the recommended laxative herbs are generally considered safe, even for children, when the dosage is reduced.

Other important food categories for overcoming excess-type constipation are: a) foods that lubricate the intestines; b) foods that help replenish and revitalize the intestinal flora; and c) foods that encourage bowel movement in general. For severe constipation, several of these foods can be emphasized until the crisis is past; in chronic constipation, one or more can be eaten every day along with a diet based on whole grains, vegetables, and those foods that clear liver excess. In either case, the laxative herbs will help speed recovery, although they should not be relied on indefinitely; for real digestive health, one must stop feeding liver excess.

2) Deficiency Constipation is caused by the lack of adequate *yin* fluids and/or blood in the body. When the body is low in either of these liquids, too much fluid is drawn out of the food in the intestines, creating dryness and hence constipation. Taking in more water is sometimes helpful but does not solve the underlying problem. More than half a century ago Jethro Kloss, in his classic healing guide, *Back To Eden*, recommended lubricating the intestines in cases of constipation by thoroughly chewing dry grains (cooked with a minimum of water), and taking no liquids with meals.

If food is chewed thoroughly and not diluted, this not only lubricates the intestines with well-insalivated food but strengthens the spleen-pancreas, which in turn releases more pancreatic enzymes into the intestines. These add further lubrication and improve digestion, increasing the available nutrients for building more and richer blood. Another result is greater *qi* energy for distributing fluids in the body. Eating this way teaches one to chew well because dry food is otherwise difficult to eat. Including some exceptionally dry foods in the diet such as whole-grain crackers or rice cakes is helpful.

Deficiency constipation is more difficult to treat than the liver-excess type, because rather than simply purging excess, it requires the more lengthy process of building up the *yin* fluids and/or blood. Deficiency constipation may exhibit a mixture of blood and *yin* deficiency signs: fresh red or pale tongue, pale face and lips with possible red cheeks, little or no tongue coating, thin body type. It is most frequently seen in women. Recommendations for increasing the *yin* fluids include foods such as millet, rice, seaweed, black beans, beets, potatoes, cheese, and pork (see "Deficient Yin," page 65). Treatment methods for deficient blood are given later (page 387).

The laxative herbs listed in the following chart are bitter and therefore should be used carefully, since they can further weaken those with *deficiencies*. Of the other food categories, the most important for deficiency constipation are those that moisten and lubricate the intestines. Similar to these foods in function are the demulcent herbs, which lay down the mucilaginous intestinal coating discussed earlier. Flax, fenugreek, and psyllium are highly nourishing demulcent seeds that swell when taken, providing bulk while cleaning and moving the bowels. These seeds are soaked and then eaten, or consumed after using them in a tea. Taking equal parts of all three seeds is the most effective method, and the dosage is three tablespoons of the combination once or twice a day. Any one seed can be helpful by itself, especially flax seed; the single-seed dosage is also three tablespoons once or twice daily.

In stubborn cases, black sesame seed excels; up to one tablespoonful can be cooked into or sprinkled on food twice daily. It is commonly available through East Asian food and herb suppliers. During a crisis, a tablespoon of castor oil taken at bedtime is effective, but unlike the seed remedies, this does little to address the cause of deficiency constipation. Castor oil should be avoided during pregnancy as it can induce miscarriage.

Bran and Enemas: The bran from various grains is often used to treat constipation, and while it is helpful for overcoming the symptoms, the consumption of whole grains is superior for long-term preventive use. The phytic acid of grains is located in the bran; therefore, even moderate amounts of bran will cause a sizeable concentration of phytic acid in the body, which depletes zinc and other minerals. Phytic acid is neutralized in the sourdough bread-making process and in soaking whole grains before cooking. (Both processes are described in the recipe section.)

Enemas and colonics are valuable during constipation resulting from excess *heat* of the intestines (signified by thick yellow tongue coating). Persons who are very deficient (with pallor, weak pulse, thin or stripped tongue coating) should avoid or use these water treatments only during crises; habitual use will eventually weaken anyone. For several days after an enema or colonic, it is important to ingest foods which enhance the intestinal flora (see chart below).

Exercise: Sluggish digestion and a sluggish body in general will result from a sedentary lifestyle. Regular physical activity tones up the muscles and reflexes, keeping peristalsis active. Exercise also burns off liver excess and improves fluid metabolism.

Foods to avoid in all types of constipation: all products with baking soda/powder, alcohol, tea, yeasted breads (use sourdough or sprouted "Essene" breads), and refined "white" foods, such as all white-flour products, white sugar, and white rice.

Foods Which Treat Constipation

Foods that Lubricate the Intestines	Foods that Promote Bowel Movement	Demulcent Herbs	Flora-Enhancing Foods
spinach	cabbage	marshmallow root	miso
banana	papaya	flax seed	sauerkraut*
sesame seed/oil	peas	fenugreek seed	dairy yogurt
honey	black sesame seed	psyllium seed	seed yogurt
pear	coconut	licorice root	rejuvelac
prune	sweet potato		acidophilus†
peach	asparagus		kefir
apple	fig	**Laxative Herbs**	chlorophyll-rich
apricot	bran from oats,	dandelion root	foods, e.g.,
walnut	wheat, or rice	rhubarb root	wheat-grass
pine nut	castor oil	cascara bark	products, dark
almond		barberry bark	greens, micro-
alfalfa sprouts			algae (wild
soy products			blue-green and
carrot			spirulina) and
cauliflower			alfalfa greens
beet			
okra			
whole fresh milk§			
seaweed			

*Raw sauerkraut and unpasteurized pickles are beneficial for improving the intestinal flora. (See "Pickles" in the recipe section.)

†In addition to *Lactobacillus acidophilus*, other bacterial organisms help renew the intestinal bioculture, among them *L. bifidus, L. bulgaricus, S. faecium, L. rhamnosus, L. Sporogenes,* and *B. laterosporus*. One or more of these are often included in commercial "acidophilus" cultures. *L. sporogenes* and *B. laterosporus,* becoming more available at stores carrying dietary supplements, are the most effective of these bacteria for treating constipation.

§Overconsumption of poor-quality milk products is a primary cause of constipation; however, a moderate amount of milk which has not been pasteurized, homogenized, skimmed, or denatured in other ways can benefit those suffering with constipation from dryness, if they are not allergic to dairy products.

Blood Disorders

Blood Deficiency

In traditional Chinese medicine, the concept of blood includes an understanding of the inherent energy within the blood. Blood is created in part from nutrients extracted in the digestive tract as a result of the action of the spleen-pancreas; blood is formed when this extract is combined with the kidney essence known as *jing*. Much of the body's *jing* is stored in the bone marrow, which correlates with the contemporary Western knowledge that blood is generated in the marrow.

Signs of blood deficiency: paleness of the lips, nailbeds, tongue, and complexion in general, thinness, spots in the field of vision, unusual hair loss, premature graying and thin, dry hair, dry skin, and trembling or numbness in the arms or hands. Disorders associated with blood deficiency are anemia, nervousness, low back pain, and headache; menses that are painful or lacking often result from blood deficiency.

Blood deficiency is caused by inadequate intake of nutrients, by the inability to absorb nutrients, or by the loss of blood through gastro-intestinal bleeding or excessive menstrual flow. Chronic diseases and stagnant blood that inhibits formation of new blood are additional causes.

To enrich and build the blood through nutrition, there are two general approaches: increase the digestive absorption of nutrients, and add those specific nutrients which generate healthy blood. To encourage absorption, build the *qi* energy of the spleen-pancreas and reduce any *damp*/mucus conditions (pages 342 and 344). The nutrients most often needed to cure blood deficiencies are iron, folic acid, and vitamin B_{12}. Adequate protein is also essential. Of these nutrients, insufficient iron is the most prevalent cause of anemia, but it is not always cured simply with the addition of iron. In order to absorb iron, one needs adequate copper and B vitamins, as well as vitamin C.

Good sources of iron are distributed widely among plant foods, including vegetables, legumes, grains, nuts, and seeds. Moreover, when a variety of these foods is consumed in their unrefined states, abundant protein, copper, and B vitamins necessary for iron absorption will be available. Sufficient vitamin C is also available from certain of these foods (see page 396). For the first stages of the treatment of blood deficiency, one may want to add to the diet the richest sources of iron. These are the algae, including both seaweeds and micro-algae such as spirulina.

Folic acid is found in abundance in micro-algae, sprouts, leafy greens, and chlorophyll-rich foods in general, but it is easily lost in prolonged cooking. Eating raw or lightly steamed greens or sprouts regularly ensures ample folic acid in the diet.

One way to obtain high levels of B_{12} is to use bacteria-derived tablets of B_{12} (discussed on page 141). Most blood deficiencies will quickly improve with the addition of even moderate amounts of the above key blood-building foods, which are primarily grains, legumes, sprouts, green foods, and vegetables.

Grains and greens in particular are important as blood tonics for other reasons. First, they are good sources of manganese, which has properties beneficial to the formation of blood. In addition, manganese may itself transform into iron, if the theories of Biological Transmutation are correct. These concepts, although controversial, seem to have validity; they were discussed earlier in connection with "Calcium via Silicon" in Chapter 15. Secondly, the green chlorophyll-rich foods have been used successfully for centuries to overcome anemia and to build the blood. This healing relationship may be a result of the structure of the chlorophyll molecule, which is nearly identical to that of hemin, the pigment which forms hemoglobin when combined with protein. The major difference between chlorophyll and hemin lies in the central atom—chlorophyll has magnesium in this position, whereas hemin has iron. Anemia is characterized by a reduction in the total hemoglobin in the bloodstream or by a reduction in the red blood cells themselves. Since chlorophyll foods contain substantial amounts of iron and manganese, they are clearly excellent nutritional resources for blood production.

Certain of the green and grain blood-builders have a long history of use. The Japanese combine pounded sweet rice (mochi) with the herb mugwort (*Artemisia vulgaris*) as a blood builder; this combination also eliminates parasites, a common cause of blood deficiencies. "Mugwort mochi" is available as a prepared commercial product in many parts of the United States; it can also be easily made by adding powdered mugwort leaf to mochi (see "mochi" in the recipe section). The Japanese variety of mugwort is much less bitter than American mugwort, and better for tonifying the blood, but it is not as effective for removing parasites. (If mugwort is not available, the common herb nettles *[Urtica urens]* can be substituted.)

When blood deficiency is severe, animal products may be necessary: try royal jelly, gelatin, carp soup, mussels, oysters, the liver of beef, lamb, or chicken; also chicken gizzard. If there are signs of kidney weakness such as fatigue, *coldness*, and low backache, lamb or beef kidney may also be beneficial. The daily dosage for gelatin is 10–15 grams ($\frac{1}{3}$–$\frac{1}{2}$ ounce). (Please refer to the properties, preparation, and dosage of meat, pages 155–158.) Other effective general blood tonics are the foods and herbs for building liver blood, page 328.

Hair and Blood Quality

Hair is one indicator of blood quality. In Eastern medicine, hair is said to be an extension of the blood and therefore is influenced by the health of the spleen-pancreas and kidneys. In addition, the head hair is directly affected by the kidneys in other ways, as discussed in the *Water Element* chapter. Healthy hair is lustrous and thick. Hair loss and prematurely gray hair can be treated by improving blood quality and strengthening the spleen-pancreas and kidneys.

Certain foods have traditionally been used to prevent gray hair: hijiki seaweed, blackstrap molasses (too much may have the opposite effect), nettles, and wheat grass. These four foods are especially rich in the blood-building nutrient iron, and nettles and wheat grass are concentrated in chlorophyll as well. The eating of nettles, hijiki, and wheat grass is also thought to help keep hair from falling out. The famous Chinese herbal blood tonic *Polygonum multiflorum (ho shou wu)* has been used to darken gray hair, but this black root is far too warming and tonifying to the liver for most Westerners, causing depression and anger in many cases. Therefore it is not recommended except for those who were raised on low-meat, low-fat diets and do not have signs of an excessive liver. Another Chinese remedy for prematurely gray hair is black sesame seed, which is also quite laxative and should not be used if it causes loose stools.

Americans have the greatest incidence of baldness of any people; this is understandable since hair loss is tied to high-fat, high-protein diets, which damage the kidneys and create acidic blood. Meat and dairy, besides being high in fat and protein, are also generally considered "sweet" in Eastern medicine. Considering the additional sweets, desserts, and sugar-laced foods and drinks in which Americans indulge, we can see that the sweet flavor dominates the typical diet. The *Inner Classic* cautions that too much sweet-flavored food makes the head hair fall out. A further caution from this ancient text: "Too much salt damages the blood [and therefore the hair]." As discussed in the *Salt* chapter, excessive salt is consumed by Americans, nearly all of it highly refined.

The Current "Age of Anxiety"

Worry and anxiety, examples of excessive thinking, greatly injure the spleen-pancreas and its blood-producing, nutrient-assimilating functions. (Recall that the emotion of worry, in excess, is detrimental to the spleen-pancreas and Earth Element.) It is commonly known in China that worry causes gray hair. Much the same is said in the Western adage about hair—"Grass doesn't grow well on a busy street."

However, gray and falling hair is not the worst effect of worry. Worry accelerates aging in general because it weakens the blood, which carries nutrients necessary for cell regeneration. Also, since worry damages the pancreas and its enzyme production, nutritional problems of every sort are more likely.

Worry and other forms of excess thought are not necessarily the same as the unfocused mind symptomatic of a weak heart-mind. Worry can be focused, but it is nevertheless repetitious, compulsive thinking. The motivation behind worry is an attempt to "figure things out" from every perspective because of doubt and insecurity. But when one has faith in a unified life process—for example, that life proceeds according to its own perfection—then real acceptance of the "suchness" of life becomes possible, and the busy mind can relax. In relaxed awareness, there exists naturally a greater understanding, even wisdom. In this way the knowledge so keenly sought after through worry finally arrives when worry stops. Eating meals with simpler combinations of foods supports deeper, less busy thinking.

Bleeding

From a Western medical point of view, many problems with hemorrhaging and bleeding in general originate from weak blood vessels and from blood that clots poorly. Chinese traditional medicine asserts that one central function of the spleen-pancreas is to "keep the blood in its channels." Bringing these two views together is not difficult: the spleen-pancreas influences the extraction of nutrients from food which are essential to the health of the blood and its vessels. For example, nutritionists have identified vitamins C, K, and bioflavonoids as three key nutrients that help arrest bleeding.

Some foods which arrest bleeding (known as hemostats) contain large amounts of these nutrients. Cayenne pepper is perhaps the best example. Consumption of hemostatic foods seems to work much more effectively than taking the three vitamins in isolation, because there are other principles and nutrients bound in synergism that contribute to the power of hemostatic plants.

The following are the most common bleeding disorders, and these are generally *heat*-induced: 1) gastro-intestinal bleeding (stomach bleeding manifests as dark, tarlike blood in the stools, while intestinal bleeding is progressively less dark and more red the closer it is to the anus); 2) urinary-tract bleeding (hematuria); 3) bleeding gums; 4) nosebleed (epistaxis); 5) spitting up or coughing up blood from the lungs or bronchial tubes (hemoptysis); 6) vomiting blood (hematemesis); 7) uterine hemorrhage (metrorrhagia); and 8) menstrual hemorrhage (menorrhagia) which, along with other bleeding in the lower part of the body, may be caused by *heat* but is just as often a direct result of *deficiency* or *cold* conditions.

Major Causes of Bleeding

Hot Blood is caused by *heat* that has penetrated deep within the body, agitating the blood and therefore increasing the possibility of hemorrhage. Signs of hot blood include scarlet tongue, skin rashes or red skin eruptions, fever, thirst, and fast pulse; the bleeding in cases of hot blood is bright red. When bleeding from hot blood is chronic, the diet needs to include more cooling foods and fewer foods that contribute to *heat* (meat, alcohol, tobacco, coffee, hot spices, and other warming foods).

Hot blood can also be caused by a deficiency of *yin*, indicated by fresh red tongue, night sweats, and fast, thin pulse. In this case, *yin*-building foods such as millet, mung bean, seaweed, tofu, and barley should be added to the diet (for further examples, see page 65).

Deficiency Bleeding has either pale or dark-colored blood, and the person has signs of general weakness, *coldness,* and/or *deficiency*. It occurs when there is insufficient *qi* or warmth, which can be improved by correcting deficiencies of the spleen-pancreas *qi* or digestive fire. In this type of bleeding, the blood and its vessels are malnourished and therefore weak, so blood can easily leak out. Hemostats that are warming or at least neutral are preferable for deficiency bleeding.

Stagnant blood (discussed later) can also cause bleeding. In such cases, the hemostats listed below are useful.

Using hemostats: Except where noted, the following remedies will retard bleeding from any part of the body, but many are particularly useful in the specific types of bleeding noted. For chronic bleeding conditions, hemostats are taken two or three times a day. In a crisis, they can be taken as often as needed; every half-hour in small amounts is usually adequate. For bleeding from hot-blood conditions, the foods can be eaten raw or lightly cooked by simmering or steaming; they can be moderately cooked in cases of deficiency bleeding. Unless specified differently, prepare the herbs according to the instructions in the "Standard Herbal Preparations" section, page 110.

Remedies for Bleeding

Cooling Remedies for Hot-Blood Bleeding:
- Spinach has general hemostatic properties.
- Nettle leaf and/or root *(Urtica urens)* taken as a tea—especially effective for bleeding in the lungs, nose, gastro-intestinal tract, and kidneys. Apply the boiled leaves directly on wounds to stop bleeding.
- Raspberry leaf *(Rubus ideaus)* is a general hemostat that also specifically treats excessive menstrual bleeding.
- Eggplant is especially effective for anal and urinary tract bleeding.
- Swiss chard has general hemostatic properties.
- Persimmon is especially effective for urinary bleeding, vomiting blood, and spitting up blood from bleeding in the throat area.
- Brush teeth with fine salt to stop bleeding gums.
- Lemon juice is diluted by half and drunk as cold as possible as a general hemostat.
- Celery and lettuce both treat blood in the urine, but have no other hemostatic properties.

Neutral and Warming Remedies for Deficiency Bleeding:
Note: Neutral remedies, marked with "†," may also be used for hot-blood bleeding.
- Shepherd's purse† *(Capsella bursa-pastoris)* is a common herb that grows wild all over the continental United States and is one of the best general remedies for bleeding of the stomach, bowels, kidneys, and lungs; it is also a useful treatment for vomiting blood, spitting up blood, menorrhagia, metrorrhagia, and vaginal bleeding.
- Olives† are helpful for treating coughing up of blood.
- Gelatin† is considered the most effective remedy for deficiency bleeding, particularly for menstrual and uterine bleeding. It is often used in difficult cases such as uterine hemorrhage resulting from fibroid tumors. For an even better result, take it with mugwort-leaf tea (below). Prepare gelatin by stirring 3–15

grams (¹⁄₁₀ to ½ ounce) in warm water. Gelatin is available in most grocery stores. The "gelatin" *(Equus asinus;* Mandarin: *a jiao)* of Chinese herbology is a better hemostat.

- Leek has general hemostatic properties.
- Cayenne pepper is an excellent internal first-aid remedy for internal or external bleeding from injuries and is also used for uterine hemorrhage, menorrhagia, bleeding from the lungs, as a prevention against strokes, and for hemorrhages in general. For bleeding injuries, apply cayenne directly on the wound and take it internally as well. For internal use, the dosage is a relatively small amount: 1 fluid ounce of tea (prepare by pouring 1 cup boiling water over 1 teaspoon cayenne); 400–500 milligrams in capsules; or 10–15 drops of tincture.
- Mugwort leaf *(Artemisia vulgaris)* is a specific herb for uterine bleeding when there are signs of *coldness* and *deficiency.*
- Chestnut is especially useful for vomiting of blood, nosebleed, and blood in the stools.
- Guava has general hemostatic properties.
- Vinegar is especially helpful for treating anal bleeding, vomiting of blood, and nosebleed. Dosage: 1 teaspoon stirred in cup of water.

Stagnant Blood: Gynecological and Other Disorders

Stagnant blood is blood that coagulates or congeals, and is brought about either by injuries to the tissues of the body or by *qi* energy insufficient to push the blood through the vessels. Signs of stagnant blood include stabbing pain that is fixed in one place, frequent bleeding, bleeding with dark purple clots, dark purple tongue with red spots, and unnaturally dark complexion. When blood is stagnant, clots tend to develop; chronic stagnation generates tumors, cysts, nodules, and hard, immobile lumps.

Women are often afflicted with stagnant blood, particularly in the lower abdominal (reproductive) area. In fact, a large portion of all gynecological problems, especially those of a painful nature, are related to stagnant blood. Examples of women's diseases commonly caused by stagnant blood are amenorrhea (absence of menstruation), dysmenorrhea (painful menstruation), uterine hemorrhage, uterine tumors including fibroids and cancer, and ovarian cysts. (Amenorrhea and dysmenorrhea are discussed in the next section, "Menstrual Disorders.")

Clearing stagnant blood is easiest in the early stages, before masses form. In all cases, one must improve the circulation of *qi* energy; when the liver is the cause of stagnation, the remedies outlined earlier for stagnant liver *qi* are appropriate (page 324).

Another approach to treating stagnant blood involves improving the quality of the blood itself. Blood filled with toxins, waste matter, and fat is much more likely to become stagnant and congealed. For healthy, vital blood, the spleen-pancreas must be maintained at peak performance, since its function has a great effect on blood formation.

In the West, *dampness* and mucus are the two main factors which weaken digestion and the spleen-pancreas, thereby causing turbid blood; in *damp*/mucus conditions, one should restrict the cold (in temperature), very sweet, and highly mucus-forming foods including meat, dairy, eggs, ice cream, and the others listed earlier in the *Earth Element* chapter.

In every case of stagnant blood, regardless of its cause, proper eating habits such as thorough chewing and preparation of simple meals are essential. Furthermore, those foods and spices which disperse stagnant blood should be added to the diet (see below). Adding one such item to each meal is an effective dietary aid in conjunction with herbal, acupuncture, or other treatments. For milder conditions, these dietary remedies may be sufficient by themselves.

Precautions and notes:

1. Each food and spice in the following list is warming, with the exception of eggplant (cooling), white pepper (cooling), aduki bean (neutral), and peach seed (neutral). The warming remedies, particularly garlic and ginger, should be used carefully, if at all, in cases marked by signs of *heat* (aversion to heat, sensation of feeling too hot, flushed face, bloodshot eyes, deep red tongue with possible yellow coating, and/or great thirst for cold fluids) or signs of *deficient yin* (tidal fevers, hot palms and soles, fresh red cheeks and tongue, frequent, light thirst, and/or night sweats).
2. Eggplant specifically relieves stagnant blood conditions of the uterus, but may weaken the uterus when blood is not stagnant.
3. Butter is most useful where there is emaciation, weakness, and a dietary history low in animal products; it is contraindicated in cases of liver excess, *dampness*, and mucous conditions, and therefore is rarely prescribed for blood stagnation in countries where a rich diet prevails.
4. Vinegar and sweet rice are contraindicated in patterns of deficient digestive fire (watery stools; pale, swollen, wet tongue; and feelings of *coldness*).

Foods and Spices Which Disperse Stagnant Blood

turmeric	scallion	nutmeg	spearmint
chives	leek	kohlrabi	butter
garlic	ginger	eggplant	
vinegar	chestnut	white pepper	
basil	rosemary	aduki bean	
peach seed	cayenne	sweet rice	

Common Conditions of Stagnant Blood

In deciding whether a condition involves stagnant blood, check the diagnostic features above. When the condition includes pain, the pain is invariably fixed in one place; pain that moves around is not caused by stagnant blood.

- Heart pain and heart disease in general frequently exhibit symptoms of blood stagnation, especially when there is blood clotting. Aduki beans, peach-seed tea, scallions, and chives are specific remedies for vascular-related blood stagnation and can be added freely to the diet for this purpose. Cayenne and other red peppers are also very useful. If the stomach objects to peppers, ginger may be substituted.

- Tumors of the uterus, including uterine fibroids and cancers, very often involve blood stagnation. Ovarian cysts can also be placed in this category. Turmeric in the diet helps dissolve these growths. Since the uterus and ovaries are not a well-circulated area, and growths there resist treatment, the following herbal decoction is invaluable for speeding the reabsorption of tumors, cancers, and similar growths in the lower abdominal region:

    turmeric* *(Curcumae long;* Mandarin: *yu jin)* (1 part)
    licorice root* *(Glycyrrhiza glabra;* Mandarin: *da zoa)* (1½ parts)
    cinnamon bark* *(Cinnamomum cassia;* Mandarin: *rou gui)* (4 parts)
    peach seed *(Prunus persica;* Mandarin: *tao ren)* (5 parts)

Notes: The preparation and dosages of all herbs in this section follow the guidelines in the *Dietary Transition* chapter (page 110). Herbs denoted by "*" are commonly available through both Western and Chinese herb suppliers. Peach seeds are usually carried only by Chinese herb outlets; they can also be collected from inside peach pits, and sun-dried. Black fungus (below) is typically found in both Chinese food shops and herb stores.

Black fungus (wood ear) and seaweeds are also especially helpful for dissolving fibroid and other uterine tumors, and these can be added to the diet for this purpose. In addition, black fungus goes well in the above herbal decoction (use 4 parts), especially when *heat* or *deficient yin* signs are present, in which case cinnamon bark, a very warming herb, should be removed from the formula. The entire cancer program which appears later should be followed not only for cancer in the feminine organs, but also for any kind of tumor in this area.

- Intestinal obstructions that occur with signs of blood stagnation respond to the above herbal formula when it is modified by replacing the turmeric with three parts rhubarb root* *(Rheum palmatum).*

- Injuries such as bruises, contusions, broken bones, and sprains (torn ligaments and tendons) often cause blood stagnation. These types of conditions will normally heal with remarkable speed when a comfrey-vinegar poultice is applied. To prepare, simply mash fresh or dried comfrey-leaf herb *(Symphytum officinale)* with a pestle in a mortar containing enough apple cider or other non-distilled vinegar to soak the comfrey thoroughly. If a mortar is not available, either a suribachi or bowl and spoon work well. Then apply the comfrey-vinegar mash at least one-half inch thick directly to the injured area and bind it on with a clean cotton cloth. The properties of comfrey penetrate through the skin to help heal the injury, while the vinegar disperses blood stagnations. This poultice should be used daily and left on at least three hours, though it is often most convenient to retain it all night while sleeping. Although not as effective as comfrey, most other greens such as plantain leaf, cabbage, spinach, and chard can be substituted when comfrey is not available.

Chives and cayenne are additional excellent remedies for injuries with signs of blood stagnation. They work internally when added generously to the diet. For external use, chive greens and/or roots are cut finely, then juiced by wringing the pulp through muslin or similar cloth, or by expressing with a juicer. The juice can then be soaked into cotton cloth and applied as a compress, or rubbed on directly as a liniment.

A cayenne-vinegar liniment is also very effective. To prepare, simmer 1 tablespoon cayenne pepper in 1 pint apple-cider or rice-wine vinegar for 10 minutes in a covered container; bottle hot and unstrained. Apply on the injured site without rubbing too much. This liniment is also useful for lung congestion, and for pains of arthritis and rheumatism.

Menstrual Disorders
Prevention and Good Habits

Women who eat a balanced diet, get adequate exercise and sunshine, and work toward emotional clarity seldom have menstrual problems. At the time of menstruation, the deeper hormonal/emotional qualities surface, while their physical corollary is discharged—the heat-bearing blood that results from a natural purification. This is a fragile state—surfacing aspects from the interior, *yin*, hormonal parts of the being are delicate and sensitive, and need protection from the *yin* climates (cold and damp) and physical and emotional extremes. During the menses, it is therefore important to avoid heavy physical work, emotional stress, and overexposure to cold and damp conditions; for example, keep the legs and feet warm, keep covered when in cold places and during the cool seasons, and avoid working with the hands in cold water. Also avoid constipation, get plenty of rest, and abstain from sex during menstruation.

Dietary Restrictions: To support health during the entire menstrual cycle, these should be avoided: alcohol, tobacco, coffee, cold-temperature foods, refined sugar, hydrogenated fats such as shortening and most margarines, polyunsaturated cooking oils (see *Oils and Fats*, Chapter 10, for options), and overconsumption of fruit or raw food. Fluoridated water suppresses thyroid activity, which upsets the hormonal system in general; chlorinated water destroys vitamin E, an essential nutrient for menstrual ease. Commercial red meats and poultry have residues of steroids composed of female animal sex hormones, which interfere with human menstruation. Over time, oral contraceptives and IUDs (intrauterine devices) also cause difficulties.

General Nutrition

- *Iron* and *iodine* need to be abundant in the diet to help replace blood lost in the menses. Legumes, most vegetables and whole grains, and the common micro-algae such as spirulina contain significant amounts of iron. Seaweeds, including kelp, dulse, wakame, and hijiki, are exceptional sources of both iron and iodine. Those with weak digestive *qi* (loose stools, chronic fatigue) need to use seaweeds cautiously. Follow the suggestions given in "Blood Deficiency," page 387, for more complete methods of blood tonification.

- *Vitamin C* increases iron absorption: cabbage, bell peppers, broccoli, sprouts, parsley, and rose hip tea are excellent sources. Additional sources are nearly all fresh fruits and vegetables. When vitamin C is taken in the form of whole foods such as these, bioflavonoids are also ingested. The combination of bioflavonoids and vitamin C is helpful for excessive bleeding in menorrhagia and for the bruising and varicose veins of menopause. Tomatoes, citrus fruits, and most other fruits, which are very cooling, cleansing sources of C, should be used sparingly, if at all, by persons with *coldness* (e.g., aversion to cold, sensation of feeling too cold, facial pallor) or general *deficiency* (weakness, frailty, little or no tongue coating).

- *Calcium* and *zinc* levels in the body begin to decrease ten days before the period starts. Use whole grains, legumes, and seeds for zinc and magnesium (magnesium needs to be adequate for calcium absorption—see *Calcium* chapter). Seaweeds, green vegetables, and legumes are good sources of usable calcium.

- Sufficient *B vitamins, vitamin A,* and *protein* are also necessary for a harmonious menstrual cycle. These nutrients help the liver convert powerful hormones present before menstruation into less provoking substances. Vitamin B_6 and folic acid are especially important; B_6 is found abundantly in whole grains; folic acid as well as vitamin A (in the form of provitamin A) are concentrated in green vegetables. Provitamin A is also richly supplied in the deep yellow vegetables—carrots are especially helpful for hormonal regulation. Sufficient vitamin B_{12} is essential to menstrual cycle health. (See pages 136–142 for deficiency signs and other pertinent information on the vitamin.)Adequate protein is available in diets based on unrefined grains and vegetables if too many sweets, alcohol, and denatured foods are not eaten. Those who are weak, thin, blood-deficient, and without mucus problems generally benefit from good-quality dairy products. Fermented products such as yogurt, soured milk, and kefir are the most digestible. In extreme *deficiency,* small amounts of other high-quality organic animal products may be necessary. (See the properties and preparation of animal foods, pages 151–158.)

- The fatty acids *alpha-* and *gamma-linolenic acid* are important for producing the hormone-like prostaglandins PGE_1 and PGE_3. These help overcome the cramping and pain associated with excess arachidonic acid and the prostaglandin PGE_2, which are usually overabundant in those with a history of heavy meat-eating. Alpha-linolenic acid, an omega-3 fatty acid, is found in green vegetables, chlorophyll foods such as chlorella micro-algae and wheat- or barley-grass concentrates, flax seed, and cold-pressed flax oil; the omega-3s EPA and DHA, metabolites of alpha-linolenic acid, are likewise valuable and are concentrated in certain kinds of fish (e.g., salmon, tuna, sardine, eel, trout, mackerel, anchovy, and butterfish) as well as omega-3-rich fish oils. Major sources of gamma-linolenic acid (GLA) include evening primrose oil, black currant oil, borage oil, and spirulina micro-algae. Please refer to *Oils and Fats,* Chapter 10, for further examples and usage.

- *Honey* appears to encourage production of the same PGE_1 prostaglandin as GLA (above), which may explain its value as a folk remedy for general menstrual problems. However, compared with GLA, the action of honey is mild. The daily dosage is one tablespoon of honey in one cup of hot water or herbal tea.
- *Vitamin E* is essential for keeping blood "slippery" and flowing, thus helping reduce blood stagnation and clotting. This vitamin also quells painful inflammations and common breast lumps caused by leukotriene production from arachidonic acid. In this respect, vitamin E has effects similar to the two fatty acids mentioned above. Vitamin E is helpful in the treatment of several menstrual disorders: excess or scanty menses, the hot flashes of menopause, and irregular cycles.

Sources of vitamin E are whole grains, especially wheat, rice, oats, and quinoa; the outer leaves of cabbage, broccoli, and cauliflower (the parts that are seldom eaten); sprouts, spinach, dandelion greens, carrot tops, and mint. Nuts and seeds such as almonds, filberts, and sunflower seeds are also excellent sources, but must be used carefully to avoid burdening the liver with fats. The richest food sources of E are wheat germ and wheat-germ oil. These are prone to rapid deterioration, and should be refrigerated in a dark, airtight container after opening. The complete vitamin E complex is present in this form. The standard daily dosage of one tablespoon of wheat-germ oil supplies 30 I.U., which is much more effective than the same amount from supplements. Most vitamin E supplements, even those extracted from foods, contain less than the complete complex.

Nevertheless, supplemental vitamin E extracted from natural sources can be beneficial, particularly in extreme menstrual difficulty. Fifty to 150 I.U. is a typical and usually effective daily dosage from supplements, although much greater amounts are sometimes used for specific conditions.

Vitamin E in the body is destroyed by chlorinated drinking water, rancid oils (most polyunsaturated oils), oral contraceptives (estrogenic compounds), and pollution. Those living in highly polluted areas or ingesting E-destructive products need higher than normal amounts of the vitamin. After harmful circumstances and bad habits are eliminated and the body is balanced, vitamin E from whole-food sources will be sufficient.

- *Herbs and spices* are still taken for menstrual difficulty by women throughout the world. In the disorders below, a number of common seasonings and spices such as dill, marjoram, and ginger are recommended. These can be used in food and also as herbs in teas, capsules, or tinctures; all herbs in this section, except for those specified otherwise, should be used according to the standard preparation and dosages given in the *Dietary Transition* chapter, page 110. Herbs can be used regularly throughout the month to balance the entire hormonal cycle, but stronger doses are helpful starting six days prior to the onset of the period in cases where there is discomfort.

The "Mixture of Four Herbs" is an invaluable Chinese formula for a variety of menstrual and other complaints. It contains:

3 parts *dang gui** root *(Angelica sinensis;* Mandarin: *dang gui)*

3 parts prepared rehmannia root *(Rehmannia glutinosa;* Mandarin: *shu di huang)*

2 parts peony root *(Paeonia lactiflora;* Mandarin: *bai shoa)*

1.5 parts ligusticum root *(Ligusticum wallichii;* Mandarin: *chuan xiong)*

The herbs in this formula are some of the most widely available Chinese herbs; the entire formula is also a part of various Chinese and Western herbal preparations (testing with *dang gui* began in Europe in the 1920s). It is particularly effective when weakness, pallor, and *deficiency* exist, but is not recommended where there are signs of *excess* (robust, extroverted personality, reddish complexion, thick tongue coating, strong voice and pulse). Uses of the formula include irregular menses, dysmenorrhea, amenorrhea, late or scanty menses, traumatic injuries with stagnant blood signs, abdominal pain from stagnant blood, stagnant liver *qi* conditions, abnormal uterine bleeding (add mugwort leaf and gelatin to the formula), and stagnant blood in general. (See "Bleeding" section, pages 391–392, for preparation of gelatin.)

Dang gui root is often taken alone for menstrual problems with signs of blood deficiency (anemia, pallor, insomnia, nervousness, emaciation). It is sometimes cooked into soups by Chinese women; if the whole root (rather than the powdered, cut, or rolled variety) is used, it can be cooked several times because of its unusual density. After it softens, it is customarily eaten with rice. The common Western herb angelica root *(Angelica archangelica)* is a related plant and can be substituted for *dang gui,* but it is less helpful when there are signs of blood deficiency.

Specific Menstrual Disorders

Pain and Cramps (Dysmenorrhea). The preceding dietary restrictions and suggestions help prevent pain and cramping occurring at any point in the menstrual cycle. Three of the nutrients—calcium, magnesium, and the essential fatty acids—are

---

*The spelling of *dang gui* is Romanized in several ways, including "dong quai" and "tang kuei."

helpful for treating acute menstrual pain. Such pain occurs from several causes:

Cold/Deficiency Dysmenorrhea. *Coldness* and/or *deficiency* in the body can cause the blood to stagnate, resulting in pain. Symptoms of *coldness* are: scanty, purplish-black menses; cramps that are eased by hot compresses; abundant, clear urine; attraction to warmth and warm food and drinks. Symptoms of *deficiency*: pale-colored, scanty menses, weakness, weak pulse, pale tongue with no coating, facial pallor. For either *coldness-* or *deficiency*-induced pain, avoid raw, cold-temperature foods and cooling fruits (especially citrus), and choose more warming food and spices such as oats, sweet rice, black peppercorn, dill, caraway, basil, black beans, and butter. Small amounts of dairy or other animal products may be necessary. Helpful herbs are angelica root *(Angelica archangelica),* mugwort leaf *(Artemisia vulgaris),* spearmint *(Mentha virides),* and *dang gui* root *(Angelica sinensis).* The "Mixture of Four Herbs" formula is also useful for this type of dysmenorrhea.

In *cold* and/or *deficiency* dysmenorrhea, it is essential to keep the body and extremities warm and dry.

Heat/Excess-Type Dysmenorrhea. Symptoms of *heat:* early, heavy, bright red or dark red menses, dark scanty urine, red tongue with yellow tongue coating, thirst, constipation, desire for cold and aversion to heat. Symptoms of *excess:* scanty menses with dark purple clots, bluish tongue, painful, expanded breasts, forceful, tight pulse, thick tongue coating. The woman with symptoms of *heat* and/or *excess* needs to reduce her consumption of red meat, dairy products, eggs, sweet foods, and other foods which build *excess* and *heat.*

For these types of dysmenorrhea, consume more cooling vegetal foods such as spinach, lettuce, celery, chard, kale, collard greens, parsley, carrots, mung beans, tofu, spirulina, and millet. Helpful herbs: flax seed *(Linum usitatissimum),* black cohosh *(Cimicifuga racemosa),* lobelia *(Lobelia inflata),* motherwort *(Leonurus cardiaca),* and wormwood *(Artemisia apiacea).* Black cohosh, motherwort, and wormwood can be used singly, but more effective is the following combination: an infusion of equal parts flax seed, black cohosh, and motherwort, with one-half part lobelia. Honey is especially useful when dysmenorrhea is accompanied by constipation (it lubricates the intestines).

Absence of Menstruation (Amenorrhea). [This section also applies to women with suppressed, scanty, or delayed menstruation.] Amenorrhea is often associated with a low-fat diet.[33] Strict vegetarians frequently go through cycles of amenorrhea until their system is accustomed to assimilating nutrients from plant food. Excessive exercise, stressful, competitive work, and other greatly *yang* activity can also damage the feminine hormones and cause amenorrhea.[34] Many sportswomen fall into this category. In addition, women who are too thin (a deficient-blood sign) often have little or no menstrual period; if they gain weight, the period usually normalizes. Following are two major patterns of amenorrhea.

Deficiency Amenorrhea, caused by insufficient blood and *deficiency* in general, has these symptoms: hot palms, nervousness, pale or sallow complexion, dryness, low body weight, intermittent fever, weak pulse, little or no tongue coating, dizziness, spots in the vision, and weak limbs.

To tonify women with this type of deficiency, build up the blood and energy. Appropriate foods include sweet rice, brown rice, oats, mugwort mochi and, if tolerated, quality dairy products; gelatin and small amounts of eggs, fish, or animal meats may also be necessary in extreme cases (see "Blood Deficiency," page 388, for suggested animal products). Very bitter, sour, or salty foods should be restricted. Too much carotene, a bitter substance, can induce amenorrhea:[35] women with deficiency amenorrhea should avoid consuming large amounts of green and yellow vegetables such as carrots, dark leafy greens, and common micro-algae.

Use equal amounts of all herbs in these herbal formulas for *deficiency* amenorrhea: 1) *dang gui (Angelica sinensis)* or angelica root *(Angelica archangelica)*, combined with motherwort *(Leonurus cardiaca)*; 2) mugwort *(Artemisia vulgaris)* combined with licorice root *(Glycyrrhiza glabra)* or molasses. These two formulas can be combined for even greater effectiveness. 3) "The Mixture of Four Herbs" described earlier is also of exceptional benefit here. In addition, see the note after the second paragraph below.

Excess-type Amenorrhea is a condition of stagnant energy and blood in which the blood flow is blocked. Symptoms may include painful, swollen lower abdomen, upset stomach, purplish tongue, bitter taste in the mouth, and emotional depression. This condition is often brought on by long-term over-consumption of animal foods. Avoid heavy meats and all dairy products; also avoid cooling fruit—especially citrus—and raw vegetables. The beta-carotene-rich green and yellow vegetables and micro-algae, contraindicated in *deficiency* amenorrhea above, are actually helpful in the excess type.

In *excess*-induced amenorrhea, one can add foods, spices, and herbs which circulate the *qi* and help overcome blood stagnation. Especially good are certain foods and seasonings: chives, eggplant, turmeric, nutmeg, garlic, rosemary, oregano or sweet marjoram, and ginger; effective herbs include pennyroyal *(Hedeoma pulegiodes)*, rhubarb root *(Rheum palmatum)*, motherwort *(Leonurus cardiaca)*, black cohosh *(Cimicifuga racemosa)*, chamomile *(Anthemis nobilis)*, and tansy *(Tanecetum vulgare)*. All these items, except for eggplant, work most efficiently as hot teas for promoting menstruation. The foods and seasonings, of course, are also beneficial taken in meals. The six herbs listed are generally a little more powerful and can be taken for stubborn, prolonged conditions. Overuse of tansy, however, is toxic—take only for a few days at a time. Rhubarb root is useful when constipation accompanies amenorrhea. In amenorrhea with mild symptoms, hot ginger/turmeric or marjoram tea is usually sufficient.

Note: For both *excess* and *deficiency* amenorrhea, hot sitz or foot baths are helpful. Also, the legs and feet should be kept warm.

Irregular Cycle. An irregular menstrual cycle can result from: a) a change in diet, b) great changes in physical and emotional activity, c) seasonal changes in the monthly cycle—going into the cooler seasons, for example, the menses at the full moon may change to the new moon, or vice versa. However, when the cycle is irregular with no apparent reason, it usually indicates a chaotic or otherwise poor diet causing liver stagnancy and accompanying nutritional deficiency.

In liver stagnation, there is often thyroid weakness and iodine deficiency; in these cases kelp and other seaweeds are helpful, as well as the general program for energizing a stagnant liver. Vitamins B_6, B_{12}, and zinc are often used for an irregular cycle—these nutrients help overcome liver stagnancy and are abundant in a varied diet of whole foods (see "General Nutrition" above).

Blood stagnation causing pain and dark purplish clots also causes irregularity (see "Stagnant Blood" section, page 392, for basic remedies). A specific remedy for irregularity from either blood or liver stagnation is rose-petal tea. The "Mixture of Four Herbs" is likewise very helpful for both these types of irregularity in the frail and *deficient* woman.

Chlorophyll foods are regulators of the menstrual cycle, undoubtedly because of their anti-stagnancy effect on the liver. Green vegetables, spirulina, chlorella, or chlorophyll liquid extract are useful. These also build the blood and establish the proper intestinal flora for the transformation and assimilation of all nutrients.

Black beans are a blood tonic, and because they strongly nurture the *yin*—the supporting and stabilizing principle—they are useful for correcting an irregular cycle. For this purpose, they can be included in small, regular amounts in the diet for ten weeks or so. Black bean juice, taken in one-cup doses twice daily, is likewise effective. To prepare, simmer six parts water to one part black beans for one and one-half hours, then remove the juice. (Do not discard the beans—add more water and finish cooking them.)

Menstrual Hemorrhage (Menorrhagia). According to Chinese tradition, excessive menstrual bleeding is often associated with a liver that no longer stores the blood, or a spleen-pancreas that no longer keeps blood in the channels. We now look at why these organs malfunction.

Specific Causes of Menorrhagia:

1) Stagnant liver *qi* is the most common cause of menorrhagia and is signified by a dark, possibly blue-, green- or purple-tinged tongue, swellings and lumps, distended abdomen, rigid, inflexible body, wirelike pulse, and many other physical and mental signs—please refer to "Liver Stagnation," pages 319 and 324, for further symptoms and general dietary recommendations. Especially helpful are kelp and other seaweeds, foods that stimulate the *qi*, and the avoidance of liver-damaging foods and habits (poor-quality oils and fats, too much food, excess meat and rich food in general, too many spices, alcohol, drugs, and chemical ingredients).

In this and all types of menorrhagia, general hemostats such as shepherd's purse and raspberry leaf can be used. (See "Bleeding," beginning on page 390, for other specific hemostats.)

2) *Deficiency* and *coldness* also cause menorrhagia; signs include weakness, chills and feelings of coldness, pallor, weak and slow pulse, and clear urine. This type of menorrhagia is often related to a weak spleen-pancreas that no longer

"keeps the blood in the channels." In this case, one must eat a simple, strengthening, warming diet to increase digestive efficiency, so that nutrients which improve the arteries and stop bleeding are absorbed and then transformed (metabolized). Avoid cooling and cold-temperature foods; bitter, very salty, or too many sour foods; citrus and other cooling fruits; and raw foods. Appropriate warming foods: oats, quinoa, pine nuts, parsnip, butter, black beans, cinnamon, anise, fennel, dried ginger, black peppercorn, molasses, and possibly animal meats in extreme cases. For further examples, please refer to the guidelines for "Deficient Spleen-Pancreas *Qi*" and "Deficient Digestive Fire," page 342. For *deficiency-cold* menorrhagia, the remedy of choice is gelatin with mugwort leaf tea. (Mugwort tea or gelatin alone is also useful.) The combination given earlier in the "General Nutrition" section—gelatin, the Mixture of Four Herbs, and mugwort—is even more effective.

The aduki bean, which tonifies the spleen-pancreas, is also a remedy. Herbalist Naboru Muramoto, who often uses Japanese folk remedies, recommends the daily consumption of five raw aduki beans at once as a treatment for excessive and prolonged menstruation. The beans must be chewed very thoroughly for this purpose.

3) Stagnant blood can also cause menorrhagia. This is particularly true when there are uterine tumors or cancer induced by stagnant blood. Gelatin is often effective in these serious cases to stop bleeding, along with the methods given earlier for clearing stagnant blood (beginning on page 392). Signs of stagnant blood-induced menorrhagia include a fixed, stabbing pain in the lower abdomen, purple-clotted menses, and dark purple tongue with red spots.

4) *Heat* and *excess* can bring on early, heavy menstruation, signified by abundant, bright-red blood. More cooling foods are needed: spinach, swiss chard, seaweed, celery, cucumber, and red raspberry-leaf tea; restricted are red meats, alcohol, coffee, and warming foods in general.

Premenstrual Syndrome (PMS). The mood swings, fatigue, tension, backache, abdominal cramping, and other imbalances that can occur at ovulation or any time prior to the period are due to unbalanced hormonal fluctuations. As discussed in the *Oils and Fats* chapter, too much of the prostaglandin PGE_2 from excessive consumption of animal products is one factor that disturbs hormonal balance, causing PMS. Another reason for hormonal imbalance is the energy stagnation that occurs when the liver is upset, causing stagnant blood, clots, and the painful physical and psychological symptoms of PMS. Remedies which control PGE_2 include omega-3 and GLA oils (see sources on pages 164 and 173).

Stagnant liver *qi* is discussed in the "Menorrhagia" section above. Chaste berries *(Vitex agnus-castus)* are a specific herbal treatment for most symptoms of PMS. This herb is also thought to help smooth out the anxiety surrounding sexual desire in some women.

Balanced nutrition is crucial for overcoming PMS. The guidelines of "Dietary Restrictions" and "General Nutrition" starting on page 395 need to be followed for long-term results.

Menopausal Difficulty. Menopause is the natural termination of the menstrual cycle and reproductive years and usually occurs somewhere between the ages of forty-two and fifty-two. At this time, the female sex hormone estrogen, produced primarily by the ovaries, gradually decreases, while the adrenals begin making estrogen and androgen to replace it. In the healthy woman, this process is smooth and easy. However, when the menopausal transformation is not harmonious, there can be various symptoms; among the more common are "hot flashes," headaches, irritability, depression, insomnia, nervousness, leg cramps, night sweats, nose-bleeds, frequent bruising, and varicose veins. In addition to sufficient exercise and a good diet, a relaxed, unstressful life will greatly help overcome symptoms. For the many women who have menopausal problems, it is of some consolation to know that most symptoms usually pass within a few months, or possibly a year or so.

A standard medical prescription for menopausal difficulties has been estrogen from animals, which relieves some of the symptoms. Estrogen therapy also tends to help with the diminished calcium absorption of menopause. Nevertheless, supplementing with estrogen has been shown to increase the risk of various imbalances, among them gall bladder disease and cancers of the breast, uterus, and liver.[36] Moreover, taking estrogen discourages the adrenals from fully developing their estrogen-producing capacity. Fortunately, there are safer remedies which promote the natural production of hormones by the adrenals, as we shall soon see.

In Chinese medicine, the symptoms of menopause imply a deficiency of *yin* fluids, particularly those *yin* fluids which calm and relax the liver. A helpful dietary approach, then, is to add foods that especially "build the *yin*": wheat germ and its oil, mung bean, mung bean sprouts, string bean, seaweed, spirulina, millet, black bean, tofu, kidney bean, barley, and black sesame seed. At the same time, one should observe the dietary restraints listed earlier against alcohol, cigarettes, coffee, excessive and poor-quality meat, et cetera.

Of the food-source nutrients recommended in "General Nutrition" (page 396), the most important for treating menopausal discomfort are vitamins E, B-complex, C, and A, and the mineral calcium. Because of decreased calcium absorption in the first stages of menopause, dietary factors which maximize calcium absorption need to be followed. Adequate magnesium and vitamin D from sunshine are necessary cofactors in calcium metabolism. Vitamin E is also a key nutrient, because it stimulates the production of estrogen. Wheat germ and wheat germ oil are especially good sources of this vitamin because they also tonify the *yin*. Whole wheat itself is helpful in additional ways—its properties include the ability to calm the spirit (sedate nervousness) and strengthen the kidney-adrenal function. If menopausal difficulties persist in spite of a good diet containing abundant vitamin E, then large doses of supplemental vitamin E usually will eliminate hot flashes and other major problems. For this effect, one must take approximately 300 I.U. of vitamin E three times a day, preferably at meal times.

Herbal therapy is also very helpful. We have seen *dang gui (Angelica sinensis)* bring relief from all symptoms, even in severe cases. Precautions and further information on using *dang gui* are given on page 221. Other beneficial herbs are motherwort *(Leonurus cardiaca)* and the costly spice saffron *(Crocus sativus)*; both are effective when used singly, although their potential for soothing menopausal distress is accentuated when combined with *dang gui.* Saffron must be taken in very small amounts; about 300 milligrams (approximately one-third of a gram or one-tenth teaspoon) once daily is a typical dosage. In large doses, saffron is highly toxic, sometimes deadly. In India, this bright yellow spice is traditionally mixed with rice and vegetables, with heated milk and honey, or with *ghee* (clarified butter). It is a wonderful spice for encouraging the *yin,* receptive, compassionate, and devotional temperament, a precious remedy for those whose menopause is fraught with irritations. To preserve its medicinal virtue, saffron is not cooked with herbal teas or food but is stirred into them after cooking and while they are still hot.

The cooling, soothing, *yin*-tonifying effects of aloe vera gel have been traditionally used for menopausal difficulty in India and Latin America. It is too cooling, however, for those who are *cold* or who have a tendency to loose stools. Dosage: 2 teaspoons gel stirred into 1 cup of water, two or three times daily.

Royal jelly, the food of the queen bee, can greatly tonify the feminine hormonal system. Chinese herbalism classifies it as a food that builds the *yin* (the body, its tissues, and fluids) and improves *qi* energy. Royal jelly prolongs the life span of the queen bee to thirty times that of other bees, and also makes her extremely fertile and prolific. These properties are often used to improve women's hormonal and reproductive capacities as well.

It has been postulated that menopause can be postponed through optimum nutrition and other health practices, perhaps for one or two decades.[37] This idea is one facet of longevity theories which suggest that people in general are living foreshortened lives, and that bodily functions such as hormonal secretions are drying up too soon. When royal jelly is added to a life-enhancing diet, most hormone-deficient people notice increased hormonal activity in terms of an improved sense of well-being and more energy.

Dosage and further information on royal jelly are given on page 152.

Cancer and the Regeneration Diets

At one time, cancer was not prevalent in America and was considered a disease of old age. Cancer now afflicts more than twenty-five percent of the population and is found among people of all ages, including infants. Evidence suggests that the recent spread of cancer to all quarters of the population is due to the increase in sedentary lifestyles, overeating of rich food, depletion of the soil, modern food processing, omnipresent low-level radiation, increased susceptibility to infections, and environmental toxins. Better diagnostic methods also account for part of the statistical increase in cancer cases.

Dietary therapy for cancer has taken many forms over the centuries, although in the early twenty-first century a consensus has arisen in established medicine that certain chemicals, smoking, too much fatty food, and insufficient vegetables, fruits, whole grains, and beans contribute to cancer.[38]

Anyone studying modern cancer treatment by diet must consider the work of Max Gerson (d. 1959). In this text we refer to his discoveries repeatedly, as he had more than thirty years of successful and extensive clinical experience in the treatment of advanced cancer solely by diet. Albert Schweitzer, the renowned philanthropist, physician and Nobel laureate, called Max Gerson "one of the most eminent geniuses in medical history." Gerson's complete cancer theory and step-by-step recommendations are recorded in *A Cancer Therapy and The Cure of Advanced Cancer by Diet Therapy: Results of Fifty Cases*.[39] Gerson's treatments were developed from his experience. He drew from ancient and modern therapies, but applied only those methods clinically proven to lead to renewal of the internal organs. In this way, the degenerations that cause cancer are eliminated and the body heals itself.

Gerson suggested that every detail of his therapy be followed for maximum effectiveness. A number of treatment options in this text, however, extend beyond his original therapy: indigenous and foreign herbs; sprouted seeds, grains, and legumes; seaweeds, micro-algae, cereal grasses, principles of simple food combining, hyper-oxygenation methods, and others. Perhaps the most striking difference between Gerson's recommendations and ours is the use of traditional Chinese diagnosis to closely match foods and their preparation to the condition and constitution of the individual. Also, certain foods are emphasized here because of their specific anti-cancer properties in the Chinese and Ayurvedic systems. The recommendations in this text are substantially different from the Gerson therapy, but a good portion of the treatments are based on his discoveries.

One of Gerson's discoveries was the value of non-specific treatment; his therapy was to rejuvenate the entire human organism. Thus, all different forms of cancer are treated in this way. He also found through clinical experience that this approach, with minor adjustments, also cured most other degenerative diseases. Many others working holistically with degenerative diseases have also applied basic rejuvenative principles to a variety of conditions. Likewise, our program for treating cancer, with its various options for adapting to individual needs, can be modified to treat other serious degenerations. It also serves as an excellent dietary foundation for further therapies that may be indicated, such as acupuncture, homeopathy, herbology, or established Western medical therapies. Individuals who fit any clearly defined organ syndrome described in the Five Elements chapters will benefit from integrating specific remedies found there with the general program in this section.

In people who are still active and vital, cancer is sometimes cured fairly easily. However, where there is serious degeneration and a collapse of vitality, cancer is difficult to cure by any means. Like Gerson, other successful pioneers in the dietary treatment of advanced cancer (most notably Jethro Kloss in America, and a host of Europeans) advocated a cleansing diet of fresh vegetables and fruits, particularly in the form of juices. Oats and other whole grains were also usually included. Meats and animal products were prohibited except in cases of extreme deficiency, although the Gerson diet included both an extract and the juice from calf liver. They have also used other cleansing methods, particularly the enema.

Several factors that influence cancerous conditions have changed since Gerson's time. During the decade of the 1960s, red meat consumption in affluent countries continued to rise, then plummeted twenty-five percent over the next fifteen years. At the same time, major increases occurred in vegetable oil consumption as well as in the quantity of chemicals, hormones, and antibiotics added to food. Soils became more depleted, causing poorer-quality animal and vegetable products; the number of cities with fluoridated and otherwise questionable water increased dramatically; parasitic infections spread aggressively throughout the population; and the saturation of the environment with various forms of radiation from televisions and computer terminals (extra-low-frequency [ELF] radiation), telecommunications equipment, and appliances multiplied several times. Ever-increasing numbers of families have all their adult members working outside the home, with no one left at home to prepare wholesome food with care.

Of the changes above, perhaps the least recognized problem is the widespread increase in the consumption of rancid and poor-quality polyunsaturated vegetable oils, some of which are made even worse through hydrogenation into margarine, shortening, and other synthetic fats. (See *Oils and Fats* chapter.)

Everyone diagnosed with cancer goes through this health challenge in a unique way. Since the National Cancer Institute finally acknowledged that diet plays a major role in the development of cancer, many people have attempted dietary reform. Even cancer specialists who use chemotherapy and other radical treatments are starting to recommend dietary changes as well. Sometimes a blend of these treatments with diet and other holistic, biologic therapies is successful. Clearly, the radical therapies are best utilized on the strong person with *excess* signs (robust constitution, ruddy complexion, strong pulses, and active, outward personality), whose cancer is growing rapidly. Gerson and many others have observed that x-rays, chemotherapy, and surgery further weaken the organism, and those with *excess* conditions can better afford this.

The traditional Eastern approach is to build up the system so that it can naturally overcome the cancer. However, because many Americans are overly built-up already, with layer upon layer of excess, extreme therapies that tear down the organism in general at the same time that they destroy the heart of the excess—the cancerous growth—are sometimes successful. Certainly the fruit- and vegetable-juice therapies have a reducing effect as well. When oxygenation therapies and purgative herbs are added, the net result is a nontoxic type of chemotherapy that destroys the cancer in stages by gradually reabsorbing it into the blood (parenteral digestion). Tumors in the digestive tract may simply break up and be excreted. Thus, cancer therapies should not only be seen in terms of dualities such as "natural" versus "unnatural." A more accurate view is a continuum of therapies, starting with the gentlest and progressing to the most drastically purging. The diets and treatments below follow this progression.

Regeneration Diets for Cancer and Degenerative Diseases

The following three diets are outlines; the specific recommendations listed later in this section should be used in making appropriate choices of grains, vegetables, legumes, fruits, herbs, cereal grasses, animal products, and other pertinent factors.

DIET A: Primarily grains, vegetables, seaweeds, legumes, sprouts, herbs, micro-algae, omega-3 and GLA foods and oils, and small amounts of spices. This diet includes some raw vegetables or sprouts if desired by the patient, but most food is cooked, either moderately for those with signs of severe *coldness* or *deficiency,* or lightly cooked for all others. Recommended herbs (specified later) are mildly cleansing, yet tonifying and immunity-enhancing. Seaweeds are taken unless there is diarrhea. Whole fruits (not their juices) are taken in moderation; they can be stewed in cases of extreme weakness, and should be avoided if they exacerbate candida symptoms or cause loose stools. Supplementation with fish or other animal products may be necessary. Proportions of foods in the daily diet: 45% grains; 35% vegetables; 10% fruit; 5% beans and other legumes; 5% other recommended foods.

Actions: This diet gently reduces the toxic excess that feeds cancer, pathogenic organisms, and degenerative diseases in those who are weak, frail, anemic, *cold,* or otherwise *deficient.* Diet A provides balance when using the more powerful treatments (D, E, and F below).

DIET B: Fruits and vegetables and their juices, wheat-grass juice, seaweeds, and the sprouts of seeds, grains, and legumes; also includes omega-3/GLA foods and oils, and appropriate micro-algae, spices, and herbs that eliminate toxins and enhance immunity. Cooked grain is eaten once a day, and lightly cooked vegetables and sprouts as well as raw vegetable-sprout salads are on the daily menu. Enemas are given when there is pain from toxic overload. Juice dosage: up to 6 cups (48 ounces) of fruit and vegetable juice daily. Wheat grass: 1 ounce of juice three times a day, or 1 heaping teaspoon of wheat- or barley-grass juice powder three times a day. Proportions of foods in the daily diet: 35% sprouted grains, legumes, and seeds; 45% vegetables and fruits and their juices; 10% cooked grain; 10% other recommended foods.

Actions: This diet eliminates disease-producing toxins more quickly than DIET A and is appropriate for those who show strength, strong pulses, and have neither loose stools nor signs of *coldness* (chills, aversion to cold, pallor, and great attraction to warmth).

DIET C: Same as DIET B above, except for the following: All grains are sprouted and all foods are raw except for a daily vegetable soup; purgative, highly cleansing herbs and frequent enemas are also given. Juice dosage: up to 10 cups (80 ounces) of fruit and vegetable juices daily. Wheat grass: 2 ounces of juice three times a day, or 2 heaping teaspoons of wheat- or barley-grass juice powder three times a day.

Actions: This diet reduces excess and toxins very rapidly and is most appropriate for the often-constipated, relatively strong individual who exhibits *excess* signs such as thick tongue coating, loud voice, strong pulses, extroverted personality, and who also may have signs of *heat*—aversion to heat, red face, great thirst, deep red tongue, and/or yellow tongue coating.

Factors in the Regeneration Diets

1. The dietary outlines A, B, and C above are not meant to be rigid. Various parts of each may need to be combined according to individual needs. Cancer and other degenerations are usually a complex mix of excesses and deficiencies, so the level of cleansing most acceptable to the patient is apt to be the best choice. Very often the patient can withstand more extreme cleansing at the beginning for a few weeks, and needs DIET A after that. In successful treatment of advanced cancer cases, total remission and revitalization can take as long as two years. Revitalization, of course, may take much longer when the diet and other healing factors are less than optimal.

    In all cases of constipation, including both "excess-" and "deficiency-types," specific foods and herbs for treating constipation should be taken (page 383).

2. In choosing remedies for constipation or for the conditions listed below that may accompany degenerative disease, it is best to select those foods that fit within the boundaries of the regeneration diet being followed.

3. Those who suffer a long-term illness frequently develop a "deficient *yin*" syndrome (fresh red cheeks and tongue, insomnia, hot palms and soles, intermittent fever, night sweats); in these cases, foods that build the *yin* are emphasized: millet, barley, seaweeds, black beans, mung beans and their sprouts, soy sprouts and, in severe cases, the animal products recommended on page 422. (See "Foods Which Tonify the Yin," page 65, for other examples.)

4. Those with stagnant blood signs (purplish tongue with red dots, stabbing pain fixed in one place, tendency to hemorrhage [occurs most frequently when the feminine organs are affected], blue or purple coloration of the lips or other skin areas) should add foods and herbs for clearing blood stagnation (see "stagnant blood," page 392). Note that several remedies for blood stagnancy appear in the following pages as well, and stagnancy in general is addressed from several perspectives.

5. The Parasite Purge Program (beginning on page 654), which purges a wide variety of pathogens, should be followed. This program works with the Regeneration Diets to cleanse toxic and *damp* excesses from the body.

6. In Chapter 5, all material on immunity is recommended for awareness of the most vital dimensions of the immune system, particularly the mental/spiritual aspect. Recalling the Fire Element principles, we know that those with degenerative conditions need to strengthen their *shen*, or heart-mind spirit. Knowing that physical and mental discomforts accompany successful healing fosters perseverance to complete the entire process of renewal. (See "Healing Reactions," page 106.)

7. In the most extremely *deficient* conditions (debility, withdrawal, shallow breathing, pale or sickly yellow complexion), the "Guidelines for Treating Severe Deficiencies," beginning on page 93, should be followed.

8. Those who take no animal products with the regeneration diets should add approximately 25 micrograms of vitamin B_{12} three times a week with meals. Sometimes this dosage is difficult to obtain, in which case pills of larger dosages can be cut up. Even though B_{12} in large amounts is nontoxic, great excesses may stress the system. Vitamin B_{12} in supplements is derived from microorganisms and is one of the few common whole-food supplements in pill form. Adequate B_{12} helps keep cellular structures free of distortions that occur from cancer, aging, injuries, or degenerative diseases.

9. Except where noted otherwise, all herbs are used according to the standard dosages and preparation methods (see page 110).

Other Treatments

TREATMENT D: Oxygenation therapies such as oral or intravenous hydrogen peroxide (H_2O_2) and ozone treatments. These therapies are best taken with antioxidant nutrients as a safeguard, for example, foods rich in vitamins A (beta carotene), C, and E; flavonoids—grape seed extract and pycnogenol, which are anticarcinogenic and among the most powerful antioxidants known, also reduce swelling and inflammation from degenerative disease processes; and wheat- or barley-grass juice powders, which are concentrated in the antioxidant superoxide dismutase (SOD) (see "Hyper-Oxygenation," page 79, for more on oxygen therapies).

TREATMENT E: Chemotherapy and radiation. The minerals and algin in kelp and other seaweeds protect against some of the devastating after-effects of these therapies. Wheat- or barley-grass juice powder can also be taken to counteract the effects of radiation and detoxify the residues of chemotherapy. Aloe gel can help heal skin inflammation resulting from radiation. Fennel seeds, made into tea, or a few seeds consumed after thorough chewing, effectively soothe an upset stomach caused by either therapy. According to studies in China, the herb astragalus improves recovery time from both chemotherapy and radiation. For this purpose it can be taken alone or, for greater effectiveness, taken in the formula provided later in this chapter. See page 412 for pertinent information on vitamin C.

TREATMENT F: Surgery. DIET A is substantial enough to facilitate recuperation after surgery, and contains sufficient antioxidants and other nutrients to inhibit tumor regrowth. (Malignant cells are often released into the blood stream in the process of surgery.[40]) Aloe gel speeds the healing of surgical scars.

TREATMENTS D, E, and F are sometimes successful without dietary improvements; however, in order to ensure long-term health, a foundation of good dietary habits is necessary.

Traditional and Modern Perspectives

The following perspectives show contrasts as well as some surprising agreements among Eastern remedies, modern nutrition, and the central features of Gerson's dietary plan.

- Advanced cancer and other serious degenerative disorders involve the total person, and all systems are affected. In cures we have observed, the successful individuals have unwaveringly focused their spirit on their diet, emotions, and awareness. Often the deciding factor is whether or not family and friends are supportive—this is especially true of those with cancer who choose non-standard therapies which neither their physician nor friends find acceptable. The stress of opposing one's customary support group may outweigh the benefits of an otherwise useful therapy. Part of this problem is avoided by choosing a holistically oriented physician and simultaneously getting support and advice from other health practitioners—for instance, experienced herbalists, naturopaths, and therapists skilled in emotional transformation.
- Cancer can result from overnutrition, especially from excessive amounts of growth-promoting foods such as meats, fats, dairy products, sweets, and rich foods in general. Overeating of these foods can be seen as a metaphor of the excessive life in general: more growth is available than the body can healthfully incorporate; therefore perverted growth (cancer) is forced to occur. Excess in degenerative disease is often associated with various forms of *dampness*—obesity, mucus, edema—although there is usually an accompanying *deficiency*.

    The Chinese classics describe cancer as a form of water stagnation or *dampness;* additional related etiologies of cancer are stagnant blood, stagnant *qi,* stagnant mucus—always some form of stagnancy. As discussed in the *Wood Element* chapter, it is essential to resolve old, stagnating resentments and other repressed emotions. Emotional extremes, including stress, adversely alter the functioning of the internal organs.

- Oxygenation of the cells dries out *damp* conditions and is perhaps the most important biologic factor in the cure of cancer and many other degenerations. Since malignant cells live anaerobically, supplying oxygen kills cancer and creates *qi* flow (oxygen stimulates the body's *qi*). According to Gerson, "oxidizing enzymes are at a low level of function in cancer patients." Tissue oxygen is maximized by moderate exercise, living where there is clean air, eating freshly prepared, lightly cooked or raw food, and emphasizing chlorophyll- and germanium-rich foods. If flour or cracked cereals are used, they should be freshly milled. Overeating must be avoided. (See "Oxygenation," page 78.)

- Symptoms of interior *dampness* such as cancer are aggravated by living in a damp space such as a basement room. The living space should be dry, and residing in a dry climate is also helpful.

- Cancer and other serious degenerations sometimes result from a vegetarian diet, particularly an ovo-lacto-vegetarian diet in which the dairy and eggs are of poor quality, and the vegetal food is denatured: refined sugar and flour, rancid oils, and chemical additives.

- Degenerative diseases can be brought on not only by too much rich and denatured food but by the ghastly combinations in which these foods are often eaten. In many homes, every meal contains five or more food groups, e.g., meat, milk/cheese, sugar, bread/pastries, coffee or alcohol. Even those with strong digestive systems eventually suffer major disorders with such complexity—the resulting intestinal fermentation feeds viruses, yeasts, fungi, and ultimately carcinogenesis (healthful digestion is enzymatic, not fermentive). In degenerative diseases, it is essential to give the digestive organs a rest several times a week with some mono-diet meals of only fruit, or vegetables, or sprouts. Other meals should follow the strict "Plan B" food combining given in Chapter 19. Those who are *deficient* may also use "Plan C" (one-pot) meals, which are most appropriate when meats or fish are taken.

- In advanced cancer cases, Gerson found that most vitamin and mineral supplements were either unnecessary or detrimental. Exceptions were niacin and vitamin B_{12}, and a special combination of potassium compounds. He recognized that nutrients in the context of food are essential to healing but, when concentrated into pills, are irritating to the severely ill person. More specifically, he discovered that pills of vitamins A, E, D, and certain calcium supplements had negative effects. Research indicates that specific foods with these nutrients may enhance immunity and prevent cancer; however, similar research using vitamin pills supports Gerson's findings: isolated vitamins are often not effective against cancer and may even contribute to it.[98,99,100]

Gerson discovered vitamin C to be another exception to the above observation, and recommended it in small (100 mg.) doses four times daily in the first few days of the treatment when pain relief was needed. Not a true vitamin, vitamin C is sometimes considered a liver metabolite which lowers cholesterol and helps the liver metabolize protein and fats. Supplemental vitamin C has proven useful in cancer therapies[41] and has an effect similar to that of oxygenation—it increases hydrogen peroxide in the system and detoxifies the blood. Substantial amounts of synthetic vitamin C are used in some cancer treatments—often five grams or more in the course of the day.

It is now known that the common forms of synthetic vitamin C may be only one-fifth as effective as the newer "esterified" forms of the vitamin. However, the ideal form of C is found in whole food. This form may be, according to our earlier estimate in the *Vitamins and Supplements* chapter, at least ten times as potent as common synthetic C. Thus, 5 grams of synthetic C may be no more effective than 500 milligrams ($\frac{1}{2}$ gram) of C from whole foods. Three or four times this quantity of vitamin C is easily obtained daily with a diet rich in sprouts, fresh fruits, vegetables, and their juices.[42] Not all food has to be raw to supply vitamin C—most of the vitamin survives steaming or simmering for ten minutes or so.

Determining whether or not a given individual should fortify the three anti-cancer diets above with supplemental vitamins and minerals requires the advice of an experienced nutritional counselor. (One should bear in mind Gerson's experience with certain supplements in *advanced* cancer.) It can be said, however, that individuals with cancer and similar degenerations who most often need supplemental vitamin C are: those who continue to eat denatured foods and substantial amounts of meat, eggs, cheese, or poultry; robust persons with signs of *excess* or *heat* who may have reduced animal-food consumption but do not eat enough fresh vegetables, juices, sprouts, and other sources of vitamin C; and those undergoing chemotherapy or radiation therapy—vitamin C in massive amounts helps the liver to neutralize the resulting enormous quantities of toxic by-products.

Beta carotene and other carotenoids have been shown to play key roles in retarding the progress of cancer.[43-45] Therapeutic doses of these are available in a variety of green and yellow vegetal foods (see *Green Food Products,* Chapter 16).

Healing any degenerative disease requires a balanced mix of all nutritional factors, although any nutrients that contributed to the disease should be restricted. Thus, diets low in animal protein, fat, and refined foods but rich in vitamins, minerals, fiber, and enzymes are usually the most successful.

- Excessive amounts of foods classified as having a "sweet" flavor (see *Five Flavors,* Chapter 23.) may contribute to cancer because they are moistening and promote dampness and mucus. Otto Warburg, twice winner of the Nobel Prize in Medicine, stated that "The prime cause of cancer is the replacement of the respiration of oxygen in normal body cells by a fermentation of sugar." Tibetan medicine warns against sweet, white foods in cancer, especially white sugar.[46]
- Salt and excessive sodium in general, according to Gerson, is a major cause of

cancer. His theory claims that all chronic disease starts with loss of potassium from cells and a resultant invasion of sodium plus water (edema), causing loss of electrical potential, improper enzyme formation, and reduced cell oxidation. From a Chinese healing arts perspective, salt is moistening and will eventually cause moisture *(dampness)* to accumulate, which, as discussed earlier, contributes to cancer. A low-salt or saltless diet withdraws water from the cells and thus may help prevent cancer, particularly in the *damp* person.

- To accelerate the withdrawal of water, potassium foods can be added. These "push" salt and therefore water out of the cells of the body. This is another reason that Gerson recommended fruits and vegetables, the richest food sources of potassium. To further enhance internal drying, he prescribed iodine and animal thyroid extract, which increase the cellular metabolism, causing the cells to pick up more potassium and oxidizing enzymes.

- Freshly pressed calf-liver juice is the best source of oxidizing enzymes, according to Gerson. It is also a rich source of omega-3 oils. However, mainly because it is difficult to find sources of unadulterated animal liver, the use of plant sources for oxidizing enzymes has increased since his time: sprouts, cereal-grass products, and raw unsalted sauerkraut.

- Gerson believed the liver to be the central organ to heal. One remarkable quality of the liver is its ability to almost completely regenerate. Gerson witnessed liver renewal in one-and-a-half to two years, or fifteen new generations of liver cells (cells regenerate every four to five weeks).

- The liver is greatly imbalanced in the majority of modern people, and the use of iodine as well as animal-liver extract by Gerson corresponds with Western and Eastern remedies for general liver stagnancy. Instead of iodine supplements, however, kelp and other seaweeds (naturally rich iodine sources) are used for cancer in traditional Chinese medicine. (Seaweed use is described later in this section.)

- Saturated animal fats, hydrogenated fats (e.g., margarine), and excessive protein place a burden on liver metabolism, and are often not completely broken down in those with degenerative conditions. Partially digested substances enter the blood stream and can cause abnormal formations such as cancer, especially in previously weakened or injured areas. Fats from animals contain arachidonic acid, which transforms in the body into prostaglandin PGE_2. This substance stimulates cell division and therefore, in excess, encourages the growth of cancer, which is basically unchecked cell proliferation. PGE_2 can be countered with oils rich in omega-3 and GLA fatty acids.

- Oil-Rich Products: As explained in the *Oils and Fats* chapter, a crucial factor in the prevention and treatment of cancer and all degenerative diseases is the avoidance of fats that cause massive free-radical production: margarines, shortenings, and polyunsaturated cooking and salad oils such as safflower, sunflower, corn, cottonseed, soy, and others. The best quality oils are contained in whole foods. In the case of cancer, however, a daily teaspoon of oleic-rich oils—either extra virgin olive or unrefined sesame—is acceptable as an option, and these should not be heated above 240°F. See "water-oil sauté" method, page 451. According to studies cited in the Journal of the National Cancer Institute, oleic acids seem to have tumor-inhibiting effects, although to a lesser extent than GLA and omega-3 sources (recommended below).[47]

Nuts and oil-rich seeds need to be used carefully because of their high oil and protein content. According to Gerson as well as Ayurvedic observations, those with cancer do better in general without foods rich in oil or fat. If nuts are craved, only the almond is thought to have some value in cancer, and only if not overeaten—a safe limit is usually six almonds daily. Peanuts must be avoided because they often contain the carcinogenic compound aflatoxin, and they also retard general metabolism. In Chinese medicine, the peanut is contraindicated wherever there is stagnancy or *dampness.*

However, there are several major exceptions among oil-bearing seeds. One of the most important is flax seed, because of its immune-enhancing omega-3 content. Flax is also one of the best sources of vegetable lignins; these compounds have antitumor, antiestrogenic, and antioxidant properties.[48, 49] Thus flax appears to have value in treating cancer in general, but particularly colon and breast cancers because the cells of these cancers, which have estrogen receptors,[50] can be inhibited by the antiestrogenic compounds in lignins.

Flax seed is available at stores which carry herbs and/or whole foods, and the organic variety should be requested. Dosage: Three to four tablespoons of soaked or crushed seeds per day, chewed thoroughly; or take the unrefined, recently cold-pressed oil twice daily in one-tablespoon doses. Flax oil should not be used as a cooking oil but goes well on food. The seeds are demulcent and helpful for constipation, especially of the dry *"deficiency"* type. Gerson found late in his life that the addition of flax oil greatly facilitated the dissolution of his patients' tumors. Several studies indicate that omega-3 oils from the body tissues of fish, which tend to be less contaminated than liver oils, have anti-tumor properties, but it is safest to use the omega-3 remedy with the greatest number of clinical successes—flax oil.

In some respects similar to the omega-3-rich oils, the GLA (gamma-linolenic acid) oils (according to evidence cited earlier in *Oils and Fats*) may also strengthen immunity and be useful against cancer. Sources and dosage of GLA are given in the *Oils and Fats* chapter, page 173. Although GLA and omega-3 oils have certain effects in common, they function differently in the body; it is wisest to include both oils in the diet for treating cancer and, when indicated, for other degenerative diseases. Once significant regeneration has been attained, GLA no longer needs to be taken because the liver will be healed sufficiently to form it from common linoleic fatty acids. However, flax seed or its fresh oil should be continued at an immunoprotective dosage of half that given above—the omega-3, alpha-linolenic fatty acids of flax are essential fatty acids in short supply in most modern foods, and cannot be synthesized in the body from other fatty acids.

- Synthetic hormones in commercial meat, though present in minute amounts, may have a bad effect. Gerson tried a highly recommended sex-hormone treatment for cancer and at first saw remarkable progress; eventually, however, the hormones seemed to cause cancer to spread. He then found that royal jelly balanced and tonified hormones with no negative effects. Recent research suggests that excess sex hormones, especially estrogen, may be responsible for certain cancers: "Breast cancer is linked to, if not caused by, the female sex hormone, estrogen."—Dr. Louise Brinton, National Cancer Institute. Estrogen is in most birth-control pills and has been the center of hormone replacement therapy in menopausal women for fifty years. Kelp is sometimes given as a protection against cancer in women who take birth-control pills and other estrogen compounds.

- Detoxification is brisk with Gerson's fruit- and vegetable-juice regimen, and can be deadly without enemas. So much toxin is released into the blood during the healing process that it blocks and poisons the liver, causing pain in any number of areas of the body (the healthy liver supports smooth *qi* flow throughout the body, and *qi* flow disruption results in spasms and cramps). To stimulate the liver (and therefore unblock *qi* flow), Gerson used coffee enemas every six hours throughout the day and even at night; in severe pain, every two to four hours. Coffee enemas have since become a standard therapy for cancer—they open the bile ducts, allowing toxins to flow from the liver, and also encourage dialysis of toxic products from blood, across the colonic wall. Directions for the coffee enema: Simmer three tablespoons of regular ground coffee in one quart of pure water for 20 minutes. Then strain and cool to body temperature; take the enema lying on the right side, with the knees drawn up to the abdomen. The fluid should be retained for fifteen minutes.

- Practitioners of Chinese medicine in the West have generally prescribed a more moderate diet for cancer, based on cooked grains and vegetables, with fewer raw foods, fruits and juices, supplemented by herbs and/or acupuncture. This causes a slower release of toxins, and enemas are used less and sometimes not at all. Since this therapy is similar to DIET A, it is most useful for those who are greatly debilitated.

- Massage styles such as Swedish should not be given to cancer patients because they might spread the cancer. However, holding pressure points (acupressure) and acupuncture treatments are often useful; Gerson recommended rubbing the surface of the skin daily with wine vinegar and rubbing alcohol (two tablespoons of each, in a glass of water). This helps the skin to release toxins.

Recommended Food Groups

As much as possible, all vegetables, fruits, grains, and other foods should be organically grown on rich soil. Also, only pure water should be consumed and used in recipes (see *Water* chapter). Water can be drunk according to thirst; however, there is more therapeutic value in satisfying thirst with juices, teas, and soups.

Sprouts: Even more important than the high nutrient profile of sprouts is the bio-availability of their nutrients. The sprouting process puts their fats and proteins into readily digestible forms which compensate for the incomplete digestion characteristic of degenerative diseases. Sprouts initiate *qi* flow in a stagnant liver; they also are rich in nitrilosides, substances that break down in the body into chemicals (benzaldehydes) that selectively destroy only cancer cells.[51]

Examples of sprouts that may be used include mung, alfalfa, aduki and other bean sprouts; all grain sprouts, cabbage, and clover; young buckwheat and sunflower greens, also beneficial, are appearing more frequently in markets alongside the sprouts. (See "Sprouts" in recipe section for directions on making your own sprouts.) Garbanzos and other large sprouts are best cooked, and all sprouts should be at least lightly cooked for those with signs of *coldness* or severe *deficiency*.

Legumes: All except soybeans can be used, but since legumes have a high protein content and do not digest easily, they should be taken in small amounts. The most easily digested legumes—mung and aduki beans (and their sprouts)—may be taken regularly. Except as a sprout, soy is not recommended in cancer because of its extremely high protein and growth-promoting properties.

Algae have been valuable remedies for the treatment of cancer in various Oriental and Western cultures, and researchers are now finding validity in these traditions.[52] Kelp and other seaweeds are used by the Chinese to soften and reduce hardened masses in the body; they contain the range of minerals, including trace minerals, often deficient in people with degenerative diseases. Without minerals, vitamins and enzymes in the body serve no function.

Seaweeds are also concentrated sources of iodine, discussed earlier as one of Gerson's remedies for speeding thyroid activity and oxidation of the cells. Seaweeds are high in sodium, however, and should be taken in regular but small amounts. If kelp is taken, the dosage is three grams in the form of tablets or capsules, or one rounded teaspoon of granules, per day. The use of other seaweeds is listed in the recipe section. Seaweeds are contraindicated in cases of weak spleen-pancreas *qi* or deficient digestive fire (signs include loose or watery stools).

In cancer therapy, it is safest to get all of one's salt from seaweeds and other foods. No salt should be added to food; very salty products such as miso and soy sauce are also best avoided. This applies to other serious disorders that call for the regeneration diets, unless otherwise noted.

Wheat- and barley-grass concentrates have exceptional detoxification value in degenerative diseases. In cancer, healing crises are reduced and detoxification goes more smoothly when either of these products are taken. Their chlorophyll helps oxygenate tissues and promotes healthy intestinal flora; they are also rich in the antioxidant enzyme SOD (superoxide dismutase), one of the best defenses against the free radical pathology of degenerative diseases. These grasses are cooling and cleansing, so they must be used cautiously by those with loose stools or signs of *coldness* or general *deficiency*. Cereal grass is especially good for treating candida overgrowth and those with *heat* signs such as red complexion, fast pulse, red tongue, aversion to heat, fever, and inflammatory degenerations such as arthritis.

Wheat- or barley-grass juice powders, mixed into water or vegetable juice, can be used in place of the fresh juices. (Those with candida overgrowth symptoms should use the powders.)

Dosage and administration: Start with 1 ounce of juice (or 1 heaping teaspoon of juice powder) daily and gradually increase to 1 or 2 ounces of juice (or 1 or 2 heaping teaspoons of juice powder) three times a day, one hour before or three hours after meals. Sip slowly and insalivate. Directions for growing wheat grass are given in *Green Food Products,* Chapter 16.

Some **micro-algae** have very favorable nutritional profiles for cancer and immune therapies. Spirulina, chlorella, and wild blue-green *(Aphanizomenon flosaquae)* provide cellular protection with exceptional amounts of beta carotene (provitamin A) and chlorophyll; dunaliella is the highest known natural source of beta carotene. Chlorella, the alga to emphasize in those with the greatest deficiency, stimulates immunity in the treatment of all degenerative diseases by means of the "Chlorella Growth Factor" (CGF). Spirulina is rich in phycocyanin, a pigment with anti-cancer properties. Spirulina is also the highest plant source of gamma-linolenic acid (GLA), a fatty acid which strengthens immunity and inhibits excessive cell division. Wild blue-green is slightly bitter, while dunaliella is very bitter; bitterness makes them good for drying moisture from tissues which support viral, bacterial, and fungal growths. Either of these bitter micro-algae often work well with chlorella or spirulina. (See "Micro-Algae Dosage" and "General Guidelines," pages 237 and 242, for help in selecting the appropriate micro-algae.)

Vegetables in general are helpful in the treatment of cancer. They are low in fat and protein, yet abundant in minerals, vitamins, and other vital nutrients. Perhaps the vegetable used most often in cancer treatment is the carrot. Quality carrots are very rich in the antioxidant beta-carotene, have an essential oil which kills parasites and unhealthy intestinal bacteria and, according to the Chinese, have the property of reducing accumulations (such as tumors). Mary C. Hogel of Salt Lake City, Utah, "terminally ill" with cancer, was one of the first to be cured with carrot juice.[53] This was in the days before juicers, and all the juice—at least one quart per day—was made by grating the carrots and then squeezing them in a cloth.

Carrots also make a good foundation juice; they are often juiced together with smaller amounts of other vegetables such as parsley, celery, beets, cabbage, bell pepper, collard, beet and turnip greens, romaine lettuce, sprouts, radishes, garlic, and others. All juices must be consumed fresh, within three hours of pressing, in order to maximize their oxidizing enzymes. Juices that are stored for two or three hours need to be kept in a refrigerated, closed container; they should be allowed to warm to room temperature before drinking.

Carrot and other juices may not have sufficient oxidizing enzymes to be effective if they are juiced in centrifuge-type juicers or liquifiers. The quickly rotating metal parts of the most common high-speed electric juicers whip air through the juice and also build a static charge that degrades the juice value. Gerson's patients did poorly when these electric juicers were used instead of a grinder and separate press. Electric juicers that grind the food by means of a rotating non-metallic shaft are acceptable. However, the best are hand juicers and presses.

Mushrooms: Early investigators were skeptical of mushrooms because they appeared to have properties similar to those of cancer—parasitical, fungus-like, and fast-growing. It now seems that these qualities may be an indication that mushrooms are useful for treating cancer. Mushrooms are often rich in germanium, an element which oxygenates. The Chinese ling zhi (*Ganoderma lucidum:* "reishi" in Japan) and the Japanese shiitake *(Lentinus edodes)* and maitake *(Grifola frondosa)* are the mushrooms used most often in the treatment of cancer and other serious immune degenerations. These traditional applications of mushrooms are now being scrutinized by researchers, who find the that polysaccharides of mushrooms exhibit anti-tumor potential.[54, 55] Mushrooms in general neutralize toxic residues in the body from meat-eating.

Chinese herbalist Moashing Ni assigns even the common button mushroom anti-tumor properties. The familiar "turkey tails" *(Coriolus versicolor)* that grow on the sides of rotting trees have recently proven to have value in cancer therapy. These can be dried, powdered, and taken in one-ounce doses twice a day. For medicinal use, mushrooms can be eaten or used as an herb and made into a tea.

Beets, both roots and tops, have the property of cleansing the liver and the blood, and are often prescribed in cases of cancer. In addition, beetroot is valued for its ability to strengthen the heart and calm the spirit. The juice of beets is very concentrated and can be mixed with carrot juice in a one-to-three ratio. Beets pickled in apple cider or wine vinegar are also excellent. Since beets lubricate the intestines, they are recommended for the constipation that often accompanies cancer.

Onions and garlic are rich sources of the potent anti-cancer bioflavonoid quercetin.[56] One onion daily inhibits malignant cell growth, and cooking does not destroy the effectiveness of quercetin. Garlic also contains large quantities of antiviral, antibiotic, and antifungal/anti-yeast compounds such as allicin.[57, 58] Thus it is especially useful in the treatment of cancer with concurrent candida proliferation. Garlic compounds also appear to be effective against leukemia.[59]

However, because of its extreme pungency, garlic can damage the stomach and liver if too much is consumed. This particularly applies to those with *heat* signs.

For maximum benefit from all of its properties, garlic should be eaten raw. Most people tolerate its burning pungency best by taking it with food at meal time. One-half clove, twice daily, is effective and a safe dosage for extended use. To reduce the odor, chew up a few fennel seeds and take chlorophyll foods such as wheat grass or parsley afterwards. Persons who cannot bear raw garlic can still receive some benefit from soups and teas containing lightly cooked garlic. Aged and fermented garlic products as well as high-quality garlic powders, liquids, and capsules are often not as effective as the fresh clove.[57] Garlic is an exceptional source of germanium. One should recognize the negative effect on the mind of extensive garlic use (page 210).

Radishes, both common and daikon, cleanse the thick toxic mucus residues of animal products that feed tumors and cancers.

Asparagus has been used in treating cancer. It is detoxifying and a valuable diuretic for removing cellular edema and *dampness* as well as increasing blood circulation. It contains an abundance of the antioxidant vitamin E; just two ounces daily is an effective dosage.

Each vegetable of the nightshade family is useful in different respects. Gerson emphasized the potato because of its high potassium content. In general, the potato is useful for balancing red-meat consumption and is thought to draw out toxins associated with meat-eating. The skin of the potato is reputed to contain an acidophilus culture beneficial in the renewal of intestinal flora.

Tomatoes are very cooling and rich in vitamin C. Their sour flavor benefits those with over*heated* conditions caused by liver excess (outward signs are red face, tongue, and eyes). Tomatoes are detoxifying and resolve food stagnation resulting from low stomach-acid secretion.

Eggplant treats stagnant-blood conditions of the uterus such as uterine tumors.

Bell peppers improve the appetite and resolve stagnant food in cancer cases where digestion is very poor; they also reduce swellings, promote circulation, and are rich in vitamin C.

These last three nightshades—tomato, eggplant, and bell pepper—are too cooling and weakening for those with loose stools (deficient spleen-pancreas *qi* or deficient digestive fire).

Brassica-genus vegetables—cabbage, turnip, kale, cauliflower, broccoli, brussels sprouts—have been recommended in general by the National Cancer Institute for cancer prevention. These contain dithiolthiones, a group of compounds which have anti-cancer, antioxidant properties; indoles, substances which protect against breast and colon cancer; and sulphur, which has antibiotic and antiviral characteristics. This family of vegetables also mildly stimulates the liver and other tissues out of stagnancy. Cabbage and its juice are particularly useful because they help clear mental depression. Another therapeutic use of cabbage is in the form of raw saltless sauerkraut (see "Pickles" in recipe section), which promotes better nutrient absorption as well as the growth of healthful (acidophilus) intestinal flora. In the context of such a beneficial ferment, gastro-intestinal renewal is enhanced; in addition, all the properties of cabbage become more effective.

Cucumbers should not be used for cancer patients because they tend to promote *dampness*, especially in the severely weak.

All other vegetables can be used in treating cancer, depending on their compatibility with the individual patient. The very sweet vegetables such as yams and sweet potatoes must be avoided when candida symptoms are severe.

As a dressing for salads, a little wine vinegar (at most one tablespoon) can be used. Vinegar quickly stimulates *qi* flow, which is helpful in stagnant conditions.

Fruit is even more cleansing than vegetables, but at the same time can promote yeast infections and weaken the digestive energy. Nevertheless, fruit and fruit juice have traditionally been recommended in large amounts for cancer and other degenerative diseases. This could be due to the fact that in the past the majority of people with these conditions needed such cleansing—they were constipated and over*heated*, and they had robust, *excessive* constitutions. Now there are many with cancer and other serious disorders (such as AIDS) who have a far different condition. They show *deficiency* in the sense of frailty, weakness, and weak digestion with loose stools. In these cases fruit, especially the juices, should be eaten sparingly, if at all. When candida symptoms are prevalent, fruit must be avoided. Certain fruits should be restricted in cases of cancer and other degenerations marked with *dampness* because they are too watery and *damp*-inducing (all melons, pineapple [strictly avoid], pear, peach, fresh fig, and all citrus); too fatty (avocado and coconut); too sweet (raisins and other dried fruit—dried figs are an exception); or because they contain aggravating acids (berries and plums).

Especially recommended fruit: Apples eliminate mucus, relieve depression, and tonify the "heart-mind," which is usually depressed and weak in degenerative diseases; for those who tolerate fruit, organic apples can be recommended as the primary fruit and juice source in therapy for cancer and other such conditions (the highly sprayed "Delicious" variety must be strictly avoided). Mulberries have two important properties: they calm the spirit and detoxify the body. Papaya has enzymes which help break down undigested protein; it also destroys parasites and dries *dampness* in general. Other generally beneficial fruits are cranberry, pomegranate, persimmon, cherry, fig (dried), grape, and mango.

Fruit and fruit juice should ideally be meals by themselves. They often interfere with the digestion of other foods. Those who use fruit and vegetable juice therapy throughout the day should take the fruit juices in the morning and vegetable juices during the afternoon and evening. If a carbohydrate meal is eaten, juices ought to be drunk at least one hour before, or three to four hours afterwards.

Grains in their whole state are generally beneficial in the treatment of cancer and other serious degenerations. Whole grains are an important source of vegetable lignins, a group of compounds mentioned earlier (found in flax seed), with anti-tumor and antioxidant properties. The rich fiber in grains produces short-chain fatty acids, including butyrate, acetate, and propionate, which inhibit candida yeast growth. Butyrate in particular has been shown to suppress the growth of cancer in the colon of humans, and cancer in general in animals.[60-62]

Oats were recommended to those with cancer and general debility by American herbalist Jethro Kloss, as a daily breakfast cereal in many health clinics in Europe, and also by Max Gerson. One beneficial action of oats is their nervine property, which helps relax the patient; the high fiber content of oats cleanses the arteries and other areas of the body of mucoid deposits; they also strengthen and regulate the *qi* energy, which is often stagnant in cancer. Oats were used in the early days of this century to boost resistance to disease. Kloss attributed this action to their antiseptic property, which discourages invading microorganisms. During the early phases of detoxification, oat water or a thin oat porridge, because of its mucilaginous properties, can soothe an inflamed and overly sensitive digestive tract.

After oats, rye is considered one of the most beneficial grains in cancer therapy because of its bitter principle and its ability to dry *dampness.* A very digestible form of rye is sourdough bread. (Omit salt from rye bread in recipe section—dulse powder may be substituted.) Yeasted breads must not be used.

Wheat is generally not emphasized in the treatment of cancer because it often causes allergic reactions and also promotes tissue growth. Nevertheless, its ability to nourish the heart and calm the spirit recommends it to those who are unsettled, restless, and insomniac. It also treats night sweats and other forms of sweating that result from *deficiency.* In these conditions, even if wheat allergy exists, one may benefit from its hypoallergenic forms: fresh wheat germ, presoaked, cooked kamut or spelt berries, cooked wheat sprouts, and "Essene" sprouted-wheat bread. Rejuvelac wheat drink (page 613) promotes healthful intestinal flora.

Corn has diuretic properties which relieve water stagnation; Ayurvedic medicine suggests corn stimulates metabolism and oxidation.

Millet and roasted buckwheat groats (kasha) are the only alkaline-forming grains. Since carcinogenic and degenerative diseases frequently arise from the over-consumption of acid-forming foods, these two grains are particularly recommended. Both are also rich sources of fiber and silica, which detoxify the intestines and form butyrate.

Brown rice tonifies the body and mind, and is beneficial for those with *deficiency,* loose stools, weakness, pallor, and mental depression.

Barley is sometimes used in Chinese medicine for reducing tumors. In general it strengthens digestion and treats diarrhea; however, it is not good in cases of constipation. Barley goes well in soups. A similar but more effective plant for treating cancer[63] (and rheumatoid arthritis) is the herb "Job's tears" *(Coix lachryma-jobi),* known in Chinese medicine by its Mandarin name *yi yi ren.* These seeds, sometimes sold in packages incorrectly labeled "pearl barley," are found in all Chinese and some Western herb stores and are prepared as a tea. The sprouts of barley (as well as rice and millet sprouts) are especially beneficial for treating weak digestion with food stagnation and candida symptoms. They also promote the flow of *qi* in stagnant liver patterns.

Amaranth, a grain-like seed, is quite bitter and one of the best "grains" for eliminating excesses associated with degenerative diseases. Quinoa, a related seed, is rich in fat and protein content, and can be used moderately.

Grains must be thoroughly chewed to activate their healing properties.

Animal products are not recommended during the cleansing phases of treatment unless there is severe *deficiency,* in which case one of the most easily digested animal foods is goat's milk. The fat in goat milk is easier to digest than that in cow's milk. Goat milk also has a mildly astringent property, and therefore does not cause mucus like other dairy or meats. This does not mean that goat milk is a specific food for cancer and other serious degenerations, but that it can be counted as one of the least damaging of the animal products, and is the animal product of choice for those who have recovered but are weak and *deficient,* or have a *deficient yin* syndrome. If animal meats seem called for because of severe weakness, fresh "omega-3 fish" can be eaten: sardine, anchovy, trout, herring, salmon, cod, butterfish, and eel. (See page 158 for preparation and dosage.)

Sweeteners: Sweeteners must be used moderately; otherwise, they can cause infections and growths to spread. The best sweetener during cancer therapy is stevia leaf and its products, and this is the only sweetener tolerated by those with candida overgrowth symptoms. The most robust and *excessive* persons (DIET C) should use only stevia and/or raw (unpasteurized) honey.

Those with *deficiency* or weakness (DIET A), or with signs of strength (DIET B) may, in addition to stevia and raw honey, take with care certain other sweeteners: maple syrup, barley malt, rice syrup, and molasses. Choose the highest quality, organic varieties if possible.

Spices: Certain aromatic spices are helpful for clearing liver stagnancy, drying up virus-feeding *dampness,* and adding variety to meals. Too much spice, however, especially of the fiery variety, can aggravate the liver and encourage cancer and other serious diseases to spread. The following mildly aromatic spices, if taken in small amounts, favorably stimulate the *qi* energy of the liver and thus remove stagnation: anise, dill, fennel, coriander, marjoram, sage, saffron, thyme, rosemary, bay leaf, sorrel, turmeric, mace, allspice. Turmeric is especially valuable (see page 210). Parsley and chives can be used moderately as spices; they contain sulfur and other antiviral compounds.

Herbs: Effective herbs for the treatment of cancer, serious virus-related conditions, and most degenerative diseases include those that are antiviral and antifungal, oxygenating, immune-enhancing, and stagnancy-clearing, *viz.,* stagnations of the blood, mucus, moisture, or *qi.* Often these herbs are bitter or aromatic in nature; such substances remove moisture. More than twenty years ago, a Native American healer from Lava Hot Springs, Idaho, traveled the Rocky Mountain West, successfully treating cancer patients with chaparral as the primary remedy. Chaparral, extremely bitter, contains NDGA (nordihydroguaiaretic acid), an anticancer substance. It is also thought to possess more of the antioxidant enzyme SOD than any other plant.

Herbs used widely in South America for cancer, even by medical doctors, are pau d'arco *(Tabevulia)* and Suma *(Pfaffia paniculata).* These herbs are less bitter than chaparral, and work by tonifying immunity. Suma is traditionally used in nearly all chronic disorders. Note: "Suma" is a both a trade name and the most common name for *Pfaffia paniculata*, which is sometimes—and more properly—called "pfaffia." A broad immune-enhancing formula is a decoction of equal parts of:

- Chaparral leaf
- Pau d'arco (inner bark)
- Suma root
- dried Ling Zhi (Reishi), Maitake, or Shiitake mushrooms
- Peach seed

Each herb in this formula is useful for cancer and viral diseases taken singly; the combination is even more effective. It is composed of herbs commonly used in the treatment of AIDS, candida proliferation, cancer, rheumatoid arthritis, multiple sclerosis, and frequent colds and flus. Peach seed *(Prunus persica;* Mandarin: *tao ren)* is the kernel inside the peach pit, and is especially effective where there are signs of stagnant blood. It is also a common anti-cancer herb used by the Chinese. To determine which mushroom is best to take: ling zhi targets the liver and heart-mind, maitake is the most cleansing, and targets the liver and lungs, whereas shiitake is the most tonifying, especially for weak digestion and assimilation. All three stimulate protective *qi* immune functions.

Because of the extreme bitterness of chaparral, it may be best taken in capsules or tablets. Pau d'arco and Suma are most commonly marketed as extracts, tablets, or capsules, and the mushrooms are also available in these forms, as well as fresh. An important consideration when using the various options is to take all herbs at the same time, to create the synergetic effect. This formula is suitable for those following DIET B or similar plans. For persons needing greater tonification and who follow treatments such as DIET A, Suma and the mushrooms in the above formula are added to more tonic herbs, all in equal parts:

- Suma root
- dried Ling Zhi (Reishi), Maitake, or Shiitake mushrooms
- Job's-tears seeds
- American Ginseng root
- Astragalus root

Astragalus *(Astragalus membranaceus et al.*; Mandarin: *huang qi)* builds energy, strengthens digestion and resistance to disease, and is useful in wasting conditions. American ginseng *(Panax quinquefolium)* also builds energy while it rejuvenates the body; it treats the *deficient yin* syndrome in which the fluids and tissues of the body are depleted. This formula of tonic herbs is often most acceptable to the debilitated person when cooked into soups or grain porridges such as rice congee. (Add herbs to the soup or porridge in the amounts that provide the standard dosage.) Following is an herbal formula to be taken as an adjunct to highly cleansing programs such as DIET C.

The root of the common herb dandelion *(Taraxacum officinalis)* has antiviral and antifungal properties and has often proven effective in cancer. Poke root

(Phytolacca acinosa; Mandarin: *shang lu),* another important anti-cancer herb, has purgative effects but is toxic if overconsumed. This herb has been used in both China and America to treat cancer as well as lymphatic and glandular swellings. The late herbalist Dr. John Christopher recommended an important cancer formula of two parts poke root and one part each of dandelion root and gentian root *(Gentiana lutea).*[64] Because of the potency and toxicity of poke root, this decoction is taken in one-tablespoon doses three times a day. If too much is taken, fever and nausea and, in extreme cases, delirium may occur. These symptoms may be reduced by eating mung beans or mung bean sprouts. Licorice *(Glycyrrhiza glabra)* tea also relieves the symptoms.

Gentian, according to Christopher, feeds oxygen to the tissues. This formula is most useful in the first few weeks of detoxification by those with excess-type constipation (dry, hard stools and *heat* signs such as red, dry tongue with yellow coating). Those who continue to have general *excess* and *heat* signs (red face, loud voice, constipation, robust personality, thick, yellow tongue coating, strong pulse, etc.) may use it for longer periods. If the flavor is unacceptable, stir in one-quarter teaspoon of stevia powder per cup, or add one-half part licorice root to the formula.

Preserving Health

After cancer or other degenerative conditions subside, it is essential to continue a high-quality diet and all the recommendations in this section against impure water, poor-quality oils, refined foods, excessive animal foods, and so on. Degenerative diseases have a tendency to re-establish themselves whenever there is renewed stress from poor diet or lifestyle extremes. Of course, after recovery, one need not continue to emphasize such strong or cleansing foods as garlic, papaya, tomatoes, mushrooms, radishes, and purgative herbs; if the cleansing diet had been primarily raw foods, cooked foods can gradually be added until a balanced diet is attained.

Other Degenerative Disorders

The list of degenerative diseases prevalent in highly developed countries is long. Some of the more common, besides cancer, include AIDS, multiple sclerosis, arthritic and rheumatic disorders, chronic fatigue (immune dysfunction) syndrome (CFS or CFIDS), Epstein-Barr virus, Alzheimer's disease, alcoholism and other intoxicant abuses, asthma, schizophrenia, severe skin diseases, and kidney failure. Similar to cancer but far less dangerous are cysts and benign tumors. These are treated in the same way as cancer, but take much longer to dissolve. This is particularly the case with uterine and fibroid tumors.

As discussed earlier, a totally separate dietary program for each degenerative condition is unnecessary. Rather, it is more practical to treat personal differences with some combination of the three wide-ranging regeneration diets: DIETS A, B, and C (page 407). These can be supplemented with other options to balance specific conditions not fully addressed by the diets. The three diets are designed to treat the major problems common to many degenerative diseases:

1. degeneration of the entire system
2. impaired immunity
3. *excess* signs often coexisting with severe *deficiencies*
4. slow and difficult healing, requiring treatment of all organs and systems
5. *dampness*-related syndromes such as viral, yeast, fungal, and parasitic infections and/or other stagnations including edema, mucus, and stagnant energy and/or blood (for a valuable perspective on the interplay between "pleomorphic" microbes and the bodily environment, see note 8 for Chapter 26 on page 696).
6. oxygen debt

A successful dietary program for these conditions usually requires some level of cleansing/reducing therapy, parasite purging, fresh vegetarian food, few or no animal products, and immune-enhancing treatments including appropriate herbs, omega-3 and GLA oils, chlorophyll-rich foods, moderate regular exercise, undereating, simple food-combining—in short, the entire program for DIETS A, B, and C. Thus the choices for dietary and herbal options depend on the patient's strength or weakness, as outlined in the regeneration diet section in terms of *excess, deficiency,* and other diagnostic factors. Following are features that need to be emphasized when applying the regeneration diets to each degenerative disorder.

Rheumatic and Arthritic Conditions

Rheumatism is characterized by pain in the bones, joints, muscles, tendons, or nerves, and is often seen as including such disorders as rheumatoid arthritis, gout, bursitis, neuritis, and sciatica. (Arthritis is more specifically defined as joint inflammation.) All of these conditions are marked by mineral imbalances in the affected tissues, with calcium status being a good indicator of mineralization in general.

Thus, in every form of these diseases, avoid calcium inhibitors: excess meat or protein from any source; intoxicants (alcohol, tobacco, coffee, marijuana, and all others); refined sugar and too many sweets; and excess salt. Also restrict foods high in oxalic acid, such as rhubarb, cranberry, plum, chard, beet greens, and spinach.

Nightshade family vegetables—especially tomato, but also eggplant, bell pepper and potato—frequently cause problems. To determine whether they are primary allergens, one can avoid them for six weeks, then add each one to the diet for a few days, one at a time. If symptoms of pain and swelling increase, then the offending nightshade(s) should be avoided. If they cause no noticeable problems, it is still wise to use these vegetables sparingly because they contain solanine, a calcium inhibitor.

From the *Calcium* chapter, we know that calcium-deficiency problems call for a balance of all minerals, and that magnesium and silicon play key roles. We also know that dairy products, because of their high fat content (49% of the caloric value of whole milk is fat), are sometimes the cause of, not the cure for, calcic disorders. We have known patients who enjoyed relatively wholesome diets but found that they could not be free of rheumatism or arthritis until they stopped eating dairy foods. In many cases, however, fresh goat milk is beneficial because of its more digestible fat, abundant fluorine, and broad mineralization.

Also important are chlorophyll-rich foods, adequate sunshine and moderate exercise. Barley- and wheat-grass products, because of their many anti-inflammatory and detoxification properties, excel in the treatment of nearly all types of arthritis and rheumatism. Alfalfa, in tablets or tea, is also of exceptional benefit in most cases; neutral in thermal nature, alfalfa is effective in these conditions with either *cold* or *heat* signs.

The appropriate regeneration DIET A, B, or C (beginning on page 407) is useful for healing damaged tissues. These diets are also excellent sources of the minerals and chlorophyll foods recommended above. Among the specific foods in these diets (see "Recommended Food Groups" beginning on page 416), it is best to avoid the above-mentioned oxalate vegetables and fruits, and restrict nightshade consumption. Otherwise, all other recommended vegetables and fruits, sprouts, algae/micro-algae, cereal grasses, grains, sweeteners, and animal products are generally beneficial (unless contraindicated by syndromes specific to the individual). Restrict consumption of all nuts, oil-rich seeds, nut butters, and similar products; these tend to promote *damp* stagnation. Almonds (5 or 6 daily maximum) and the omega-3/GLA-rich seeds are the exceptions.

Further Causes and Remedies:

1) *Wind* and *dampness* are part of the usual rheumatic/arthritic diagnostic picture. Internally generated *wind* is frequently a feature of a stagnant liver, in which the *qi* is not smoothly distributed, causing nervousness and fluctuating symptoms. The *dampness* is usually generated by toxic mucus-like residues from the incomplete digestion of dairy foods, meats, refined sugars (including alcohol), and poor-quality fats and oils. (Note that some of these items are also the calcium inhibitors listed above.) *Dampness* and *wind* obstruct the nerves and other channels of energy transport, including the acupuncture meridians. Such chronic obstruction leads to nerve, bone, and sinew pain and inflammation.

In many cases, *dampness, wind,* or other influences are combined, with none predominating. In other cases, one influence is most pronounced. For example, if *dampness* is the most prominent influence, there will be swelling and edema, obesity, a feeling of heaviness in the extremities, sluggishness, and dull pain. *Damp* excesses are reduced by each of the regeneration diets; of special benefit are the pungents listed under "Deficiency-type" below.

If *wind* is the major influence, there is pain that moves around in the body or that comes and goes; frequently there is also dizziness. *Wind* also is reduced by each of the regeneration diets, although buckwheat should be omitted because of its tendency to increase *wind*. Specific foods, spices, and herbs that quell *wind* are given in the *Wood Element* chapter, pages 328–329.

When *heat* signs (fever or inflamed, swollen joints) are pronounced, DIETS B or C are best until *heat* has been subdued, then DIET A. Individuals with arthritic and rheumatic complaints are particularly sensitive to adverse climates, and should avoid overexposure to wind, dampness, and any other influences that correspond to those they harbor internally. Climatic wind drives all external influences, including dampness, into the body.

2) A diet rich in animal fats not only promotes *wind/damp* obstructions as mentioned above, but also contributes directly to tissue pain and inflammation in another way. Animal fats are the primary sources of arachidonic acid, which through various metabolic pathways in the body initiates the production of pain-inducing, inflammatory prostaglandins (PGE_2) as well as leukotrienes (discussed in *Oils and Fats* chapter). Leukotrienes are the most powerful sources of inflammation yet discovered in the body, and their production can be inhibited by ingestion of omega-3 and GLA fatty acids, recommended as part of the regeneration diets. In clinical trails, a majority of rheumatoid arthritics either stopped or reduced by half their anti-inflammatory medication after using combinations of omega-3 and omega-6 fatty acids.[65] Flax oil (53% omega-3) and GLA-rich oils (80% omega-6) are often used together for this purpose. All forms of arthritis and rheumatism seem to benefit from the anti-inflammatory, immune-enhancing "omega-3" fish or plant oils and "GLA" oils.[66-69] Other oils, if unrefined monounsaturates, may be used sparingly (see "Oil-Rich Products," pages 413–415, for guidelines on using the above oils).

3) Internally generated *damp* toxins sometimes enter the blood stream through a "leaky gut," a condition in which partially digested foods penetrate through weakened areas in the intestines and are absorbed by the blood. In response, the immune system triggers inflammations as it attempts to counteract these food-borne antigens. The leaky-gut syndrome seems to be made worse by frequent use of nonsteroidal anti-inflammatory drugs (NSAIDs),[70] which are taken by many arthritis sufferers. A diet with insufficient fiber is a primary cause of poor intestinal integrity.

Herbal Therapy. To reduce *wind/damp* excesses and other toxins more quickly than with diet alone, as long as there is not severe *deficiency*, specific "antirheumatic" herbs work more efficiently than the regeneration diet herbal formulas. Such herbs should include those that dry *dampness* (e.g., chaparral and burdock), reduce inflammation (e.g., devil's claw, burdock, black cohosh), produce sweating to excrete *exterior* toxins lodged in the tendons and joints (e.g., sassafras and black cohosh), quell *wind* with antispasmodic properties (e.g., black cohosh and ginger), and stimulate circulation to penetrate blockages (e.g., prickly ash and ginger).

The resulting formula is composed of herbs traditionally used in the West for arthritic and rheumatic disorders.

4 parts Chaparral leaf *(Larrea divaricata)*
2 parts Devil's Claw root *(Harpagophytum procumbens)*
2 parts Sassafras root bark *(Sassafras albidum)*
2 parts dried Ginger root *(Zingiber officinale)*
1 part Black Cohosh root *(Cimicifuga racemosa)*
1 part Burdock root *(Arctium lappa)*
1 part Prickly Ash bark *(Xanthoxylum americanum)*

Note: If the bitterness of this formula proves to be unacceptable, add 1 part licorice root; or take the chaparral—the most bitter component—in capsules or tablets. Another option is to encapsulate all herbs of the combined formula. (Follow the standard herbal dosage and preparation [page 110] throughout this section.)

The above formula is best for those with pronounced signs of *dampness, heat,* or general *excess* (strong, robust constitution, loud voice and thick tongue coating); it should be taken only until these signs are no longer present.

***Deficiency*-type.** The above formula is not appropriate, however, for individuals who are generally *deficient* (weak, frail constitution, pale complexion, little or no tongue coating, introverted personality), or who have weak digestion and loose stools, or pronounced *cold* signs (constant, sharp joint pain that improves with applications of heat; pale complexion; aversion to the cold and cold foods). In these cases, DIET A is the best choice, and the foods should be moderately or well cooked. Specific foods to emphasize: pungents which remove *damp* or *cold* obstructions, such as black peppercorn (freshly ground), dill, fennel, coriander, marjoram, sage, saffron, thyme, rosemary, bay leaf, onion, chives, garlic, horseradish (best if pickled in vinegar), and ginger root; grains, vegetables, and legumes with warming or neutral thermal natures including oats, spelt, quinoa, rice, corn, mustard greens, parsley, parsnip, and black beans. Of these foods, garlic and/or horseradish are often highly effective after a few weeks of regular (twice-daily) use. The bioflavonoid quercetin, abundant in onions and garlic, reduces the formation of inflammatory prostaglandins and leukotrienes mentioned above.[71, 72]

Pine or fir tree pitch is a useful folk remedy for rheumatic complaints: eat a pea-sized piece once or twice daily, but for no longer than five weeks (long-term use may cause mild toxicity). Fish with warming or neutral thermal properties and ample omega-3 oils, including trout, anchovy, sardine, salmon, tuna, and butterfish, can be used in treating *cold* or *deficient* individuals. Chicken may also be helpful. Small amounts of cereal grasses and seaweeds, though cooling, are beneficial, unless stools are loose or watery. Appropriate herbs create warmth and circulation (angelica, cinnamon bark, prickly ash), dry *dampness* (motherwort and Suma), reduce *wind* (osha/ligusticum and angelica), promote perspiration (angelica and osha/ligusticum), and enhance immunity (Suma and Siberian ginseng):

4 parts Suma root *(Pfaffia paniculata)*
4 parts Motherwort *(Leonurus cardiaca)*
4 parts Prickly Ash bark *(Xanthoxylum americanum)*
4 parts Osha/Ligusticum root *(Ligusticum-related species)*

2 parts Angelica root *(Angelica archangelica)*
1½ parts Siberian Ginseng *(Eleutherococcus senticosus)*
1½ parts Cinnamon bark *(Cinnamomum cassia)*

Although generally most effective in a formula such as the above, Suma, osha/ligusticum, angelica, motherwort, and Siberian ginseng are also beneficial when taken singly. The formula with American ginseng (page 423) may be used when there is severe *deficiency*. Osha *(Ligusticum porteri)* is more powerfully acting than its sister plant, *Ligusticum wallichii* from China (Mandarin: *chuan xiong*). Nevertheless, the Chinese variety is effective, and can be found at all Chinese and many Western herb outlets, and may be substituted if osha, a wildcrafted herb, is not available.

Various salves, liniments, and other external applications with such ingredients as camphor, peppermint oil, eucalyptus oil, wintergreen oil, cinnamon oil, tea oil (from *Oleum camelliae,* a common tea plant), cayenne, wormwood, and lobelia may increase the healing rate as well as reduce symptoms in rheumatic and arthritic conditions (see "cayenne liniment," page 395).

*   *   *

Like other degenerations, rheumatoid arthritis is often thought to be accompanied by the proliferation in the body of various harmful microbes,[73] which in some cases can be controlled by prescription drugs (e.g., hydroxychloroquine sulfate and clotrimazole[74]). Since there are side effects to all drugs, we recommend using them as a last resort, and working first with the above herbal formulas and the suggestions accompanying the regeneration diets, especially the hyper-oxygenation methods and garlic, both of which destroy a wide range of pathogenic microbes.

Beta-carotene helps prevent tissue destruction in rheumatoid arthritis.[75] Rich beta-carotene food sources with anti-inflammatory properties include cereal grasses and wild blue-green and spirulina micro-algae. Periodic use of a vegan diet is also a beneficial treatment.[76] (In fact, we have yet to know—or even hear of—a case of arthritis in which painful symptoms persisted more than a few months after the start of a high-quality grain and vegetable-based regime such as DIET A.) Avoid alfalfa seeds and sprouts; these contain the amino acid canavanine, which may promote inflammatory reactions in rheumatoid diseases (including *lupus erythematosus*).[77] However, alfalfa leaf and other sprouts are generally useful.

Alcoholism and Other Intoxicant Abuses

Desires for strong substances that lead to addictions originate with imbalance, usually in the form of mental/physical/spiritual stagnations and blockages. The diets that support these stagnations are generally too heavy and *yin,* containing great excesses of such items as salt, meats, fats, poor quality and synthetic hydrogenated oils, and chemical ingredients—which help generate accumulations of *heat*, *wind*, and *damp* excesses with accompanying depression, anger, pain, and inflammation. Most intoxicants temporarily relieve the distressing symptoms of these obstructions in the body-mind. Clearly, one should avoid obstructive dietary and lifestyle habits which make intoxicants appealing.

A plethora of intoxicants and other substances can become addictive; among the more prevalent are alcohol, marijuana, cocaine, LSD, amphetamines, heroin, and methadone; even the most commonly abused stimulants such as tobacco, coffee, and refined sugar can present withdrawal problems equal to those of more dangerous drugs. Once intoxicant addictions become rooted, the whole being degenerates, and various disorders arise, especially:[78]

- liver *qi* stagnation (swellings, lumps, distended abdomen and chest, tension, thyroid problems, repressed emotions, frustration, anger, impatience), which over time leads to liver *heat* (red face, eyes, and tongue, insomnia, splitting headaches, constipation, aggression, violence), liver *wind* (moving or fluctuating pain, pulsating headache, spasms, cramps, dizziness, manic/depression) and/or deficient liver *yin* (dry eyes, weak vision, night blindness, dry brittle nails, and other general *deficient yin* signs). For remedies see "Summary of Common Liver Syndromes" beginning on page 324.
- kidney-adrenal stress, resulting in deficient kidney *yin* (ringing in the ears, dry throat, dizziness, low backache, weak legs, red tongue, insecurity, agitation), deficient kidney *yang* (cold extremities, aversion to cold, weak knees and low back, frequent urination, edema, enlarged, pale tongue, lack of will power), and deficient *jing* (poor physical and/or mental development, inadequate brain function, early senility, impotence, dizziness, loose teeth, loss of head hair). Many drug "highs" consume massive amounts of *jing* essence. For remedies see "Common Syndromes of the Kidneys" beginning on page 356.
- lung *yin* deficiency (dry cough, periodic fever, frequent thirst, fresh-red cheeks, night sweats, hot palms), especially resulting from smoking addictions to marijuana or tobacco. For remedies see "*Deficient Yin* of the Lungs," page 350.
- heart-mind spirit derangements (lack of mental focus, forgetfulness, poor sleep patterns, mental illness, speech problems, and agitation during detoxification). For remedies see "Calming and Focusing the Mind" beginning on page 336.
- general *deficiency* (frailty, weakness, faint voice and shallow breath, little or no tongue coating, lack of motivation) and blood deficiency (pale lips, nailbeds, tongue, and complexion; thinness; thin, dry hair; spots in the field of vision; irregular menstruation). To treat general *deficiency,* see page 91; for blood *deficiency,* page 387.

If two or more of the above syndromes are present, avoid remedies that are contraindicated by any syndrome. All remedies can be integrated into the regeneration diets, beginning on page 407.

Addictions to strong substances and drugs—including prescription drugs—that result in substantial toxicity and stagnation can be treated with the appropriate regeneration diet. The main consideration is to match the dietary and herbal program to the specific condition of the person. Because intoxicants sometimes cause unusual patterns of simultaneous strengths and weaknesses in the body, dietary flexibility is important. Those taking prescription drugs should stop only with the advice of a physician.

One of the primary aims in addiction work is a smooth, obstruction-releasing *qi* flow throughout the body-mind so that intoxicants are no longer craved. This entails clearing the liver, which directs smooth *qi* flow in general. Imbedded in the liver are chemical residues representing the life history of unresolved problems, denials, resentments, and repressions that have been masked by intoxicants.

The regeneration diets, with their emphasis on cereal grasses, seaweeds, sprouts, light, metabolism-enhancing GLA/omega-3 oils, chlorophyll foods, and their restriction of heavy, greasy, stagnation-producing foods, are optimal for clearing liver stagnancy and the attendant emotional and physical problems.

In the regeneration diet's "Recommended Food Groups," there are no restrictions *per se* on any item for persons overcoming addictions, so any grains, vegetables, fruits, or legumes can be eaten as long as these foods are suited to the constitutional condition and syndromes involved. The suggestions for "Oil-Rich Products" (page 413), however, should be followed rigorously. Too many fats, nuts, and oil-bearing seeds, or insufficient omega-3/GLA oils, will have a pronounced negative effect on rejuvenation. If needed for overcoming *deficiency* and weakness, some of the best animal products for clearing stagnation are the omega-3-rich fish (page 422) and raw goat milk products.

As discussed elsewhere in this book, many individuals with severe addictions are hypoglycemic (see pages 375–377), and have extreme nutrient deficiencies in general. The regeneration diets supply an abundance of vitamins, minerals, enzymes, amino acids, and other necessary nutrients in their freshest, most assimilable form. If these or similar diets are not followed, simply adding nutrient-rich foods such as micro-algae, kelp or other sea vegetables, cereal grass, herbs, and fresh flax oil to the present diet will help. If the diet remains poor, supplements containing individual nutrients may be useful.

Herbal Therapies. The first two herbal formulas (beginning on page 422) recommended for the regeneration diets work very well for most intoxicant addictions. The formula containing chaparral is appropriate for the majority of addiction patients. Chaparral is extremely efficient at detoxification and is thought to extract the residues of all intoxicating substances, including those of marijuana, LSD, and cocaine. The most debilitated individuals should choose the formula with American ginseng. Individuals with definite *excessive* signs (robust, strong body, thick tongue coating, reddish complexion) and constipation will benefit from the formulas below containing golden seal.

Two remedies are based on golden seal root *(Hydrastis canadensis)*, an intensely bitter, cooling, anti-inflammatory, antibiotic, laxative herb. Golden seal is most appropriate for relatively strong persons with *excessive* conditions that may include infections, digestive problems, liver stagnancy, and/or general *heat* signs (red face, yellow tongue coating, constipation, aversion to heat, aggression). The first remedy, golden seal combined with cayenne *(Capsicum frutescens)* in equal parts, is used to treat alcoholism; it stimulates *qi* flow to push through obstructions, reduces liver excesses, and dries most forms of *dampness* including mucus, obesity, edema, parasites, and arterial plaque.

Another golden seal-based formula for treating cocaine, heroin, and methadone addiction includes herbs that detoxify the liver and remove stagnation and *dampness* (golden seal and spearmint), decrease stress by moistening lung and kidney *yin* (marshmallow root *[Althea officinalis]*), clear obstructions (orange peel or other citrus peel *[Citrus reticulata;* Mandarin: *chen pi]*), cleanse the lungs and lymphatic system (mullein leaf *[Verbascum thaspus]*), calm the mind, soothe digestion and open consciousness with an aromatic quality (spearmint leaf *[Mentha virides]*). The proportion of herbs in this formula is 2 parts each of golden seal, mullein, and marshmallow root, and 1 part each of orange peel and spearmint. Both of the above formulas can be powdered and taken in capsule form to avoid their bitter taste. For those wanting a tasty, simple, mildly therapeutic tea to drink during the day to calm the nerves, settle digestion, and gently reduce liver stagnation, one of the mint-related herbs is a good choice—lemon balm, spearmint, peppermint, or catnip.

A more gradually acting herbal therapy than the golden seal or chaparral formulas is the Chinese herb bupleurum root. It is useful for reducing general *excess* but is not as radically cleansing as golden seal or chaparral; it also does not share these herbs' laxative properties. Thus bupleurum is better in cases of less extreme *excess,* or after initial cleansing has eliminated constipation and substantially reduced *excess* signs.

Bupleurum is a specific remedy for liver stagnancy, *heat,* and *wind* conditions. As it regulates the total liver complex of emotional and physical imbalances, it relaxes stressed body tissues while harmonizing the often angry, discordant liver emotions. Bupleurum directs energy higher in the body, and therefore treats organ prolapse as well as mental depression.

An important formula for many of those with addictions is "Bupleurum Sedative Pills," also known as "Free and Easy Wanderer" *(Xiao Yao Wan)* pills in China; the following herbs in this formula are used to: overcome liver-caused stress, relax the nerves, soothe the emotions, and detoxify poisons (bupleurum, peony, licorice, peppermint), improve circulation (ginger and *dang gui*), build the blood *(dang gui* and peony root), strengthen digestion and reduce hypoglycemia (atractylodes), increase *qi* (licorice and atractylodes), and calm the mind (poria cocos and peppermint). The pills are commonly available through herbalists carrying Chinese herbs. For those who prefer to obtain the individual herbs for tea or capsules, the proportion of herbs in "Free and Easy Wanderer" is:

> 5 parts Bupleurum root *(Bupleurum falcatum;* Mandarin: *chai hu)*
> 5 parts *Dang Gui* root *(Angelica sinensis;* Mandarin: *dang gui)*
> 5 parts Peony root *(Paeonia lactiflora;* Mandarin: *bai shao)*
> 5 parts Poria Cocos mushroom *(Poria cocos;* Mandarin: *fu ling)*

5 parts Atractylodes root *(Atractylodes alba;* Mandarin: *bai zhu)*
5 parts Ginger root *(Zingiber officinale;* Mandarin: *gan jiang)*
4 parts Licorice root *(Glycyrrhiza glabra;* Mandarin: *gan coa)*
1 part Peppermint leaf *(Mentha piperita;* Mandarin: *bo he)*

Exercise and Activity. Regular exercise stimulates *qi* circulation and thereby clears blockages, burns up toxins, helps food to digest, and reduces depression. Involvement in groups (e.g., yoga, prayer/meditation) with lofty purposes in life is often helpful for developing new attitudes and inspiration for changing an addictive, abusive lifestyle.

Alcoholism: The physical symptoms of this addiction may involve any of the disorders common to intoxicant addictions, listed earlier. In addition, it is nearly always characterized by *heat* combined with toxic *dampness,* and so cooling foods that dry *dampness* must be emphasized. DIET A is effective, although DIETS B or C, if the person shows signs of strength, are often better because of their more cooling and cleansing nature. Ideally, B or C is used until *heat* signs diminish—typically during the first few weeks of detoxification.

Certain cooling, detoxifying foods are commonly prescribed by Chinese medicine in the treatment of alcoholism: tofu, mung bean sprouts, mung beans, fresh wheat germ, romaine lettuce, banana, either sugar cane or dried unrefined cane juice (e.g., Rapadura™), pears, and spinach. Honey eaten by the spoonful until satiation during a hangover reduces the desire for more alcohol. GLA fatty acids (discussed in the *Oils and Fats* chapter) help reduce the desire for alcohol. Soups are helpful and provide a good medium for tofu, mung beans, romaine lettuce, and spinach in the diet. The herb American ginseng *(Panax quinquefolium)* is prized in East Asia for the treatment of alcoholism, and may be used in conjunction with the golden seal or chaparral formulas given earlier. In the event of extreme weakness, American ginseng is indicated as part of the regeneration diet herbal formula containing it (page 423). (Because of its warming nature, do not use Chinese or Korean *Panax ginseng.*) Avoid warming spices such as ginger, cinnamon, and black pepper.

After a cleansing program that purges *heat* and other signs of *excess,* high protein sources can be added for one to two years to rebuild the liver. Especially beneficial is spirulina or other green micro-algae; in cases of weakness, small amounts (1–3 ounces) of omega-3-rich animal products also may be necessary three or four times per week: sardine, mackerel, tuna, pork liver, and pork or beef kidney.

Tobacco addiction: Ingestion of lobelia herb is of specific benefit. The chemical lobeline, found in lobelia, closely resembles nicotine, and therefore reduces cravings for it. Several times daily and during cravings, drink ¼ cup lobelia tea, or take 10–20 drops of the tincture.

Regular consumption of oats has been shown to curb the desire for cigarettes.[79] This may be due to their sedative properties. Nicotine spreads through all body tissues, damaging them like other powerful drugs; cellular renewal with the pure food and herbal nutrition in the regeneration diets is indicated.

Asthma

According to both Eastern and Western diagnostic measures, asthma involves disharmony in one or more organ systems: 1) the digestive center (spleen-pancreas, stomach, and intestines), 2) the kidney-adrenals and liver/gall bladder, and/or 3) the heart and lungs. Most often, all these systems malfunction, with one of them most imbalanced. These organ imbalances are corrected by following the specific guidelines for treating the major types of asthma, listed below. Note: The regeneration DIETS A, B, and C are given beginning on page 407; all herbs should be used according to the standard preparations and dosages (page 110).

Cold-type asthma: characterized by white, clear, or foamy mucus, cold extremities, pale face, and a frequent feeling of coldness. Use DIET A, but modify it by cooking all food moderately to well. Foods and spices which are especially helpful: garlic, mustard greens, anise, sweet marjoram, basil, fresh ginger, blackstrap molasses, almond, sunflower seed, walnut, Chinese or Korean ginseng *(Panax ginseng),* black bean, and oats. The nuts and seeds may be eaten regularly, but only in small amounts. Walnuts are the most useful for cold-type asthma.

Heat-type asthma: characterized by fast, heavy breathing, red face, sensation of heat in the body, yellow mucus, dry stools, and scanty urine. Especially helpful foods and herbs: daikon radish, sprouts, apricot (a maximum of five daily), lime, lemon, tofu, nettle leaf *(Urtica urens),* horehound *(Marrubium vulgare).* Follow DIETS B or C until *heat* is reduced, then shift to DIET A.

Mucus-type asthma: characterized by copious mucus; mouth is often held open; breathing is difficult when lying down; tongue coating is thick and greasy. Especially helpful foods and spices are: horseradish, lemon, lime, raw honey, aduki bean, alfalfa sprouts, slippery elm tea *(Ulmus fulva),* and the herbal formula below for all types of asthma. If mucus-type asthma is accompanied by *deficiency,* then use the modified DIET A given below; otherwise use DIET B or C.

Deficiency-type asthma: characterized by a weak pulse, little or no tongue coating, pale complexion, shortness of breath, head needing to be propped up in order to sleep, and breathing becoming difficult with slight body exertions. Especially helpful foods are: oats, rice, barley, pollen (start with very small amounts and increase to several teaspoons daily), black beans, nuts (especially walnuts and almonds), buckwheat, figs, and Chinese or Korean ginseng. DIET A is recommended but is modified in this way: the food should be well-cooked.

Note: Of these four types, the mucus-type asthma is the most prevalent in the West, and it often is found in combination with some degree of the *deficiency* type. Thus DIET A is the most suitable for these types. As long as no symptoms of *heat* exist, those with *deficiency-* or mucus-type asthma also benefit from the remedies listed under *cold-*type asthma.

For all types of asthma: Simple food combining (see "Plan B" in *Food Combinations* chapter), deep breathing exercises, outdoor activity, and regular warm baths followed by quick cold showers that cool just the body surface. Avoid breathing chemical fumes, smoke, dust, and becoming chilled. Ice cream, cow's milk, and other bovine dairy must be strictly avoided, but raw goat's milk is usually well-tolerated. Chlorophyll and vitamin-A foods (spirulina and wild blue-green micro-algae, apricot [not more than five per day], pumpkin, carrot, mustard greens, and green vegetables in general) protect the lungs and support cellular renewal. Omega-3 and GLA fatty acids are exceptional for alleviating the constrictions and spasms that frequently accompany asthma. (Food sources and dosages of these oils begin on pages 164 and 173, respectively.)

Emesis (vomiting) therapy is often useful in asthma, especially when symptoms worsen soon after eating. To produce emesis, drink a cup of mint tea or hot lemonade followed by 2 cups of lobelia herb tea (2 cups warm salt water may be substituted), and, if necessary, trigger regurgitation by sliding the middle finger down the throat. To treat the convulsions that may occur with asthma attacks, a little lobelia tea or 10–20 drops of lobelia tincture can be taken.

Asthma is frequently related to low blood sugar. (See symptoms and suggestions in "Hypoglycemia" section, page 375.) Asthma attacks may also be caused by allergies (see "Allergies and Food Combining," page 272). When asthma symptoms match one of the "syndromes of the lungs" (page 349), the appropriate remedies given there may be integrated into the treatments in this section.

A valuable herb/seed tea for treating cold-, mucus-, and deficiency-types of asthma consists of equal parts of

Fennel seed *(Foeniculum officinalis)*
Flaxseed *(Linum usitatissimum)*
Fenugreek seed *(Trigonella foenumgraecum)*
Licorice root *(Glycyrrhiza glabra)*
Lobelia seed and/or leaf *(Lobelia inflata)*
Mullein leaf or flower *(Verbascum thaspus)*

This formula, minus the warming ingredients (fennel and fenugreek), is beneficial for *heat*-type asthma. Because of the tiny hairs on mullein leaves, the tea should be strained through muslin or cotton fabric before drinking.

AIDS

Contrary to popular medical thinking, people with AIDS can recover in response to good nutrition and a balanced lifestyle.[80] Understandably, most AIDS researchers and patients exert tremendous effort in search of a miracle drug cure. When this is the sole focus, the essential work with nutrition and attitudinal healing is easily neglected.

As in any degenerative disease, success is greater the sooner a renewal program is begun. If treatment is begun in the later stages of AIDS when there is extreme *deficiency* characterized by diarrhea, emaciation, fever, night sweats, yeast infections, loss of appetite, and persistent cough: 1) regeneration DIET A is indicated, and the food should be at least moderately cooked or, if desired by the patient, well-cooked (regeneration diets begin on page 407); 2) the *"deficient yin"* food options (page 408) should be included; 3) the herbal formula with astragalus root (page 423) is used with great benefit in all such wasting diseases.

Correct diet may be a deciding factor in healing AIDS and other related viral diseases. The membrane of the human immunodeficiency virus (HIV) associated with AIDS is rich in cholesterol. Therefore it is not surprising that cholesterol-lowering diets show promise as a therapy for AIDS.[81] The high-fiber, low-fat regeneration diets are effective for reducing cholesterol and the saturated fats that contribute to it. Certain features of these diets—the omega-3/GLA fatty acids, the various mushrooms, seaweeds, sprouts, and cleansing herbs—lower cholesterol excesses further, and thereby further inhibit HIV activity.

Traditional Chinese medicine offers a broader view of the value of the regeneration diets: pathogens proliferate best in moist, stagnant, *damp* environments. The regeneration diets with included parasite plan not only destroy pathogens, but are low or absent in such *damp,* stagnancy-producing items as refined foods, heavy fats, dairy products, and meats, and rich in whole fresh foods as well as the features listed in the above paragraph, all of which speed up the metabolism.

People who contract HIV do not always develop AIDS symptoms, even for years afterward in some cases. Evidently, their immune system is sufficiently strong to keep HIV in check. Once AIDS symptoms manifest, rebuilding immunity to the point where HIV is no longer a threat—or even no longer exists in the body—should be the treatment goal. Good immune function is supported by sufficient rest and exercise, healthy food habits, awareness and spirit-strengthening practices, and the avoidance of draining activities such as stress, intoxicants, and promiscuity. (For further insights, see the "Immunity" sections, pages 71–87.)

Because of the likelihood of infections caused by bacteria, viruses, parasites, yeasts, and fungi that proliferate in those with weak immunity, some AIDS patients have benefited from garlic.[82] Garlic inhibits most of the pathogenic types of the above organisms, sometimes more effectively and safely than drugs.[83] HIV rapidly infects cells in the body by spreading via aggregated lymphocytes; the ajoene complex in garlic breaks down these aggregates.[84] Dosage: 10 grams ($\frac{1}{3}$ ounce [approximately three medium-size cloves]) once daily, or 5 grams twice daily, 6 days a week. Note that this dosage for AIDS is much higher than that listed in the "Recommended Food Groups"—see this section (page 419) for the methods and options for consuming garlic. The 10-gram dosage is appropriate only for those following the regeneration diets or similar programs. When a diet of much rich, fatty food is consumed, an effective garlic dosage is often 60–80 grams daily.

Garlic exhibits an extremely warming thermal nature and can therefore deplete the *yin* fluids which, as mentioned earlier, may be already diminished in those with long-standing infections such as occur in AIDS. When *deficient yin* signs (emaciation, periodic low-grade fevers, frequent thirst, night sweats) are present, garlic may still be tolerated if it is balanced by consumption of *yin*-nurturing foods and herbs on a daily basis. An especially helpful *yin* tonic in most of these cases is the gel of the aloe plant, which also possesses substantial antiviral and immune-enhancing activity as a result of a compound it contains known as acemannan (Carrisyn™).[85] In addition, aloe gel has broad anti-fungal and anti-bacterial activity, which proves useful in many of the AIDS-related infections; the cooling nature of the gel counteracts inflammation and its associated pain.[86] Only unrefined, bitter-tasting aloe gel has the healing properties described above. Similar anti-microbial and yin-preserving properties are available from colloidal silver, which is discussed in Appendix A, page 661.

Of special interest to persons with AIDS (and Epstein-Barr virus [EBV])is the herb St. Johnswort *(Hypericum perforatum),* which contains the blood-red volatile oil "hypericin," effective against retro-viruses such as HIV and EBV.[87] (A property of hypericin, rarely encountered in other medicinal herbs, enables it to penetrate the blood/brain barrier[87] and thus treat "brain fatigue" in EBV patients.) The herb also supplies an antidepressant dye which acts on the nervous system to reduce anxiety, hysteria, and depression. Before the twentieth century, St. Johnswort was used to rid the body of "bad spirits," a term associated with serious diseases. Terminology aside, St. Johnswort was correctly identified as having great healing potential in the treatment of difficult conditions. The recent scientific discovery of antiviral properties in St. Johnswort reaffirms the value of our ancestral healing awareness. St. Johnswort can be taken by itself or added to other herbal formulas, including those recommended here.

Another frequently indicated herb is licorice root *(Glycyrrhiza glabra;* Mandarin: *gan cao).* This extremely sweet root harmonizes the liver and greatly helps detoxify the body. It treats sores and carbuncles, improves digestion (strengthens spleen-pancreas *qi,* especially when pan-roasted), moistens dry lungs, stops coughing, reduces inflammation, and relieves sore throats. Research indicates it may counteract various viruses, including herpes simplex I and HIV.[88] Licorice is best taken in small doses and can be added to other herbal formulas, such as those suggested for the regeneration diets, in ½-part quantities. It should not be used in cases of hypertension or edema (watery swelling), and should be discontinued if these conditions develop. If there is diarrhea, use licorice only after pan-roasting. This herb is not to be confused with common "licorice" candy, which often contains no true licorice whatsoever.

Like garlic, oregano oil and citrus seed extract provide unusual broad-spectrum antimicrobial activity against germs, fungi, amoebas, and viruses (see pages 619 and 661), and have therefore been helpful in AIDS therapy. Those with garlic intolerance may find these powerful concentrates particularly valuable.

Other regeneration diet items to be emphasized include: 1) Algae: In addition to their anti-cancer properties, the sulfated polysaccharides in Irish moss, kelp and possibly other common seaweeds appear to have activity against HIV.[89] Kelp,

Irish moss, and edible seaweeds in general are soothing to the lungs and digestive tract, where they cool inflammations. The detoxification properties of seaweeds are indicated in most degenerative diseases unless diarrhea is present.

2) The herbs of the regeneration diets are among the strongest immune tonics—maitake, shiitake, and/or ling zhi mushrooms, astragalus, American ginseng, Suma, and pau d'arco; also included are powerful cleansing remedies for those with substantial *excess:* poke root is an exceptional lymphatic cleanser in addition to possessing cathartic and potential anti-cancer/HIV properties;[90] chaparral, dandelion, and gentian are extremely bitter and antiviral, reduce *dampness* in the form of excessive fats, cholesterol, mucus, and poisons, and increase tissue oxygen.

3) Bee pollen counteracts wasting and *deficiency,* and its energizing nature balances strong cleansing measures. It helps form the body's *jing* essence, which acts as a reservoir of resistance against chronic disease states. Turmeric is also useful in that it inhibits HIV-1 replication (see page 210).

AIDS patients with an extensive background of antibiotic use normally benefit by improving the intestinal flora with chlorophyll-rich foods such as micro-algae and cereal grasses, fermented foods such as saltless sauerkraut, rejuvelac, and *Lactobacillus sporogenes, Lactobacillus acidophilus,* or *Bacillus laterosporus* cultures.

Strategies for treating chronic fatigue syndrome (CFS) can generally parallel those for treating AIDS.

Multiple Sclerosis (MS)

MS and similar nerve-damaging conditions such as Parkinson's Disease are extremely difficult to completely cure if severe nerve degeneration has occurred; however, the progression of the disease can usually be stopped, and even reversed in less extreme cases.

Those with MS frequently suffer from *Candida albicans* overgrowth, which must be addressed first; they also tend to have various allergies, especially to gluten. Allergy-inducing gluten is found in wheat, rye, barley, and sweet rice. These cereals should be omitted from the regeneration diets (page 407) to determine whether the condition improves. (See "Celiac Disease" for symptoms of gluten sensitivity.) Foods to emphasize in these diets are those that strengthen and soothe the nerves, such as soaked, raw oats, sprouted wheat (if there is no gluten sensitivity), rice, and raw goat's milk.

MS patients have a severe deficiency in various fatty acids,[91] particularly the most common polyunsaturated fatty acid—linoleic acid. One explanation is that an inflammation occurs, possibly from free-radical-induced oxidation in the absence of adequate antioxidants, and/or from proinflammatory prostaglandins from fatty acids of animal origin. In any event, the myelin nerve sheaths—and finally the nerve tissues themselves—become damaged.

Polyunsaturated fatty acids in their natural state act as cooling *yin* tonics for the nerves, and so a lack of them may predispose certain individuals to MS. Conversely, the inflammation of MS may also deplete these fatty acids. Cooling oil-rich products such as fresh wheat germ or wheat-germ oil have proven beneficial. Likewise, the anti-inflammatory oils—flax-seed and those rich in gamma-linolenic acid (GLA) are helpful. As discussed in the *Oils and Fats* chapter, GLA-rich oils added to the diet greatly increase the healing rate of persons with MS. When taking both wheat-germ and flax oils, it is best to take them on alternating days. (See pages 165 and 133 for dosages of flax and GLA oils.) Other polyunsaturated oils may be used, but all such oils (as well as wheat-germ oil) should be recently cold-pressed, unrefined, kept cool, and shielded from light.

Lecithin is often deficient in those with MS and is usually helpful when taken daily (3 tablespoons of granules). Soybean products such as tofu, tempeh, soy sprouts, and soy milk, as well as cabbage and cauliflower, are rich lecithin sources which contain polyunsaturated fatty acids. Eggs are another good lecithin source, but are not as beneficial due to their high saturated fat content.

In Chinese medicine, the nerves are ruled by the liver and Wood Element, and nerve inflammations respond not only to anti-inflammatory oils but to other liver *yin*-building foods and herbs. The most useful liver *yin* tonics for treating MS include: leafy green vegetables, mung beans, mung sprouts, millet, seaweeds, cereal-grass concentrates, micro-algae, and in cases of marked *deficiency*, gelatin or organic animal liver may be helpful. An interesting correspondence between Chinese medical theory and modern science is that the green foods and liver of this *yin*-nurturing group are some of the best sources of the free-radical controlling, anti-inflammatory enzyme superoxide dismutase (SOD).

The spasms and paralysis of MS are indicative of nerve weakness or *wind* according to Chinese healing traditions. Foods and herbs which calm *wind* (and the nerves) are given in the *Wood Element* chapter, page 328. An anti-*wind*, antispasmodic herb specific to MS treatment is Saint Johnswort *(Hypericum perforatum)*. All such herbs can be added to the regeneration diet herbal formulas. The first two of these formulas (beginning on page 422) are appropriate for MS therapy; however, the third formula with poke root, which is very bitter and drying, may deplete *yin* nutrients to the point of irritating the nerves of persons with MS.

Genital Herpes

This highly contagious, sexually transmitted disease does not necessarily belong in the category of degenerative diseases but is discussed here because it requires the same continuous, in-depth treatment. In order for lesions and other symptoms to disappear permanently, one must strictly follow a pure diet such as the modified DIET A (below) for at least six months.

Herpes is characterized in traditional Chinese medicine as *dampness* combined with *heat* in "the lower burner," the reproductive and eliminative area of the body. In place of the herbs recommended for DIET A, use a decoction of the roots of sarsaparilla *(Smilax officinalis),* dandelion *(Taraxacum officinalis),* and gentian

(Gentian officinalis) in equal parts. If the stools become loose, use only sarsaparilla. During outbreaks, a remarkably effective external remedy for most herpes sufferers is a bath in strong black tea. Add at least six ounces of common black tea leaves to very hot bath water, allow it to cool to a safe temperature, then soak in the water for approximately one hour.

Areas of regeneration DIET A (page 407) to modify or emphasize: avoid all intoxicants (including coffee and tobacco), all concentrated sweeteners (stevia leaf may be used), all fruits (including tomatoes), all nuts (especially peanuts), and oil-bearing seeds except flax seed and its cold-pressed oil. Also avoid sesame oil (small amounts of olive oil are acceptable). Spirulina provokes *dampness* in the lower burner region in those with herpes, but chlorella and wild blue-green are often helpful (see guidelines in Chapter 16.)

After six months and if herpes lesions have not emerged for at least six weeks, DIET A may be expanded, if desired, to include fruit, goat-dairy products, and small amounts of other animal products. This program generally succeeds when it is followed consistently. Whether the herpes virus itself is completely purged from the system is not known, but in many cases all symptoms are relieved permanently. Hyperoxygenation, particularly with ozone, has been shown to help in stubborn cases. Supplements of the amino acid lysine may suppress the frequency of external symptoms; however, lysine use inhibits the formation of arginine, an amino acid essential to the manufacture of white blood cells, which play a vital role in immunity.[92]

Except for the external use of black tea, the dietary and herbal treatment of many other sexually transmitted diseases is the same as the herpes treatment, as nearly all involve some form of *damp heat* in the "lower burner." The same approach can be applied to syphilis, gonorrhea, genital warts caused by the human papilloma virus, and chlamydia trachomatis (a bacterial parasite). Treatments recommended in this section can usually complement standard medical remedies for these conditions, but should not replace them except under the guidance of a physician or other qualified health counselor.

Severe Skin Diseases

In some disorders of the skin, the internal organs are debilitated as they are in the degenerative diseases; in other instances the organs are relatively healthy. In either case, excesses such as *dampness, heat,* and/or *wind* are typically present. DIETS A, B, and C (beginning on page 407) are nearly always indicated because they remove these excesses. DIET A should be used when there is frailty or other signs of *deficiency,* and DIET B or C when the person is stronger and more robust, with greater signs of *excess* (thick tongue coating, excess weight, loud voice, extroverted personality).

Most skin diseases result to a large degree from faulty fat metabolism. Foods rich in omega-3 and GLA fatty acids help remedy this situation. Sesame seeds, rich in oleic fatty acids, are also of benefit in the diet; unrefined sesame oil is the oil of choice and can be used moderately as a salad or cooking oil.

The beta-carotene/provitamin A foods are beneficial in the treatment of skin diseases, particularly if the condition is of an inflammatory nature. Yellow and green beta-carotene foods to emphasize include carrots, winter squash, pumpkin, leafy greens such as dandelion greens, beet greens, spinach, kale, chard, and watercress. The deep blue-green micro-algae such as spirulina and wild blue-green are also beneficial. All greens are rich in chlorophyll, which purifies the blood of the toxins that cause skin eruptions. Seaweeds, because of their cooling, detoxifying nature, are recommended for regular use.

Other foods to be added freely to the diet are mung beans, aduki beans, and unpeeled cucumber slices. Alfalfa and soy sprouts are also emphasized in cases of acne. Goat milk products are the best animal product to use during skin diseases. Eliminate foods which are spicy, fatty, or greasy; also avoid all sweets, citrus fruits, and certain fish—oysters, herring, and shrimp.

Since skin conditions reside on the exterior of the body, diaphoresis (sweating) is useful to encourage elimination of toxins through the pores. The diaphoretic herbs commonly used for skin eruptions include:

Sarsaparilla root *(Smilax officinalis)*

Sassafras root bark *(Sassafras albidum)*

Burdock seed *(Arctium lappa)*

Yarrow leaves and flowers *(Achillea millefolium)*

Even though the vitality of the skin is related to the lungs, eruptions surface because of faulty blood cleansing by the kidneys and liver. These two organs purify the blood, and when they are overburdened toxins in the blood are excreted through the skin. To purify the blood, one can emphasize the chlorophyll-rich foods mentioned earlier. In addition, blood-purifying herbs, which include the diaphoretic herbs listed above, are useful. Other important blood-cleansing herbs:

Dandelion root *(Taraxacum officinalis)*

Golden seal root *(Hydrastis canadensis)*

Chaparral leaves *(Larrea divaricata)*

Pansy flowers *(Viola tricolor)* (for children)

Echinacea root *(Echinacea angustifolia and spp.)*

Yellow dock root *(Rumex crispus)*

Burdock root *(Arctium lappa)*

Red clover blossoms *(Trifolium pratense)*

Horehound leaves *(Marrubium vulgare)*

Poke root *(Phytolacca spp.)* (use at most 1 tablespoon of poke tea twice daily)

These herbs cleanse and cool *heat* toxins and dry *damp* mucoid accumulations in the blood and lymph system. For acute skin eruptions, often just one herb is sufficient, for instance, dandelion root, burdock root, or chaparral leaves. Except for red clover blossoms and the diaphoretic herbs, they all promote bowel movement; if constipation persists in spite of these herbs, rhubarb root is useful (also see "Constipation," page 383).

People with the most serious chronic skin conditions suffer a depletion of *yin* fluids and blood, marked by signs of weight loss, frequent thirst, insomnia, night sweats, and hot palms and soles. When such a condition exists, add *yin* and blood-building foods and herbs (pages 65 and 387), especially marshmallow root, slippery elm bark, and yellow dock root; these can be combined with any of the herbs listed above. A traditional Western tea for chronic skin diseases that combines all the previous treatment principles is: equal parts of sarsaparilla root, yellow dock root, sassafras root bark, marshmallow root, and red clover blossoms.

External Treatments

To assist internal remedies, certain external applications can be used to cleanse or nourish the skin; others destroy disease-producing bacteria on the skin surface.

Psoriasis: Wash the area with sarsaparilla tea or seawater; apply garlic oil or walnut oil; bathe in seawater or mineral water; add several cups of unrefined sea salt to bath water; avoid excessive exposure to the sun. To prepare garlic oil, soak several sliced, mashed cloves of garlic in 4 ounces of sesame oil for 3 days, then strain the oil by squeezing it through a cloth.

Eczema: Apply raw honey, or teas of golden seal or poke root; rub with slices of fresh papaya; apply a poultice of grated, crushed daikon radish or raw potato—the juice of the radish or potato can also be applied as a wash.

Acne: Apply lemon juice; wash with castile or other pure soaps that contain no detergents; apply a paste of bentonite, green, or any other clays moistened with apple cider vinegar as the only fluid—leave on at least one half-hour, then wash off with water.

Psoriasis, eczema, and urticaria: Rub with sliced cucumber, dab with vinegar several times a day; avoid soap and shampoo and wash with plain water.

Schizophrenia and Other Mental Illness

In this text, "schizophrenia" refers to the wide range of severe mental disorders defined by therapist Dr. Carl Pfeiffer as "disperceptions of unknown cause." Mental illnesses (including schizophrenia) with symptoms of nervousness, anxiety, depression, delusions, and other disperceptions benefit from the recommendations given in the *Fire Element* chapter. In addition, when these conditions become debilitating, they often involve a degeneration of the entire system. In these cases, fundamental cleansing and rebuilding with the appropriate regeneration DIET A, B, or C (beginning on page 407) is a wise decision.

A generally helpful treatment has been devised by practitioners of "ortho-molecular" medicine. Dr. Carl Pfeiffer, a veteran of this technique, has overseen the treatment of more than 25,000 patients, many of them schizophrenic. His successful and rather simple treatment protocol for various types of schizophrenia (described in *Nutrition and Mental Illness* [Healing Arts Press, 1987]), includes substantial doses of several nutrients including zinc, manganese, vitamins B_3, B_6,

B_{12}, C, and folic acid. Additionally, orthomolecular therapists often find that schizophrenic symptoms vanish when the patient's hypoglycemic, allergic, and/or candida-yeast overgrowth conditions are relieved.

By following a regeneration program, schizophrenics may become less dependent on drugs and synthetic nutrients. In DIETS A, B, and C, generous quantities of the nutrients listed above are available from grains, sprouts, fruits, vegetables, seaweeds, chlorophyll-rich foods, fresh oils, and legumes. Nutrients from whole foods, moreover, occur in a natural matrix of enzymes, minerals, fatty acids, and other beneficial factors. Those who follow the orthomolecular treatment while simultaneously rejuvenating with a wholesome diet can expect greater success than with the nutrients alone.

Interestingly, the two nutrients prescribed by Pfeiffer and his colleagues in every type of schizophrenia are manganese and zinc, which are sometimes given to flush excess copper from the system. Schizophrenia most often involves an excess of copper in the body, and a deficiency in manganese and zinc. However, even schizophrenics who are low in copper can safely be given manganese and zinc because they too are usually deficient in these minerals.

This suggests that the mineral deficiency is related to an additional problem: Schizophrenics are often lacking in the prostaglandin PGE_1.[93] The synthesis of linoleic acid into gamma-linolenic acid (GLA) as well as GLA into PGE_1 are both absolutely dependent on zinc.[94] Manganese is additionally helpful because it assists in the synthesis of fatty acids in general. Taking GLA fatty acids in the diet also increases PGE_1 in the schizophrenic.[95] (See GLA recommendations, page 173.)

Excessive tissue copper can result from copper water pipes, copper IUDs, or copper cooking ware; according to Pfeiffer, contraceptive pills and deficiencies of vitamins C or B_3 alter body chemistry and cause copper to be retained. Those whose drinking water comes through copper pipes should switch to a pure natural water or purified, remineralized water (see "Purified Water as Cleansing Agent," page 127).

Histadelia, which is often accompanied by copper deficiency, accounts for about 20% of all cases of schizophrenia, with such symptoms as obsessions, compulsions, and tendencies to suicidal depression. Histadelics can obtain copper from such sources as unrefined grains, green vegetables, and legumes. Copper from inorganic sources, for example, from copper pipes and copper IUDs, may not act as healthfully in the body as copper from food sources.

Because of the great likelihood of celiac disease (allergy to gluten) in schizophrenics, it is best to avoid the glutinous grains (wheat, rye, barley, and sweet rice). Instead, use rice, millet, buckwheat, corn, oats,* quinoa, and amaranth. Allergies to corn are common for other reasons—it too must be avoided if

---

*As discussed in the "Celiac Disease" section (page 381), oats are glutinous but do not aggravate conditions of gluten intolerance.

it provokes reactions. For further causes of allergies and their remedies, see "Allergies and Food Combining," page 272.

Hypoglycemia and systemic candidiasis also frequently contribute to schizophrenia. (See symptoms and recommendations in the "Candida Overgrowth" and "Hypoglycemia" sections, pages 71 and 375.)

Discussed in the *Fire Element* chapter are "Common Syndromes of the Heart-Mind" and other patterns which involve mental imbalance. Remedies given there can be added to the suggestions in this section. The range and causes of mental disorders seem vast from a psychological perspective, but most "mental problems" are supported by chemical and physical imbalances that can be healed with the appropriate whole foods.

The following herbal formula replaces the herbs recommended with the regeneration diets: an infusion of 1 part scullcap *(Scutellaria laterifolia)*, ½ part lobelia *(Lobelia inflata)*, and 1 part calamus root *(Acorus calamus* and related species). Dosage: 2–3 cups daily. Each of these has traditionally been used singly as a remedy for mental disorders. Calamus has a long history of use in India and China for improving cerebral function; it also helps to restore brain tissue damaged by drugs, injury, or stroke.[96, 97]

Part V

Recipes and Properties of Vegetal Foods

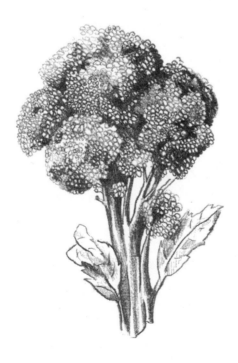

Vibrational Cooking

Different kinds of cooking and temperatures produce different vibrations in the food. For a lighter taste, cook quickly with little or no salt. The quality of the food will be activating yet relaxing and more suitable for a stagnant, tense person. Children who are naturally active and joyful with inexhaustible energies have a fast metabolism, which is supported by this quality of food. It stimulates their mental processes and nerves and helps them apply their will power.

For a more harmonious and sweeter taste, cook on a low heat for a longer time without disturbing. The food will have a patient quality and can calm an angry person and slow down an impatient one.

More cooking, the use of pressure, salt, oil, more heat and time—all make the energy of the food more concentrated. The quality of the food will be hearty and strengthening with a savory flavor. This is healing for inactive or weak people and for those who have lost their interest in food and life. They need human warmth and empathy as well as a variety of interesting foods. Activities such as tossing, mashing, puréeing, stirring, and kneading help to blend and energize the food. And when done with love and mindfulness, these can stimulate a weak digestive system and the desire for a more enjoyable and active life.

For a varied and balanced quality of food use a combination of the above and adapt them to the seasons and the needs of those for whom you are cooking. Everyone has different temperaments and health conditions at different ages. Balancing the relaxing and energizing qualities of food can attune one to nature's cycles and spark immediate changes, especially in children.

Proper attitudes are as important as the quality of food and cooking techniques. The art and practice of cooking good food with good judgment metabolizes the quality of your life. There is an invisible energy imparted to the food by the cook that affects everyone who partakes of it. It is helpful to be aware of what your intentions are. The appearance, taste, balance, and presentation of food and the way everyone feels after eating are reflections of your physical, mental, emotional, and spiritual state.

- Food prepared in anger imparts anger.
- If the cook is being too thrifty and not meeting everyone's nutritional needs there can be a feeling of deprivation and then excessive bingeing (on not-so-nutritious food), leading to even more expense.
- When the cook is feeling rejected, the food will most likely be rejected, too.
- Cooking in a hurried or chaotic manner can result in anxious, chaotic thoughts and actions.

Cooking can be a time of self-reflection. When you feel yourself becoming unbalanced, you have an opportunity to change your condition simply through the cooking process. Just be mindful of what you want to accomplish and concentrate on the food and how you want to prepare and serve it. Most likely, you will change and enjoy cooking, and the meal will be quite pleasurable.

Other Suggestions for the Enjoyment of Cooking

- Respect what you are doing and be pleased with your cooking, no matter how simple.
- Be grateful for the opportunity to cook for the nourishment and well-being of yourself and others.
- Relax and put aside your troubles. Devote your time to the preparation of the meal.
- Tidy up the kitchen and yourself. Roll up your sleeves, tie back long hair, put on an apron, cut out loud music, and eliminate odors that overpower the sounds and smells of cooking. Let the sounds of sizzling, steaming, bubbling, etc., make music as the aromas of food fill the air.
- Plan your meals before beginning to cook.
    1. Consider everyone's condition and mood, the time of day and weather, and tomorrow's events (are there plans for travel, exams in school or a holiday?). The food of today prepares one for tomorrow. Does someone feel melancholy? You may want to bake a spice cake to add sweetness and zest to their day. At social functions, eating more variety and lighter, sweeter foods helps one be more harmonious and sociable. When studying, however, simple concentrated food helps one to focus.
    2. Be intuitive. Let the colors, tastes, shapes, and smells be your guide.
    3. Plan the cooking flow: when to put on beans, soak seaweeds, make sauces, steam vegetables, and so on, so everything is ready at mealtime.
    4. Have all ingredients, cookware, and serving dishes ready beforehand. As soon as the food is ready, arrange it attractively on the table. Bring in the hot soups and dishes last.
- Be simple. Have a beginner's mind. Allow plenty of time and don't overload yourself with complicated recipes. Cookbooks and measurements are good guides, but use your own creativity and trust yourself to cook well without them.
- Maintain an orderly atmosphere in the kitchen by cleaning up as you cook or before the meal is served. Return things to their proper place.
- When using the stove, learn to listen internally for when food is done.
- Avoid eating or tasting the food while cooking. A full stomach interferes with creativity and deprives you of the ceremony of the first taste at the meal.
- Avoid tasting from a utensil and putting it back in the food. The enzymes from saliva will cause spoilage and change the vibration of the food. (This is also true of mixing in food from earlier meals.)
- Certain refined foods such as cornstarch, white rice, and the white-flour versions of noodles, spaghetti, and bread take almost twice as long to digest as whole grains and give one a feeling of being full or having something that

"sticks to the ribs." This creates the delusion of being nourished and warm. However, these foods form a sticky mucus that accumulates in the intestines causing coldness, constipation, and stuffiness. Nevertheless, it is important for some people to maintain this feeling of fullness until they can accept the light, clear experience resulting from eating whole grains.

- Get to know the effects and healing powers of each food and then strive to bring out its natural taste and life force without changing it very much. Use simple combinations and delicate spices to create variety. Mixing too many things together usually results in strange tastes and confusion for the taste buds and digestive system. One may notice his or her own confused, chaotic thinking after such a meal.
- Learn to cook individual grains. The essence of vibrational cooking is mirrored in the simplicity of a single food.
- To learn to cook well, cook for someone who inspires you . . . someone you care for.

COOKING METHODS

All methods of cooking break down food for easier assimilation. Each method also adds a warming quality to the food such that after eating, the food contributes relatively more warmth to the body than in its raw state. Cooking does not, however, change a cooling food to a warming one. In addition, each cooking method contributes moisture, dryness, or has other attributes listed below.

Steaming

Adds a moist, *yin* quality; brings out the flavor of each vegetable; involves short cooking time.

- Put ½ to 1 inch water in a pot. Bring to boil.
- Place vegetables in a steamer. Lower heat and cover.
- Steam until vegetables are crisp. Do not overcook, or they lose their potency. Try 10 minutes and check for tenderness. (Green beans take about 10 minutes; beets, 30 minutes.)
- The cooking water contains minerals and water-soluble vitamins, and should be used in cooking or preparing other foods and drinks.

Suggestions:
- Cut vegetables into small pieces or slices for faster cooking.
- Roll greens together and stand up so steam can penetrate.
- Small squashes, string beans, and small potatoes can be steamed whole.
- Sauces can be served on the side or poured over vegetables.

Water Sauté

Contributes a watery *yin* quality; shorter cooking time than steaming; uses less water; vegetables can be cut into large pieces or left whole.

- Place a small amount of liquid in a pot. Bring to a scald, just below boiling.

- Add seasonings, then ingredients.
- Reduce heat and simmer until bright-colored and verging on tenderness.
- Save any remaining cooking water for later use.

Waterless Method

One of the best methods. Vegetables cook in their own juices. The flavor, vitality, and appearance are greatly enhanced.

- Preheat a heavy pan and put in 2 tablespoons water to provide steam until the vegetables release their own juice.
- Bring water to a scald. Add seasonings and vegetables. Reduce heat.
- Cover and cook slowly until just tender and bright-colored.

"Waterless" and "vapor control" cookware are excellent to use for this.

Stir-frying or Sautéing

A tasty, quick method of cooking using oil to seal in the natural flavors and juices. Be careful not to overcook oils. They become acidic and have a tendency to thicken the blood. This method benefits those who often feel chilly since stir-frying is one of the warming methods as a result of hot oil and vigorous cooking. (People who have a liver problem should avoid cooking with oil.) A longer, more gentle method of sautéing can also be tried using little or no oil.

Fast Sauté
- Heat a heavy skillet and brush lightly with oil.
- Keep a high heat and add vegetables.
- Toss from side to side gently with chopsticks or a wooden spoon for 5 minutes.
- Cover and let cook over medium heat for about 10 minutes for a softer vegetable.
- Or stir constantly another 8 minutes for a crisper vegetable.
- Sauce or seasonings can be added at end of cooking. Cover for a minute or so to let flavors permeate.

Long Method (Nituhe—Japanese Sauté)

You can cook a larger volume and vegetables cut into larger pieces. The vegetables simmer slowly without any disturbance, giving them a soothing quality with a sweeter taste and softer texture.

- Preheat a heavy pan. Brush lightly with oil.
- Add vegetables. Cover and cook on low heat 30–35 minutes. (Or add about $\frac{1}{2}$ cup liquid, cover, return to boil, and simmer 30–45 minutes.)
- Periodically hold pan by its sides or handles and shake in a counter-clockwise motion to prevent burning.
- Add seasonings 5 minutes before end of cooking.

Sautéing Without Oil

Method 1 Rub bottom of pan with a 3-inch piece of soaked kombu. Leave it in pan while sautéing to prevent sticking. Use medium heat. (Remove kombu at end.)

Method 2 Heat skillet and toss vegetables gently on a low to medium heat. (Add a little water, if you like.)

Water-Oil Sauté
- Cover bottom of skillet with water. Heat.
- Add a little oil on top of water.
- Sauté by the usual method, being careful not to overheat oil.
- Has the flavor of stir-fry without over-heating the oil.

Chinese Stir-frying (3 steps)

1. Rapid searing
- Heat a heavy skillet or wok until hot (30 seconds).
- Add 1 tablespoon oil and swirl the pan to cover entire surface. Do not let it smoke.
- Add ingredients such as scallions, garlic, and ginger and toss to flavor oil.
- Add main ingredients, but not all at once so temperature doesn't drop.
- Toss, flip, and swish with long chopsticks or a wooden spoon to coat with oil so the natural flavors are seared in and to prevent scorching. These motions make stir-fried dishes spirited.

2. Vigorous steaming
- Quickly add seasonings and liquid.
- Bring to boil. Cover. Reduce heat.
- Simmer vigorously 1–4 minutes. Crackling from the pan will tell you when liquid has cooked off.

3. Final seasoning
- Uncover pan and add kuzu or arrowroot (dissolved in liquid) or a few drops of sesame oil for an aromatic sheen.
- Give ingredients a few fast turns over high heat to glaze them well.
- A stir-fried dish is never watery except those meant to be saucy.
- Remove from wok immediately so food doesn't turn dark or have a metallic taste.
- Serve in a heated dish.

Oven Use

Adds a drying, more warming quality than steaming, water sautéing, or simmering; enhances sweet flavor; reduces moisture. Most basic methods of cooking can be carried out in the oven. Simply place ingredients in the oven on medium heat and serve them in their own baking dish.

Baking Cook without liquid (uncovered usually).

Oven-fry Brush with oil and bake.

Steaming Preheat oven and casserole dish. Pour a small amount of hot liquid over vegetables. Cover to hold in the steam.

Braising Food is half-covered with liquid and simmered, covered.

Pressure Cooking

Concentrates nutrients and juices; fast cooking; saves time and fuel.

Pressure-cooked Vegetables:
- Bring a few tablespoons of water to a boil, uncovered, in a pressure cooker.
- Put in vegetables. Cover and bring up to pressure.
- Reduce heat to low and cook for a short time, or remove from heat. (Cooking time varies with different vegetables.)
- Cool down immediately by placing pressure cooker under cold running water.
- Remove vegetables at once.

Broiling

Quick cooking; high, dry heat makes food more warming than cooking in water. Food cooks in its own juices, but the moisture is greatly reduced. Brush vegetables with a sauce to retain nutrients and to keep them from drying out. Serve immediately or vegetables will shrivel and not be as attractive when cooled.

COOKWARE

Some of the best cookware is made from ceramic, glass, or lead-free earthenware. It is totally non-reactive to the foods cooked in it. Electrochemically speaking, unstable ions react with other organic materials. The enzymes in food, raw or cooked, are very chemically active and react with the metallic ions in metal cookware, creating unpleasant metallic tastes and making the food toxic, to the degree that the cookware contains any toxic substances. If you choose to cook with metal, use high-density cast iron (without a graphite coating) and heavy-gauge stainless or surgical steel, or good quality enamel.

- When cooking with metals, remove the food immediately after cooking so it won't retain as much of a metallic taste.
- Do not add lemon, pineapple, tomatoes, vinegar, or other acidic food to cast iron or it will create a strong metallic taste and turn the food a blackish color.
- Avoid cooking with aluminum, poor-quality stainless steel, thin enamel on flimsy pots, Teflon, and other cookware coated with synthetic materials. They contain toxic substances that react and/or chip off into the food. Aluminum cookware and aluminum foil are especially harmful.
- The best pots are thick-bottomed. They prevent burning over high heat and distribute the heat evenly.
- Use glass or ceramic containers for herbal teas.

Clay Baker

A clay pot made from a special porous unglazed clay that allows the pot to breathe during cooking. The clay pot is soaked in water before cooking. During cooking, water particles are released, penetrating and blending with the natural food juices to increase flavor and tenderness. Can cook soups, casseroles, bread, cakes, vegetables, and fruit.

To use:
- Soak clay baker in water 10–15 minutes.
- Add ingredients.
- Place in cold oven and cook to your preference.

Ohsawa Ceramic Cooking Pot

Designed especially for use with pressure cookers.
- Avoids metallic taste and reaction to metal.
- Can cook vegetables and fruit without water.
- Cooks soups, grains, and beans and steams bread.

To use:
- Add ingredients to ceramic pot. Cover.
- Place pot in pressure cooker. Add water halfway up the side of the pot. Secure lid.
- Bring to normal pressure and cook for recommended time.

Note: The lid holds firmly in place so water from container will not go into food. The pot can be used in other containers.

Waterless Cookware

Made from multi-ply stainless steel. Contains a moisture seal designed to cook vegetables without water or oil and with less heat.

Vapor Control

Made from heavy-gauge stainless steel with an air space between a double-wall construction. Fill the air space partially with water and heat. Keeps a constant temperature.

Kitchen Utensils

- Use chopsticks and wooden spoons rather than metal utensils if you need to add a more relaxed, *yin,* earthy quality to your cooking.
- Use a clean cutting board and knife that you enjoy using and keeping sharp.
- Use a mortar and pestle or Japanese suribachi for grinding and mashing.
- Use a bamboo or pottery steamer.

Cleaning Cookware, Dishes, and Kitchen

- Wash in warm soapy water and rinse in cold water to remove soap.
- Use soap made only from biodegradable ingredients.
- Avoid using harsh cleansers and metal scouring pads that scratch surfaces of cookware. Use only natural brushes or plastic scouring pads.
- For burned food on bottom of pans: Add water and baking soda or wood ash, and bring to a boil.
- Porcelain: Wash in boiling water with wood ash to season and restore whiteness.
- Before washing, soak containers with sticky oatmeal on them in cold water.
- For lingering smells: Soak in boiling water with mustard powder, salt, lemon juice, or baking soda.
- Clean greasy walls, floors, and cabinets with boiling water and a little ammonia.

GLOSSARY

Arrowroot: Powdered tropical root; thickener; nutritive; high in calcium.

Carob: Powdered pod; tropical; rich in natural sugar, calcium, and minerals; alkaline; conditions bowels; use as chocolate.

Kuzu (Kudzu): Powdered tuber from Japan; thickener; cools and soothes the stomach and intestines.

Lecithin: Nutritional supplement from soybeans; breaks up deposits of fat; lowers cholesterol; sold in granules.

Mirin: A subtly sweet Japanese cooking sherry made from rice.

Soy Sauce: Shoyu—Made from wheat, soybeans, water, and sea salt. Tamari—Made from only soybeans, water, and sea salt.

Umeboshi: Salty-sour pickled plum from Japan; highly alkaline; antibiotic; regulates intestines.

Umeboshi Vinegar: The brine of the umeboshi, or pickled plum.

HEALING WITH THE RECIPES

Most of the recipes in the following sections contain purely vegetarian foods drawn from several cultural traditions, including American, European, and East Asian. The Western traditions include raw food and sprout recipes and a good selection of typical American dishes adapted to vegetarian cuisine. A number of the recipes recognize the desire of Americans to eat a varied and complex diet, and are included primarily for those in the early stages of dietary transition to high quality, whole foods. Nevertheless, as noted earlier in the food combining sections, too many ingredients in a meal can lead to poor health. Complex meals should be taken at most occasionally, and then only by those with good digestion. If a recipe contains too many ingredients for those needing therapeutic meals, one may simplify the recipe. In *Food Combinations,* Chapter 19, are examples of Plan B meals suitable for persons with weak digestion and in need of healing. With these in mind, one may gain insight into how to simplify various recipes.

Many of the more complex dishes in the recipe section are combinations of ingredients that are cooked together in a watery medium. These include soups, pasta dishes, casseroles, grain and/or bean dishes, and others. As discussed under Plan C in the *Food Combinations* chapter, such a process, particularly if there is ample water and lengthy cooking time, better joins the ingredients for digestion than if they are taken separately. Those dishes that are cooked with some but not abundant water still have this effect to a certain degree, albeit less than that intended by the Plan C "One-Pot Meal."

When using a food for treating a specific disease or syndrome, several creative dishes featuring this food can often be found in the recipe section, and the reader can, if necessary, adapt these to meet dietary needs. Changing an ingredient in a recipe sometimes entails altering other parts. With a little practice and common sense, success will prevail.

For best results in all recipes, use the highest quality ingredients, as suggested in earlier chapters:

All foods should ideally be unrefined and organically grown on rich soil. See "Resources," page 704, for mail-order sources if you lack quality foods locally.

Grains: Use unrefined grains, and whole-grain pastas, cereals, and flours.

Oils: Use extra virgin olive and other unrefined types of oleic-rich oils such as sesame, oleic sunflower, or organic peanut; clarified butter or other oils rich in saturated fat may also be used by certain individuals. Do not cook with shortening, margarine, or polyunsaturated oils such as safflower, corn, soy, sunflower, cottonseed, and others; see general guidelines for oils on page 183.

Vinegars: Use unrefined apple cider, brown rice, or other unrefined vinegars.

Salt and salty products: Use unrefined sea salt and unpasteurized, naturally fermented misos and soy sauces made from organic ingredients and unrefined salt.

Animal products: Use high-quality yogurt, cheeses, and other fermented dairy products according to food combining principles: eat them as condiments or additions to vegetable dishes and salads, especially those containing primarily green and non-starchy vegetables or acid fruits. If needed for *deficiencies,* fish and organic meats may be used; they combine best with the above vegetables, and may be marinated and included in soups or broths, as described in the *Protein and Vitamin B$_{12}$* chapter, page 158. In addition, examples of meats in "congees" are given on pages 478–479, which are the only listings of meat in the following sections.

Note: The "Recipe Locator," an index for finding recipes and the properties of vegetal foods, begins on page 636.

Grains

For thousands of years, ancient people cultivated grains from common grasses which contain nutrients essential for human development, vitality, and prevention of disease. As discussed earlier, when whole grains are complemented with a good variety of other unrefined plant foods, all the elements of nutrition necessary for human development are available. Therefore, in embracing grains as the mainstay of diet, one finds that missing nutrients and cravings are not a problem, once a level of healthy digestion has been achieved. If prepared in balance with individual needs, grains satisfy hunger and taste, provide energy and endurance, calm nerves, and encourage deep sleep. They promote elimination, quick reflexes, long memory, and clear thinking.

From the perspective of *yin/yang* analysis of food, grains are usually placed in the center. They support one in finding the "Golden Mean," the place of receptivity, relaxation, and mental focus. For modern people, these active and passive qualities do not generally combine. That is, when we are receptive and relaxed, our minds are not focused. In order to become focused, we give up relaxation and take on stress.

For several generations in America, grains were identified by the name "starch," usually with a condescending tone in the voice. We considered all starches equivalent and thought they were the basis of excess body weight. Most grains were used (and still are) for animal feed, which added to their low esteem in the minds of most people. In addition, grains were primarily known in the forms of bread, oatmeal, white rice, and either grits and cornmeal in the South, or highly processed dry breakfast cereals. The majority of North Americans still cannot correctly identify whole-wheat berries, brown rice, barley, rye, and buckwheat. And since we haven't generally eaten grain in its whole form, we don't realize that whole grains need a completely different procedure for proper digestion than processed ones do.

It usually takes a couple of weeks just to learn how to chew whole grain well, and for the salivary glands to start working correctly. For each bite, try chewing thirty-two times or more. For people who are sick, fifty to seventy times is effective. This advice also applies to other foods that have a fibrous consistency, such as legumes, nuts, and seeds, and some vegetable stems, roots, and leaves.

When people are too weak to chew well, cereal creams are appropriate. Even those should be chewed as much as possible. Individuals with no teeth can chew with their gums to release saliva.

Whole grains and other carbohydrates will not digest efficiently without a thorough admixture of saliva. The action of saliva is necessary to trigger reactions that occur further along the digestive tract.* Also, saliva is alkaline, and most grain is mildly acid-forming; since almost all disease conditions involve an overly acidic condition of the blood, thorough chewing is preventative, as it promotes an alkaline rather than acid result from grains.

In recent years, instead of the name "starch," whole grains along with legumes and vegetables have most often been referred to as "complex carbohydrates," which tells us that a more complex series of events occurs in their digestion as compared with that of simpler sugars. Complex carbohydrate digestion of whole foods is a harmonious, steady, balanced metabolism, providing a complete complement of necessary nutrients. This is quite the opposite of the rush-followed-by-depression one experiences from highly refined, nutrient-deficient grains and sugars.

Even though the complex carbohydrates have now been widely identified as the single most deficient item in the modern diet, most people are still not aware of the many qualities in grain other than fiber and carbohydrate. Nor is the unique and widely differing nature of each grain being recognized. In this section we describe the major properties of the grains as drawn from both tradition and science, to stimulate an interest in the uniqueness and beauty of this family of food.

Before delving into the rather specific properties of grains, it is first convenient to know how the actions of grains bring balance to general constitutional types. Note that the following list provides wider applications of grains than the similar Six Divisions/Influences lists in the earlier part of this book. This feature is important for those persons who emphasize a variety and abundance of grains in their diets.

Balancing Personal Constitution with Grains

Excess (robust person with strong voice and pulses, thick tongue coating, extroverted personality, and reddish complexion): this person does best with grains that reduce excess, such as amaranth, rye, whole barley (not pearled), wild rice.

Deficiency (frail person with weakness and low energy, weak voice and thin or no tongue coating, introverted personality, and sallow or pale complexion): most grains are appropriate, with rice, wheat, barley (pan-roast before cooking), spelt, well-cooked oats, and quinoa the most beneficial.

Heat (person feels too hot, thirsts for large amounts of cold liquid, has red signs such as bright- or deep-red tongue, red face or eyes, yellow tongue coating, yellow and scanty mucus): the cooling grains include millet, wheat, amaranth, wild rice, blue corn, and whole barley.

---

*The enzyme ptyalin in saliva reduces carbohydrates to maltose, which in turn is broken down in the intestines by the enzyme maltase to form dextrose, a simple sugar. Maltase will only act on maltose, which is not formed without proper insalivation of carbohydrates. Other possibilities for carbohydrate breakdown exist, but these usually involve unhealthy fermentations.

Cold (person feels cold, likes warm food and beverages, has pale complexion, dresses too warmly for the temperature or climate, is contracted and can't bend back, may have pain "frozen" [fixed] in one place): warming grains include oats, spelt, sweet rice, quinoa, and basmati rice. Neutral grains are also useful: rice, rye, corn, and buckwheat.

Damp (person feels sluggish and has pathogenic moisture such as edema, obesity, chronic mucus and phlegm problems, cysts, and tumors): the grains which dry *dampness* are amaranth, buckwheat, unrefined barley, corn, rye, wild rice, basmati rice (in small amounts), and dry roasted oats.

Dry (typically a thin person with dry mouth, nostrils, lips, skin, and stools): wheat, rice, sweet rice, quinoa, millet, barley (pan-roast before cooking), spelt, and well-cooked oats are best for regular use.

Wind (nervous person with instability and symptoms that move around and come and go such as spasms, cramps, and moving pain; certain relatively static conditions such as numbness, paralysis, and strokes are also often *wind*-induced): grains that help calm *wind* include quinoa, cooked oats, and wheat; avoid buckwheat.

Summer Heat (high fever, sweating, exhaustion, and fluid depletion): roasted barley tea or drinks quell the effects of *summer heat;* brown rice, especially the long-grain variety, helps reduce irritability which often accompanies *summer heat.*

Cooking Grains

- Gently wash.
- Soak 8–12 hours. This germinates the dormant energy, releasing nutrients and making the grains more digestible.
- Discard soak water.
- Do not fill pot more than ¾ full.
- For large quantities of grain, use less water and increase cooking time.
- Use approximately ⅛–¼ teaspoon salt to 1 cup grain.
- 1 cup of grain serves two.
- Roasting grain makes it more alkaline and *yang.*
- Cook by the waterless cookware, pressure cooker, basic or low-heat method.
- Low-Heat Method: Cook soaked or sprouted grains on low heat overnight or for several hours. Adjust water. The grains are more alkaline and certain enzymes are preserved.
- The addition of sea vegetables to grains adds a delicious full flavor and nutritional value.

After Cooking

- Remove grain from pot so it will not expand and sweat, causing grain to be wet and tasteless.
- Dig deeply into the pot so that each scoop contains grains from the top and bottom—for a more balanced dish.

- Place in a bowl or shallow bamboo basket.
- Cover with a bamboo mat or cheesecloth and store in a cool place. Don't worry if it begins to ferment a little; it will be sweeter and more digestible. However, if fermentation goes too far, the grain cannot be eaten.

Storage of Uncooked Grains

- Wheat and its relatives spelt and kamut have hard, thick outer layers and have been known to store for dozens of years under the right conditions.
- Rice and other grains with a less thick layer will store for about two years.
- Millet has a very thin outer layer and often gets scratched in milling, thus rendering it more prone to rancidity.
- Store grains in clean, closed containers in a dry, cool place.
- Put in a mint tea bag or a bay leaf to keep critters out if the storage container is not tightly closed.

AMARANTH

Used by the ancient Aztecs as a valuable food and in their worship rituals, amaranth has recently come to the attention of world health workers with the discovery that in areas of Africa and Latin America where it is consumed, there exists no malnutrition. Because of its high nutritional value and ability to thrive in poor soil and during drought conditions, amaranth and plants with similar properties (such as quinoa) are considered part of a "beneficial lost storehouse" of the world's agriculture and diet.

Amaranth can be used to help fulfill protein and calcium requirements. It is especially helpful for people with consistently elevated needs, such as nursing or pregnant women, infants, children, or those who do heavy physical work. Even when it is used alone, amaranth has protein complexes that are more than adequate for most individuals; however, amaranth is also unusually high in lysine, an amino acid that is low in wheat and most other grains. A combination of amaranth and low-lysine grain then presents a very high amino-acid/protein profile, even higher than found in meats and other animal products (although such a profile is not necessary for most people).

The value of this combination is that high levels of both protein and calcium are available for those individuals mentioned above as well as for people in transition to vegetarian food. Although amaranth is a costly little seed (in recent years six to ten times the price of wheat), it is a concentrated food and may actually be more palatable in a combination that dilutes its intense flavor.

Healing properties: Cooling thermal nature; bitter and sweet flavor; dries *dampness;* benefits the lungs; high in protein (15–18%), fiber, amino acids (lysine and methionine), vitamin C, and calcium. It contains more calcium and the supporting calcium cofactors—magnesium and silicon—than milk. Its calcium is utilized efficiently in this form. Use in breads, cakes, soups, and grain dishes. Pop like popcorn or toast for a nutty flavor. Sprout and use in salads.

AMARANTH PILAF WITH ALMOND SAUCE

    1 cup amaranth
    2 cups bulghur wheat
  ¾ cup lentils, soaked
    1 small onion, minced
    1 teaspoon oil (optional)
  7–8 cups boiling water
    1 teaspoon sea salt
Almond Sauce:
    2 cups bechamel sauce (p. 602)
  ½ cup almonds, toasted and ground
    1 tablespoon mint

- Sauté onion.
- Add amaranth and bulghur and sauté 5 minutes longer.
- Add lentils.
- Pour boiling water over grains, lentils, and onion. Add salt. Cover and cook ½ hour over low heat.
- Prepare sauce.
- Pour grain-lentil mixture into oiled casserole dish and cover with almond sauce.
- Bake at 375°F 15 minutes.
- Serves 6–8.

AMARANTH DUMPLINGS IN CABBAGE SOUP

  ¼ cup amaranth seed or flour
  ¾ cup whole-wheat flour
  ¼ cup boiling water
    2 cups cabbage, shredded
    1 quart stock or water
  1–2 tablespoons miso
    Parsley

- Mix amaranth and whole-wheat flour together. Add boiling water. Knead 5 minutes. Mold dumplings into any form of ½-inch thickness (square, triangle, round).
- Cover cabbage with stock and simmer in a covered pot until tender.
- Add remainder of stock and bring to boil.
- Drop dumplings into soup. When they rise to the surface, they are cooked.
- Dilute miso with a bit of stock and add to soup. Allow to simmer a few minutes.
- Garnish with parsley.
- Serves 4.

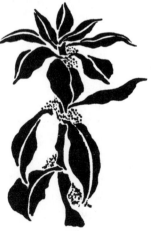

BARLEY

Healing properties: Cooling thermal nature; sweet and salty flavor; strengthens the spleen-pancreas, regulates the stomach, and fortifies the intestines; builds the blood and *yin* fluids and moistens *dryness;* promotes diuresis; benefits the gall bladder and nerves; very easily digested—a decoction of barley water (2 ounces pearled or roasted whole barley to a quart of water) is traditionally used for convalescents and invalids; treats diarrhea (pan-roast before cooking); soothes inflamed membranes; alleviates painful and difficult urination; quells fever (use in a soup); helps reduce tumors, swellings, and watery accumulations such as edema. Whole barley, sometimes called "sproutable," is mildly laxative and contains far more nutrition than the commonly used "pearl" variety, including more fiber, twice the calcium, three times the iron, and 25% more protein. To remove the laxative property, roast whole barley until aromatic before cooking. This also makes barley, which is considered the most acid-forming grain, more alkalizing.

In addition to its use as a cereal or cereal cream (from flour), roasted barley can be ground to a powder and stirred into hot water as a drink, or decocted as a tea in its whole berry form. Both the tea and drink relieve *summer heat* and fatigue, and act as digestive aids and coffee substitutes.

Sprouted barley is a common Chinese herb; it is slightly warming and has a sweet flavor; treats indigestion from starchy food stagnation or poorly tolerated mother's milk in infants; tonifies the stomach; alleviates stagnant liver signs including chest or upper abdominal swelling and tightness; and strengthens weak digestion and poor appetite in cases of spleen-pancreas deficiency. Also useful in candida yeast-induced digestive weakness.

Caution: Roasted whole barley or pearl barley can worsen cases of constipation.

SOFT BARLEY

    1 cup whole barley, soaked
4–5 cups water
⅛–¼ tablespoon salt

- Combine barley, water, and salt in a pot.
- Bring to boil. Cover. Reduce heat to low.
- Simmer 1¼ hours.
- Place in a serving bowl.
- Serve with gomasio, parsley, or natto miso.
- Serves 2.

BARLEY WITH VEGETABLES

1 cup barley, soaked
½ onion, diced (optional)
½ cup carrot, diced
¼ cup burdock root, sliced, or
1 shiitake mushroom, soaked 15
  minutes and sliced
1 teaspoon sesame oil
3 cups water
¼ teaspoon sea salt

- Sauté vegetables (optional).
- Dry-toast barley lightly.
- Place barley and vegetables in a pot with water and salt.
- Cover and bring to a boil.
- Reduce heat to low. Simmer 40 minutes.
- Place in a serving bowl.
- Serves 4.

BARLEY LOAF WITH LENTILS

1 cup barley, soaked
½ cup red lentils, soaked
¼ cup sunflower seeds
4½ cups water
¼ teaspoon sea salt
1 bay leaf
Parsley

- Preheat oven to 350°F.
- Place all ingredients in a pot except parsley. Bring to boil.
- Reduce heat, simmer 2 minutes.
- Pour mixture into a greased loaf pan.
- Cover and bake 1 hour.
- Serve in slices with parsley.
- Serves 4.

BUCKWHEAT

Healing properties: Neutral thermal nature; sweet flavor; cleans and strengthens the intestines and improves appetite. Is effective for treating dysentery and chronic diarrhea. Rutin, a bioflavonoid found in buckwheat, strengthens capillaries and blood vessels, inhibits hemorrhages, reduces blood pressure, and increases circulation to the hands and feet. Rutin is also an antidote against x-rays and other forms of radiation.

Buckwheat is used externally for skin inflammations, eruptions, and burns—apply a poultice made of roasted buckwheat flour mixed with vinegar.

If toasted, buckwheat is known as "kasha" and becomes one of the few alkalizing grains. Commercial kasha is thoroughly toasted and is a dark, reddish brown; by purchasing "raw" buckwheat (which has an almost white color), one can choose to toast it less or not at all for the warmer seasons.

Young buckwheat greens, grown from sproutable buckwheat seeds (with a hard, indigestible black covering that drops off after sprouting), are excellent sources of chlorophyll, enzymes, and vitamins.

Insects do not attack it, and like ginseng, buckwheat will die when grown with most chemicals.

Cautions: Not recommended for those with *heat* signs such as high fever, thirst, red face, deep-red tongue color, and high blood pressure, or for those with *wind* conditions including dizziness, disorientation, nervousness, spasms, or emotional instability.

KASHA CEREAL

1 cup buckwheat groats
4–5 cups boiling water
½ onion, diced (optional)
A few grains sea salt

- Place all ingredients in a pot with the boiling water. Bring to boil again.
- Cover. Reduce heat to low. Simmer 30 minutes until soft.
- Place in bowl.
- Serves 2–4.

TOASTED KASHA WITH CABBAGE GRAVY

2 cups buckwheat groats
5 cups water
A few grains sea salt
1 teaspoon oil (optional)
Gravy:
  1 onion, minced
  1 cup cabbage, shredded
  ½ cup carrot, diced
  ½ cup whole-wheat flour
  2 cups water
  2 tablespoons soy sauce
  2 tablespoons sesame butter
  1 teaspoon oil (optional)

- Preheat oven to 350°F.
- Dry-toast groats or sauté in 1 teaspoon oil until brown. Let cool.
- Add water and salt. Bring to a boil. Reduce heat to low. Cover and simmer 5 minutes. Place in baking dish.
- Sauté onion, cabbage, and carrots in 1 teaspoon oil for 5 minutes or steam.
- In a deep saucepan, dry-toast whole-wheat flour lightly. Cool. Add 2 cups water. Bring to boil.
- Add soy sauce, sesame butter, and sautéed vegetables.
- Turn down heat when mixture begins to thicken. Simmer 15 minutes.
- Pour gravy over kasha and bake 30 minutes.
- Serves 4–6.

KASHA STUFFED SQUASH

2 acorn squash, baked and halved
2 cups buckwheat groats, cooked
2 cups bechamel sauce (p. 602)

- Remove seeds from squash. Fill centers with buckwheat.
- Top with bechamel sauce.
- Bake 20–30 minutes.
- Serves 4.

BUCKWHEAT CROQUETTES

2 cups cooked buckwheat
1 cup whole-wheat flour
1 small onion, grated (optional)
1 teaspoon sesame oil (optional)
1 scallion, minced (optional)
½ cup parsley, chopped
¼ cup sunflower seed meal
Sea salt to taste

- Sauté onion.
- Mix ingredients together.
- Form into small balls. Dip into seed meal and fry, or form into patties and bake at 350°F for 30 minutes.
- Serves 4–6.

BUCKWHEAT RAISIN LOAF

1 cup buckwheat flour
1 cup plain cooked buckwheat
1 cup roasted cooked buckwheat
¾ cup raisins or currants
2 tablespoons ginger, minced
1½ teaspoons anise seeds
3 cups water
½ teaspoon salt
2 teaspoons oil (optional)
2 teaspoons lecithin

- Preheat oven to 350°F.
- Combine first 3 ingredients.
- Simmer raisins, ginger, and anise in water 30 minutes.
- Add raisin mixture, (oil), lecithin, and salt to buckwheat mixture. Knead until it holds together.
- Bake in oiled baking dish 30 minutes or until golden.
- Serves 8.

KASHA VARNITCHKES (Jewish noodle dish)

2 cups buckwheat groats
8 cups boiling water
½ teaspoon sea salt
1 onion, minced (optional)
1–2 teaspoons sesame oil (optional)
½ pound whole-wheat noodles, cooked and drained
¼ cup sunflower seeds, toasted

- Dry-toast groats until brown and nutty.
- Add salt and water. Cook 20 minutes.
- Sauté onion until golden.
- Mix onions, kasha, and noodles together.
- Serve hot sprinkled with sunflower seeds.
- Serves 4–6.

CORN

Corn, also known as maize, is the only commonly used native grain of the Western Hemisphere.

Healing properties: Neutral thermal nature; sweet flavor; diuretic; nourishes the physical heart; influences the stomach, improves appetite, and helps regulate digestion; promotes healthy teeth and gums; tonifies the kidneys and helps overcome sexual weakness. Drink a tea decoction made from the whole dried kernels to treat kidney disease.

Corn was traditionally cooked by Native Americans with lime. When cultures in Africa, the American South, and elsewhere first began using the grain as a staple in the late nineteenth and early twentieth centuries, there resulted an epidemic of pellagra, an often-fatal wasting disease involving skin lesions, diarrhea, and nerve deterioration. The cause was discovered to be niacin deficiency. Corn is very low in niacin, but when lime is cooked into it, niacin absorption in the body increases. Eating corn regularly poses no problem for people who have a varied diet of other wholesome foods. However, when corn predominates in a narrow diet, the ancient tradition of adding lime makes sense. (Good sources of niacin are wheat germ, peanuts, nutritional yeast, whole wheat, and most meats.)

Fresh corn on the cob has properties similar to dried corn but also acts like a fresh vegetable—it contains more enzymes, more of certain vitamins, and is better suited to the warmer seasons and the robust person than the dried variety.

Corn silk is highly diuretic and can be used as a tea infusion for urinary difficulty, high blood pressure, edema, kidney stones, and gallstones. It is neutral in thermal properties and sweet and bland in flavor.

Blue corn is an open-pollinated variety (not hybridized) indigenous to southwestern America; the Hopi and Navajo people use it as a staple food. It is cooling and has a sweet and slightly sour flavor; influences the stomach and tonifies the kidneys; contains 21% more protein, 50% more iron, and twice the manganese and potassium of yellow or white varieties. When ground, its beautiful blue sheen gives a special quality to any recipe.

INDIAN CORN OR HOMINY

4 cups whole dry corn, soaked 24
hours
8 cups water
½–¾ cup sifted wood ash (optional)
1 teaspoon sea salt

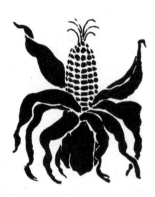

- Combine all ingredients except salt in a pressure cooker. Bring to full pressure and cook 30 minutes.
- Remove from heat and let pressure come down.
- Drain in a colander. Rinse 3–4 times to remove ash. (The skins should be loose and float off in the water. If they are still intact and tough, add a little more ash and cook 10 minutes more.) Ash varies in alkalinity, therefore the amount needed to soften the hulls will vary also.
- Return corn to pressure cooker. Add salt and recover with fresh water. Bring to pressure, and cook for 50–60 minutes.
- Serves 8.

ZUNI INDIAN BOILED CORN DUMPLINGS

1 cup cornmeal
1 cup corn flour or whole-wheat
flour
½–1 cup boiling water
¼–½ teaspoon salt

- Mix cornmeal and corn flour.
- Add boiling water and salt. Knead for 5 minutes.
- When dough is stiff and smooth, pinch off small pieces and shape into balls.
- Drop into boiling water or broth.
- Boil 30 minutes.
- Serve with root vegetables, squash, or beans.
- Yields 1–1½ dozen.

Variation   Knead mashed beans into corn mixture before boiling.

POLENTA (Coarsely ground corn)

1 cup polenta
3 cups water
⅛–¼ teaspoon sea salt

- Mix ½ cup water with polenta. Boil remainder of water and gently pour in polenta. Stir while pouring. Bring back to boil. Add salt and cover. Simmer 30–40 minutes. Stir occasionally.

Variation   Mix with vegetables or raisins and nuts; pour into molds. Cut into squares when cool and fry.

IROQUOIS CORN WITH CHILI BEANS AND SQUASH

4 cups cooked polenta
1 sautéed onion (optional)
4 cups cooked kidney beans
  seasoned with
2 teaspoons chili powder
2 medium winter squash, cooked
  and puréed

- In a glass casserole dish, make layers of polenta, onion, beans, and squash.
- Cut into squares and serve cold or bake 30 minutes at 350°F.

MILLET

Healing properties: Cooling thermal nature; sweet and salty flavor; diuretic; strengthens the kidneys; beneficial to stomach and spleen-pancreas; builds the *yin* fluids; moistens *dryness;* alkalizing—balances over-acid conditions; sweetens breath by retarding bacterial growth in mouth; high amino acid (protein) profile and rich silicon content; helps prevent miscarriage; anti-fungal—one of the best grains for those with *Candida albicans* overgrowth.

Also useful for diarrhea (roast millet before cooking), vomiting (millet soup or congee), indigestion, and diabetes. Soothes morning sickness—eat millet soup or congee regularly. Millet is known as "the queen of the grains."

Due to its alkali-forming nature, millet is often cooked with little or no salt.

Sprouted millet can be used for digestive stagnation caused by undigested starch, for checking lactation, and other applications similar to sprouted rice (see below).

Caution: Millet is not recommended for those with signs of very weak digestive functions such as consistently watery stools.

COOKED MILLET

1 cup millet, soaked
3 cups water
A few grains sea salt

- Place millet and salt in a pot of water. Cover.
- Bring to a boil. Reduce heat to low.
- Simmer 30 minutes or pressure cook 20 minutes.

- Serves 2.

Variations Toast millet in a little oil before cooking. For softer millet, add more water.

MILLET WITH ONIONS, CARROTS, HIJIKI

2 cups millet, soaked
½ onion, diced (optional)
2 carrots, diced
¼ cup hijiki, soaked and cut
6 cups water
½ teaspoon sea salt
Toasted sesame seeds

- Layer vegetables on bottom of pot in order given.
- Add millet, water, and salt. Cover.
- Bring to boil. Reduce heat to low.
- Simmer 30 minutes or pressure cook 20 minutes.
- Stir and serve sprinkled with sesame seeds.
- Serves 4.

MILLET WITH SQUASH

5 inches kombu, soaked
2 cups millet, soaked
1 cup acorn, butternut, or summer squash, diced
¼ cup burdock root, sliced
5–6 cups water
½ teaspoon sea salt

- Place kombu on bottom of pot. Layer with squash and burdock.
- Add millet, water, and salt.
- Bring to boil. Reduce heat to low.
- Simmer 30 minutes or pressure cook 20 minutes.
- Serves 4–6.

MILLET-MUSHROOM CASSEROLE

4 cups cooked millet
Sauce:
½ cup whole-wheat flour
½ onion, finely diced (optional)
¼ pound mushrooms, sliced
1 teaspoon oil (optional)
1½–2 cups water
2–3 tablespoons soy sauce
Parsley

- Preheat oven to 350°F.
- Place millet in an oiled casserole dish.
- Sauté onions and mushrooms until soft.
- Add flour and coat vegetables well.
- Add water, stirring constantly to keep from lumping. Bring almost to a boil. Reduce heat and simmer 5–7 minutes.
- Add soy sauce. Cover and simmer 10 minutes. Stir occasionally to prevent sticking.
- Poke holes in millet with a chopstick so sauce can be absorbed.
- Pour sauce over millet and bake 20 minutes.
- Serve hot or cool and cut into slices. Garnish with parsley.
- Serves 4–6.

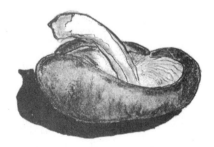

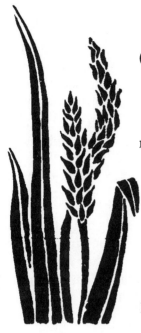

OATS

Healing properties: Warming thermal nature; sweet and slightly bitter flavor; soothing; restores nervous and reproductive systems; strengthens spleen-pancreas; builds and regulates the *qi* energy; removes cholesterol from the digestive tract and arteries; strengthens cardiac muscles. Can be used in cases of dysentery, diabetes, hepatitis, nervous and sexual debility, indigestion and swelling including abdominal bloating. One of the richest silicon foods, oats help renew the bones and all connective tissue. Oats also contain phosphorus, required for brain and nerve formation during youth. Useful as a poultice to relieve itching; they also heal and beautify the skin when used as a pack.

If drunk regularly, oat water acts as an internal antiseptic to strengthen immunity and ward off contagions. It and oat porridge are excellent for people who are weak and *deficient*. To prepare oat water, simmer 2 tablespoons oat groats or flakes in 1 quart water for 30 minutes to two hours (longer cooking increases thickness and nourishing qualities). Strain or drink it as it is, either warm or at room temperature, according to thirst. Oats in any of its more common forms—oatmeal, steel-cut oats, or whole oat groats—are also ideal for preventing infections and contagious diseases, especially in children.

Oat flakes are nearly as nutritious as whole oat groats, as they have been only lightly processed by rolling and steaming; they are the only whole-grain cereal that many people eat. Oats can be used in soups, puddings, breads, crusts, toppings, and desserts.

WHOLE OATS

1 cup whole oats, soaked
5–6 cups water
⅛–¼ teaspoon salt

- Place in a pot with salt and water. Bring to boil.
- Reduce heat to very low and simmer overnight.
- Or simmer 2–3 hours in 2 cups water.

Variations Cook with dulse or raisins. For a nuttier, less bitter flavor, dry-toast unsoaked oats, then cook as above.

QUINOA

A member of the *Chenopodium* family and a cousin of amaranth, quinoa (pronounced keen wa) has some of the same outstanding characteristics. One of the ancient staple foods of the Incas, it was called "the mother grain. " (Botanically, quinoa is not a true grain, but can be used as one.) It has grown in the South American Andes for thousands of years, and thrives in high, cold altitudes.

Since 1982 quinoa has been cultivated in the United States with various degrees of success, and it is now generally available where unrefined foods are sold.

Healing properties: Warming thermal nature; sweet and sour flavor; generally strengthening for the whole body; specifically tonifies the kidney *yang* (warming and energizing function of the body) and the pericardium functions.

Compared with all grains, it has the highest protein content (since it has a protein profile similar to amaranth, please refer to the information given earlier). Quinoa has more calcium than milk and is higher in fat content than any grain. A very good source of iron, phosphorous, B vitamins, and vitamin E. An appropriate grain for recent vegetarians who crave nutrient-concentrated foods.

Prepare as a cereal like rice, or in combination with other grains because of its strength. Grind into flour and use in baking breads and cakes.

QUINOA WITH OATS

1 cup quinoa, soaked
1 cup rolled oats
¼ teaspoon sea salt
3 cups water

- Place all ingredients in pot, cover.
- Bring to boil, reduce heat to low.
- Simmer 30 minutes.
- Turn heat off and let sit 5 minutes with closed lid.
- Serve with cooked or baked fruit or squash.

QUINOA CROQUETTES

Cooked quinoa with oats
Oil to brush pan

- Cook quinoa and oats (as above) in advance and let cool off (grains must be cool to stick together).
- Cut in slices.
- Fry in lightly oiled pan on both sides until golden brown.
- Serve with salad and vegetables.

QUINOA TABOULI

1 cup quinoa, rinsed well and
   soaked
2 cups water
Pinch of sea salt
½ cup peas
1 tomato, diced
½ cucumber, sliced
6 olives, cut in rings
Chives, minced
Parsley, minced
½ teaspoon each thyme and
   marjoram
3 tablespoons lemon juice
Soy sauce to taste

- Combine quinoa, water, and salt in pot. Cover.
- Bring to boil, simmer 20 minutes.
- Steam peas 1 minute.
- Place in ceramic bowl and mix with rest of ingredients.
- Add quinoa, toss gently together.
- Serves 3.

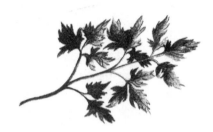

BAKED QUINOA VEGETABLE LOAF

3 cups cooked quinoa
1 cup whole-wheat flour
½ cup water
1 tablespoon miso
1 tablespoon lecithin granules
1 teaspoon each basil and thyme
1 onion, chopped
2 cups carrots, sliced
2 cups broccoli, 1-inch pieces
1 tablespoon sunflower seeds
Parsley

- Combine quinoa and flour in bowl.
- Dissolve miso and lecithin in warm water and mix with grains and herbs.
- Optional: let dough rest 4 hours to blend flavors and naturally ferment.
- Place onions, carrots, and broccoli in steamer, cook 7 minutes.
- Gently mix dough with vegetables and place in lightly oiled baking pan.
- Dry-toast sunflower seeds until golden brown and sprinkle on top of loaf.
- Bake 30-40 minutes at 350°F.
- Garnish with parsley.

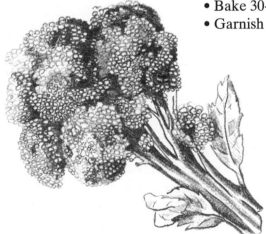

RICE

Healing properties: Neutral thermal nature; sweet flavor; strengthens spleen-pancreas; soothes the stomach; expels toxins; increases *qi* energy; is hypoallergenic; whole brown rice is concentrated in B vitamins and therefore beneficial for the nervous system—helps relieve mental depression. Used also for diarrhea, nausea, diabetes, and thirst. A handful of raw brown rice chewed thoroughly as the only food in the first meal of the day helps expel worms.

As a remedy for infants who cannot tolerate mother's milk, feed them roasted rice tea: pan-roast rice until dark brown, add water, and simmer for 20 minutes. The resulting liquid (tea) can be taken 2–3 times daily.

Rice is a tropical grain, and it alleviates the irritability associated with *summer heat.* Short-grain rice has a nuttier flavor, chewier consistency, and is better for the nervous or frail person and cooler seasons than long grain, which is less sticky. Basmati rice is slightly aromatic and is considered lighter than other rices, making it more appropriate for *damp,* overweight, or other stagnant conditions. Be sure to purchase whole-grain basmati, which is often difficult to obtain, even in natural food stores. "White basmati" is parboiled before refining, which drives a small but important percentage of vitamins and minerals into the interior of the grain. However, it is still lacking the bran and its associated fiber, the germ and its essential oils, and the majority of other nutrients found in these removed parts.

Sprouted rice is a common herb of Chinese medicine. Its properties include neutral thermal energy and sweet flavor. It is used for weak digestion and poor appetite as a result of spleen-pancreas deficiency, and for resolving food stagnation composed of undigested starches. Also helps reduce lactation and is useful for nursing mothers who have painful, swollen breasts or who are weaning their infants. Sprouted rice loses much of its therapeutic value when well cooked. Use it fresh for food stagnation and to retard lactation; to strengthen the spleen-pancreas and improve appetite, lightly toast, powder, and mix in hot water.

On two occasions earlier in this century when Master Hsu Yun, the last Zen Patriarch of China, was walking and bowing—touching knees, hands, and head to the earth every few steps—through the mountains of China in the winter, he encountered bitter storms that buried him in snow, and he awaited his death. However, each time he was saved by a Bodhisattva who miraculously appeared and offered him a bowl of brown rice, which provided him with strength to endure the storm. The Chinese at this time associated white rice with lofty rank and position, and so an elevated being such as a Bodhisattva offering brown rice seemed out of character. As a metaphor, this story suggests that spiritual essence (symbolized to the Chinese by the Zen Patriarch) as well as physical strength is preserved by brown rice. Of course, this metaphor can extend to whole foods in general. An ancient Japanese proverb has a similar message: eating grains without their skins causes people to become poor (in body and spirit) and to have no clothes (protection against coldness and disease). Refer to "Brown Rice—Rediscovered," page 12, for more information on the nutrient value of brown rice and its bran coating.

Sweet rice: Contains more protein and fat than other rice. It is easy to digest, particularly when made into the traditional Japanese food known as "mochi. " (See "Mochi" recipe.)

Healing properties: Warming thermal nature; sweet; increases *qi* energy; warms the spleen-pancreas and stomach; is mildly astringent—used for frequent and excessive urination, spontaneous sweating, and diarrhea. Also is often helpful in the treatment of diabetes.

Cautions: Sweet rice can worsen diseases marked by phlegm and mucus; in addition, it should be avoided by those with deficient digestive fire (watery stools, mucus in stools, and signs of *coldness*).

Wild rice: Not a true rice but more closely related to corn; indigenous to North America and traditionally known as *manomen* or "water grass"; a staple for the Ojibway, Chippewa, and Winnebago Indians of the Minnesota area. These people were quite tall and muscular with very red skin.

Healing properties: Cooling thermal nature; sweet and bitter flavor; diuretic; benefits the kidneys and bladder.

This slim, dark grain has more protein than other rice. It is rich in minerals and B vitamins and is a hardy food for cold climates—it cools the superficial tissues and concentrates warmth in the interior and lower body areas.

PRESSURE-COOKED BROWN RICE

    1 cup brown rice, soaked
1¼–1½ cups cold water
  ⅛–¼ teaspoon sea salt

- Place rice, water, and salt in pressure cooker and bring up to pressure.
- As soon as pressure gauge begins to hiss loudly, reduce heat to low and cook 30–45 minutes.
- Remove from heat and allow pressure to come down.
- Remove rice and serve.
- Serves 2.

SIMMERED BROWN RICE

1 cup brown rice, soaked
1½–2 cups cold water
⅛–¼ teaspoon sea salt

- Place rice, water, and salt in a heavy pot with tight-fitting lid.
- Cover and bring to a boil.
- Turn heat to low and simmer 1 hour or until water has been absorbed.
- Remove rice from pot and serve.
- Serves 2.

ROASTED BROWN RICE (has a nutty flavor)

1 cup brown rice
1–1½ cups cold water
⅛–¼ teaspoon sea salt

- Wash rice and toast in a dry skillet until golden brown.
- Cook for 40–50 minutes.
- Remove from pot and serve.
- Serves 2.

SPROUTED BROWN RICE

2 cups sprouted brown rice (p. 569)
2–3 cups water
¼–½ teaspoon sea salt or kelp

- Cook over low heat several hours or overnight.
- Remove from pot and serve.

FRIED RICE

4 cups cooked brown rice
1 teaspoon oil
½ cup carrot, diced
1 green onion, chopped (optional)
1–2 tablespoons soy sauce

- Sauté onion 2 minutes in oil.
- Add carrots, sauté 3 minutes.
- Add rice on top plus a few drops water.
- Cook on low heat 10 minutes.
- Add soy sauce. Cook 5 minutes.
- Mix and serve.
- Serves 4.

BAKED RICE

1 cup brown rice
2–3 cups boiling water
⅛–¼ teaspoon sea salt
½ teaspoon sesame oil (optional)

- Preheat oven to 350°F.
- Dry-toast or sauté rice in oil until slightly brown.
- Place in a baking dish.
- Pour boiling water over rice. Cover.
- Bake 45–50 minutes (until water is absorbed).
- Serves 2.

BAKED RICE PILAF

Add ½ cup diced vegetables (raw or sautéed) to rice before cooking. Follow above recipe.

SWEETENED RICE

Add raisins and ⅛ teaspoon each: coriander, cinnamon, ginger, cumin, and turmeric to rice, and cook by any method above.

BROWN RICE WITH WHEAT BERRIES

1 cup brown rice
¼ cup wheat berries
2½–3 cups water
¼ teaspoon salt

- Soak rice and wheat separately overnight. Cover wheat with 1 cup water and rice with 1½ to 2 cups water.
- Cook wheat 30 minutes. Drain well.
- Add to rice with salt and cook 50–60 minutes.

Variation Replace wheat berries with rye berries, dry corn, aduki beans, black beans, or lentils.

BROWN RICE WITH MILLET

1 cup brown rice
¼ cup millet
2½ cups water
¼ teaspoon sea salt

- Soak together overnight and cook 45–60 minutes.

Note: Millet or the grains in the variation below can be toasted instead of soaking for a more nutty flavor. Adjust amount of water for more or less dryness.

Variation Replace millet with buckwheat, barley, or sweet rice.

RICE, GARBANZOS, AND CARROTS

2 cups brown rice, soaked
½ cup garbanzo beans, soaked
2 carrots, in large chunks
½ teaspoon sea salt
Water

- Pressure cook garbanzos 45 minutes, in advance.
- Place carrots on bottom of pot, next add garbanzos, rice, salt, and water.
- Cook together 45–60 minutes.
- Serves 4.

RICE BALLS

Shape cooked brown rice into balls the size of ping-pong balls. (Dip hands in cold salted water to prevent sticking.) Roll balls in toasted sesame seeds, mashed and cooked beans, or chopped nuts. Wrap in toasted nori sheets.

Variation Put natto miso or a sliver of umeboshi plum in the center, or use vinegar according to the directions for nori rolls (p. 592). (Will not spoil for days. Great for traveling.)

WILD RICE

1 cup wild rice (soaked)	• Place rice, water, and salt in a covered pot.
4 cups water	• Bring to a boil.
⅛–¼ teaspoon salt	• Turn heat to low and simmer 30–45 minutes. Rice is ready when the black grains have split open.
	• Fluff with a fork and simmer 5 more minutes.
	• Drain off excess liquid and save for soup stock.
	• Serves 4.

FESTIVE WILD RICE

1 cup long-grain brown rice	• Preheat oven to 350°F.
1 cup wild rice	• Wash and rinse rice.
½ cup pine nuts	• Dry-toast pine nuts in skillet or oven until golden.
6 cups water	• Place rice and water in casserole.
½ cup mushrooms, sliced	• Layer rest of ingredients over rice. Do not stir.
½ onion, diced (optional)	• Cover and bake until all water has been absorbed—about 1–1½ hours.
1 block tofu, cubed small	• Garnish with fresh parsley.
2 tablespoons soy sauce	• Serves 6.
½ teaspoon each: basil, thyme	
Parsley for garnish	

MOCHI

Widely used in Japan as a medicinal food, mochi is easy to digest and is excellent during convalescence; it is used for anemia, for strengthening weakened conditions in general, and it aids breast-feeding mothers in supplying abundant, high-quality milk. Mochi is made by pounding 'sweet' or 'glutinous' rice; it is necessary to use an unbreakable bowl (e. g., stainless steel). A large wooden pestle, traditionally called a *kien,* is used to pound the rice. The end of a baseball bat, a board, or a large wooden mallet work equally well.

MOCHI

3 cups sweet rice
5 cups water
½ teaspoon sea salt

- Simmer rice in salted water for 2–3 hours, or pressure cook for 20 minutes (until very soft).
- Place in a large sturdy bowl and pound until all grains are broken (a paste will form).
- Sprinkle the rice mass and bottom of pestle with cold water occasionally to prevent sticking.
- With moistened hands, shape dough into balls, patties, squares, etc.
- Serve fresh or pan-roasted. Makes one pound.

Note
- Refrigerate or dry to store. Mochi will harden in about 12 hours, at which point try baking, toasting, frying, or boiling into soups before eating.

Variations
- Add fresh or dried mugwort* leaves the last 5–10 minutes of cooking the sweet rice. Fresh or dried nettle leaves may be substituted.
- Pound and shape, etc., as above.

Suggestions
- Top with grated daikon and shoyu.
- Roll mochi balls in toasted, ground walnut meats.
- Wrap nori strips around mochi squares.

CONGEE

Traditionally known as *hsi-fan* or "rice water," congee is eaten throughout China as a breakfast food. It is a thin porridge or gruel consisting of a handful of rice simmered in five to six times the amount of water. Although rice is the most common grain for congees, millet, spelt, or other grains are sometimes used. Cook the rice and water in a covered pot four to six hours on warm, or use the lowest flame possible; a crockpot works very well for congees. It is better to use too much water than too little, and it is said that the longer congee cooks, the more "powerful" it becomes.

---

*Mugwort *(Artemisia vulgaris)* is an herb valued as an organic source of iron. Primary uses: expels worms, helps intestinal troubles, and is effective against internal bleeding. Most weak conditions benefit from it. In combination with mochi it becomes an excellent food for anemia and leukemia patients. Mugwort mochi builds the blood and provides outstanding nourishment for pregnant women. Mugwort tops are best picked in the spring. Boil the leaves in salted water and dry them by spreading them out in a well-ventilated dark place (store them dried). The dried leaves may also be obtained at Western or Chinese herb shops (Mandarin: *ai ye*). Nettles *(Urtica urens)* also build the blood, remove parasites, and stop bleeding.

Healing Properties: This simple rice soup is easily digested and assimilated, tonifies the blood and the *qi* energy, harmonizes the digestion, and is demulcent, cooling, and nourishing. Since the chronically ill person often has weak blood and low energy, and easily develops inflammations and other *heat* symptoms from *deficiency* of *yin* fluids, the cooling, demulcent and tonifying properties of congee are particularly welcome; it is also useful for increasing a nursing mother's supply of milk. The liquid can be strained from the porridge to drink as a supplement for infants and for serious conditions.

Other therapeutic properties may be added to the congee by cooking appropriate vegetables, grains, herbs, or meats in with the rice water. Since rice itself strengthens the spleen-pancreas digestive center, other foods added to a rice congee become more completely assimilated, and their properties are therefore enhanced. Listed below are some of the more common rice-based congees and their specific effects.*

THIRTY-THREE COMMON CONGEES

Aduki Bean: Diuretic; curative for edema and gout

Apricot Kernel: Recommended for coughs and asthma, expels sputum and intestinal gas

Carrot: Digestive aid, eliminates flatulence

Celery: Cooling in summer; benefits large intestine

Chestnut: Tonifies kidneys, strengthens knees and loin; useful in treating anal hemorrhages

Water Chestnut: Cooling to viscera; benefits digestive organs

Chicken or Mutton Broth: Recommended for wasting illnesses and injuries

Duck or Carp Broth: Reduces edema and swelling

Fennel: Harmonizes stomach, expels gas; cures hernia

Ginger: Warming and antiseptic to viscera; used for deficient *cold* digestive weakness: diarrhea, anorexia, vomiting, and indigestion.

Kidney from Pig, Sheep, or Deer: Strengthens kidneys; benefits knees and lower back; treats impotence (use organic kidney)

Leek: Warming to viscera; good for chronic diarrhea

---

*Adapted from *Chinese Medicinal Herbs*, translated and researched by F. Porter Smith and G. A. Stuart; San Francisco: Georgetown Press, 1973, p. 470.

Liver from Sheep or Chicken: Benefits diseases of the liver; very powerful (use organic organ meats)

Mallow: Moistening for feverishness; aids digestion

Mung Bean: Cooling, especially for *summer heat;* reduces fevers; thirst relieving

Mustard: Expels phlegm; clears stomach congestion

Salted Onion: Diaphoretic; lubricating to muscles

Black Pepper: Expels gas; recommended for pain in bowels

Red Pepper: Prevents malaria and *cold* conditions

Pine Nut Kernel: Moistening to heart and lungs; harmonizes large intestine; useful in *wind* diseases and constipation

Poppy Seed: Relieves vomiting and benefits large intestine

Purslane: Detoxifies; recommended for rheumatism and swellings

Radish: Digestant; benefits the diaphragm

Pickled Radish (salt): Benefits digestion and blood

Brown Rice: Diuretic; thirst-quenching; nourishing; good for nursing mothers

Sweet Rice: Demulcent; used for diarrhea, vomiting, and indigestion

Scallion Bulb: Cures *cold* diarrhea in the aged

Sesame Seed: Moistening to intestines; treats rheumatism

Shepherd's Purse: Brightens the eyes and benefits the liver

Spinach: Harmonizing and moistening to viscera; sedative

Taro Root: Nutritious; aids the stomach; builds blood

Wheat: Cooling; used with fevers; clears digestive tract; also calming and sedating due to wheat's nourishing effect on the heart

Yogurt and Honey: Beneficial to heart and lungs

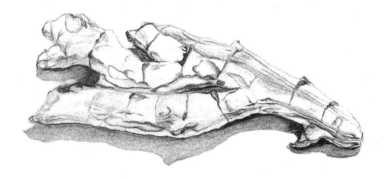

RYE

Healing properties: Neutral thermal nature; bitter flavor; affects liver, gall bladder, and spleen-pancreas; diminishes *damp*, watery conditions in the body; clears liver stagnancy; increases strength and endurance; aids muscle formation; cleans and renews arteries; aids fingernail, hair, and bone formation.

Eat in its raw, sprouted state or as soaked flakes to benefit from its fluorine, which increases tooth enamel strength. Rye broth or congee are often helpful for treating migraine headache. Good for cold, harsh climates and seasons.

Rye is a very hard grain and is ideally suited to sourdough baking, which adds sourness to its natural bitter flavor, making it even more effective for the liver. For breadmaking with rye and further insights into its healing attributes, see "The Bounty of Rye," page 501.

RYE CEREAL WITH NUTS

1 cup whole rye berries
2½ cups water
½ cup ground peanuts or sunflower seeds
¼ teaspoon salt
¼ cup raisins
1 tablespoon molasses (optional)
2 tablespoons wheat germ or bread crumbs

- Dry-toast rye and crack in electric blender or grain mill.
- Bring water to boil and stir in rye.
- Add nuts, salt, and raisins. Reduce heat to low. Cover. Simmer 30 minutes.
- Add molasses and wheat germ. Serve warm.
- Serves 2–4.

ONIONS STUFFED WITH RYE AND GARBANZOS

4 onions, peeled
1 cup whole rye berries, soaked
2 cups water
½ cup cooked garbanzo beans, mashed
Soy sauce to taste
1 cup herbal sauce with thyme and sage (p. 602)
Parsley

- Place rye and water in pot. Cover and bring to boil. Simmer on low heat 1 hour.
- Preheat oven to 350°F.
- Parboil onions. Cool and cut off tops. Scoop out insides. Finely chop the cut-out onion and add to rye, garbanzos, and soy sauce. Mix together.
- Stuff onions with mixture.
- Pour on herb sauce and bake 30 minutes.
- Garnish with parsley.
- Serves 4.

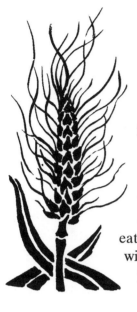

WHEAT

Healing properties: Cooling thermal nature; sweet and salty flavor; tonifies the kidneys; builds the *yin;* one of the few foods which Chinese medicine attributes with directly nourishing the heart-mind: calms and focuses the mind and can be used for palpitations, insomnia, irritability, menopausal difficulty, and emotional instability. Encourages growth, weight gain, and fat formation—it is especially good for children and the frail person. On the other hand, it should be eaten in small amounts, if at all, by the obese as well as those with growths and tumors. Mildly astringent, wheat is used for juvenile bed wetting, spontaneous sweating, night sweats, and diarrhea; quenches thirst, moistens dry mouth and throat. Charred wheat, ground to a flour and mixed with sesame oil, can be applied to treat burns.

Wheat sometimes provokes allergic reactions. This is particularly the case with flour that is rancid from oxidation. Wheat flour should ideally be used right after grinding. Otherwise, it needs to be kept in an air-tight container, refrigerated, and used within two weeks. Some people are allergic to only processed-flour products and can eat pre-soaked whole berries (cooked), sprouted wheat, or wheat germ. If eating wheat causes bloating and gas, stomach pain, indigestion, excessive mucus or increased pulse rate, it is best avoided, especially during pregnancy.

Wheat absorbs a wider range of minerals from rich soil than other grains. In addition, its nutrient profile—the comparison of its nutrients with one another—is similar to that of the human body. For this reason and because it nurtures the heart-mind, wheat is sometimes considered an ideal food for human growth and development. The fact that people have greatly overeaten refined and rancid wheat products that have been genetically altered for smut resistance continuously since 1926, partly explains the many common allergies to this vital food.

SPELT

Healing properties: Warming thermal nature; sweet flavor; strengthens the spleen-pancreas; moistens dryness; nurtures the *yin* fluid and structural aspect of the body; and benefits the frail and *deficient* person. It is often used for treating diarrhea, constipation (use whole berry), poor digestion, colitis, and various other intestinal disorders.

A relative of wheat with origins in Southeast Asia, spelt was brought to the Middle East more than 9,000 years ago, and has since spread over the European continent. Very recently, spelt has enjoyed renewed popularity in Europe as a result of translations of mystical writings of 12th-century healer St. Hildegard of Bingen, who praised spelt as the grain best tolerated by the body. Until the last few years, spelt in America has been fed mostly to race horses and livestock as a replacement for oats.

Today it is used in the West in much the same way as wheat; the main distinction is that people with allergies to wheat frequently do not react to spelt. Although spelt contains gluten, those with gluten sensitivity—even celiacs—can usually tolerate it. In addition, spelt is appreciated as much for its hearty nut-like flavor as for its healing qualities.

The grain berry grows an exceptionally thick husk that protects it from pollutants and insects. It is stored with its husk intact, so it remains fresher. Thus, unlike other grains, it is not normally treated with pesticides or other chemicals. The strong, protective husk may also be a metaphorical signature of this grain's capacity to strengthen immunity.

Spelt is richly supplied with nutrients. In general, it is higher in protein, fat, and fiber than most varieties of wheat. An important feature is its highly water-soluble fiber, which dissolves easily and allows for efficient nutrient assimilation by the body. To use spelt in baked goods, cereals, and other dishes calling for wheat or other grains, substitute it one for one. Spelt is becoming widely available in the form of pastas, cereals, breads, flour, and whole-grain berry. When using spelt for healing debilitated conditions, it is often best in a thin porridge or congee. At the Hildegard Practice, a clinic in Konstanz, Germany, spelt has been used as an adjunct in the treatment of many disorders, especially chronic digestive problems of all kinds, chronic infections (herpes, AIDS), nerve and bone disorders (Parkinson's disease, Alzheimer's disease, arthritis), cancer, and antibiotic side effects.

KAMUT

An ancient form of durum-related wheat, "kamut" (*Triticum polonicum;* pronounced "kuh moot," an antiquated Egyptian name for wheat) flourished in Egypt more than 5,000 years ago. Although nearly replaced by other strains about 2,000 years later, it was nonetheless continuously grown until the mid-twentieth century by farmers in the area who prized its rich flavor. Soon after World War II, however, it became virtually extinct when growers switched to higher-yielding—but sometimes less flavorful—hybridized wheat. (Plant breeders often place higher value on yield than taste and nutrition.) Fortunately, a few seeds reportedly recovered from a burial crypt made their way to America, where organic kamut now thrives in Montana.

Kamut has many of the properties of common wheat with far less of its allergenic component: in some tests, approximately two-thirds of those with wheat allergy will have less or no allergy to kamut. Like all wheat, it is glutinous, yet the majority of gluten-sensitive individuals can eat it without adverse side effects (celiacs and others with gluten intolerance, as well as those with general allergies to wheat, should first test for reactions with very small portions). Its berry more than twice the size of modern wheat, this heirloom grain is also richer in unsaturated fats and protein. Noted for making excellent pastry, noodles, cereals, and baked goods, it has a lighter and more delicate flavor and finer texture than standard wheats, yet is pleasantly rich and substantial. Clearly, these qualities explain why this grain is becoming highly sought after.

WHEAT BERRY TURNIP STEW

2 cups wheat berries, soaked
6 cups water
2 medium turnips, diced
½ onion, diced (optional)
5 inches wakame, soaked and cut
1 clove garlic, minced
1–1½ teaspoons savory
½ teaspoon sea salt

- Bring wheat and water to boil.
- Simmer on low heat 2 hours (until berries make a gruel).
- Add turnips, onion, wakame, and salt. Simmer 30 minutes.
- Add garlic and savory and cook 15 minutes longer.
- Serves 6–8.

BULGHUR WHEAT

Made from wheat berries that are boiled, then dried and cracked. To reduce oxidation, either prepare your own, or purchase it in a sealed package, and store in an air-tight container.

TABOULI

1 cup bulghur
2 cups water
1 cup parsley, chopped
¼ onion, diced (optional)
1 tomato, diced
Juice of 1 lemon
1 teaspoon olive oil
¼ teaspoon sea salt
2 tablespoons fresh mint, chopped, or 1 teaspoon dried mint

- Bring water to a boil. Add bulghur and salt.
- Cook on low heat, covered 15 minutes. Cool.
- Gently toss the rest of the ingredients with the bulghur.
- Serves 4.

ROASTED BULGHUR WHEAT

1 cup bulghur wheat
2½ cups boiling water
½ teaspoon sea salt

- Dry-toast bulghur until it has a nutty aroma.
- Transfer to a bowl. Pour boiling water and salt over bulghur.
- Cover bowl and allow to sit 1 hour.
- Serves 4.

GREEK PILAF

1 cup cooked bulghur wheat
1 cup cooked rice
½ onion, minced (optional)
1 clove garlic, minced
1 stalk celery, minced
¼ cup sunflower seeds
1–2 teaspoons olive oil (optional)
1–2 teaspoons mint
Juice from 1 lemon
¼ cup parsley, chopped
½ teaspoon sea salt
½ cup Sesame Butter-Lemon Sauce
    (p. 603)

- Sauté onion, garlic, celery, and sunflower seeds until onion is soft, or cook in a little water.
- Mix with remainder of ingredients.
- Serve topped with Sesame Butter-Lemon Sauce.
- Serves 4–6.

STUFFED GRAPE LEAVES

Use preserved imported leaves or pick leaves in early June and use them fresh or preserve in salt water in tightly closed jars.

- Preheat oven to 350°F.
- To fill:
  Place leaf down flat.
  Put 1–2 tablespoons Greek Pilaf near the stem end.
  Roll tightly, folding in sides.
- Bake 20–25 minutes.
- Top with Sesame Butter-Lemon Sauce.

NOODLES

Fun to eat, easy to chew and digest, plus quick to prepare. There are Japanese noodles (soba) made from buckwheat flour; Chinese cellophane noodles, made from mung beans; American and European noodles such as spaghetti, lasagna, and macaroni made from whole wheat, spinach, artichoke, corn, kamut, soybeans, rice, spelt, and so on.

Noodles oxidize quickly and easily become rancid, compared with unmilled grain seeds. Noodles bought in sealed packages are usually less rancid. Better yet are "fresh" whole-grain noodles, which are usually made within the week; these are sometimes available refrigerated in stores carrying wholesome foods. Of course, the best option is homemade noodles, not only for nutritional value, but flavor.

Another problem with a diet rich in whole-grain noodles is the phytic acid they contain, which tends to bind minerals in the body. Of course, this problem is neutralized in a sourdough process, and so the home noodle-maker should use such a natural leavening process.

BASIC METHOD OF COOKING NOODLES

1 pound noodles
3 quarts water
1 teaspoon salt

- Bring water and salt to a rolling boil. Add noodles and bring back to boil. Reduce heat to medium-low and cook until done.
- To test: break in half—if the center and the outside are same color, it is done.
- Rinse under cold water to prevent clumping.
- Add noodles to broth or serve with sauce.

SOBA (BUCKWHEAT NOODLES) WITH VEGETABLES

2 cups soba, cooked
1 cup mushrooms, sliced
1 cup broccoli
½ cup mung sprouts
1 teaspoon corn oil
1 tablespoon soy sauce

- Sauté mushrooms 3 minutes.
- Add broccoli and sauté 3 minutes.
- Add sprouts and sauté 2 minutes.
- Add soba and soy sauce and mix gently.

SPAGHETTI WITH PESTO SAUCE

Pesto Sauce:
3 cups fresh basil leaves
½ cup almonds, chopped
¾ cup parsley, chopped
1 clove garlic (optional)
¼ cup olive oil or water
Salt to taste
1 pound spaghetti, cooked

- Prepare sauce by combining all ingredients with fresh basil and blend on low speed until a smooth paste.
- Toss with hot spaghetti.
- Serves 6.

Note: To replace fresh basil, soak 1 cup dried basil in olive oil or hot water for several hours to soften.

NOODLES IN BROTH

1 pound noodles, cooked
15 flowered carrots, lightly steamed
1 cup shredded cabbage, lightly steamed
5–6 cups hot broth, seasoned with soy sauce to taste
Parsley

- Place noodles in a bowl. Arrange carrots and cabbage attractively around noodles.
- Pour in enough broth to almost cover.
- Garnish with parsley.
- Serves 6–8.

TOFU ALMOND STROGANOFF WITH SPINACH NOODLES

Sauce:

    1 onion, chopped (optional)
    1 cup mushrooms, sliced
    ½ cake tofu, ¼-inch cubes
    ½ teaspoon oil
    5 tablespoons flour
    3 cups almond milk or seed yogurt
      (pp. 612–613)
    ¾ teaspoon dill weed
    1 teaspoon sea salt
    1 pound spinach noodles, cooked

- Sauté onion.
- Add mushrooms and tofu. Sauté 5 minutes or steam.
- Dilute flour in almond milk. Add with dill and salt to sautéed vegetables.
- Heat gently 30 minutes. Stir occasionally.
- Serve over noodles.
- Serves 6–8.

SEITAN

Made from the gluten in wheat flour and a smaller amount of whole-wheat flour; very high in protein; produces strength and vitality; sometimes referred to as wheat meat; a good substitute for animal food. It can be added to soups, stir-fry dishes, salads, stews, dressings, etc.

SEITAN

    3 cups gluten flour (1 pound)
    ¾ cup whole-wheat pastry flour
1½–2 cups water
Sauce:
    4 cups water
    1 cup soy sauce
    ¼ cup ginger, minced

- Mix flours together.
- Slowly add water to form a kneadable dough. Knead 15–20 minutes until smooth.
- Shape into a 2-inch thick disc. Steam 20 minutes. Cool. Cut into 1-inch squares.
- Sauce: Mix water, soy sauce, and ginger together. Bring to a boil. Drop in gluten. Simmer 3 hours (or cook in crockpot 8 hours). Stir occasionally.

Note: Liquid should cover gluten at onset of cooking.

LENTIL STEW WITH SEITAN

1 cup lentils, soaked
5 inches kombu, soaked
3–4 cups water
½ onion, cut in crescents (optional)
1 clove garlic, minced
2 large carrots, wedges
2 medium potatoes, sliced
1 cup seitan
2 bay leaves
½ teaspoon thyme
1 tablespoon miso
1 tablespoon oil

- Prepare lentils and cook 30 minutes with kombu.
- Sauté onion and garlic 2 minutes.
- Add carrots and potatoes and sauté 5 minutes.
- Add sautéed vegetables, bay leaves, and seitan to lentils. Cover and simmer 30 minutes.
- Add thyme. Dilute miso in some broth and return to stew. Cover and simmer 15 minutes.
- Serves 6.

CHOW MEIN WITH SEITAN

1 pound noodles, cooked and drained
Oil for frying (frying optional)
Sauce:
5 cups broth or water
1 onion, crescent moons (optional)
5 shiitake mushrooms, soaked and sliced
3 cups seitan, cubed
1 cup celery, sliced diagonally
1 cup Chinese cabbage, shredded
2 cups mung sprouts
2 kale leaves, sliced
2 tablespoons kuzu dissolved in
⅓ cup water
Soy sauce to taste

Prepare sauce:
- Bring broth to boil.
- Add onion and mushrooms. Reduce heat to low. Simmer 7 minutes.
- Add seitan. Bring back to boil. Reduce heat and simmer 5 minutes.
- Add celery, cabbage, sprouts, kale, kuzu, and soy sauce. (Taste should not be salty.) Simmer until thickened—about 10 minutes.
- Slice cooked noodles in half. Fry until golden brown. Drain on paper towels.
- Place noodles in small serving bowls and cover with sauce.
- Serves 6.

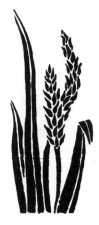

CEREALS

Cereals are grains that have been rolled, milled, or cracked. Once the grain is broken, water enters more readily. Cooking time is reduced and so is the nutritional value. It is best to mill your own cereals and use them immediately or store them in the refrigerator.

BASIC HOT CEREAL RECIPE

Use the meals, grits, or coarsely ground flours of rice, barley, rye, spelt, wheat, millet, corn, buckwheat, kamut, or oats; also cracked wheat, bulghur wheat, or steel-cut oats.

1 cup cereal (1½ cups oatmeal)
3 cups boiling water
⅛–¼ teaspoon sea salt

- Pour cereal into boiling water.
- Stir briskly to prevent lumping.
- Reduce heat to low.
- Cover and cook 20–40 minutes.
- Add more water if cereal gets too thick, and continue to cook. If cereal begins to burn, continue cooking in a double boiler.
- Serves 2.

Note: Mix cream cereal and corn meal in a bit of cold water before cooking to prevent lumping. The longer cereals cook, the sweeter they taste. In warmer weather, cook cereals less, and remove lid last 5 minutes of cooking to disperse heat.

Variations   Add wheat germ, toasted seeds, chopped nuts, seed yogurt, nut butter, nut milk, raisins, dried apples, cinnamon.
Dry-toast cereal for a nutty flavor before cooking. Oat flakes are especially delicious and more hearty prepared this way.

FRITTERS

Cold or leftover cereal
Oil for frying

- Slice cereal into pieces about ¼-inch thick.
- Fry each side in a bit of oil until golden.
- Garnish with parsley and scallions.
- Serve with sauce or sautéed vegetables.

MUESLI

2 cups rolled oats
⅓ cup each: sunflower seeds, chopped almonds, raisins
3 cups water
1 apple

- Combine oats, sunflower seeds, almonds, and raisins.
- Pour water over mixture. Mix lightly. For *deficient* or *cold* persons, heat or even boil water before pouring.
- Cover. Allow to stand overnight.
- In morning—grate apple into muesli. Mix well.

Breads

The "Great Grain Spirit" is symbolized by a warm, fragrant loaf of bread. Hot from the oven, fresh bread baked with care has the mysterious power of bringing warmth and togetherness into the home and to special occasions. The breaking of bread together is a ritual practiced by many cultures to symbolize their willingness to share what one has with others.

In the West, bread has been the major medium for the consumption of grain. For people to adapt to grain in only its whole, unmilled seed state is not a practical reality, nor is it necessarily desirable. The milling of grain is itself symbolic of the analytic process that characterizes the West. The author has observed that people on a grain-and-vegetable diet are usually drawn to increase flour products during intense analytic processes. The advantage of traditionally leavened flour products is that they promote integration as well. The grinding of grain causes some loss of nutrients, but at the same time, natural leavening reunites flour into one living substance, contributing vitamins and enzymes through the action of a beneficial fermentation.

It is often heard among health advocates that breads are not as nutritious and easily digested as unmilled grains. However, leavened breads such as sourdough with wholesome, fresh ingredients are a superior product with high nutrient value. Even so, they must be chewed well and eaten in moderate amounts to digest properly. Eating bread with cheese, fruit, sweeteners, liquids, and thin, brothy soups can interfere with digestion. Bread is best eaten with hearty soups, salads, vegetable dishes, plus spreads such as flax butter and *ghee* (page 183).

Individuals with a very weakened condition usually do better without bread and can use grain in its unmilled or cereal-cream form. We find that many people with allergies to wheat and other high-gluten grains (barley, rye, and sweet rice) will not react to the hypoallergenic glutinous grains (spelt, kamut, oats) or to sprouted grain. Sprouts are cooling; if a relatively more warming quality is needed, sprouted wheat or other grain sprouts can be cooked into "Essene Bread" as described later in this section. (Such breads are also available through most natural food stores in the United States and Canada.)

For best results in baking bread

- Use freshly ground flours. Bread will rise better and be more nutritious.
- Use hard, red winter wheat; higher in protein and gluten.

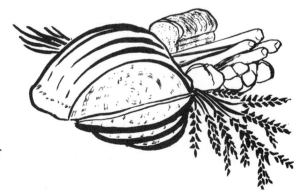

- Breads made with cooked whole grains, added to whole-wheat flour, are easier to digest.
- Use small amounts of sea salt.
- Sweeteners and oil are not necessary.

Best times for baking bread

- Make bread in the morning (*yang* or expanding time) and bake bread at night (*yin* or contracting time).
- On warm sunny days (rises better).
- When you feel vital and happy.

Different Flours and Combinations

Barley flour   Makes a sticky bread; can be combined 50–50 with whole-wheat flour for lightness.

Brown rice   Yields a sweeter and smoother bread; blends well with other flours. Use flour 20% in combination.

Buckwheat   Makes a good winter bread, dark and heavy. Use in combinations with wheat and rice flours.

Chestnut flour   Use to sweeten cakes, cookies, and puddings; adds lightness and creaminess; add to other flours or use alone.

Corn meal flour   Gives a good, light bread; good combined with small amounts of other flours.

Garbanzo flour   Can be used alone or mixed with other flours; especially good in sauces and pancakes.

Kamut flour   Light in texture; can be substituted in equal amounts for whole-wheat pastry flour in cake, pie, and muffin recipes.

Millet flour   Always combine with other flours, especially whole-wheat ($\frac{1}{3}$ millet to $\frac{2}{3}$ whole-wheat).

Oat flour   Light in texture; can be substituted for pastry flour; adds moistness to cakes and pastries; add approximately 20% to corn, whole-wheat, or rice flours.

Rye flour   Makes a sticky bread; can be combined 50–50 with rice or whole-wheat flour for a lighter bread. 100% rye bread greatly improves in flavor after several days.

Soy flour   Add small amounts to other flours for a more smooth and moist texture.

Spelt flour   Can be substituted 100% for wheat in bread recipes; usually well-tolerated by those allergic to wheat.

Sprouted wheat flour A sweet flour used in desserts, breads, wafers, and sauces; use alone or with other flours; stickier than whole-wheat flour.

To make:
- Sprout wheat (p. 569).
- Spread sprouts and dry in sun or on a screen for 2–3 days, or in a food dehydrator or oven on low temperature.
- Grind into flour using suribachi, blender, or flour mill.

Whole-wheat flour Made from hard red wheat; high in gluten; use alone or in combinations with other flours.

Whole-wheat pastry flour Made from soft white wheat berries; makes pie crusts flakier, crackers and cookies crisper, and adds lightness to baked goods.

NATURALLY LEAVENED BREAD

Natural leaveners introduce live airborne yeasts into the dough and yield a bread that is light and totally digestible with a distinctive and delicious sweet or sour taste. Some natural leavening agents are sourdough, miso, rejuvelac, fermented cooked grains, etc.

Whenever a flour and water mixture remains in a warm place, some natural leavening occurs. The use of fermented products such as sourdough merely accelerates the leavening process and provides for a certain type of fermentation to take place.

Quality sourdough products were, until the last few years, a commercial rarity in America, although with a little perseverance they can nearly always be found in Europe. Recently, however, a number of new as well as established American bakeries are offering a variety of sourdough products, made simply with ingredients such as organic whole-grain flour, whole salt, and pure water.

Sourdough and natural leavening have been with us for thousands of years. Yeast for bread is a relatively recent innovation, discovered in the chemists' lab in France about one hundred years ago.

According to some European researchers, naturally leavened bread is superior to cultured yeasted breads. Yeasted bread is linked to stomach bloat, indigestion, thin blood, and weak intestines; yeasted products seem uncannily to exacerbate conditions that occur with candida yeast overgrowth symptoms, including many degenerative diseases. Thus, various European and—more recently—certain American health clinics forbid their clients yeasted bread.

Commercial yeasted breads, even the whole-grain varieties, often have other problems. They typically contain flour bleach, which forms alloxan, a compound known to cause diabetes in animals by destroying the beta cells of the pancreas (*Clinical Nutrition Newsletter*, Dec. 1982). Flour bleach does more than bleach. It acts chemically to soften and age flour, and to repel insects.

Other benefits of naturally leavened breads:
- The long proofing allows the fermenting agents to break down the cellulose structure and release nutrients into the dough, improving its nutritional value.
- Contains lactobacillus, which helps generate the intestinal flora essential for proper digestion and elimination.
- The natural bacterial action and baking neutralize nearly all of the phytic acid which occurs in wheat and other grains. (Phytic acid reduces mineral metabolism—especially in those whose diet includes a good percentage of grains and legumes—and can contribute to anemia, nervous disorders, and rickets.) About 90% of the phytic acid remains in yeasted breads.
- It stays edible for weeks and is more delicious and nutritious in five to ten days, if stored in a cool dry place.

Working with sourdough is an art. A ferment is alive and reflects its environment. When breads don't rise or turn out the way you would like, keep experimenting, because various factors may have to be harmonized before bread will reflect what you intend. At first, bread that rises like yeasted bread may be what you prefer, but once accustomed to the more concentrated naturally leavened breads, fluffy products will seem lacking in character. However, if your naturally leavened breads turn out unusually dense, here are some helpful ideas for making them lighter: 1) use more sourdough starter, up to one cup per loaf; 2) add to the flour one or two tablespoons of wheat-gluten flour; 3) knead the bread more; 4) cut none or at most one shallow slit in top of loaf (seventh step below in "Sourdough Bread" recipe); 5) use wooden or ceramic leavening bowls—metal lessens fermentive activity.

SOURDOUGH STARTER

1 cup water
1 cup whole-wheat flour

- In a sterilized jar and with a sterilized spoon, mix flour and water together. (Sterilize in boiling water.)
- Cover with a cotton cloth. Live airborne yeasts will begin to turn it sour.
- Stir daily with a sterilized spoon for uniform fermentation.
- After 3 days your starter will be ready.
- Loosely cover with lid and store in a cool place.

To replenish: Always leave a small amount of starter in jar. Replace with more flour and water. Stir well and store.

SOURDOUGH BREAD

14 cups whole-wheat flour
5 cups water
1½ teaspoons sea salt
1 cup sourdough starter

- Mix 7 cups flour with water, salt, and starter.
- Add remaining flour slowly until dough becomes too thick to stir.
- Knead gently until smooth, uniform, and elastic.
- Cover and let rise 2 hours in non-metal bowl.
- Replenish starter.
- Knead dough again.
- Shape into 3 or 4 loaves.
- Cut shallow slits in top to keep from cracking.
- Place in oiled and floured bread pans. Cover. Let rise 4–6 hours.
- Place in a cold oven with a pan of plain water on oven floor.
- Bake at 425°F for 15 minutes.
- Lower heat to 350°F. Continue cooking until golden, about 45 minutes.
- Remove from pans to cool.
- Cut into thin slices before serving.
- Yields 3–4 loaves.

Note: The first six steps of this recipe prepare the basic sourdough batter to be used in recipes for rolls, crusts, bagels, etc. that appear in the following pages.

SOURDOUGH CORNBREAD

½ cup sourdough starter
2 cups cornmeal or corn flour; or 1 cup cornmeal and 1 cup whole-wheat flour
1½ cups water
½ teaspoon sea salt
1 teaspoon kelp powder

- In a ceramic bowl combine starter, meal and water.
- Allow to sit 6–8 hours until very bubbly with a sour aroma.
- Preheat oven to 375°F.
- Fold salt and kelp into the batter.
- Pour into a preheated oiled pan.
- Bake 45 minutes until nicely browned.
- Yields 1 loaf or 1 dozen muffins.

SOURDOUGH CAKE

½ cup sourdough starter
1½ cup whole-wheat pastry flour
½ cup sprouted wheat flour
1–1½ cup apple juice
½ teaspoon sea salt
1 tablespoon lemon juice
1 teaspoon grated orange or lemon
   rind

- In a bowl, combine starter, flours, and apple juice.
- Allow to sit 6–8 hours until very bubbly.
- Preheat oven to 350°F.
- Fold salt, lemon juice, and rind into the batter.
- Pour into a cake pan brushed with oil or lecithin.
- Bake 45 minutes until nicely browned. May also be steamed (p. 497).
- Yields 1 cake.

Variations   Replace sprouted wheat flour with rice, chestnut, millet, or oat flours. Add sweeteners, dried fruit, spices, extracts, nuts.

SOURDOUGH BREAD STICKS

- Prepare sourdough and let rise 2 hours (p. 493).
- Pinch off balls of dough and roll into sticks by hand.
- Place on a cookie sheet brushed with oil or lecithin.
- Make diagonal slits on top. Let double in size.
- Bake at 350°F for 20 minutes.

SOURDOUGH DINNER ROLLS

- Follow the above recipe, shaping dough into rolls.
- Bake 30 minutes at 350°F.

SOURDOUGH PIZZA AND PIE CRUST

- Prepare sourdough (p. 493) and let rise until double in size (4–6 hours).
- Roll out until very thin.
- Place in a pie or pizza pan that has been brushed with oil or lecithin. Trim and flute edges.
- Let rise 30 minutes.
- Add pizza or pie filling. Bake.
- 1½ cups flour yields one 9-inch crust.

SOURDOUGH VEGETABLE OR FRUIT ROLL

- Prepare sourdough (p. 493) and let rise until double in size (4–6 hours).
- Divide dough into 4 parts and roll each piece into a thin rectangular sheet.
- Spread vegetable or fruit purée or jam over the surface and roll into cylinders. Seal edges with a little water.
- Let rise 1–2 hours.
- Bake at 350°F for 30 minutes or until nicely browned.
- Cut into rounds and serve on chrysanthemum leaves.

SOURDOUGH BAGELS

- Prepare sourdough (p. 493). Knead well and allow to sit 4–6 hours.
- Punch down and divide into equal pieces doughnut size.
- To shape: Shape into round rolls, then push thumbs through the center and shape the holes.
- Drop bagels into boiling water for 30–60 seconds. They will rise to the top.
- Sprinkle with poppy or sesame seeds.
- Bake on oiled cookie sheets at 425°F for 20 minutes or at 350°F for 30 minutes.

SOURDOUGH MUFFINS (Corn Muffins)

- Follow the recipe for sourdough cornbread on page 493.
- Pour batter into muffin tins brushed with oil or lecithin.
- Bake at 350°F for 30 minutes.

Variations Add cooked rice, cooked corn kernels, sunflower seeds, etc.

SWEET MUFFINS

Replace water with apple juice. Add raisins, chopped apples, and cinnamon, blueberries, etc.

BUCKWHEAT MUFFINS

Use whole-wheat flour and cooked buckwheat.

RYE MUFFINS

Add 1 cup cooked cracked rye to 2 cups whole-wheat flour.

SOURDOUGH PITA (Arab pocket bread)

- Prepare sourdough and let rise until double, 4–6 hours (p. 493).
- Punch down and divide into equal pieces. Shape into balls and allow dough to rest 10 minutes.
- Preheat oven to 350°F.
- Sprinkle balls with flour. Roll ¼-inch thick.
- Bake on an ungreased cookie sheet on the lowest rack for 5 minutes (until bread puffs up).
- Slice in half and fill with falafel and condiments.

BATTER BREAD

2½ cups whole-wheat flour
1½ cups millet flour
1 cup rice flour
½ teaspoon sea salt
1 tablespoon oil (optional)
3 cups water

- Preheat oven to 325°F.
- Combine flours and salt.
- Rub in oil gently through your palms.
- Stir in water and mix until heavy and sticky.
- Allow to stand 8 hours or overnight in a warm place, then turn into a heated oiled loaf pan.
- Bake 1 hour or until nicely browned.
- Remove bread from pan and cool on a rack.
- Slice before serving.
- Yields 1 loaf.

Note: To test the bread to see if it is done, insert a knife into the loaf; if it comes out dry, bread is done.

Variations
- 2½ cups whole-wheat flour, 1½ cups whole-wheat pastry flour, 1 cup buckwheat flour
- 3 cups rye flour, 2 cups rice flour
- 2 cups whole-wheat flour, 2 cups rice flour, 1 cup oat flour
- Sourdough: Add ½ cup sourdough starter to batter; allow to stand overnight.

VEGETABLE BATTER BREAD

Add leftover grains or freshly cooked vegetables to batter.

SWEET BATTER BREAD

Add puréed squash, sweet potato, apples, or other fruit to batter. Flavor with raisins and nuts; cinnamon, cardamom, vanilla, anise, or ginger; orange or lemon peel.

STEAMED BREAD

Place dough in a ceramic bowl or container that will fit inside a larger pot. Cover with a plate. Fill pot with 3–4 inches water. Place a rack or chopsticks in the bottom of the pot. Place the bowl on top of the rack. Cover and simmer 3–4 hours on a medium-low flame. Replenish water as necessary. Let cool. Run a spatula around the inside of the pan to loosen the loaf. Turn upside down and thump to release loaf.

To pressure cook: Follow above directions. Steam for 1 hour.

TASSAJARA BARLEY BREAD

2 cups barley flour
4 cups whole-wheat flour
1 teaspoon kelp powder
3 tablespoons sesame seeds
3 cups boiling water
1–1½ teaspoons sea salt

- Dry-toast barley flour until brown.
- Mix flours, salt, kelp, and sesame seeds.
- Add boiling water and knead well.
- Cover with damp towel and allow to rest briefly.
- Cut and shape into round loaves. Place on oiled cookie sheet or bread pan. Cover and proof 4–8 hours.
- Preheat oven to 350°F.
- Pre-moisten top and cut shallow slits.
- Bake 1½–2 hours.
- Yields 2 loaves.

Variation   Add ½ cup sourdough starter.

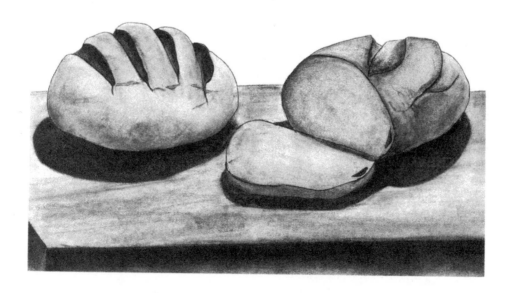

SPROUTED ESSENE BREAD

4–6 cups wheat sprouts
(The sprouts should be the same
length as the berry.)

- Grind sprouts in a food grinder.
- Knead, then shape into a loaf or rolls. Set into a bread pan or cookie sheet.
- Cover and bake at 225°–250°F for approximately 2 hours. Let cool.

Variation   Use soft white wheat, rye, or barley sprouts.

CHAPATIS

3 cups whole-wheat pastry flour
1 teaspoon oil
½–¾ teaspoon sea salt
1 cup water

- Combine ingredients in a bowl. Mix in water.
- Knead well. (Should have consistency of ear lobe and be slightly sticky.)
- Allow dough to rest at least 1 hour, or overnight.
- Shape into small balls.
- Roll into flat rounds (the thinner, the crispier).
- Heat a cast-iron skillet.
- Oil each chapati on both sides (optional), but do not oil pan.
- Cook each side for a minute, until lightly brown. Or bake at 350°F for 15 minutes, until golden brown.
- Fold in half to keep soft and warm.

CRÊPES

2 cups whole-wheat flour or rice flour
6 cups water
¼–½ teaspoon sea salt
Oil for brushing pan
Fillings: Vegetable spreads
Nut spreads
Fruit sauces

- Combine ingredients in a bowl. Whip the batter by hand.
- Allow to sit for 2 hours or overnight.
- Use a cast-iron skillet with low edges.
- Heat pan well and brush with oil.
- Reduce heat to ⅓ maximum.
- Pour batter in pan, turning it clockwise to spread evenly. (Batter should be thin.)
- Cooking time: 7–10 minutes for first side; 3–5 minutes for second side.
- Spread filling over crêpe. Roll and serve.
- Serves 4.

PANCAKES

2 cups whole-wheat flour
2 cups water
¼–½ teaspoon sea salt
½ teaspoon oil

- Combine ingredients in a bowl. Whip the batter by hand.
- Allow to stand for 1 hour or overnight.
- Heat a cast-iron skillet. Brush bottom of pan with oil.
- Pour in ¼-inch batter.
- Cover and cook over low heat 5 minutes.
- Turn over and cook 5 minutes more.
- Serve with miso toppings, spreads, sautéed vegetables.

WAFFLES

Heat waffle iron and brush with oil. Add pancake batter. Cook until golden.

Variations The following options can be used in the above crêpe, pancake, and waffle recipes.

Sourdough
Add ½ cup sourdough starter (p. 492).
Allow to sit overnight.

Buckwheat
1½ cups buckwheat flour
½ cup whole-wheat flour

Corncakes
1 cup corn flour or corn meal
1 cup whole-wheat flour

with cooked grain
1½ cups whole-wheat flour
½ cup whole-wheat pastry flour
½ cup cooked grain

FLAKY PIE CRUST—good for covered pies and pastries

3 cups whole-wheat pastry flour
⅓ cup oil or sunflower meal
1 teaspoon liquid lecithin
½ teaspoon sea salt
⅔ cup hot water

- Preheat oven to 375°F.
- Combine dry ingredients. Rub in oil and lecithin with fingers.
- Add hot water slowly. Stir as little as possible.
- Roll up into a ball. Divide in half and roll out.
- Place bottom piece into pie pan and add filling. Cover with top piece, prick with fork, and flute edges.
- Bake 40–50 minutes, until crust is browned.
- Yields 2 crusts.

Note: The more oil you add, the flakier the crust will be.

CRUMBLY PIE CRUST

½ cup buckwheat flour
½ cup brown rice flour
½ cup whole-wheat pastry flour
2 tablespoons crushed seeds or nuts
¼–⅓ cup oil (optional)
½ teaspoon liquid lecithin
¼ teaspoon sea salt
1 teaspoon cinnamon
A few tablespoons water

- Preheat oven to 350°F.
- Combine dry ingredients. Rub in oil and lecithin with fingers.
- Add just enough water so that the dough holds together, but is crumbly.
- Press into a 9-inch pie pan and bake 10–15 minutes. Or, fill with pie filling and bake.
- Extra dough can be sprinkled on top of pie before baking.
- Yields 1 crust.

LIGHT PRESSED PIE CRUST

¾ cup oat flour or oat flakes
¾ cup brown rice flour
¼ teaspoon sea salt
¼–⅓ cup oil or sesame meal
2–2½ tablespoons ice water

- Preheat oven to 400°F.
- Oatmeal may be blended in electric blender to make flour.
- Combine dry ingredients. Rub oil in with fingers.
- Add just enough ice water so that dough holds together, but is crumbly.
- Press into a lightly floured pie pan and flute the edges.
- Prick well with a fork.
- Bake 10–12 minutes. Or fill with pie filling and bake.
- Extra dough can be sprinkled on top of pie before baking.
- Yields 1 crust.

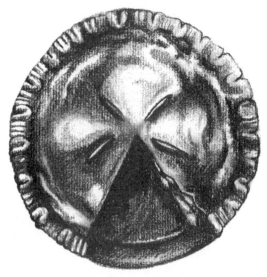

THE BOUNTY OF RYE

by Jacques de Langre

Rye is one of the neglected or forgotten cereal grains, yet it offers such unusual benefits that one should not overlook its bounties for health or just for superior taste in a loaf of bread.

Diseases such as fatty plaque in the blood vessels, or calcium deposits (sclerosis) in the smaller arteries—and the ensuing loss of elasticity coupled with high blood pressure—all affect the coronary system. Many incidences of blurred vision and progressively worsening eyesight are also traceable to arteriosclerosis, as are lameness in the legs, strokes, and brain malfunctions.

The natural remedy for all of these conditions is rye in bread form. This cereal grain in its whole form, cool-milled on stone and with all of its bran and germ kept intact, has the capability of reducing and totally eliminating vessel and plaque calcification. Rye also possesses the power to re-energize anemic bodies and rebuild the entire digestive system. This is accomplished through the rye's high carbohydrate content and its richness in nitrogenous matter.

This ability to restore suppleness and unclog the blood vessels makes rye a highly prized breadmaking element.

Rye flour is invariably hard to find in its whole form, since few bakers bother making it into bread; flour obtained from millers is old and stale and makes poor-tasting bread anyway. It's true that it requires some dexterity in dough formulation and handling, but once it has been demonstrated to an interested baker, the results of true-rye-sour-starter 100% rye bread are so outstanding that he or she will persevere in making the superior product.

Making 100% rye bread into what is called "black bread" by the natural leaven process is a challenge, but the rewards are well worth the extra effort. All Jewish rye in the U. S. is made with yeast, and therefore is of little benefit—and may even be harmful—to its consumer.

The essential condition for a totally healing rye bread begins with the choice of good quality rye berries. Since rye grows in relatively poor soil and cold weather, it is mainly a winter crop that thrives in high altitudes and has the greatest winter hardiness of all cereal grains. It is even found growing as far north as the Arctic Circle. The characteristic green-and-red intermix of the berries is a sign of a good strain, but it is also very important to secure the rye from a knowledgeable grain dealer and to get assurance that the rye is free of ergot.

Ergot is a fungus or a sclerotium that develops on grasses and especially on rye. Among the potentially harmful chemicals in ergot is lysergic acid, the active ingredient of LSD-25, and the cause of "St. Anthony's fire," a disease prevalent in northern Europe in the Middle Ages in areas of high rye bread consumption. While it is true that natural leaven completely neutralizes ergot's alkaloid substances, it may still present some danger to the consumer when, as in the case of modern-style Jewish rye, it is made improperly with yeast or with dehydrated culture substitutes sold to commercial bakers for the purpose of expediency.

It is because of its possible ergotism that rye has been neglected as a bread ingredient, but modern grain cleaning and the diligence of reputable grain dealers have almost totally eliminated the danger. Inspecting the whole rye berries yourself prior to milling it easily reveals the presence of hard fungal structures; the rye would be made safe by removing those that are shaped like rye kernels but much larger and darker. This is ergot—and since it contains several poisonous organic compounds called alkaloids, it should not be milled without a thorough cleansing and removing of the fungal infestation.

The abundant advantages of milling one's own clean rye berries in their entirety and made into bread truly warrant the conscious baker's full attention.

The benefits of rye or black bread are fully evident when the dough has been seeded with a natural starter made exclusively with rye sour. A robust rye sour will acquire a very special character and display a different kind of aroma, pattern of bubbles, and fermentation than a starter made entirely from wheat. (See "Rye Sour Starter" for Black Rye, below.)

Rye was the major ingredient of bread consumed by the poor in medieval Europe; for economic reasons it was often diluted with meal or coarse flour made from acorns, water caltrops, or horse chestnuts.

In order to become familiar with baking fermented rye products, it is fitting to try an early Middle-Age formula for "Nieules" or "Nielles." The name translates into "rye cockles" or "blight," which readily shows that in antiquity the poor people, who had to contend with the very real danger of hunger and were often forced to eat ergotized rye as the only grain available, knew full well how to clean and minimize the just-as-real threat of ergot. They even made fun of the small cakes by calling them "smuts. "

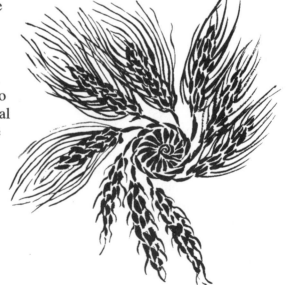

RYE NIELLES (BLIGHT RYE CAKES)—for 250 cakes

6 cups freshly milled whole rye
2 tablespoons barley malt or barley malt syrup
2 tablespoons sesame oil
2–5 whole eggs* (optional)
2 orange rinds, finely grated (to replicate the horse chestnut's bitter flavor)
1½ teaspoons natural gray sea salt
½ cup rye sour starter; more if a wetter dough is desired (use rye starter formula listed with Black Rye below)
4 tablespoons toasted and finely chopped almonds, walnuts, or chestnut meat (for sprinkling on the moist cakes before baking)

- Mix all ingredients together, except for salt and the chopped nuts. When dough begins to form, add the salt and begin to knead in earnest until a smooth dough is obtained. Place dough in a covered bowl and let it rest in a cool, draft-free place for 1 to 2 hours (longer in winter). Knead again for a few minutes and replace dough in bowl, cover with a damp towel, and allow it to rest (proof) in a cool place for another 2 hours.
- Using a roller on a floured board, shape the dough into a thin, even layer. Dust with flour to keep from sticking to the board. The stretched dough should be just under a quarter-inch thick. Lightly dust both sides with rye flour as you finish shaping.
- Cut out various small shapes 1 to 2 inches wide, using a cookie cutter, wood stamps, or a sharp knife. Prick each with a fork. Sprinkle lightly with flour and allow the raw cakes to rise slightly.
- Drop small groups of raw cakes into a pan of boiling water, and as soon as they surface fish them out with a sieve. Cool briefly and quickly under cold running water, then allow them to drain on a towel. Place on baking sheets and, while still moist, sprinkle them with grated nut meat. Bake for 10 to 20 minutes at 325°F, or until golden brown. Cool and store in tightly sealed jars.

*Note: The binding quality and rich taste of eggs can generally be replaced by lecithin. Two tablespoons of granulated lecithin stirred well into a little warm water can replace three eggs. The lecithin/egg substitution ratio is 2 teaspoons lecithin in 4 teaspoons water per egg.

BLACK RYE BREAD

Black rye bread is tricky but well worth mastering. This is the simplest method and, having succeeded with this, you may be bold enough to scale the heights of rye mastery, the seven-day-baked traditional pumpernickel. (The complicated method for baking the real old-fashioned pumpernickel takes seven days of consecutive mixing and baking to complete.)

Success with your first attempt may be achieved by following the easy method outlined hereafter. If your efforts fail, and what you take out of the oven appears inedible, take heart and allow the sticky mass to age and acquire a reputation. With patience and a few days, even a most unpromising mess will either magically change into a delicious cake-like bread, or turn into a gaudy green and pink mildewed stone made of whole rye. Either way you will have acquired notoriety for your artistry, since black bread supplies a dark and suitable backdrop for the wondrous colors of nature developing from the moldy spores.

Black bread is not at its best for taste or texture right after being baked; in fact, its very stickiness at birth ensures its survival. While other breads get devoured as they emerge from the oven, rye breads just lie there amorphous and forlorn. But after two or three days, watch out! The black rye's appeal and taste return at a gallop and pack a wallop of flavor, aroma, and healing properties. When well-done and cared for, its eating repays you a thousandfold for all of the trials and tribulations you have experienced during its baking.

With no other variety of grains does the rye baker shine. Earlier we gave you a warning that baking Black Rye was another ball game. In all truth we now give you another warning: if you succeed at baking good rye bread with rye sour starter consistently, the rest of the world will beat a path to your door.

RYE SOUR STARTER

½ cup rye flour, freshly ground
1 cup water

- Mix together in clean glass jar; cover with cotton cloth or loose lid.
- Let sit in warm place for 3 days. When ready, starter should smell sour and be bubbly.

RYE SOUR LEAVEN

3 cups rye flour, freshly ground
2 cups water
1 cup starter

- In a ceramic bowl stir flour, water, and starter.
- Let sit 8 hours or overnight until bubbly with a sour smell.
- Yields 6 cups.

BLACK RYE BREAD—to make 4 loaves in 3- by 6-inch pans

6 cups rye sour leaven
2 cups cold water
8–9 cups rye flour (freshly ground)
2 teaspoons natural gray sea salt crystals

- Pour the rye sour leaven into a bowl or kneading trough. The mixture should be of batter consistency and have a pungently sour but pleasant aroma. Mix all of the water into the rye sour, then gradually add the flour until the mix becomes smooth. Add the salt crystals and begin to knead. If it appears too hard, add 25 to 75 grams—$\frac{1}{8}$ to $\frac{3}{8}$ of a cup—of extra water. The dough should be very wet and sticky. Don't despair if the dough sticks to your hands; this is the correct consistency, so don't overknead in a futile attempt to correct this soggy mass.
- Scrape as much of the goo off your hands as time will allow, and walk away from the quagmire with dignity . . . but not finality. Here is where persistence pays off, for when you return to the rye dough an hour or two later it will dramatically have changed its texture and demeanor. (If it hasn't, take courage in remembering the name of the preceding recipe. If the former was called "Blight Cakes," this one could be dubbed "Scourge.") With just one attempt you'll learn why rye isn't popular with bakers today, but also eating it will tell you why the Middle Ages treasured it for its power to strengthen human character.
- After you've taken the time to read the preceding rumination, the rye dough is usually ready to be divided and shaped (that's a loose word) into individual loaves. Allow one to two hours proofing time in the pans or cloth-lined baskets. The proofing box or enclosure should provide moisture and, toward the end of the proofing period, a small amount of heat.
- Baking: once the oven is preheated to 450°F, place the risen loaves in the oven, preferably on a clay or ceramic hearth. Lower the temperature to 350°F after 10 minutes, and do not open the oven door during the entire baking time. Pull one loaf out at the end of an hour and test for doneness by rapping the bottom of the loaf.
- The baking is complete if, at this point, the loaf's bottom gives a sharp, dry sound when rapped soundly with the knuckles. The loaves can now be placed on a suitable rack for cooling.

(Excerpted and adapted from the book *The New Bread's Biological Transmutations,* The Grain and Salt Society, 273 Fairway Dr., Asheville, NC 28805.)

Legumes: Beans, Peas, and Lentils

Because of their high protein content, legumes are often thought to be a partial replacement for the protein from animal products. Yet the idea of complementing the protein of legumes with other foods to make it more "complete" and like that of animal protein is an idea that gains unquestioned acceptance only in a society obsessed with protein. Many of this book's recipes partially embrace this way of thinking since somewhat richer-tasting food is more appropriate for those in transition from a complex diet of extreme flavors.

Nevertheless, there are many people who do not digest legumes well and experience problems with flatulence and allergies. In many of these cases the problem may lie in improper preparation, wrong choice of legume, and poor food combining, all of which are discussed in the following pages.

The protein from legumes can help regulate sugar, water, and other aspects of metabolism, as well as promote balanced sexual activity and proper growth and development of the body, including the brain. These same activities come under the domain of the kidney-adrenal functions according to Chinese medicine, which also embraces the bean as a proper food for the kidneys.

As a rule, legumes are drying and diuretic. Thus, except for soybean products, they are not ideal foods for thin, dry, frail, or generally *deficient* persons. For those who wish to counteract this tendency in legumes, Ayurveda suggests combining them with oily foods. In cultures where there is high legume consumption, such a practice is common. For instance, Mexicans customarily fry their beans in lard or oil, and in areas of the Middle East where garbanzo beans are a daily food, they are regularly prepared as *hummus,* which contains substantial amounts of the oily sesame seed butter. Adding seaweeds and sufficient salt also creates a moistening effect in legumes that is lighter than the effect of oily foods.

On the other hand, legumes balance the *excessive*, strong, and robust person, including those with signs of overweight, *heat,* or *damp* conditions such as yeasts or edema. Once again, soybean is the exception—it reduces *heat* but is not good for yeast or overweight conditions.

In addition to acknowledging the generally beneficial effect on the kidneys, another traditional practice exists in China in which legumes are assigned healing value according to their Five Element color. For example, red legumes such as aduki bean, red lentil, and kidney bean influence the Fire Element, heart, and small intestines; yellow legumes such as garbanzo bean, yellow pea, and soybean influence the Earth Element, spleen-

506

pancreas, and stomach; white legumes such as lima bean, navy bean, and great northern bean influence the Metal Element, lungs, and large intestine; dark, black, and brown legumes such as black bean, black soybean, and brown lentil influence the Water Element, kidneys, and bladder; green legumes such as mung bean, green pea, and fresh green bean influence the Wood Element, liver, and gall bladder.

Nutrients

Legumes are not only high in protein, but also in fat and carbohydrate. They are rich sources of potassium, calcium, iron, and several B-vitamins. Sprouted legumes are an excellent source of vitamin C and enzymes.

The following section gives the unique properties of each legume.

Healing Properties of Legumes

Aduki Bean

Neutral thermal nature; sweet-and-sour flavor; influences heart and small intestine; tonifies the kidney-adrenal function; detoxifies the body; removes *heat* conditions; disperses stagnant blood; reduces swelling; diuretic and drying. Used for *damp* and watery conditions, leukorrhea, jaundice, ascites, diarrhea, edema, boils, and to promote weight loss. For prolonged menstruation, chew well five raw aduki beans daily until menses stop.

"Aduki juice" is prepared by simmering one cup of beans in five cups of water for an hour (remove the juice and continue cooking the beans). Take ½ cup juice ½ hour before meals as a remedy for nephritis and most other kidney complaints. Regular use of the juice with meals increases mother's milk.

Aduki paste can be made for external application in mumps and boils: grind raw aduki beans to a powder and mix with warm water and enough honey to form a paste. Apply directly to the affected skin areas and secure it with cotton cloth and adhesive tape. The paste is effective for five hours and can be applied as often as desired. Using aduki juice or beans in the diet is also helpful for these disorders.

Cautions: Thin, *dry* people should use this bean sparingly (combine adukis with seaweeds and sufficient salt to improve moistening effect).

Anasazi Bean

In Navajo, anasazi means "ancient one"; this unhybridized bean, indigenous to North America, has been cultivated since 1100 A.D. Sweet in flavor, containing only one-fourth of the flatulence-causing sugars of other beans and about one-third more sodium, these mottled, maroon-and-white seeds are similar in size to pinto beans and are often used interchangeably in recipes.

Black Bean (Black Turtle Bean)

Warming thermal nature; sweet flavor; beneficial to kidneys and reproductive function; builds *yin* fluids and blood; diuretic. Used for low backache, knee pain, involuntary seminal emission, and infertility.

Black bean juice is effective for hoarseness, laryngitis, kidney stones, bed wetting, urinary difficulty, and hot flashes of menopause. Preparation and dosage are same as "aduki juice," p. 507.

Hardy members of the kidney bean family, black beans are native to Mexico.

Black-eyed Peas

Also called "cowpea" or "China bean"; they originally came from Africa, where they grow in the wild. In the United States black-eyed peas are associated with Southern cuisine. Soft, quick-cooking beans, they can also be eaten fresh in the pod.

Black Soybeans

Neutral thermal nature; sweet flavor; influences the spleen-pancreas and kidneys; improves blood circulation and water metabolism; diuretic; removes toxins from the body; quells *wind* conditions. Used to treat rheumatism, kidney disease, and kidney-related conditions such as low backache, weak bones, and painful knees. Drink the juice (prepare as "aduki juice," p. 507) to relieve spasms and cramps, inflammations, and chronic cough resulting from weak kidneys.

Bolita or Pink Bean

Relative of the pinto bean, it is an heirloom seed which has escaped hybridization. Used extensively in Hispanic and American Indian cultures, it adapts to and grows in a variety of environments, which tends to vary its size and color somewhat. Contains more calcium and sodium than most other beans. Use the bolita interchangeably in pinto and/or kidney bean recipes.

Fava Bean

Neutral thermal nature; pleasing sweet flavor; diuretic; strengthens the spleen-pancreas. Used to treat edema and swelling. Fava bean juice (follow recipe for "aduki juice," p. 507) is commonly used to help cure diarrhea. Besides its pod, the bean is encased in a tough bitter skin which can be removed after soaking overnight. Also called "broad" or "horse" bean, this hearty, ancient legume grows readily on most continents, though it is not well known in North America.

Garbanzo Bean (Chick-pea)

Sweet flavor; beneficial to pancreas, stomach, and heart (shaped somewhat like a heart); contains more iron than other legumes and is also a good source of unsaturated fats. There are many varieties, varying in size and color (red, white, black, brown).

Great Northern and Navy Beans

Cooling thermal nature; sweet flavor; beneficial to the lungs; promote beautiful skin. Can be eaten as fresh green beans.

Kidney Bean

Cooling thermal nature; sweet flavor; diuretic; increases *yin* fluids; used in treating edema and swelling. Kidney beans are part of a large family of legumes including pinto, green wax, bolita, mung, and great northern varieties. Many of these have been cultivated in the Americas since prehistoric times.

Lentil

Neutral thermal nature; mild flavor; diuretic; beneficial to the heart and circulation; stimulates the adrenal system; increases the vitality ("*jing* essence") of the kidneys. Lentils cook more quickly than other beans.

One of the first cultivated crops, lentils are grown and eaten all over the planet. India produces more than fifty varieties of different colors and sizes, cooked into their traditional "dahl."

Lima Bean

Cooling thermal nature; sweet flavor; beneficial to the liver and lungs; beautifies the skin; increases *yin* fluids; highly alkalizing (equal to soybeans in alkalinity); neutralizes acidic conditions such as often arise from excessive meat and refined-food consumption. One of the best beans for most Americans.

Also known as the "butter" or "sieva" bean, it is a relatively new member of the kidney bean family. Thriving in warm climates, limas are a favorite in South America. Starchier and less fatty than most other beans.

Mung Bean

Cooling thermal nature; sweet flavor; detoxifies the body; beneficial to the liver and gall bladder; produces *yin* fluids in general as well as specific *yin* fluids for the liver; alleviates *damp-heat* in the body; diuretic; reduces swelling. Used as a cure for food poisoning (drink liquid from mung soup), dysentery (cook with garlic), diarrhea, painful urination, mumps, burns, lead and pesticide poisoning, boils, heat stroke, conjunctivitis, and edema—especially edema in the lower extremities. Also useful in the treatment of high blood pressure, acidosis, and gastro-intestinal ulcers marked by *heat* signs. Consume mung soup to treat inflamed (red) skin outbreaks, *summer heat,* thirst, restlessness, impatience, and urinary difficulty accompanied by *heat* signs.

A member of the kidney bean family and originally from India, mung beans have become a traditional part of Chinese cuisine. One of the most important beans therapeutically, they are particularly useful because of their capacity to cleanse the heart and vascular system and reduce toxicity (according to author Hong-Yen Hsu, they remove all toxins).

Sprouted mung beans are commonly available in grocery stores. They are very cooling with a sweet flavor, used to detoxify the body, treat alcoholism, build the *yin* fluids, and to improve the "triple heater" function of Chinese medicine.

Cautions: Use the bean in small amounts if at all in conditions of *coldness.* Excess mung sprouts can exacerbate cases of deficient digestive fire (loose, watery stools, low energy, and signs of *coldness*).

Peas

Neutral thermal nature; sweet flavor; tonify the spleen-pancreas and stomach; harmonize digestion and reduce the effect of an overworked, excessive liver on the stomach and spleen-pancreas; reduce counter-current *qi* (for example, vomiting, hiccups, belching, coughing); diuretic; mildly laxative. Also used for spasms, edema, constipation, and skin eruptions such as carbuncles and boils.

Soybean

Cooling thermal nature; sweet flavor; strengthens the spleen-pancreas; influences the colon; moistens conditions of *dryness;* supplements the kidneys; cleanses the blood vessels and heart, improving circulation; helps restore pancreatic functioning (especially in diabetic conditions); promotes clear vision; diuretic; lowers fever; highly alkalizing and eliminates toxins from the body; boosts milk secretion in nursing mothers. Also used as a remedy for dizziness, childhood malnourishment (especially in the form of tempeh and soy milk), skin eruptions, constipation, edema, excessive fluid retention and toxemia during pregnancy, and food poisoning. For the imbalances during pregnancy and for food poisoning, drink soybean juice (prepare as "aduki juice" above). Soybeans are a natural source of lecithin—a brain food.

Unless well-cooked, soybeans inhibit the digestive enzyme trypsin, making them difficult to digest. The fermentation process, such as used in tempeh, tofu, miso, and soy sauce, also eliminates the beans' trypsin-inhibiting effect.

Soybean sprouts are cooling with a sweet flavor. They are diuretic and used to treat spasms, arthritis, food stagnation, *heat*-type coughs and other *heat* conditions marked by one or more signs such as yellow tongue coating, yellow mucus, and scanty, dark yellow urine.

First described in Chinese manuscripts in 2800 B.C., the soybean is called the "beef" of China due to its extensive use and high protein content (38%). It is concentrated in essential fatty acids (including omega-3) and contains more protein than milk without the saturated fat or cholesterol.

Recent research suggests soy products may protect against atherosclerosis, PMS, bone loss, and menopausal difficulty. Most research indicating a positive effect from soy has utilized fermented soy products such as Japanese "natto." Natto is quite similar to tempeh (see pages 522–526). Soy sprouts and virtually all varieties of beans also feature the above protective attributes. Soy milks, infant soy formulas, soy protein powders, soy concentrates, and soy isolates often contain denatured proteins and/or isolated proteins without the necessary nutrient cofactors of digestion and metabolism; thus they generally do not promote enduring health.

String Bean

Neutral thermal nature; sweet flavor; strengthens the spleen-pancreas and kidneys; increases *yin* fluids. Used for diabetes and the frequent urination and thirst accompanying this condition. Also used to treat involuntary seminal emission, diarrhea, and leukorrhea.

Caution: String beans can worsen constipation.

Improving the Digestibility of Legumes

Some people have difficulty digesting beans and other legumes and develop gas, intestinal problems, irritability, and unclear thinking. The gas from legumes is generated by trisaccharides they contain. Enzymes are present in healthy intestines to break down the trisaccharides into simple sugars. Eating small amounts of legumes encourages formation of the necessary enzymes. However, before digestive excellence occurs, there are techniques for preparing and eating legumes that alleviate most problems.

- Chew them thoroughly. Realize that small amounts—a few tablespoons of legumes—have nutritional and healing value.
- Avoid giving legumes to young children (under approximately 18 months of age) before they develop gastric enzymes to digest them properly. Too many legumes can cause weak legs, a bulging stomach, and gas pain. Except in the case of soy allergy, soybean products such as tempeh, tofu, and soy milk usually digest more easily than other dried legume preparations for infants and children. Fresh peas and green beans are also usually well tolerated.
- Make the right choice of legume.
    1. Aduki beans, lentils, mung beans, and peas digest most easily and can be eaten regularly.
    2. Pinto, kidney, navy, black-eyed peas, garbanzo, lima, and black beans are harder to digest and should be eaten occasionally.
    3. Soybeans and black soybeans are the most difficult to digest. However, soy products (tofu, tempeh, soybean sprouts, soy milk, miso, and soy sauce) are easily digested. Too much soy, especially in the form of tempeh, tofu, and soy sprouts, can weaken both the digestion and kidney-adrenal function. To reduce these effects, lightly cook soy sprouts and cook tofu and tempeh thoroughly.
- Use proper combinations, ingredients, and seasonings.
    1. Legumes combine best with green or non-starchy vegetables and seaweeds; combinations with grains or cooked fruits for desserts are acceptable for those with strong digestion. Otherwise, when legumes cause digestive problems, follow plan A, or in severe cases, plan B food-combining methods given in the *Food Combinations* chapter.

2. Season with sea salt, miso, or soy sauce. Add salty products such as these near the end of cooking. If added at the beginning, the beans will not cook completely and skins will remain tough.

   Suggested salt: ¼ teaspoon unrefined salt or 1 teaspoon soy sauce to 1 cup dry legumes. The above salt recommendation is moderate and can be increased if salt is used sparingly in other foods. More salt can be used for legumes than other foods since salt is a digestive aid to high-protein products; the use of the salty flavor in legumes can also be inferred from Five Element theory (the salty flavor enters the kidneys, and beans are the beneficial "grain" for the kidneys). Thus one may picture salt as directing the products of legume metabolism to the kidneys.

3. Cook legumes with fennel or cumin to help prevent gas. Mexicans prize the herb *epazote* or "wormseed" leaf for dispelling gas associated with bean consumption. Epazote *(Chenopodium ambrosioides),* related to the common weed "pigweed," is now available in America from several herb distributors. It works best freshly picked, then cooked into legumes when they are almost done. It grows readily in most soils (see Resources Index under "Herbs" for seed source of wormseed). Epazote also helps rid the body of worms.

4. For improved flavor and digestion, more nutrients, and faster cooking, place soaked kombu or kelp seaweed in the bottom of the pot. Add 1 part seaweed to 6 or more parts legumes. Use seaweed soak water to cook grains and vegetables.

5. Soak legumes for 12 hours or overnight in four parts water to one part legume. For best results, change the water once or twice. Lentils and whole dried peas require shorter soaking, while soybeans and garbanzos need to soak longer. Soaking softens skins and begins the sprouting process, which eliminates phytic acid, thereby making more minerals available. Soaking also promotes faster cooking and improved digestibility, because the gas-causing enzymes and trisaccharides in legumes are released into the soak water. Be sure to discard the soak water.

6. After bringing legumes to a boil, scoop off and discard foam. Continue to boil for 20 minutes without lid at beginning of cooking to let steam rise (breaks up and disperses indigestible enzymes).

7. If problems with gas persist, this step and number 8 below are very useful. Pour a little apple-cider, brown-rice, or white-wine vinegar into the water in the last stages of cooking legumes. For salad beans, marinate cooked beans in a solution of two-thirds vinegar and one-third olive oil at least one-half hour before serving. Combining vinegar with legumes softens them and breaks down protein chains and indigestible compounds; it is often an effective remedy for those who suffer after eating them.

8. Sprout legumes to break down their protein into amino acids, the starches and trisaccharides into simple sugars, and to create valuable enzymes

and vitamins. Sprouting legumes until they have rootlets maximizes their digestibility. Lentils, mung, and aduki beans sprout most easily. However, sprouts are somewhat cooling and most useful in the spring and summer; they do not strengthen and warm the *yang* energy of the body sufficiently for those who are very weak and *cold*. To add a more warming quality to bean and all other sprouts, they can be steamed, sautéed, or lightly simmered. In contrast, people who are aggressive and over*heated* will do well with regular use of sprouts; others may find moderate use best.

Techniques for Cooking Legumes (Beans, Peas, and Lentils)

Water and Cooking Time				
Legumes (1 cup dried)	**Simmer**		**Pressure**	
	cups water	time	cups water	time
Aduki bean	2–3	1½ hrs.	2–3	45 mins.
Black bean	2–3	2½ hrs.	2–3	1¼ hrs.
Lentils	3–4	1 hr.	3	20 mins.
Green split peas	3–4	1 hr.	3	20 mins.
Whole peas	3–4	3 hrs.	3	1 hr.
Pinto-Kidney bean	2–3	2–3 hrs.	2–3	1 hr.
Garbanzo bean	3–4	4–5 hrs.	3	2–3 hrs.
Limas and Black-eyed peas	2–3	1 hr.	2–3	35 mins.
Mung bean	3–4	1 hr.	3	20 mins.
Yellow or black soybean	4	4–6 hrs.	3	2 hrs.

Note: The above guidelines represent minimum cooking times. In many traditional cultures, simmering legumes, especially the larger beans, all day, ensured digestibility.

Herbal Combinations

- Coriander, cumin, ginger (lentil, mung, black, aduki)
- Sage, thyme, oregano (black, pinto, lentil, kidney)
- Dill, basil (lentil, garbanzo, split pea)
- Fennel or cumin (pinto, kidney)
- Mint, garlic (garbanzo, lentil)

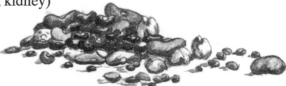

All Methods

Sort through for dirt and stones. Then wash and rinse thoroughly.

Basic Method

1. Place soaked kombu in bottom of pot. Add soaked legumes and cold water.
2. Bring to boil. Reduce heat to low.
3. Cover and simmer until almost done.
4. Add seasonings and salt.
5. Continue to cook, about 15 minutes, until soft.
6. Uncover. Turn to medium if you want to cook off excess liquid.

Pressure-Cooked Method

Requires less cooking time, water, and soaking.
1. Place soaked kombu and legumes in pressure cooker with cold water.
2. Cover and bring to pressure. Reduce heat to low and cook required time.
3. Allow pressure to come down.
4. Remove cover. Season and simmer for about 15 minutes or until excess liquid is cooked off.

Ceramic Pot Method

1. Place soaked kombu on bottom of ceramic pot. Add soaked legumes and water. Cover.
2. Place pot in pressure cooker or pan. Add water halfway up the sides of ceramic pot. Secure lid.
3. Cook according to Basic Method or Pressure-Cooked Method.
4. Add seasonings and simmer 15–20 minutes.

Baking Method

1. Place soaked legumes in pot with cold water and soaked kombu.
2. Add 4–5 cups water to each 1 cup of beans.
3. Place pot on stove. Bring to boil for 15 minutes to loosen skins.
4. Pour legumes into baking dish.
5. Cover and place in oven at 350°F for 3–4 hours.
6. Add more water when needed.
7. Bake until 80% done.
8. Add salt and seasonings. Cook until soft.
9. Remove cover to brown.

Variation   Add diced onions, kale, or other vegetables when legumes are 50% done.

BEAN BURGERS OR CROQUETTES

2 cups cooked beans
1 carrot, diced
¼ onion, diced (optional)
1 tablespoon herbs (see above)
½ cup bread crumbs, whole-wheat flour, or cooked grain
Sea salt to taste
Toasted nuts or seeds

- Mash beans.
- Mix ingredients together and form patties or small balls.
- Fry or bake at 350°F until browned (approximately 30 minutes).

CROQUETTES OF LENTILS

2 cups cooked lentils
4 tablespoons whole-wheat flour
¼ onion, chopped fine (optional)
1 tablespoon parsley
Soy sauce to taste

- Follow directions for Bean Burgers, above.

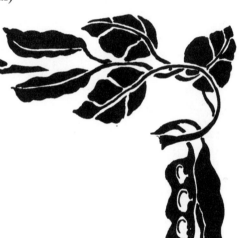

CROQUETTES OF GARBANZOS OR GREEN PEAS

2 cups cooked garbanzos or green peas
4 tablespoons whole-wheat flour
½ clove garlic, minced (optional)
1 tablespoon parsley
1 tablespoon lemon juice
½ teaspoon each cardamom, coriander

- Follow directions for Bean Burgers, above.

DOSA (pancakes from India)

1½ cups brown rice
⅔ cup mung beans
2 cups water
¼ teaspoon sea salt

- Wash and soak 12 hours or overnight. Soak rice in 1½ cups water and beans in ½ cup water.
- Grind mung beans finely and rice less so, using a mortar and pestle, blender, or processor.
- Combine with salt. Allow to sit overnight or 8 hours in a warm place so yeasts can turn the mixture into a light, fluffy batter.
- Pour batter, which should be thin, into hot skillet.
- Cook like pancakes (cover pan so you don't have to turn them).
- Serves 4.

REFRIED BEANS

2 cups cooked beans (aduki, black, pinto)
½ cup bean juice or water
½ onion, chopped (optional)
¼ teaspoon coriander
¼ teaspoon cumin
1 tablespoon oil (optional)
Sea salt, if needed

- Sauté onion.
- Add seasonings. Sauté 1 minute.
- Add ½ cup beans at a time.
- Mash with the back of a wooden spoon or a potato masher.
- Add bean juice. Simmer until enough liquid has cooked off.
- Serves 4–6.

Variations Tostadas—toasted tortillas topped with refried beans, salsa, avocado slices, and lettuce.
Tacos—a soft tortilla wrapped around refried beans with guacamole, salsa, and shredded cabbage.

BAKED SWEET BEANS

2 cups soaked beans (aduki, lima, navy, kidney)
8–10 cups water
½ onion, chopped (optional)
1 tablespoon molasses
1 teaspoon dry mustard
¼–½ teaspoon sea salt

- Use the Baking Method (p. 514).
- Add ingredients when beans are 80% done.
- Continue to cook as directed.
- Serves 6–8.

GARBANZOS AND BECHAMEL SAUCE

2 cups cooked garbanzos
Sauce:
 2 tablespoons whole-wheat flour
 1 tablespoon sesame butter
 ½ teaspoon sea salt
 ½ onion, chopped (optional)
 1 teaspoon oil (optional)
1½ cups water
 1 teaspoon mint

- Sauté onion.
- Add flour, sesame butter, and salt diluted in the water.
- Bring to a boil, simmer 15 minutes.
- Fold in garbanzos and mint at end of cooking.
- Serve over grain.
- Serves 4–6.

BEANS WITH CARROTS AND ONIONS

5 inches kombu, soaked
2 cups beans, soaked
¼ onion, diced (optional)
1 carrot, diced
6–8 cups water
½ teaspoon sea salt

- Place kombu on bottom.
- Place vegetables on top of kombu (encourages flavors to blend with beans).
- Add beans and water.
- Use Basic, Crock-pot, or Baking Method (p. 514).
- Stir before serving.
- Serves 6–8.

ADUKI, RAISINS, AND APPLES

5 inches kombu, soaked
2 cups aduki beans, soaked
1 cup dried apples, soaked
1 cup raisins, soaked
5–6 cups water (including raisin and apple soak water)
¼–½ teaspoon sea salt

- Follow directions for Beans with Carrots and Onions, above.

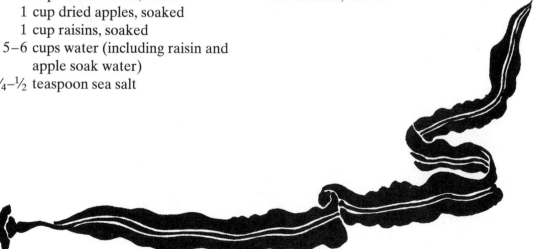

LENTIL-WALNUT LOAF

2 cups lentils, cooked and drained
¼ onion, diced (optional)
½ teaspoon oil (optional)
½ cup wheat germ
½ cup whole-wheat bread crumbs
½ cup walnuts, chopped, or
   sunflower seeds
½ teaspoon sage or thyme
½ cup vegetable or lentil broth
1 tablespoon vinegar
Sea salt to taste

- Preheat oven to 350°F.
- Sauté onion until soft.
- Mix all ingredients. Place in large oiled loaf pan.
- Cover. Bake 30 minutes.
- Uncover and cook 10 minutes.
- Serves 6–8.

LENTIL CURRY (DAHL)

1 cup lentils, soaked
4 cups water
1 tablespoon curry powder or
   ¼ teaspoon each: coriander,
   cayenne, ginger, cinnamon, and
   turmeric
¼ teaspoon salt

- Cook lentils until soft.
- Add salt and seasonings.
- Cover and cook 5–10 minutes.
- Serve over rice.
- Serves 4.

HUMMUS

2 cups cooked garbanzos
¼ cup sesame butter or sesame meal
1 clove garlic, minced (optional)
6–8 tablespoons lemon juice
   Dash of hot pepper
1 tablespoon olive oil (optional)
Sea salt to taste

- Mash or purée garbanzos with rest of ingredients.
- Spread on plate and garnish with parsley and a drizzle of olive oil.
- Serve as a dip with pita bread.

FALAFEL

2 cups cooked garbanzos
½ cup bread crumbs
½ cup whole-wheat flour
1 clove garlic, minced (optional)
2 tablespoons parsley
¼ teaspoon each: cumin, basil,
   marjoram, cayenne
1 tablespoon sesame butter

- Mash or purée garbanzos (add enough water for blender).
- Combine with rest of ingredients.
- Form into 1-inch balls or patties.
- Deep-fry or bake in 350°F oven until crisp and golden.
- Serve in pita bread, garnished with tomatoes, lettuce, olives, and Sesame Butter-Lemon sauce (p. 603).

HEARTY BLACK BEANS

2 cups black beans, soaked
3½ cups water
¼ onion, chopped (optional)
1 clove garlic, minced (optional)
1 teaspoon ground coriander
1½ teaspoons ground cumin
1 teaspoon oil (optional)
½ teaspoon sea salt
Pinch of cayenne
Juice of ½ lemon

- Place beans in water. Bring to boil. Cover.
- Reduce heat and simmer 1 hour.
- Sauté onion, garlic, coriander, and cumin.
- Add to beans.
- Add salt, cayenne, and lemon juice.
- Continue cooking until beans are done.
- Serves 4.

MISO

Miso is a fermented soybean paste thought to have originated in China some 2,500 years ago. It is made by combining cooked soybeans, mold *(koji)*, salt, and various grains, then fermenting for six months to two or more years. There are three basic types of miso: soybean *(hatcho)*, barley *(mugi)*, and rice *(kome)* and forty to fifty other varieties. Miso ranges in color from tans and russets, deep ambers and clarets, cinnamon reds, rich chocolate browns, and loamy blacks to some of the modern varieties of sunlight yellow and creamy beige. Each type has its own distinctive flavor and texture ranging from meaty and savory to sweet and delicate. Many quality misos are now made in the United States.

Recommendations

- Darker and longer-fermented miso—colder climates
- Lighter and less fermented—warmer climates
- Red and moderately fermented—moderate climates or year round

It is best for those raised on a high salt and animal diet to partake of the less salty, lighter, and red varieties. However, those raised as vegetarians may tolerate the more salty and darker miso.

Healing Properties

13%–20% protein; contains an amino acid pattern similar to meat along with a trace of vitamin B_{12}; a live food containing lactobacillus (the same in yogurt) that aids in digestion and assimilation; adds flavor and thus can help reduce the large amounts of fat and oil usually used for seasonings; creates an alkaline condition in the body promoting resistance against disease. According to tradition, miso promotes long life and good health; treats and prevents radiation sickness; has been used to treat certain types of heart disease and cancer; neutralizes some of the effects of smoking and air pollution.

Miso may be used in place of salt and soy sauce as a seasoning. The same saltiness can be obtained with the following measurements: $\frac{1}{2}$ teaspoon salt = 2 tablespoons soy sauce = 1 tablespoon salty miso = $1\frac{1}{2}$ tablespoons mellow miso = $2\frac{1}{2}$–3 tablespoons sweet miso.

Always obtain unpasteurized miso. Such miso is a live food, and prolonged cooking kills the beneficial microorganisms. Add unpasteurized miso to preparations just before removing from heat. Like salt, miso is better assimilated when combined with foods due to its concentrated nature.

Miso has the ability to absorb toxins from plastic containers and should be transferred into glass, wood, or enamel for prolonged storage. The same holds true for other fermented foods and all oils. Discard the miso that is stuck to the plastic. Store in a cool place.

Words of Caution

When making a transition from a meat-based diet to one of vegetarian foods, many people begin to use miso in quantity. This is partially due to miso's hearty flavor which is as concentrated as the taste of meat. In some ways, however, because of aging and high salt content, miso is stronger than meat. Overuse will bring on all the same problems of excess salt use, including weakened heart and nervous system. In addition, some individuals with *Candida albicans* yeast overgrowth and similar fungal conditions must use miso sparingly, since its ferment can promote the growth of yeasts. (Much the same can be said of the excessive consumption of soy sauce.) When used moderately by most people, miso provides excellent nutrition.

Uses

May be used like bouillon, soy sauce, and Worcestershire sauce; used as a flavorful, stout ingredient in stews, soups, gravies, sauces, dressings, stuffings, dips, casseroles, and in various toppings for grains, tofu, vegetable dishes, hot cereals, sweet and Irish potatoes, toast, pancakes, and so forth.

SWEET SIMMERED MISO

3 tablespoons miso
2 teaspoons rice syrup
$\frac{1}{2}$ cup water, or
1 cup applesauce

- Combine all ingredients in an earthenware pot or skillet.
- Simmer for 2–3 minutes over a low flame, stirring constantly with a wooden spoon until mixture thickens.
- Serve as a spread or butter on toast in small amounts.

Variations   Reducing or omitting sweeteners makes a more savory flavor. Add grated ginger, raisins with grated lemon or orange rind, grated daikon radish, grated carrot, or vary your herbal combinations between thyme, parsley, rosemary, coriander, cumin, basil, oregano, mint, cinnamon, garlic, and onion. To make a sauce, dip, or spread from a miso topping, just add enough water to make the right consistency.

LEMON-WALNUT SAUTÉ

10 mushrooms (or 5 soaked shiitake mushrooms), thinly sliced
1 tablespoon lemon rind, grated
¼ cup walnuts, chopped
1 teaspoon oil
1 tablespoon miso
3 tablespoons water
1 teaspoon sweetener (optional)

- Sauté mushrooms, lemon rind, and walnuts over medium heat until tender.
- Reduce heat to low.
- Dissolve miso in water.
- Add miso and sweetener to the sauté and cook, stirring constantly, until all ingredients are coated evenly with the miso.
- Allow to cool before serving.

MISO IN GUACAMOLE

1 avocado
¼ tomato, diced
1 clove garlic, minced (optional)
1 teaspoon miso
1 tablespoon onion, minced (optional)
1 chili pepper, diced
Dash of cayenne pepper

- Combine ingredients and mash with a fork until smooth.

SPINACH AND MISO SAUCE

1 pound spinach, cooked and drained
1 tablespoon white miso
1 tablespoon sesame butter
Water

- Combine ingredients and purée in a blender with enough water to make a creamy sauce.

Variation Use carrots, squash, broccoli, cauliflower, etc., with, or instead of, spinach.

MISO-SESAME BUTTER DIP OR SAUCE

1 tablespoon miso
1 tablespoon sesame butter
¼ cup lemon juice
¼ cup water

- Purée with a mortar and pestle.
- Serve as a dip. Add ¼ cup more water to make a sauce.

BASIC MISO SOUP

½ cup wakame or kombu, cooked
and cut into small pieces

2–3 tablespoons miso

1½ cups chopped vegetables

4 cups water (soup stock or
seaweed soak water)

1 teaspoon sesame oil

- Sauté seaweed and vegetables.
- Add water and bring to a scald.
- Reduce heat to low and simmer covered 15 minutes.
- Cream miso in a little broth, return to soup.
- Bring soup back to scald and remove from heat. Garnish.
- Serves 4–6.

Vegetables

Daikon, leek, onion, burdock root, eggplant, mushrooms, turnips, carrot, cabbage, potatoes, spinach, lotus root, sweet potatoes, bean sprouts, wild vegetables, chrysanthemum, tofu, wheat gluten, and seaweeds.

Garnishes and seasonings

Nut butters, seeds and nuts, toasted nori and dulse, deep-fried tofu pieces, croutons, white wine, sake, arrowroot thickener, ginger, garlic, seven-spice, mustard, parsley, chives, pepper, mint, and grated lemon rind.

NATTO MISO

The traditional chutney of rural Japan, made from soybeans, barley, barley malt, kombu, ginger, and sea salt, is becoming widely available in the West. It is delicious as a condiment or chutney in soups, sweet and sour sauces, stir-fried dishes, or rolled up in rice balls. Use and prepare the same as regular miso.

TEMPEH

Tempeh (TEMpay) is a fermented food from Indonesia made from cooked soybeans bound together by a mold *(Rhizopus)* into patties or cakes. Different varieties are obtained by combining soybeans with wheat, rice, millet, peanuts, or coconut and allowing it to ferment for different lengths of time. (There are up to thirty varieties available.)

Healing Properties

Highly nutritious; can be used to benefit the frail *deficient* person; 19.5% protein; low in saturated fats, rich in unsaturated fats, and contains substantial omega-3 oils; Rhizopus mold produces a medicinal antibiotic to increase the body's resistance to infections; free of chemical toxins.

Asian tempeh is an exceptional source of vitamin B_{12}. Unfortunately, tempeh produced in the West is fermented in an environment too clean to spawn B_{12}, and therefore is virtually devoid of this necessary nutrient. Some tempeh manufacturers, however, have now inoculated their product with B_{12}-producing micro-organisms.

In recipes with meat, poultry, or fish, tempeh makes an excellent substitute for these animal products. The flavor of tempeh often reminds people of various chicken and fish dishes.

For best results in preparation

- Tempeh is available fresh, frozen, dried, or precooked. Can be steamed, baked, fried, or broiled. (Same as tofu.)
- For crispy tempeh with a savory flavor, slice thin and fry.
- Serve in small quantities when fried. This improves digestibility.
- Store in a cool place or freeze. Do not worry if it gets grayish and has an ammonia smell (because of sporulation). However, discard when smell becomes unpleasant.
- Do not eat tempeh raw; it needs to be cooked thoroughly.

SEASONED TEMPEH (Fried)

8 ounces tempeh, sliced or cubed
½ cup water and 1 tablespoon salt
   or
½ cup lemon juice and ½ teaspoon salt
Herbs (see suggested seasonings, below)

- Soak in liquid, salt, and herbs 15–20 minutes.
- Drain well.
- Fry until golden.

SEASONED TEMPEH (Boiled)

8 ounces tempeh, sliced or cubed
¼–½ cup water
½ tablespoon soy sauce
Herbs

- Place tempeh in water, with soy sauce and herbs. Bring to boil.
- Simmer uncovered until liquid is absorbed.
- Drain.

Suggested seasonings

- 1 teaspoon cumin powder
- 1 teaspoon curry powder
- ½ teaspoon each coriander, cumin, and ginger
- ½ teaspoon grated ginger

Variations Tempeh french fries: Cut into french-fry shape and deep-fry. Serve with grain burgers and salad.

Tempeh shish kebab: Cut into 1-inch cubes and skewer with marinated vegetables.

Tempeh pancakes: Serve topped with applesauce.

TEMPEH IN STIR-FRIED RICE

1 teaspoon oil
1 clove garlic, minced (optional)
1 carrot, diced
2 cups cooked rice
1 cup green peas, cooked
8 ounces tempeh, cut into cubes,
  cooked and seasoned
2 tablespoons soy sauce

- Sauté garlic and carrot in oil for 3 minutes.
- Add rice and sauté 2 minutes.
- Add peas, tempeh, and soy sauce. Mix well. Cook 5 minutes.
- Serve immediately.

NOODLES WITH TEMPEH

1 teaspoon oil
½ onion (optional)
½ cup carrots, sliced
1 cup cabbage, chopped
1 cup green peas
4 ounces noodles, cooked and
  drained (p. 485)
¼ teaspoon curry powder
2 tablespoons soy sauce
¼ teaspoon salt
8 ounces tempeh, cubed, seasoned
  and fried

- Stir-fry onions and carrots 3 minutes.
- Add cabbage and peas, stir-fry 2 minutes more.
- Add seasonings and stir-fry 1 minute more.
- Mix in tempeh and noodles.
- Serve hot or cold.
- Serves 4.

TEMPEH IN SAUCE

8 ounces tempeh, cut in ¾-inch
  cubes and cooked
3–4 cups sauce:
  Miso-Sesame Butter (p. 521)
  Mushroom (p. 602)
  Sweet and Sour (p. 605)

- Prepare sauce.
- At end of cooking, stir in tempeh.
- Serve as an entrée or over pasta or grains.

TEMPEH BURGERS

1 clove garlic, minced (optional)
2 red chilies, minced
1 teaspoon coriander seeds
½ teaspoon lemon rind, grated
1 tablespoon miso or 2 tablespoons
  soy sauce
8 ounces tempeh (small pieces)

- Combine all seasonings.
- Grind in a mortar until smooth.
- Add tempeh pieces and grind until well mixed.
- Shape into patties.
- Fry or bake at 350°F until golden brown.
- Garnish and serve on a bun.

BREADED TEMPEH CUTLETS

8 ounces tempeh, cut into
  1½ x 2 x ½-inch cutlets
2 teaspoons salt in ½ cup water
¼ cup whole-wheat flour
7 tablespoons whole-wheat
  bread crumbs or corn meal
Toppings:
  Chinese Ginger Sauce
  (see "Sauces" p. 604)
  Bechamel Sauce
  Miso Gravy

- Soak tempeh in salt water 15–20 minutes.
- Drain.
- Dust with flour and bread crumbs.
- Set on a rack to dry.
- Deep-fry or bake at 350°F until crisp and golden brown.
- Serve with a topping.

Variations   Same as Seasoned Tempeh, above.

BROILED TEMPEH SHISH KEBAB

½ teaspoon coriander seeds
1 clove garlic, minced
1 tablespoon molasses
2 tablespoons miso
8 ounces tempeh, cut into
  ½-inch cubes
Dipping sauce:
  4 tablespoons soy sauce
  1 teaspoon lemon juice
½ teaspoon chilies
  1 teaspoon grated ginger
½ cup water

- Grind first 2 ingredients in a mortar until smooth.
- Mix in molasses and miso.
- Coat tempeh with mixture and marinate overnight.
- Next day, prepare dipping sauce.
- Skewer cubes and grill for 7–8 minutes over an open fire or broil in the oven.
- Serve with dipping sauce.

TEMPEH WITH TORTILLAS AND GUACAMOLE

8 corn tortillas
1½ cups guacamole (p. 521)
8 ounces tempeh, cubed, cooked
  and seasoned
5 lettuce leaves, shredded
1 tomato, diced
1 cup alfalfa sprouts
Salsa (p. 604)

- Warm tortillas by placing a fresh tortilla on the bottom of a heated pan until warm. Then place another one under it, on the bottom, until there is a stack—or—heat oil and fry on each side until warm.
- Spoon a dollop of guacamole on tortilla.
- Top with a sprinkling of tempeh cubes.
- Then add lettuce, tomato, or sprouts.
- Top with salsa.

TEMPEH MOCK-TUNA

8 ounces tempeh	• Steam tempeh.
1 tablespoon water	• Add water and mash.
¼ cup mayonnaise (p. 579)	• Cool.
1 tablespoon onion, minced (optional)	• Add other ingredients and mix well.
½ teaspoon salt	• Serve in sandwiches, or as a salad or spread.
2 tablespoons parsley or celery, minced	

TOFU

Tofu is a processed soybean curd that originated in China thousands of years ago to improve the digestibility of the highly valued soybean. Making tofu is an involved process of soaking, blending, and cooking soybeans and mixing them with a natural solidifier (nigari or lemon juice). Some commercially made tofu is solidified with chemical nigari, alum, or vinegar and its quality is inferior.

Nutrients

Contains easily digested protein; B-vitamins and minerals including calcium, phosphorus, iron, sodium, and potassium; inexpensive; low in calories (eighteen per ounce). Depending on how it is made, tofu's calcium content can equal that of milk.

Healing Properties

Cooling thermal nature; benefits the Metal Element including the lungs and large intestine; moistens *dry* conditions in the body; relieves inflammation of the stomach; neutralizes toxins—used in cases of alcoholism, chronic amoebic dysentery, healing reactions, dietary changes, etc.; also traditionally applied to concussions as a thick tofu poultice.

Tofu is a concentrated protein and can be beneficial when eaten in moderate amounts, especially in warmer weather and by those with *heat* signs (red tongue, red face, aversion to heat, or sensation of being too hot); it is sometimes used to reduce *heat* signs accompanying heart disease and high blood pressure. For most people, its *yin,* cooling quality needs to be altered by thorough cooking; adding warming spices such as ginger is particularly helpful for *cold* persons.

Tofu is quite versatile. Its subtle bland nature balances extreme flavors and adds contrast to salty and pungent foods. It can be baked, steamed, broiled, deep-fried, sautéed, boiled, or even eaten raw—ideally only when a person feels hot and dry.

Store tofu in a cool place in an airtight container or sealed jar, covered with water. Change water daily.

Caution: Eating massive amounts of tofu regularly (as some Americans do) can contribute to kidney-adrenal weakness, loss and graying of hair, impotence, frigidity, and decrease in sexual sensitivity.

BAKED TOFU WITH LEMON SAUCE

1 cake tofu, sliced ¼-inch thick
Creamy Sauce:
   1 tablespoon miso
   2 teaspoons lemon juice
   1 teaspoon sesame butter
   ⅓ cup water
   Parsley

- Preheat oven to 350°F.
- Stack slices of tofu on end in a shallow baking dish, slightly tilted and leaning on each other (//////).
- Blend ingredients together to make a creamy sauce.
- Spoon over top of tofu.
- Bake 15–20 minutes covered.
- Garnish with parsley.
- Serves 4.

BROILED TOFU

1 cake tofu, sliced
2 tablespoons soy sauce
1 teaspoon ginger, grated
Parsley, chopped

- Turn oven to broil.
- Mix soy sauce and ginger together.
- Sprinkle over tofu.
- Place in casserole dish.
- Broil until slightly brown on both sides. (Tofu broils quickly; be careful not to burn it.)
- Garnish with parsley.
- Serves 4.

TOFU MEATLESS BALLS

1 cake tofu
¼ cup walnuts, chopped
¼ cup bread crumbs or wheat germ
⅛ cup whole-wheat flour
1 tablespoon parsley, chopped
½ teaspoon each oregano and basil
½ onion, minced
1 tablespoon soy sauce

- Thoroughly mix everything together.
- Form into 2-inch balls.
- Deep-fry or bake at 350°F until golden.
- Serve as an hors d'oeuvre with a dip, or place in a casserole dish and cover with a sauce. Cover and bake an additional 20 minutes. Serve over grain or noodles.
- Serves 4.

STEAMED TOFU ROLLS

2 cakes tofu
½ cup carrot, grated
½ onion, chopped fine (optional)
¼ cup fresh parsley, chopped
2–3 tablespoons soy sauce
4 sheets nori
½ teaspoon oil (optional)

- Sauté onions and carrots.
- Crumble tofu and mix with carrots, onion, parsley, and soy sauce.
- Spread tofu mixture ¼-inch thick over nori. Leave 1½ inches at the end uncovered.
- Roll nori up.
- Gently place nori rolls seam down in a steamer. Steam 15 minutes.
- Allow to cool and slice into ½-inch-thick pieces. (If sliced while still hot they will crumble.)
- Serves 6–8.

TOFU CASSEROLE

1 cake tofu, crumbled
1 cup bread crumbs
1½ cups almond bechamel sauce (see p. 602)
¼ onion, chopped fine (optional)
¼–½ teaspoon salt
¼ teaspoon oil (optional)

- Sauté onion.
- Mix all ingredients together.
- Pat into an oiled baking dish.
- Bake in a pan of water in a 375°F oven for 45 minutes.
- Serves 4.

TOFU WITH SHIITAKE MUSHROOMS

3 shiitake mushrooms
1 cup water
1 cup green peas
1 carrot, minced
1 teaspoon sesame oil (optional)
1 cake tofu
¼–½ teaspoon salt
1 teaspoon soy sauce

- Soak mushrooms in water 20 minutes. Drain. Reserve water. Chop mushrooms fine. (Save tough stems for soup stock.)
- Sauté mushrooms 2 minutes, add peas and carrots, and sauté 2 more minutes.
- Add ⅓ cup reserved water and salt. Cover and cook 20 minutes.
- Add soy sauce.
- Purée tofu in blender with ⅓ cup reserved liquid.
- Add to cooked vegetables and stir with chopsticks. Cook for 5 minutes.
- Serves 4.

DEEP-FRIED TOFU

1 cake tofu
Arrowroot flour
Sesame oil

- Place tofu on a cutting board with a small dish under one end, so that it is tilted. Then place a weight or plate on top of the tofu for about an hour—or wrap it in a terry cloth towel, folded into fourths, 1½–2 hours or overnight. This will drain off the excess liquid.
- Cut tofu into cubes ⅓ inch by ½ inch.
- Lightly coat each piece with arrowroot flour.
- Deep-fry until golden brown. (Putting too much in at one time will lower the temperature of the oil and tofu will not cook properly.)
- Drain on paper towels or drop into boiling water to remove remaining oil.
- Add to soups, sauces, stews, sandwiches, pasta sauces, etc.

SCRAMBLED TOFU

1 cake tofu
2 cups cooked millet or rice
1 onion, chopped (optional)
1 clove garlic, minced (optional)
1 tablespoon curry powder
1 teaspoon oil
¼–½ teaspoon salt

- Sauté onion and garlic in oil until onion turns transparent.
- Add curry and salt. Sauté 1 minute.
- Crumble tofu and mix well with rice or millet.
- Add to curry mixture and sauté 10 minutes.
- Serves 4.

TOFU EGGLESS SALAD

2 cakes tofu
½ cup dill pickles
2 tablespoons nutritional yeast (optional)
⅛ cup mustard
½ teaspoon salt
½ cup mayonnaise or salad dressing
Dash of turmeric (adds color)
1 green onion, chopped (optional)

- Option: Simmer tofu in water for 5 minutes to make it more digestible and encourage the flavors of the remaining ingredients to blend.
- Crumble tofu into a bowl.
- Add all the other ingredients.
- Mash and mix it together.
- Chill before serving as a salad or sandwich spread.
- Serves 6–8.

Nuts and Seeds

In this section we consider the properties and healthful use of nuts and oil-rich seeds. These fatty foods are typically the best sources of vitamin E, which acts as a nerve protector and immune-enhancing antioxidant; common nuts and seeds also contain the greatest quantity of fats of all unprocessed foods—much of it in the form of essential fatty acids. Both fats and the fat-soluble nutrient, vitamin E, play an crucial role in liver function and its attendant emotions of anger, depression, and impatience. People who eat isolated fats such as refined seed oils have a greater need for vitamin E as an antioxidant to protect against the oxidation of these oils. On the other hand, if large amounts of isolated vitamin E is ingested, more fat is craved. By eating vitamin E as a component of the oils it naturally occurs in, for instance, in nuts, seeds, unrefined oils, and whole grains, there is less need to be concerned about taking supplemental vitamin E for protection.

Vitamin E and essential fatty acids are but a sampling of the nutritional power of seeds. (Nuts, grains, and legumes are also seeds.) Certainly the many additional nutrients in seeds, including a wealth of vitamins, minerals, amino acids, carbohydrates, minerals, and others, play synergistic roles in the creation of their remarkable properties. Looked at in total, the seed is the spark of life, a living and perfect food with all the elements necessary for vitality.

The problem of rancid seeds and nuts

- Nuts and seeds become rancid and lose their nutrients when they are hulled or shelled. Deterioration begins immediately and continues, somewhat, even when vacuum-packed without oxygen.
- Rancidity causes irritation to the linings of the stomach and intestines.
- The pancreatic enzymes that digest oils in these foods are retarded. Thus the oils cannot be digested or assimilated efficiently.
- Can contribute to poor immunity, cancer, and other chronic diseases.
- Destroys vitamins A, E, and F in the food, plus those stored in the body.
- A cause of gall bladder and liver complaints. (Results in anger and indecision.)

It is better not to eat nuts and seeds at all than to eat rancid ones.

Selection and storage

- Buy nuts only in the shell. They will last up to one year.
- Store hulled seeds in dark bottles in cold places. Heat and light speed oxidation. Do not store in plastic. Oil-rich food combines with plastic to form plasticides.
- Taste seeds and nuts before buying.
- Poisons and toxins tend to accumulate in all seeds, so it is important to buy organic non-sprayed ones.

Preparation and eating of nuts and oil-rich seeds

- The best way to eat seeds or nuts is to soak them overnight to initiate the sprouting process, which makes fats and proteins more digestible. Then dry and eat raw or roast or cook them.

  They can also be cooked into cereals and broths, ground into meals or butters, or liquefied (see "Grain and Seed Milks" and "Rejuvelac and Yogurt" recipes).
- Roasting reduces the effect of rancidity and cuts down on the oiliness, making nuts and seeds easier to digest. Lightly roast—overheating makes the oils in them harmful.
- People with sensitive digestion should follow simple food-combining principles, i.e., eat nuts and seeds alone or with acid fruit or green and non-starchy vegetables (see *Food Combinations* chapter).
- It is best to eat nuts and seeds that grow in your climatic region.
- Roasting increases their warming qualities for the fall and winter and the *cold* or *deficient* person; sprouting improves their cooling and fresh qualities for the spring and summer and for the *hot* or *excessive* person.
- The medicinal value is greatly increased when chewed well.
- Eaten in large amounts, they can cause problems in digestion, with blemishes and pimples, and are notorious for producing foul-smelling flatulence.

Guidelines for Using Nuts and Seeds

Most nuts and seeds (especially the oil-bearing seeds) tonify the body and add weight and strength. They are rich sources of protein and fat, and are best consumed in small amounts. The thin, dry, unstable, nervous, and generally *deficient* individual benefits most from these heavy, grounding foods. Unfortunately, this type of person cannot metabolize substantial amounts of dense food and so must eat nuts and seeds in moderation.

On the other hand, the individual with signs of *excess* (robust body and personality, ruddy complexion, strong voice and pulse, thick tongue coating) should use nuts and seeds very sparingly, if at all.

The *damp,* sluggish person with conditions such as edema, mucus, overweight, candida overgrowth, tumors, or cysts should avoid nuts and oil-rich seeds. An exception are certain seeds concentrated in omega-3 fatty acids, which increase the metabolic rate, helping to overcome sluggishness. Common examples include flax seeds, chia seeds, pumpkin seeds, and unsalted pistachios. If used with restraint, these seeds are also the best for the

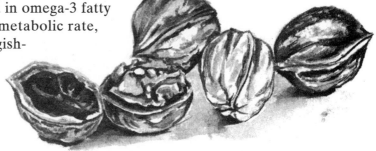

excessive-type person described above.

Because their specific healing properties are not clearly defined, or in some cases, not known, several popular nuts are omitted from the following list of properties: cashews, filberts (hazelnuts), pecans, and Brazil nuts. In general, these nuts all follow a pattern of being rich in fat and protein and therefore should be used according to the above general guidelines to tonify the *deficient* person; avoid them in cases of *excess* and *dampness.*

Healing Properties of Nuts and Seeds

Almond

Slightly warming thermal nature; sweet flavor; relieves stagnant *qi* energy of the lungs; transforms phlegm; alleviates cough; lubricates the intestines. Used for lung conditions including coughing and asthma; also helps in cases of fluid-dryness types of constipation. For lung conditions, use almond drink; prepare by grinding almonds to a powder and mixing with water.

Ayurveda considers almonds one of the best of all nuts, useful for building *ojas,* an essence that vivifies intellection and spirituality as well as reproductive ability. Ayurveda also advises not eating the skin of the almond because it may irritate the gut lining, and avoiding almonds that are blanched in hot water. To remove the skins and to begin the germination process of the almond (which improves digestibility and adds nutrients), soak them overnight and peel in the morning. However, almond skin contains a bitter principle, while not desirable for healthy individuals, is actually beneficial for resolving moist lung conditions. Almond is the only nut to alkalize the blood; all others acidify.

Caution: Almonds can exacerbate phlegm and sputum if the person has *damp* signs such as sluggishness, thick, greasy tongue coating, and edema.

Black Sesame Seed

Neutral thermal nature; sweet flavor; tonifies the *yin* fluids and blood; strengthens the liver and kidneys; has general demulcent properties—lubricates the intestines and the five *yin* organs (heart, liver, kidney, spleen-pancreas, and lungs); acts as a general tonic. Used to relieve rheumatism (reduces *wind* obstruction), constipation, dry cough, blurry vision, ringing in the ears, blood in urine, low backache, weak knees, stiff joints, nervous spasm, headache, insufficient mother's milk, and dizziness, numbness, or paralysis caused by deficient blood or *yin.* Also useful to darken prematurely gray hair. Very helpful in conditions of the elderly as well as chronic wasting diseases where constipation and deficient body fluids exist. In India, used as a special food for the cool, damp season.

Caution: Avoid in cases of deficient spleen-pancreas marked by diarrhea or watery stools.

Note: Common tan sesame seeds exhibit the same properties as black seeds but are milder-acting. Sesame seeds should be ground up before eating or cooking to make them more digestible. They become even more digestible with soaking overnight then lightly pan-roasting before grinding. This helps to reduce the effects of their substantial oxalic acid content, which ties up calcium and other minerals. "Sesame butter" sold in stores is whole sesame seeds milled into a butter; "sesame tahini" is made of sesame seeds with their hulls removed before milling. Thus tahini, a refined food to avoid, lacks fiber, many minerals and metabolic cofactors necessary for complete digestion. In our clinical experience, tahini contributes to liver stagnancy issues along with attendant emotional imbalances, namely, anger, depression, and irritability.

Chia Seed

An energy tonic that lubricates dryness. Next to flax, they are the highest source of omega-3 fatty acids. The Southwest American Indian ate chia for sustenance during endurance contests. Latin Americans use them to treat constipation.

Coconut

Warming thermal nature; sweet flavor; strengthening; quells *wind;* hemostatic; tonifies the heart. Used for weakness, emaciation, nosebleed, and childhood malnutrition.

Coconut is a good source of saturated fat for vegetarians; however, it can be dangerous when used by those with excess saturated fat and cholesterol in the diet (for example, a diet concentrated in heavy meats, eggs, and dairy).

Coconut milk is warming, sweet, clears the effects of *summer heat,* quenches thirst, increases semen, and builds the *yin* fluids. It is often helpful in treating edema resulting from heart weakness and diabetes.

Flax Seed

Neutral thermal nature; sweet flavor; laxative; mucilaginous; relieves pain and inflammation; influences the spleen-pancreas and colon. The richest source of omega-3 fatty acids, which have vitally important properties for strengthening immunity and cleaning the heart and arteries. Useful in many degenerative disorders (see *Oils and Fats* chapter).

Peanut

Warming thermal nature; sweet flavor; affects lungs and spleen-pancreas; lubricates the intestines; harmonizes the stomach. Used to increase the milk supply of nursing mothers (add roasted peanuts to rice or millet soup), to stop bleeding including hemophilia and blood in the urine (eat raw peanuts), to treat deafness (eat raw peanuts), and to lower blood pressure (drink tea of shells).

Note: In the above remedies, use the whole peanut, including the thin brown skin.

Caution: Peanuts can cause skin outbreaks. They also greatly slow the metabolic rate of the liver. Therefore they should be avoided by overweight, *damp,* sluggish, yeast-infected, or cancerous persons. If eaten moderately, peanuts can benefit the person with fast metabolism such as the thin, nervous person who digests large amounts of food rapidly. Peanuts are often heavily sprayed with chemicals and grown on land saturated with synthetic fertilizers. In addition, they are subject to the carcinogenic fungus aflatoxin. Organic peanuts should therefore be used—they contain fewer chemical residues, and are less subject to aflatoxin.

Pine Nut

Warming thermal nature; sweet flavor; influences the lungs, colon, and liver; lubricates the lungs and intestines; increases body fluids; mildly laxative; quells *wind* conditions. Helpful in treating dizziness, dry cough, spitting up blood, *wind* obstruction (rheumatism), and constipation. Pine nuts are highly susceptible to rancidity and should be refrigerated in a sealed container after shelling.

Pistachio

Neutral thermal nature; sweet, bitter, and slightly sour flavor; influences the liver and kidneys; purifies the blood; lubricates the intestines. Used for constipation; Ayurveda considers them an important tonic for the whole body. They are most commonly available salted. However, in this form, they should not be used by those with *damp* conditions.

Pumpkin and Squash Seeds

Neutral thermal nature; sweet-and-bitter flavor; influence the colon and spleen-pancreas; diuretic; vermifuge (expels worms—especially effective for round worm and tapeworm). Used for motion sickness, nausea, impotency, and swollen prostate with signs of difficult or dribbling urination. They are valuable sources of zinc and omega-3 fatty acids. They can be taken as a tea decoction or broth (blend with water and strain), or eaten raw or roasted. Lightly pan or oven roast to remove harmful *E. coli* from their surface. Dosage is 1–2 ounces daily.

Sunflower Seed

Warming thermal nature; sweet flavor; influences the spleen-pancreas; acts as a *qi* energy tonic; lubricates the intestines; hastens the eruption of measles (prepare as a tea decoction). Used to treat constipation of the *dryness* type. Because of their high polyunsaturated fatty acid content, these seeds go rancid quickly once their protective shell is removed—it is best to shell them just before eating.

Walnut

Warming thermal nature; sweet flavor; walnuts can reduce inflammation and alleviate pain. This effect may be due to their omega-3 oils content (5% of its total oils). They also moisten the lungs and intestines, and help relieve coughing and wheezing accompanied by signs of coldness (e.g., chills and watery mucus), nourish the kidney-adrenals and brain, and enrich the sperm. They treat involuntary seminal emission and impotency, cold and painful back and knees, and other kidney yang deficiencies (page 358), and constipation from dryness in the elderly. Avoid taking walnuts in cases of loose stools and heat signs (e.g., red face, anger, tendency to canker sores, yellow mucus, or strong thirst). Walnuts may harbor parasites; roasting and other methods of cooking make them safe to eat.

Vegetables

Vegetables are a vital part of the daily diet and are ideally chosen from what is available in your area according to your needs. Some are more highly recommended than others because they are more nourishing and easier to cook and digest.

- Serve vegetables with grain for complete nourishment. In general, grains build, while vegetables cleanse the body of toxins and purify and renew the blood. The combination is healing and soothing.
- Vegetables contain special enzymes that aid in the cleansing process. Those in the raw state or those grown in warmer climates have stronger cleansing tendencies and are especially beneficial to those who include animal foods in their diet. Included are mushrooms, green peas, cucumbers, yams, okra, peppers, summer squashes, lettuce (which has some narcotic effects), the nightshades, and vegetables that contain oxalic acid—spinach, chard, beet greens, etc. Others are: beets, which purify the blood; artichokes, which benefit the liver; and asparagus, which has a diuretic effect on the kidneys.

Even though these vegetables can have a somewhat strong nature of their own, they will usually not cause a problem if eaten in season and in the region in which they are grown. However, some are very eliminating and need to be used with caution by certain individuals. For example, people with calcic disorders (arthritis, heart disease, tooth decay, etc.) would do well to avoid the vegetables high in oxalic acid or solanine (see "Nightshade family," below), since these chemicals inhibit calcium metabolism. People with a weak digestive center and watery stools may wisely choose to eat sparingly of cucumbers, summer squash, and okra—such vegetables promote *dampness* in the digestive tract and/or bowel movement.

- Vegetables such as carrots, parsnips, turnips, rutabagas, watercress, parsley, the cabbage family (cauliflower, broccoli, bok choy, etc.), winter squash, kale, and certain other dark leafy greens have milder properties. They grow in temperate-to-cold climates and contain minerals and other elements that make it possible for some of them to survive harsh weather and even live under snow all winter. When eating these regularly, we take on their qualities and build resistance to cooler weather and disease. In storage, several of them keep their vitality a long time. Cabbage contains high amounts of vitamin C, mostly concentrated in the core of the plant, that is not destroyed in storage, by moderate cooking, or in sauerkraut.
- Onions, scallions, chives, leeks, garlic, and shallots have medicinal value and otherwise are too strong for daily use. When cooked, they stimulate excess desires; when raw, they give rise to anger, according to major East Asian teachings on spiritual development.

- Garlic, carrots, the cabbage family, and some other vegetables contain sulphur, which expels worms and intestinal parasites.

Healing Properties of Vegetables

It is important to recall that the healing value of food is influenced by its flavors and thermal properties. Examples: Bitter food dries *damp* body conditions including edema, mucus, cysts, or yeasts. Food with a cool nature diminishes *heat* conditions with signs such as yellow mucus, yellow tongue coating, red eyes, sore throat, and the sensation of being too hot, whereas warming food encourages circulation of energy and treats the sensation of feeling too cold. Some vegetables have neither a warming nor cooling property, and in these cases, their thermal nature is considered neutral.

Except where specified differently, the quantity of a vegetable to use for therapeutic value in chronic conditions should, first of all, be an amount that is moderate and satisfying; that portion is then eaten regularly, perhaps four to six times a week. If more than one vegetable is used, they can be combined in a meal or alternated daily. For example, one could alternate between beets, onions, and shiitake mushrooms as part of a program for treating hardening of the arteries and excess cholesterol. Supporting this program with a high-fiber/low-fat grain-and-vegetable diet is essential.

In acute ailments, vegetables may be used more frequently according to the need. Thus, as a remedy for a sore throat, one could consume cucumber or spinach soup two or three times a day until symptoms subside.

The following list of common vegetables highlights those which have prominent qualities and special healing value. Vegetables that are listed as high in silicon have the ability to increase calcium absorption and renew the arteries and all other connective tissue (see *Calcium* chapter). The nightshades are grouped together because of the strong properties they share. Likewise, the onion family is discussed as a group.

Asparagus

Slightly warming thermal nature; bitter and mildly pungent flavor. Contains the diuretic asparagine, which explains its capacity to eliminate water through the kidneys. Treats many types of kidney problems but should not be used when there is inflammation. Helps to cleanse the arteries of cholesterol and is useful in vascular problems such as hypertension and arteriosclerosis.

Caution: Too much asparagus can irritate the kidneys.

The underground tubers of asparagus used in Chinese herbology tonify the *yin* fluids of the kidneys and moisten the lungs; it is a cooling remedy used to treat lung congestion, spitting up blood, coughing up blood-tinged sputum, chronic bronchitis, and the wasting stage of diseases such as diabetes and tuberculosis. It also improves the feminine principle, especially in the aggressive person, and is used to ease menstrual difficulties, promote fertility, and increase one's receptive and compassionate nature. The root of the common asparagus can be substituted.

Caution: Avoid in *cold*-type diarrhea (watery stools) and in lung congestion when chills predominate.

Beet

Neutral thermal nature; sweet flavor; strengthens the heart, sedates the spirit, improves circulation, purifies the blood, benefits the liver, moistens the intestines, and promotes menstruation. Used with carrots for hormone regulation during menopause; treats liver stagnancy and liver ailments in general, as well as constipation—especially the type resulting from fluid dryness; also treats nervousness and congestions of the vascular system. A silicon-rich vegetable.

Caution: The greens contain abundant oxalic acid, and if eaten excessively, inhibit calcium metabolism.

Broccoli

Cooling thermal nature; pungent, slightly bitter flavor; diuretic; brightens the eyes; treats *summer heat* conditions. Used for eye inflammation and nearsightedness. Contains abundant pantothenic acid and vitamin A, which benefit rough skin; has more vitamin C than citrus; a high natural source of sulfur, iron, and B vitamins. If lightly cooked, broccoli will retain its rich chlorophyll content, which will counteract gas formation resulting from its sulfur.

Caution: Broccoli has five goitrogenous chemicals which disrupt the body's ability to use iodine. Avoid in cases of thyroid deficiency and low iodine.

Cabbage

Green and purple varieties: slightly warming thermal nature; sweet-and-pungent flavor; mucilaginous; moistens the intestines; benefits the stomach; improves digestion; and is used in many cultures to beautify the skin. Is also used for treating constipation, the common cold, whooping cough (cabbage soup or tea), frostbite (body-temperature wash of cabbage tea), mental depression and irritability; helps rid the digestive system of worms (take cabbage with garlic for greater effectiveness against parasites). Contains vitamin U, an ulcer remedy. For either stomach or duodenal ulcers, drink one-half cupful of freshly made cabbage juice two or three times a day between meals. Continue for at least two weeks even though symptoms may disappear sooner. If too pungent-tasting, mix with celery juice.

Cabbage owes many of its healing properties to its abundant sulfur content (sulfur is warming, destroys parasites, and purifies the blood).

When eaten and simultaneously used as a poultice, cabbage treats skin eruptions, leg ulcers, varicose veins, arthritis, and wounds; eating cabbage regularly helps overcome chronic cold feet. To make a poultice, grate the cabbage, mix it with water, and wrap it onto the affected area with a cloth. Another method is to bruise the leaves and wrap these on directly. This method of application was used by a yoga teacher we know in Switzerland who severely cut her leg in a skiing accident; gangrene set in and her doctors recommended amputation. Instead she used continual cabbage poultices and ate a great deal of raw cabbage daily. The wound healed rapidly.

Cabbage contains iodine and is a rich source of vitamin C (more C than oranges); the outer leaves are concentrated in vitamin E and contain at least a third more calcium than the inner leaves. Cabbage in the form of raw sauerkraut is excellent for cleansing and rejuvenating the digestive tract, improving the intestinal flora, and treating difficult cases of constipation (see "Sauerkraut" recipe).

Compared with round-head cabbage, Chinese (Napa) cabbage has neither a pungent nor warm thermal nature; it is cooling with a sweet flavor and is useful for many kinds of inflammations, yellow mucus discharges, and all other ailments that have *heat* symptoms. It also moistens the intestines and treats constipation. Chinese cabbage contains just 20% of the sulfur of round-head types. Studies indicate several of the cruciferous vegetables (cabbage, broccoli, and brussels sprouts) inhibit cancerous growth in the large intestine.

Caution: Chinese cabbage should to be used carefully during nausea and by those with chronic weakness (*qi* deficiency).

Carrot

Neutral thermal nature; sweet flavor; benefits the lungs; strengthens the spleen-pancreas; improves liver functions; stimulates the elimination of wastes; diuretic; dissolves accumulations such as stones and tumors; treats indigestion including excess stomach acid and heartburn; eliminates putrefactive bacteria in the intestines that cause poor assimilation; used for diarrhea and chronic dysentery; contains an essential oil that destroys pinworms and roundworms.

Carrots are alkaline-forming and clear acidic blood conditions including acne, tonsillitis, and rheumatism; they are also one of the richest sources of the anti-oxidant beta-carotene (provitamin A), which protects against cancer (carrots are a traditional Western folk remedy for cancer) as well as treats night blindness, ear infections, earaches, and deafness. Beta-carotene/vitamin A benefits the skin and is anti-inflammatory for the mucous membranes. Therefore carrots are useful for skin lesions and lung, digestive tract, and urinary tract infections. They ease whooping cough and coughs in general. The juice heals burns when applied directly. Carrots increase the milk supply of nursing mothers and help regulate all hormones. They help ripen measles and chicken pox. They also contain large amounts of silicon and thereby strengthen the connective tissues and aid calcium metabolism. Their silicaceous fiber and ability to liquefy the bile make them useful in treating constipation.

For the above conditions, eat at least 6 ounces of carrots a day or drink a cup or two of the juice. Eating carrot sticks daily helps strengthen children's teeth, and in some cases, reduces overcrowding of the teeth by encouraging the development of the lower jaw. Grated carrots are best for parasites and dysentery and have been used as a poultice over cancerous growths to reduce inflammation and odor. Carrots are cooked in cases of diarrhea; when cooked and puréed or as a soup, they benefit infants with weak digestion. For a concentration of vitamin A and other nutrients, juice is ideal—it should be taken only on an empty stomach and should be diluted with water for infants. Carrots make a good foundation juice for adding other juices.

Caution: Carrot juice is very sweet, and regular overconsumption may lead to weakened kidneys with symptoms such as head hair loss. More than four cups daily is not recommended.

Carrot tops are bitter. They serve as a mineral-rich addition to soups and broths. The stems can be removed before serving. Adding a little of the tops when juicing carrots makes the juice less sweet and a better remedy for cancer prevention, liver stagnation, and *damp* conditions.

Celery

Cooling thermal nature; sweet-and-bitter flavor; benefits the stomach and spleen-pancreas and calms an aggravated liver; improves digestion; dries *damp* excesses; purifies the blood; reduces *wind* conditions such as vertigo and nervousness; and promotes sweating. Also used for *heat* excesses such as eye inflammations, burning urine, blood in the urine, acne, and canker sores and to cool internal *heat* in the liver and stomach, which often contributes to headaches and excessive appetite, among other maladies.

For appetite control, raw celery can be eaten between and during meals (see "Overeating," page 251). To slow down and encourage more thorough chewing of food, eat celery with a meal. Celery is one of the few vegetables (lettuce is the other) that combines well with fruit, as it has an ability to dry *damp* conditions, including those associated with eating fruit and concentrated sweeteners.

Celery juice combined with a little lemon juice is a remedy for the common cold when fever is more prominent than chills. This combination is also helpful in headaches caused by high blood pressure or by *heat* conditions (red face, head feels hot, red tongue, and/or irritability). Celery juice alone or in combination with lemon is useful for diabetes and helps clear the acidosis commonly caused by diabetes. For this purpose, drink 2–4 cups of the juice daily.

Very high in silicon, celery helps renew joints, bones, arteries, and all connective tissues. Because of these effects and the capacity of celery to clear digestive fermentation *(dampness)* and acidic blood that frequently accompany tissue inflammations, it is useful in the treatment of rheumatism, arthritis, gout, and nerve inflammations.

Both the stalks and roots are used in the East and West to treat high blood pressure and are a safe remedy for high blood pressure during pregnancy.

Cucumber

Cooling thermal nature; sweet flavor; diuretic; counteracts toxins and lifts depression; cleanses the blood; influences the heart, spleen-pancreas, stomach, and large intestine; quenches thirst, moistens the lungs, purifies the skin; acts as a digestive aid, especially in the form of pickles. Helpful during the hot or dry times of the year—treats the effects of *summer heat.* Apply the juice from cucumbers to relieve all burns, especially sunburn; drink the juice to help treat kidney and bladder infections. Consuming whole cucumber or its juice cools most other inflammatory or *heat* conditions, including stomach inflammation, conjunctivitis, sore throat, acne, inflamed skin diseases and discharges. Its cooling property is active even when cooked. In East Asia, cucumbers are often added to soups.

A pack of grated cucumber placed on the face beautifies the skin. If placed over the eyes, it relieves hot, inflamed, swollen, dry, or irritated eyes.

Cucumber contains erepsis, a digestive enzyme that breaks down protein and cleanses the intestines. This property also enables cucumber to destroy worms, especially tapeworms. (See "Parasite Purge" formula and add cucumber if tapeworms are suspected.)

Caution: Cucumber is not recommended for those with watery mucus or diarrhea.

Dosage: 6 ounces whole cucumber daily or 1 cup of juice.

Cucumber skin is rich in silicon, chlorophyll, and is bitter. Eating cucumber with skin enhances its medicinal virtue in the above applications. A tea of the skin alone is used for swelling in the hands and feet.

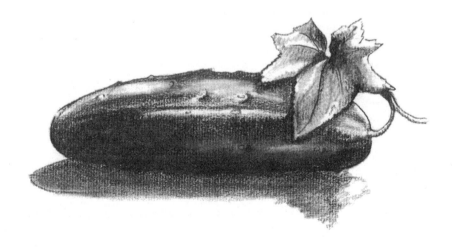

Jerusalem Artichoke

Sweet flavor; nourishes the lungs, relieving asthmatic conditions; treats constipation; stimulates insulin production and contains inulin, thereby reducing insulin needs (good for diabetic conditions). Also known as "sunchoke," these sunflower-related tubers are indigenous to North America and were a staple in Native American diets. They are a fall and winter vegetable with crisp white flesh, excellent raw or lightly cooked (they become rubbery if cooked more than 10–15 minutes).

Kale

Warming thermal nature; sweet and slightly bitter-pungent flavor; eases lung congestion; benefits the stomach. An ancient member of the cabbage family, it also has abundant sulfur and its juice can be used to treat stomach and duodenal ulcers. Kale is a hardy cold-weather green whose flavor becomes sweeter with a touch of frost. It is an exceptional source of chlorophyll, calcium, iron, and vitamin A during its growing season in the fall, winter, and early spring.

Kohlrabi

Neutral thermal nature; pungent, sweet, and bitter flavor; improves *qi* energy circulation and eliminates blood coagulations and stagnancies; reduces *damp* conditions of the body. Treats indigestion and blood sugar imbalance—used for hypoglycemia and diabetes; relieves painful or difficult urination; stops bleeding in the colon; reduces swelling of the scrotum; alleviates the effects of intoxication from drugs or alcohol. The juice is drunk as a remedy for nosebleed.

Lettuce

Cooling thermal nature; bitter and sweet flavor; diuretic; sedative; dries *damp* conditions including edema and digestive ferments and yeasts; contains the most silicon of common vegetables. Used for starting or increasing the production of mother's milk; also useful in the treatment of hemorrhoids. Its diuretic, cooling nature treats scanty urine and blood in the urine. Combines well with fruit at the same meal. Lettuce contains the sedative lactucarium, which relaxes the nerves without impairing digestion.

Leaf lettuce is much richer than head lettuce in nutrients, especially chlorophyll, iron, and vitamins A and C.

Cautions: Not to be used if eye diseases exist. Excess lettuce in the diet can cause dizziness.

Mushroom: Common Button Variety

Cooling thermal nature; sweet flavor; decreases the fat level in the blood; helps to rid the respiratory system of excess mucus; has antibiotic properties and can be used to treat contagious hepatitis; increases white blood cell count and thereby bolsters immunity against disease-producing microorganisms; has anti-tumor activity and can help stop post-surgery cancer metastasis; promotes appetite; improves recovery time from measles by causing them to ripen. Most mushrooms, including the button variety, have the ability to reduce the "*heat* toxins" from meat-eating (toxic reactions with *heat* signs).

Shiitake Mushroom

Neutral thermal nature; sweet flavor; beneficial to the stomach; said to be a natural source of interferon, a protein which appears to induce an immune response against cancer and viral diseases. Used in the treatment of cancer, especially cancers of the stomach and cervix. It decreases both fat and cholesterol in the blood and helps discharge the excess residues of accumulated animal protein.

Mushrooms are a good source of germanium, an element that improves cellular oxygenation and enhances immunity. The Chinese *Ganoderma (ling zhi)* mushroom is thought to tonify immunity best and appears to have a strong effect against tumors and cancers.

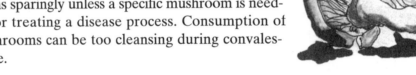

Cautions: Long-term vegans should use all mushrooms sparingly unless a specific mushroom is needed for treating a disease process. Consumption of mushrooms can be too cleansing during convalescence.

Mustard Greens

Warming thermal nature; pungent flavor; influences the lungs; tonifies and moistens the intestines; clears chest congestion; improves energy circulation and dissolves stagnant or congealed blood. Reduces *cold* mucus (mucus that is clear or white and copious) associated with lung infections. For colds and coughs, use mustard greens in a tea.

Cautions: Not for those with inflamed eye diseases, hemorrhoids, or other *heat* signs.

Nightshade Family

The beloved potato, tomato, eggplant, and all peppers except black pepper belong to the nightshade family whose primary toxin is solanine, an alkaloid which has been known to produce diarrhea, heart failure, headache, and vomiting. Extreme reactions are rare but do occur in instances in which an allergic or otherwise very sensitive individual overindulges. Those who are sensitive may notice an expanded and light feeling several hours after eating the nightshades; they may also find it more difficult to focus mentally. The expansive effect can be beneficial for those who become tense from work, stress, or activity which takes great concentration, provided one has no other reaction to these plants. The mildest effect comes from the potato, especially the red potato.

Americans seem to crave the nightshades. Of the three largest cash vegetable crops, potatoes rank first and tomatoes third. It seems these indigenous South American plants provide balance for a meat-based diet. Both the tomato and egg-plant can alleviate meat-induced liver and blood stagnancy. Potatoes also play a unique nutritional role in the "meat and potatoes" diet to be described later.

For those with sensitivity (including many vegetarians), solanine and other strong components of nightshades can be neutralized somewhat by baking, roasting, frying, or cooking these vegetables with salt or miso. Serve with parsley or seaweeds.

Each nightshade has specific properties:

Eggplant

Cooling thermal nature; sweet flavor; reduces swelling; clears stagnant blood by dissolving congealed blood and accumulations such as tumors resulting from stagnant blood; specifically treats congealed blood affecting the uterus; also has hemostatic action (reduces bleeding). Used for bleeding hemorrhoids, blood in the urine, and bleeding in general; a rich source of bioflavonoids which renew arteries and prevent strokes and other hemorrhages. Treats dysentery, diarrhea accompanied by *heat* signs such as yellow tongue coating, canker sores (apply charred eggplant powder—roast until charred or use eggplant tooth powder), snake and scorpion bites (apply a pack of raw eggplant); and frostbite (use a compress of room-temperature eggplant tea). Influences the liver and uterus and is particularly helpful for resolving repressed emotions and their harmful effects on these organs.

Caution: Eggplant should be eaten sparingly by pregnant women. In Japan, women are advised not to eat eggplant during pregnancy because it can cause miscarriage.

Actually a fruit, eggplant combines with other foods like a non-starchy vegetable.

Potato

Neutral thermal nature; sweet flavor; mildly diuretic; tonifies the spleen-pancreas and the *qi* energy; harmonizes the stomach; lubricates the intestines; fortifies the *yin* aspect of the kidneys; contains an abundance of carbohydrates that are already in the form of sugars. This sweet flavor can favorably influence the spleen-pancreas, particularly in those individuals who do not chew other carbohydrates well enough to obtain a satisfying amount of sugars. Potato neutralizes body acids, which helps relieve arthritis and rheumatism; and its rich potassium content is good for those who have used too much salt and high-sodium food, including meat.

The potato reduces all inflammations. Its juice is applied externally to heal burns, and is drunk to lower blood pressure and to treat stomach and duodenal ulcers. For ulcers, follow the same dosage as given above for cabbage juice. Potato can be juiced most easily in a juicer; juice can also be squeezed from grated potato by twisting it in cloth. The fresh juice is considered to have antibiotic properties. It also helps establish beneficial intestinal flora and is a rich source of vitamin C, enzymes, and minerals.

In nineteenth and early twentieth-century America, a poultice of grated raw potato was a common remedy for drawing out external abscesses, carbuncles, and eczema and for relieving swelling and soreness of the eyes. Today this kind of poultice still finds use as a Bolivian folk remedy for headaches.

Potato is considered one of the most completely nourishing foods if eaten with its skin. As an experiment to test the nutritional value of potatoes, two Danish food scientists lived healthfully for three years during World War II on whole potatoes only.

Because potato increases the *yin* aspect of the body, it improves one's receptive, nurturing, and compassionate nature. *Yin* also includes the body's structure, and so potatoes can be used to help build and maintain body tissues. In addition to the expansive effect of the nightshades noted above, the potato's *yin,* earthy nature is frequently craved by those with "jet lag" and other stresses of the high-tech world.

Cautions: Green potatoes and sprouts that grow on potatoes are toxic—be sure to remove the eye of the sprout imbedded in the potato. The renowned Austrian philosopher Rudolf Steiner observed that eating too many potatoes can cause laziness. This is a reasonable claim since an excess of potatoes will create an excess of the *yin,* receptive principle in the body (receptivity taken to the extreme can cause laziness).

Tomato

Very cooling thermal nature; sweet and sour flavor; builds the *yin* fluids and relieves *dryness* and thirst; tonifies the stomach and cleans the liver; purifies the blood and detoxifies the body in general; encourages digestion and so is used in cases of diminished appetite, indigestion, food retention, anorexia, and constipation.

Tomato relieves liver *heat* and accompanying symptoms such as high blood pressure, red eyes, and headache. To treat areas of stagnant blood in the body, tomato can be used as a food and as an external pack of the raw finely sliced fruit on the stagnant site.

Even though an acidic fruit, after digestion the tomato alkalizes the blood and so is useful in reducing the acid blood of rheumatism and gout.

Vine-ripened tomatoes are best; green-picked tomatoes that are later ripened can weaken the kidney-adrenal function.

Cautions: Tomato upsets calcium metabolism and should be avoided in cases of arthritis. Large amounts of tomatoes are weakening for everyone.

Dosage: 1–2 tomatoes twice daily.

Onion Family: Basic Healing Properties

All members of the onion family share certain key qualities: they are pungent and influence the lungs (the pungent flavor "enters" the lungs); and they promote warmth and thus move energy in the body, resolve blood stagnancies, reduce clotting, and expel *coldness*. They are perhaps the richest foods in sulfur, a warming element that purifies the body, helps remove heavy metals and parasites, and facilitates protein/amino acid metabolism. Thus, those on a high-protein diet can benefit from the onion family. These plants also clean the arteries and retard the growth of viruses, yeasts, ferments, and other pathogenic organisms often proliferating in those eating unbalanced diets. In spite of their medicinal virtue, these plants are thought to foster excessive emotional desire and therefore are not recommended in the major Eastern traditions for those seeking mental and spiritual refinement.

Other specific properties of each member:
Chive

Influences the kidneys, liver, and stomach; dries *damp* conditions; increases *qi* energy circulation; noted for treating blood coagulations, bruises, and swellings, especially when these occur from injuries. It is also good for treating the pain of arthritis (of the *cold* type). The juice from either the whole crushed chive plant or its leaves can be applied to the injured or arthritic area. For best results, also eat fresh or lightly cooked chives or drink chive tea.

In addition, chives relieve weak, *cold* digestion marked by watery stools, strengthen the kidney *yang* and sexual capacity, and thus can be useful for treating leukorrhea, urinary incontinence, and spermatorrhea when such conditions result from *coldness* (typical signs may include clear and copious urine, white or clear abundant mucus discharge, pale complexion, chills, and an aversion to the cold).

Cautions: Avoid when eye diseases, skin eruptions, and *heat* signs are present.

Dosage: 2–3 cups chive tea or consume about 2 ounces of chives daily.

Garlic

The most pungent onion family member (for other basic healing properties, see previous page); promotes circulation and sweating; removes abdominal obstructions and stagnant food; inhibits the common cold virus as well as viruses, amoebae, and other microorganisms associated with degenerative diseases such as cancer. Eliminates worms, unfavorable bacteria, and yeasts including *Candida albicans;* promotes the growth of healthy intestinal flora; used for dysentery, pneumonia, tuberculosis, asthma, hay fever, diarrhea, snake bite, Lyme disease, anthrax infection, warts, abscesses, and hepatitis. In chronic conditions, garlic must be taken regularly for several weeks to initiate substantial improvement.

Garlic eliminates toxins from the body (including poisonous metals such as lead and cadmium). Poultices made with chopped garlic draw out swelling from boils; garlic tea, applied cool with a cotton cloth and also consumed, will relieve poison ivy, poison oak, and nettle stings (simmer four cloves of chopped garlic in one cup water for twenty minutes). For protection against dysentery such as when traveling in foreign countries, chew up a clove of garlic before consuming suspected food or water. For amoebic or other forms of dysentery, eat ½ clove three or four times a day for the duration. For the common cold, sore throats, and sinus headaches, hold a clove of garlic in the mouth for at least 15 minutes, then consume it. To ward off mosquitoes, eat garlic at least once daily. Garlic also helps repel fleas from dogs and other pets if combined with their food.

As a remedy for athlete's foot, sprinkle powdered garlic daily on wet feet and let dry. Socks may be worn.

A drop of garlic oil in the ear canal once a day helps clear ear infections. The oil mollifies the acrid quality of the garlic, making this a safe remedy even for children. To prepare the oil, crush several cloves of garlic and soak in three ounces of olive oil for at least three days. Then strain the oil through a cloth.

To remove some of its strong flavor and aroma, garlic can be steamed. Unfortunately, a degree of the potency is lost with any kind of cooking. Consume a few sprigs of fresh parsley or cereal grass tablets or beverage after eating raw garlic to help neutralize its odor and reduce the burning sensation in lining of the digestive tract. To make garlic acceptable for children and others who are sensitive to its fiery nature, place a slice between two thin slices of apple, or chop finely and mix with food. Garlic eaten this way is not overly hot. Though less effective than the raw variety, aged and fermented garlic with only a slight odor is commercially available. Other forms of fairly potent capsules and pills are also available that dissolve lower in the digestive tract and thereby cause less odor.

Cautions: Garlic is contraindicated in *heat* conditions (red face and eyes, sensation of feeling too hot, aversion to the heat, canker sores, and desire for large quantities of cold drinks) and when there are *heat* symptoms related to *deficient yin* fluids (dry mouth, intermittent fever, fresh red cheeks, night sweats, fast thin pulse, frequent but small thirst, etc.). Be alert to quantity and length of use—Chinese herbology claims too much garlic damages the stomach and the liver.

Dosage: Some individuals have success using large amounts of garlic—six cloves or more spread out over the day. Certainly such quantities are better tolerated when taken with wheat/barley-grass products or other cooling foods, or eaten with meals. A minimum effective dosage in most cases is approximately ⅓ clove two or three times a day. For the common cold, hold the garlic between the teeth and cheeks for 20 minutes before eating it.

Leek*

In addition to pungency, leek has a sour flavor, which is astringent and associated with the liver. Leek can be used to treat dysphagia (difficulty in swallowing). The astringent property of the leek counteracts bleeding and diarrhea.

Onion*

Lowers blood pressure and cholesterol; decreases catarrh (phlegm and inflammation of the nose and throat); treats dysentery; inhibits allergic reactions; induces sweating; and is a cure for the common cold. A traditional cough remedy consists of onions simmered in water until soft with a little honey added; one onion is eaten every four hours. Onion packs on the chest are a remedy for bronchial inflammation and other chest congestions. Juice compresses or raw onion packs are also used externally on insect bites to draw out swelling and pain. Onion tea calms the brain and acts as a general sedative.

Scallion*

In addition to pungency, scallion also has a bitter flavor, which is associated with the heart: used in cases of both chest and heart pain. Promotes urination and sweating; alleviates *exterior* conditions such as the common cold or flu if taken during the first stages, especially when the cold is a "*wind-cold* influence" (chills will predominate over fever). Is often favored in China over garlic for these disorders because its flavor is milder. Like garlic, it has antifungal and antimicrobial effects, but to a lesser degree. Can be used as a tea decoction in the treatment of measles. Relieves *dampness* and watery accumulations such as edema. Scallions are also a remedy for diarrhea, abdominal swelling and pain, and arthritis when these disorders result from *coldness* (chills, pallor, aversion to the cold).

Caution: Avoid when *heat* signs prevail, including yellow tongue coating, yellow mucus, fever, aversion to heat, and great thirst.

Dosage: 3 or more cups daily of scallion tea (infuse about 8 finely chopped whole scallions per pint of water).

*   *   *

*For basic healing properties common to all onion-family members, see page 545.

Parsley

Slightly warming thermal nature; pungent, bitter, and salty flavor; improves digestion; detoxifies meat or fish poisoning; ripens measles to hasten recovery. Parsley is a source of remarkable nutrition: it contains several times the vitamin C of citrus and is one of the higher sources of provitamin A, chlorophyll, calcium, sodium, magnesium, and iron. Promotes urination and dries watery mucoid conditions; good for the treatment of obesity, mucus in the bladder, swollen glands and breasts, and stones in the bladder, kidney, or gall bladder. Parsley is effective for nearly all kidney and urinary difficulties, although not for cases of severe kidney inflammations (since it is warming). Parsley strengthens the adrenal glands and benefits the optic and brain nerves; it is also useful in the treatment of ear infections, earache, and deafness. It is often taken as a cancer preventive. Parsley counteracts halitosis and poor digestion, and has a refreshing green color, thus making it an exceptional garnish. Parsley tea strengthens the teeth and makes a face lotion to increase circulation and bring color to the skin.

Caution: Parsley should not be used by nursing mothers since it dries up milk.

Dosage: For the internal applications above, drink 2–3 cups tea daily made from fresh or dried parsley or eat 1–2 ounces of fresh or lightly cooked parsley daily.

Parsnip

Warming thermal nature; sweet flavor (which increases if parsnips are picked after a few weeks of frosty weather); benefits the spleen-pancreas and stomach; helps clear liver and gall bladder obstructions; promotes perspiration; mildly diuretic; lubricates the intestines; reduces *wind* and *damp* conditions; analgesic (allays pain); concentrated in silicon.

Used in soups or teas for coughs, colds, and shortness of breath; also treats headaches, dizziness, rheumatism, and arthritis.

Caution: Parsnip leaves are poisonous.

Pumpkin

Cooling thermal nature; sweet and slightly bitter flavor; relieves *damp* conditions including dysentery, eczema, and edema; helps regulate blood sugar balance and benefits the pancreas—used for diabetes and hypoglycemia. Promotes discharge of mucus from lungs, bronchi, and throat; regular use has been shown to benefit bronchial asthma. Cooked pumpkin destroys intestinal worms, but not as effectively as pumpkin seeds (see "Squash" below for dosage).

Radish

Cooling thermal nature; pungent and sweet flavor; moistens the lungs; cuts mucus; removes food stagnation; and detoxifies. Regular use will help prevent viral infections such as the common cold and influenza.

Radish transforms thick mucous conditions (often resulting from past or current animal product over-consumption) as well as mucus associated with *heat* (*heat*-related mucus is yellow or green.) It is especially good for clearing the sinuses, hoarseness, phlegm, and sore throats. Radish also relieves indigestion and abdominal swelling.

The cooling nature of radish benefits these commonly *heat*-induced conditions: nosebleed, spitting up blood, dysentery, and occipital headache.

In addition to resolving mucus, the toxin-purging property of radish makes it useful for detoxifying old residues in the body during a dietary upgrade.

A traditional Western remedy for gallstones and kidney and bladder stones consists of a tablespoon of grated radish taken daily for several weeks.

Caution: People who are *deficient* and *cold* should avoid radishes.

Dosage: Several radishes 2–3 times daily or ½ cup radish juice twice daily.

Spinach

Cooling thermal nature; sweet flavor; builds the blood and stops bleeding—is a specific remedy for nosebleed; diuretic; laxative; moistens *dryness* of the body, quenches thirst, and is particularly useful in the treatment of diabetic dryness and thirst. Its cooling nature cleanses the blood of toxins that cause skin disease and discharges marked by redness and inflammation.

According to Chinese dietary theory, spinach has a "sliding" nature, which facilitates internal body movements such as bowel action and urination, and thus is a treatment for constipation and urinary difficulty.

The rich iron and chlorophyll content of spinach builds blood. Its sulfur content helps relieve herpes irritations. It also has abundant vitamin A, which makes it valuable in the treatment of night blindness. The usefulness of the exceptional store of calcium in spinach tends to be neutralized by its oxalic acid content.

Cautions: People who tend to get kidney stones should eat spinach sparingly. Because of its sliding nature, spinach is not for those with loose stools, urinary incontinence, or involuntary seminal emission.

Squash

Warming thermal nature; sweet flavor; influences the spleen-pancreas and stomach; reduces inflammation and burns (fresh squash juice is applied to relieve burns); improves *qi* energy circulation; alleviates pain. Squash and its seeds destroy worms, although the seeds are more effective. Compared with summer squash, winter squash contains greater amounts of natural sugars, carbohydrates, and vitamin A.

The watery summer squashes and zucchini have a *yin,* cooling, refreshing property; they overcome *summer heat* and are also diuretic. For overcoming edema or difficulty urinating, eat steamed summer squash or zucchini with its skin.

Cautions: Too much summer squash, especially zucchini, can diminish the "middle heater" energy and warmth necessary for good digestion.

Dosage: For parasitic worms, eat a small handful of seeds of winter squash or pumpkin (pumpkin is a variety of squash) once or twice daily for 3 weeks. To counteract *summer heat,* eat summer squash or zucchini lightly cooked or raw.

Sweet Potato and Yam

Cooling thermal nature; sweet flavor; strengthens the spleen-pancreas; promotes *qi* energy; increases quantity of milk in lactating women; removes toxins from the body; builds the *yin* fluid capabilities of the kidneys, which in turn benefits dry and inflamed conditions in the body. Is also used to treat thinness and diarrhea. Sweet potato is very rich in vitamin A and is therefore useful for night blindness; adding spirulina, and in extreme cases, organic animal liver, to sweet potato soup makes an especially effective night-blindness formula. If a child swallows a metallic object such as a coin, feed him plenty of sweet potato, which will stick to the object and allow it to come out easier in the feces.

Note: Nearly all "yams" sold in America are actually sweet potatoes with reddish flesh.

Cautions: Eating too much sweet potato will cause indigestion and abdominal swelling; the red-fleshed varieties of sweet potato ("yams") are exceptionally sweet and can cause weakness if overeaten.

Turnip

Neutral thermal nature; pungent, sweet, and bitter flavors; improves circulation of *qi* energy and removes stagnant blood; builds the blood; promotes sweating; resolves mucus and other *damp* conditions; relieves coughing; clears food stagnation and improves appetite. Turnip, a member of the mustard family, is a good source of sulfur, a warming, purifying element; because of its alkalizing nature, sulfur, and other factors, turnip detoxifies the body. It also is generally helpful for indigestion, hoarseness, diabetes, and jaundice and is most commonly used in the West and East to treat various lung-related imbalances including bronchial disorders, asthma, and sinus problems. The mildly pungent qualities of the turnip are easily destroyed through cooking. Sliced raw turnip is superior when pungency is needed to disperse lung congestion.

Turnip greens are exceptionally rich in vitamin A.

Watercress

Cooling thermal nature; pungent, bitter, and sweet flavor; diuretic; influences the lungs, stomach, bladder, and kidneys; regulates and strengthens the *qi* energy; purifies and builds the blood; removes stagnant blood; moistens the lungs and throat; helps reduce cancerous growths; benefits night vision; clears facial blemishes; stimulates bile formation and other glandular secretions; a rich source of vitamin A, chlorophyll, sulfur, and calcium. Used as a remedy in treating jaundice, urinary difficulty, "hot" lung phlegm (yellow in color), sore or dry throat, mumps, intestinal gas, and bad breath. One of the most effective ways to use watercress is in vegetable juices. It is also useful in herb teas or eaten raw, steamed, or lightly cooked in soups. A hardy green, watercress even grows in the cold winter months in flowing water sources.

Caution: Watercress can exacerbate cases of frequent urination.

Cooking Vegetables

Raw vegetables in their natural state are invaluable for their nutrition; however, proper cooking methods (not overcooking) can preserve well over 90% of their nutrients. Although some vitamin C is destroyed by heat, cooking breaks down the cellulose structure, making other nutrients more accessible than they would be otherwise.

Foods that have been chemicalized or that have been picked for a long time lose their flavor and strength. Properly cooking them down reduces the bulk; when eaten, nutrients are extracted more easily, and the flavor is concentrated and therefore improved.

Cooking destroys parasites and amoebas that enter the digestive system through raw vegetables. It also reduces the cleansing properties of food and makes it more strengthening and digestible—better for *deficiencies.*

Once cooked, leftover vegetables should be eaten in the next meal, or at least within twenty-four hours; refrigeration of leftovers reduces their flavor, aroma, and therefore their life energy, but is nonetheless a necessity if they are kept longer than six hours in a hot environment.

Ways to retain colors, tastes, and nutrients

- Cooking for a short time with little or no water with direct heat helps to retain vitamins and freshness. Cooking for a longer time on a low heat gives vegetables a sweeter taste and makes them relatively more warming.
- Leave vegetables unpeeled; one may also cook them whole. Separate leaves from roots and cook the roots separately as they take longer. Serve both at the same meal for a good balance. (Removing part of the plant destroys its natural energy balance.) When storing root vegetables, dry the leaves and store in jars.

- Garnish cooked vegetables with fresh parsley or scallions to add vitamin C and freshness.
- Avoid overcooking and excessive boiling. Nutrients and aromatic oils that give flavor are lost and the vegetables are harder to digest.
- When cooking in liquid, some nutrients leach into the water. Be sure to serve the cooking liquid with the vegetables or use it in soups, breads, grains, etc. Keep vegetables covered while cooking.
- Cooking time and method will vary with each vegetable and how it is cut. Root vegetables are harder and drier and take longer to cook.
- Vegetable roots, tubers, and gourds are cooked when a fork enters without difficulty. Leafy greens are cooked the moment their color changes to fresh, bright green.
- Wash vegetables in cold water. Scrub root vegetables lightly. Vitamins and minerals are close to the skin. Before eating raw vegetables, soak them in a solution that removes parasites (see page 572 for methods).
- It is wasteful to cook more vegetables than needed for a meal. Leftover vegetables lose their vitality.
- Shear broccoli, kale, etc., of the center stem and hard portions. Dice finely and cook them a while before adding tops.
- Cook asparagus in a narrow vessel such as a coffee pot. Stand the tough ends on the bottom, as they need to cook longer.
- To retain the red color of beets, cook whole with a beet leaf or leave on root ends and one-inch of stalk. Cook beets alone unless you prefer the foods cooked with them to be beet red.
- Cut greens off turnips and rutabagas and cook separately, but leave the stems on. The bitterness, which is a nutritious part, is in the thin colored line under the peel where the stem meets the turnip. To diminish the bitter flavor, add salt at end of cooking.
- When cooking vegetables with soy sauce or miso, dilute these salty condiments with water and add at end of cooking. They will spread more evenly.

Selection of Vegetables

- Make shopping a pleasure; have a good relationship with local farmers— they offer more nutritious and economical produce.
- Select fresh, local, seasonal, organic fruits and vegetables with crispy leaves and firm heads. Freshly picked vegetables have a livelier taste and impart better healing properties.
- Do not avoid small vegetables and fruit. They can be more nutritious and tastier and teach us patience handling and cutting them.

Storage

- Fresh greens: Keep out of sun and warm places. Store in refrigerator or cool places. Open up bundle and dry in a dark place for 3–4 hours. Store in plastic

bags or store in a paper bag to absorb moisture that causes them to mold or go limp.
- Root vegetables should be stored in a cool, damp place such as buried below the frost line in the ground. If in a root cellar, they can be put in a box of sand, a burlap bag, or plastic bag with ventilation holes. They keep for months.
- Winter squash like cool, dry, ventilated storage.

Cutting Vegetables

In the process of cutting, the energy pathways of food are subtly rearranged to make it easier to cook, more digestible, more appealing to the eye, better tasting, and to obtain a variety of appearances and flavors from one ingredient.

Let the unexpected enliven your table by cutting simple vegetables into a variety of shapes. All vegetables can be cut many ways. Each way will produce a uniquely different taste and energy and will require a different method of cooking.

1. Smaller thinner pieces take more time and energy to cut and become relatively more warming and strengthening.
   - Can be cooked for a shorter time.
   - Good for sautéing, steaming, and waterless cooking.
   - Cutting old, wilted, or frozen vegetables into small pieces energizes them. This method of cutting is beneficial in cold weather, for weaker or older people, and hypoglycemic people (blood sugar levels tend to rise from simply the visual impact of finely cut vegetables). Tall, thin people may prefer their vegetables to be cut into small or round pieces; while short or stout people often prefer them cut into thin and longer pieces.
2. Leave fresh vegetables whole or cut them into large pieces so they retain their natural vitality and sweetness.
   - Require longer cooking.
   - Good for stews and baked dishes.

Unity   Many of the following suggestions recognize that the life energy of a meal and the mental clarity of the cook are closely related. For example, keeping vegetables separate until cooked and washing off the board and knife after each vegetable contribute to the idea of uniqueness and individuality, two qualities that must be preserved in order for unity to occur.

Learn to cut with harmony in mind

- Start with a clean board and knife that you handle well.
- Each vegetable has a separate chemical balance. Wipe off the board and knife after you cut each one.
- Use the vegetables as you cut them, or keep them separate on plates.
- Cut the vegetables that are to be cooked together roughly the same size.
- Cut the vegetables with specific intention. For example: 1) Cutting from top

to bottom or on the diagonal is a harmonious way to give everyone some of different parts of the vegetable. It also tends to hold nutrients in the vegetable as it cooks; 2) If vegetables are cut horizontally, some people may receive only the upper or lower part. However, this method is good for releasing nutrients quickly into lightly cooked soups.

- Become one with your knife and vegetable. Let it tell you how it is to be cut.
- Practice patience and enjoy handling your food, and the meal will be more satisfying and energizing.

Variations in Cutting

Dicing

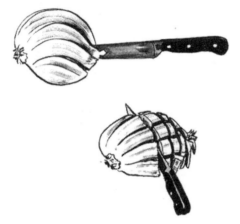

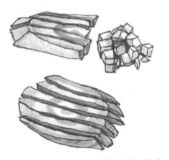

Matchsticks

Dicing: Cut thin sections to about ⅛ inch from root end. Then slice the opposite direction into small pieces.

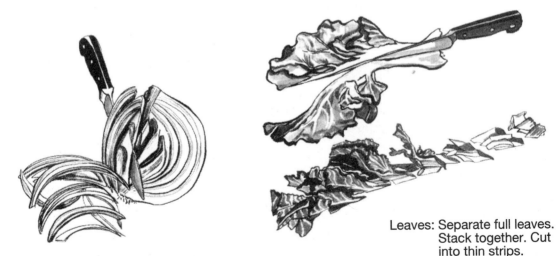

Crescent moons: Cut lengthwise into halves. Turn on axis and cut vertically into thin slices.

Leaves: Separate full leaves. Stack together. Cut into thin strips.

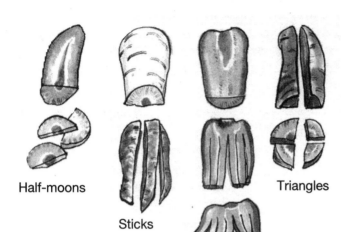

Half-moons

Sticks

Triangles

Fan Shape

Flower: Soak in ice
water to
open up.

Diagonal Cut

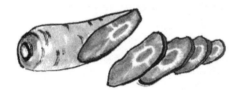

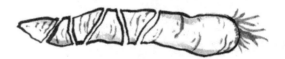

Large Diagonal Wedges

Blocks
Squares
Triangles

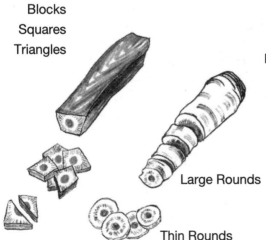

Large Rounds

Thin Rounds

Flowers: Cut 4 or 5 thin wedges
full-length around the
vegetable—then cut into
rounds.

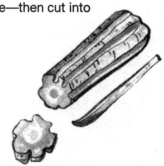

SAUTÉED, STEAMED, AND WATERLESS COOKED VEGETABLES

Most vegetables are better served alone, however, some combinations are quite harmonious and colorful. Try some of the combinations below. Vegetables should be added according to how long they need to cook and how they are cut. Examples of the order are given below.

- Radishes, cut into rounds
  Carrots and beans, cut diagonally
- Celery, cut diagonally
  Corn kernels
  Sprouts
- Potatoes and turnips, quartered
  Cabbage, chopped
- Rutabagas, diced
  Yams, cut into half-moons
  Parsley, minced
- Carrot flowers
  Fresh peas
- Carrots and turnips, cut in matchsticks

- Parsnips and carrots, cut in wedges
  Chervil, minced
- Onions and squash, diced
  Bok choy or chard cut into 1-inch squares
- Shredded cabbage
  Grated carrots
  Mung bean sprouts
- Carrots and broccoli stems, cut diagonally
  Broccoli flowerets
  Parsley, minced
- Broccoli and cauliflower flowerets

- Create a variety of special dishes by adding sauces and dressings. Examples: sweet-and-sour; tofu; sesame butter and lemon; nut; Chinese; Mexican; and arrowroot sauces. (See pages 602–605.)

JAPANESE SNOW PEAS

2 cups snow peas or green peas
½ cup broth
1 teaspoon mirin
2 teaspoons soy sauce

- Bring ¼ cup broth to a simmer.
- Add peas and cook 1 minute until tender.
- Remove peas with a slotted spoon and place on a platter.
- Add soy sauce, mirin, and remaining broth to the pot. Simmer uncovered a few minutes.
- Pour over peas.
- Serves 4.

CREAMED BEETS

2 whole cooked beets
1 cup bechamel sauce (p. 602)
½ teaspoon tarragon
1 teaspoon lemon juice

- Slice beets into rounds.
- Mix with bechamel sauce, tarragon, and lemon juice.
- Heat thoroughly before serving.
- Serves 4

CHRYSANTHEMUM ONIONS

4–6 medium onions
1 cup broth
Sea salt to taste
¾ cup grated carrots
1 tablespoon arrowroot dissolved in 2 tablespoons water
1 teaspoon mirin
¼ teaspoon umeboshi plum paste

- Cut each onion into 8 sections ¾ their depth, leaving the bottoms intact.
- Place them close together in a saucepan with broth and salt.
- Simmer about 20 minutes until tender.
- Remove onions and drain.
- Spread the cut sections apart to create a flower.
- Fill each center with grated carrots.
- Prepare sauce by adding arrowroot mixture, mirin, and umeboshi to broth.
- Heat until thick and serve with onions.
- Serves 4–6.

CABBAGE NORI ROLLS

1 medium-sized cabbage
6–8 nori sheets
Chopped parsley

- Quarter cabbage lengthwise. Cut into thin wedges.
- Steam 3–5 minutes.
- Toast nori sheets over flame until jade green.
- Roll up a few cabbage wedges in a bamboo mat and squeeze out excess water.
- Fill a nori sheet with rolled wedges and roll into a cylinder using a bamboo mat or by hand. (Directions on p. 592.)
- Allow to set for a few minutes. Cut into 1½-inch rolls.
- Garnish with parsley.

Variation   Roll up cooked carrot sticks with cabbage wedges.

EAST INDIAN-STYLE CABBAGE

1 medium cabbage, chopped
1 teaspoon sesame oil (optional)
½ teaspoon mustard seed
1 teaspoon each ground coriander and cumin, grated ginger
¼ teaspoon turmeric
¼ cup almond milk

- Heat oil. Add mustard and cover. Allow them to pop and dance inside the pot for a few minutes.
- Scatter in remaining spices and stir once.
- Add cabbage. Sauté 8 minutes.
- Add milk and cover.
- Simmer on low heat 30 minutes until tender and bright light green.

TART CABBAGE

1 cabbage, finely shredded
2–3 tablespoons water
½ teaspoon sesame oil
½ teaspoon umeboshi paste

- Heat water in skillet, then add oil and heat.
- Stir-fry cabbage 3–4 minutes until wilted and just cooked.
- Add umeboshi. Stir and mix well.
- Serves 4–6.

Variation   Sweet and Sour Cabbage— Add 1 tablespoon mirin at end.

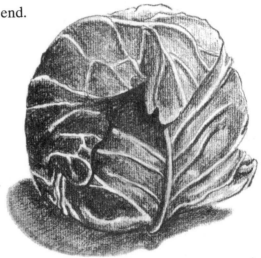

GINGER CARROTS

4 carrots sliced diagonally
1 teaspoon grated ginger
1 teaspoon sesame oil (optional)
Sea salt to taste

- Sauté carrots 3 minutes.
- Add ginger and salt.
- Cover and shake pan counterclockwise.
- Cook 30 minutes on low heat until tender.

Variation   Glazed Carrots—add 1 tablespoon arrowroot diluted in ½ cup water. Stir and simmer 1–2 minutes more.

BRUSSELS SPROUTS WITH PINE NUTS AND MUSHROOMS

1 pound brussels sprouts
4 shiitake mushrooms, soaked and sliced
½ cup pine nuts or sunflower seeds
1 teaspoon thyme
½ teaspoon ginger
½ teaspoon sea salt
1 cup water

- Steam or cook brussels sprouts by a waterless method until tender.
- Cook mushrooms, nuts, and seasonings in water until mushrooms are tender.
- Arrange brussels sprouts on a dish and pour mushroom mixture on top.
- Serves 4.

CAULIFLOWER BOUQUET WITH BECHAMEL SAUCE

1 whole cauliflower
1 cup bechamel sauce with lemon juice (p. 602)
Bread crumbs

- Trim and steam cauliflower whole for 7–10 minutes.
- Preheat oven to 350°F.
- Place upright in a casserole dish.
- Cover with bechamel sauce and sprinkle with bread crumbs.
- Bake 20 minutes until top is golden brown.
- Serves 4–6.

DUMPLINGS IN GREEN LEAF ROLLS

Dumplings:

½ cup sweet rice flour
½ cup brown rice flour
¼ teaspoon sea salt
½ teaspoon parsley, minced
½ teaspoon grated lemon peel
¼–½ cup boiling water
5–10 large leaves of cabbage, collards, chard, etc.
1 5-inch piece kombu
2 cups water
1 teaspoon miso and 2 teaspoons kuzu diluted in 2 tablespoons water

- Mix flours, salt, parsley, and lemon peel together.
- Add ¼ cup boiling water and knead 5 minutes.
- Form into dumplings 2 inches long by 1 inch wide.
- Simmer leaves in a little water until limp and vivid green.
- Squeeze out excess water and slice off hard parts of stem. (Save for soup.)
- Place dumplings in center of leaf, fold edges over, and roll into a tight bundle. (If leaves are small, lay one leaf on top of another so bases point in opposite directions.) Secure with toothpicks.
- Place kombu on bottom of pan.
- Place rolls, folded edges down, on top of kombu.
- Add remainder of water. Cover and cook over medium heat 20–30 minutes.
- Remove rolls and kombu from pan. (Save kombu for another dish.)
- Add miso and kuzu mixture to broth. Cook until kuzu is transparent.
- Pour sauce over rolls just before serving.
- Serves 4–6.

Variation   Use ½ cup cooked grain instead of sweet rice flour.

CORN TAMALES

5–7 ears unhusked corn
½ teaspoon sea salt

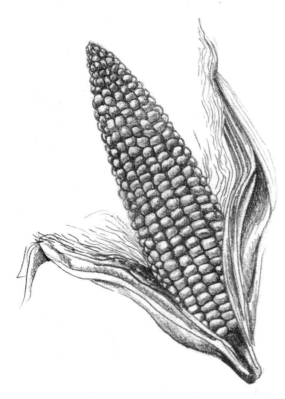

- Husk corn and save husks.
- Cut kernels from cob. Scrape cob well with a knife to remove all pulp.
- Grind corn in a food grinder or with a mortar and pestle.
- Mix with salt.
- Place 2–3 tablespoons corn filling in center of a large husk. (Or 2 small husks overlapped.) Fold edges over and roll into a tight bundle.
- Gently stack tamales, folded end down, in a steamer.
- Steam 1 hour until set.
- Open husks and serve with Salsa de la Sierra (p. 604).

Variation   Sweet Tamales—Add ¾ cup raisins, ½ teaspoon cinnamon

KNIFE AND FORK VEGETABLES

1 large onion, quartered (optional)
2 plantains, thickly sliced
2 sweet potatoes, thickly sliced
1 bay leaf
¾ teaspoon cumin
Sea salt to taste
1 teaspoon kelp powder
1 head cabbage, cut into 8 wedges
3 small crookneck squash, cut in half lengthwise
2 zucchinis, thickly sliced
1–2 cups broth
1 tablespoon rice vinegar
Lemon wedges

- In a large pot cook onion, plantains, potatoes, bay leaf, cumin, salt, and kelp, using the waterless method or by simmering in a little broth until tender.
- Add cabbage, squash, and zucchini. Simmer 7–9 minutes until colors are vivid.
- Remove vegetables and place on a large platter.
- Add vinegar to broth. Heat through and pour over vegetables.
- Serve with lemon wedges.
- Serves 10–15.

GREEN BEANS WITH ALMONDS

2½ pounds green beans, cut into
  1-inch pieces
½ teaspoon sea salt
1 teaspoon ginger, grated
1 tablespoon lemon juice
3 tablespoons slivered, roasted
  almonds
4 tablespoons parsley or cilantro,
  minced

- Combine green beans with salt and ginger. Steam or cook by a waterless method.
- Toss with lemon juice.
- Sprinkle with almonds and parsley.
- Serves 4–6.

STIR-FRIED ASPARAGUS

5 cups asparagus
1 tablespoon water
1 teaspoon sesame oil
½ teaspoon sea salt
2 tablespoons water

- Trim away the woody section of the asparagus. Cut each spear into 2-inch lengths diagonally.
- Add 1 tablespoon water to pan and heat.
- Add oil.
- Add asparagus and stir-fry 1 minute.
- Add salt and 2 tablespoons water. Bring to a fast simmer. Cover and turn to medium low. Cook 2–4 minutes until crisp and bright green.
- Serves 4–6.

WILD MUSTARD GREENS, NETTLES, DANDELION, LAMB'S QUARTERS AND OTHER WILD VEGETABLES

Can be steamed, sautéed, or cooked by a waterless method the same as regular vegetables. Add to soups and use raw in salads.

Special hints

—Gather young nettles with gloves on.
—For bitter vegetables:
- Pour boiling water over them several times and discard the water.
- Bring water to a boil before adding vegetables to pot. (Cold water sets the bitter taste.)
- Mix with mild-tasting vegetables and miso to neutralize the strong wild tastes.

Wild vegetables give us great strength and vitality, especially when we pick them ourselves.

SLIVERED BURDOCK ROOT WITH CARROTS

1 onion, cut in crescents (optional)
1 cup slivered burdock root
1 cup slivered carrots
1 teaspoon oil (optional)
1 tablespoon miso diluted in ¼
   cup water
Grated lemon peel

- Sauté or steam onion, burdock, and carrot about 8 minutes.
- Add miso mixture and lemon peel.
- Simmer 10 minutes on low heat.
- Serves 4.

NEPAL VEGETABLE CURRY

1 onion, chopped (optional)
1 tablespoon oil (optional)
1 bay leaf, broken
1 green chili, chopped
1 clove garlic, minced
1 inch ginger, grated
¼ teaspoon turmeric
Sea salt to taste
1 pound potatoes or carrots,
   cubed
½ cauliflower, broken into
   flowerets
1 cup green peas
1 teaspoon each coriander and
   cumin seeds
1 cup hot water or almond milk

- Sauté onion until golden brown.
- Add bay leaf, chili, garlic, ginger, turmeric, and salt. Stir in potatoes and sauté until browned.
- Add remaining ingredients and hot water.
- Cook gently on medium heat until vegetables are tender.
- Serves 4–6.

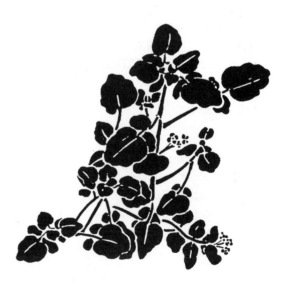

BAKED VEGETABLES

Preheat oven to 350°–400°F.

Wash and gently scrub the vegetables. Leave on roots and ½ inch of stems. Bake in skins. Arrange on baking dish and bake until fork-piercing tender. The larger vegetables and the ones with thick skins will take longer to cook. The vegetables can be baked whole or cut. To retain moisture, pour a small amount of water in the baking dish.

Baking Times

Beets, rutabagas	1½ hours	Covered or uncovered
Carrots, turnips, parsnips	40 minutes	Covered or uncovered
Eggplant	40 minutes	Uncovered
Potatoes	1 hour	Uncovered
Summer Squash	20–30 minutes	Covered or uncovered
Winter Squash	1 hour	Uncovered

Cut vegetables   Cut in half and place cut side face down in baking dish. Or baste with oil, lecithin, or sauce to seal in juices and flavors, and place cut side up on baking dish.

Slow method   Bake at 250°F for 4–8 hours depending on type and size of vegetable.

BAKED VEGETABLES IN NUT GRAVY

¼ onion, minced (optional)
1 clove garlic, minced (optional)
1 teaspoon oil (optional)
2 rutabagas, diced
4 parsnips, diced
2–3 tablespoons ground nuts or seeds
½ teaspoon kelp powder
1 teaspoon cinnamon
1 tablespoon soy sauce
½ cup water

- Preheat oven to 350°F.
- Sauté onion and garlic 1 minute.
- Add rutabagas and parsnips. Sauté 5 minutes more (optional).
- Combine nuts, kelp, cinnamon, and soy sauce with water.
- Transfer vegetables to a casserole dish that has been lightly brushed with oil or lecithin.
- Cover with gravy.
- Cover and bake 30–40 minutes.
- Serves 4.

ROASTED CORN ON THE COB

- Leave on husks. Bake at 350°F for 30 minutes.
- Soak drier corn in water before roasting.

BAKED STUFFED VEGETABLES

Stuffing:

    1 small onion, finely chopped (optional)

    1 clove garlic, minced (optional)

    1 teaspoon oil (optional)

    2 celery stalks, finely chopped

    2 tablespoons parsley, chopped

    1 cup bread crumbs or cooked grain

Salt to taste

- Sauté onion and garlic 1 minute.
- Add celery and sauté 3 minutes.
- Mix with remaining ingredients. Add liquid if necessary.
- Serves 4.

Variations Herbs, ginger, raisins, mint, toasted nuts, capers, olives, corn kernels, sesame butter, mustard, grated carrots, cooked chopped greens.

Preparation of vegetables

- Bake or steam until tender.
- Preheat oven to 350°F.
- Cut in half and remove pulp. Chop and use in stuffings.
- Fill each center half with stuffing.
- Top with bread crumbs or ground nuts.
- For beets, potatoes, and winter squash: Heat thoroughly in oven.
- Eggplants, zucchini, summer squash, and peppers: Place in a casserole with $\frac{1}{8}$-inch hot liquid and heat thoroughly in oven.

BAKED TOMATOES

- Cut off tops.
- Bake 30 minutes at 350°F.
- Sprinkle with tarragon, parsley, and coriander last 5 minutes of cooking.

CAULIFLOWER AND CARROTS IN SESAME SEED PASTE

1 cauliflower, cut into flowerets
2 carrots, cut into flowers
½ cup toasted sesame seeds
⅔ cup water
1 teaspoon mustard seed
1 teaspoon oil (optional)
½ teaspoon sea salt
1 tablespoon lemon juice
1 cup water

- Blend sesame seeds and ⅔ cup water into a paste.
- Heat skillet. Add oil then mustard seeds. As soon as they begin to pop, add the cauliflower and carrots.
- Cover and shake pan gently 1–2 minutes.
- Add sesame paste, salt, lemon juice, and 1 cup water.
- Cover and simmer 15 minutes or until vegetables are tender.

CARROT-SQUASH PIE

2 cups carrots, grated
3 cups squash purée
¼ onion, minced (optional)
1 teaspoon grated ginger
½ teaspoon each coriander and cumin
1 teaspoon Dijon mustard
1 teaspoon sea salt
¼ cup ground almonds
1 crumbly pie crust (p. 500)

- Preheat oven to 350°F.
- Sauté onion and ginger (optional).
- Mix all ingredients together.
- Place in pie shell.
- Sprinkle with almonds.
- Bake 35 minutes.
- Yield: one 9-inch pie.

VEGETABLE SHISH KEBAB

6 mushrooms
5 1-inch cubes tofu, tempeh, or seitan
6 small white onions (optional)
6 broccoli flowerets
6 chunks of carrots
Basting sauce:
½ cup soy sauce
1 teaspoon arrowroot
½ teaspoon grated ginger or lemon juice
A little water or mirin

- Slightly steam all ingredients.
- Marinate in basting sauce 30 minutes.
- Arrange vegetable pieces on skewers.
- Place under broiler 1–2 minutes.
- Baste and turn over. Baste when necessary and broil until done.
- Serves 6.

GRILLED SWEET POTATOES

4 sweet potatoes, cut into 1-inch rounds

1 cup miso-walnut sauce (Choose miso and walnut options in Basic Sauce, p. 602)

- Steam potatoes until tender.
- Arrange pieces on skewers and baste with sauce.
- Broil 1–2 minutes.
- Baste again and turn over. Broil 1–2 minutes more.
- Serves 4–6.

VEGETABLE PIE

1 sourdough pie shell (p. 494)

¼ onion, diced (optional)

1 carrot, diced

1 turnip, diced

¼ head cabbage, chopped

1 teaspoon oil (optional)

1 clove garlic, minced

1 teaspoon tarragon

¼ teaspoon sea salt

1 cup bechamel sauce (p. 602)

1 sheet nori, toasted

- Preheat oven to 350°F.
- Bake pie shell 20 minutes.
- Sauté onion, then carrots and turnips. Add a little water. Cover and steam 5 minutes.
- Add cabbage and seasonings. Steam 5 minutes more or until tender.
- Combine vegetables with sauce and place in pie shell.
- Bake 10–15 minutes.
- Sprinkle with toasted nori.
- Yield: one pie.

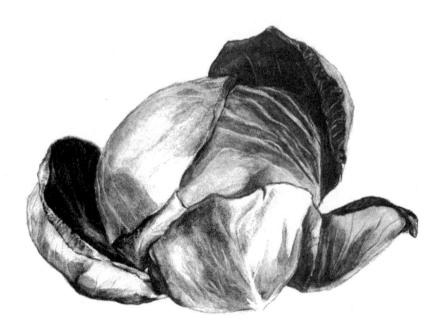

SHEPHERD'S PIE

1½ cup each turnips, carrots,
   potatoes, diced
1½ cup cabbage, shredded
  Sea salt to taste
1 tablespoon miso in 1 cup water
1 sourdough pie crust (p. 494)

- Preheat oven to 350°F.
- Cook and mash vegetables separately with salt.
- Use a 3-inch-deep casserole dish.
- Layer vegetables in pie crust. Sprinkle miso mixture on top of each layer.
- Bake 30 minutes.
- Yield: one pie.

VEGETABLE TURNOVERS

Suggested fillings:
- Sauerkraut
- Green peas
- Sautéed onion, cabbage, and potatoes

Sourdough pastry (p. 494)

- Preheat oven to 350°F.
- Roll out dough very thin.
- Cut into four 5-inch-diameter circles.
- Place one spoonful of filling in the center of each circle. Bring the edges together and pinch shut.
- Flute the edges.
- Place on a baking sheet. Prick with a fork.
- Bake 30–40 minutes until edges are lightly browned.

VEGETABLE PIZZA

1 sourdough pizza crust (p. 494)
¼ onion, diced (optional)
2 carrots, diced
½ pepper, diced
1 teaspoon oil (optional)
1½ cups bechamel sauce with miso
   (p. 602)
1 cup seitan, tofu, or tempeh,
   crumbled and seasoned with soy
   sauce
1 teaspoon each oregano and
   thyme
6 black pitted olives, cut in rings

- Preheat oven to 375°F.
- Sauté or steam onion, carrots, and pepper.
- Add to bechamel sauce and simmer 10 minutes.
- Pour evenly over dough.
- Sprinkle with seitan, tofu, or tempeh.
- Bake 20 minutes.
- Sprinkle with oregano and thyme. Dot with olives.
- Bake 10 minutes more.
- Yield: one 12-inch pizza.

Variation   Use Pasta Sauce (p. 605)

SPROUTS

Sprouts represent the point of greatest vitality in the life cycle of a plant. One clearly experiences this vitality when eating sprouts consistently. During sprouting, vitamin and enzyme content increases dramatically. At the same time starch is converted into simple sugars, protein is turned into amino acids and peptones, and crude fat is broken down into free fatty acids. Hence, the sprouting process predigests the nutrients of the seed, making it easier to assimilate and metabolize. This explains why grains and legumes, many of which are common allergens, often do not cause allergies when sprouted.

Nevertheless, the sprouting process increases the cooling attributes of the seed, which can over-cool the *cold* person and weaken digestion in those with low "digestive fire." Generally, if one is frail, feels cold often and/or tends toward loose stools, then sprouts must be eaten sparingly. Cooking makes sprouts more appropriate for these individuals. On the other hand, the *excessive* person (robust body and personality, thick tongue coating, ruddy complexion, strong radial pulse and voice) will benefit from abundant raw or lightly cooked sprouts.

Sprouts are a specific remedy for cases of stagnant liver *qi* (with signs such as swellings and lumps, mental depression, frustration, swollen abdomen and chest, purple-tinged or dark tongue, and/or greenish complexion).

During cold seasons, sprouts act as an excellent source of fresh vegetables. Cooking them at this time of the year balances their cooling nature. In fact, in China where sprouts have thousands of years of traditional use, they are routinely cooked. Raw sprouts have been desirable in the West because they more efficiently reduce the massive excesses occurring among the general population. For better digestion for every type of person, large grain and legume sprouts such as aduki, lentil, corn, green peas, soy, garbanzo, and wheat can be lightly steamed and are still vital and energizing. They need to be simmered, sautéed, or steamed longer for people who are *cold* or *deficient*.

The growth characteristics of sprouts are most appropriate for attuning one to the energetic upsurges of spring and summer.

ALFALFA

Alfalfa is America's favorite sprout and is considered more nutritionally concentrated than other sprouts, primarily because of its rich mineralization. The tiny alfalfa seed produces a root that can reach 100 feet into the earth, where it has access to minerals and trace elements untouched by other plants. Alfalfa follows the doctrine of signatures: its ability to produce exceptional roots benefits our "roots," which are often identified physiologically as our intestines and kidney/bladder functions.

Arabs were the first to discover alfalfa and found it a highly strengthening food, both for themselves and their race horses. Because of its attributes, they named it al-fal-fa, which means "father of all foods."

Healing Properties of the alfalfa plant

Neutral thermal nature; bitter flavor; dries dampness; diuretic; appetizer; benefits the urinary system and intestines; detoxifies the body. Alfalfa cleans and tones the intestines and takes harmful acids out of the blood. Also used for arthritis, edema, weight loss, bladder stones, plantar warts, chronic sore throat, fevers, gas pains, peptic ulcers, drug and alcohol addiction recovery.

Alfalfa contains eight enzymes which help assimilate protein, fats, and carbohydrates. It is safe food even for children and helps nursing mothers produce more milk. A sampling of important nutrients includes rich protein (16-31% of dry weight), carotene (equal to carrots), calcium, iron, magnesium, potassium, phosphorus, sodium, sulfur, silicon, chlorine, cobalt, and zinc. Alfalfa also contains vitamins K and P (bioflavonoids) and abundant chlorophyll.

In addition to alfalfa sprouts found in most supermarkets, alfalfa is available as a dried leaf herb, in tablets, capsules, and powders. To make tea, steep 1 tablespoon seed or 2 ounces dried leaf in 1 quart boiling water. In powder form, the pleasant taste of alfalfa is a welcome addition to soups and salads.

Daily Dosage: 2–3 cups tea; 2–4 grams (2,000–4,000 mg.) of capsules or pills 3 times daily; 6–12 grams powder; 3 ounces sprouts.

Caution: Alfalfa sprouts and seeds, rich sources of the amino acid canavanine, should be avoided in rheumatoid diseases such as rheumatoid arthritis and systemic lupus erythematosus. Canavanine can ignite inflammations in these conditions. Alfalfa leaf, however, is not a source of canavanine and may be used in rheumatoid diseases.

HOW TO MAKE SPROUTS

Use one part seed to at least three parts water. Soak in a wide-mouth jar. All measurements below yield one quart of ready sprouts. Half-gallon or larger jars are more convenient.

Seed	Soak time	Days to Sprout
2 tablespoons alfalfa or red clover	6 hours	5–6 days
¼ cup radish or mustard	6 hours	5–6 days
½ cup lentils or fenugreek	8 hours	3 days
½ cup mung beans	8 hours	3–5 days
1 cup wheat or rye	12 hours	3 days
1 cup aduki, garbanzos, soy, or other legumes or grains	12 hours	3–5 days
2 cups sunflower seeds	12 hours	2 days

- Cover the mouth of the jar with a plastic or stainless steel sprouting screen or cheesecloth, which is tied on or secured with a rubber band (sprouting jars, bags, and automatic sprouting machines are also available—see Resources Index). After soaking seeds, drain well and keep in a warm (65°F) dark place—they can be covered with a cloth or bag. Sprouting time increases with more light and cooler conditions.
- Rinse twice a day, ideally morning and evening. An exception is soy, which may rot if not rinsed four times daily. Keep jar tilted mouth down for better drainage. A dish drainer works well for this. Thorough rinsing and complete draining improve sprout flavor.
- After three days place alfalfa, red clover, radish, and mustard sprouts in a cool place with indirect sunlight to induce chlorophyll. Continue rinsing twice daily until sprouts are ready.
- Radish and mustard seed sprouts exhibit biting pungency, which adds a delightful zesty quality when mixed with other sprouts or in various dishes. During the sprouting process, the hulls on certain seeds slough off. It is important to remove hulls from alfalfa and radish sprouts since these easily rot. Hulls from mung, aduki, and fenugreek are often removed for a lighter-tasting quality, although they can be eaten and provide fiber.
- To remove the loose hulls from sprouts, place then in a large bowl of water and agitate them, further loosening and brushing them aside. Gently reach under the sprouts and lift them out of the water, without disturbing sunken hulls, which can then be discarded. Drain sprouts well. If refrigerated, they keep up to one week in a plastic bag or covered glass jar.

Note: Alfalfa may not sprout in polluted tap water. Use distilled or spring water or sprout with other seeds (mung, lentil, fenugreek) in the same jar. You will have a delicious salad. Save all rinse water for cooking, animals, or plants.

Salads

The art of salad-making lies in the arrangement of colors and shapes. A carefully tossed or arranged salad can transform the simplest meals.

Arranged Salads

- A tiny amount of color (a grated carrot or beet) can dramatize a dish of whole leafy greens.
- A simple garnish (olives or toasted seeds) can add remarkable flavor.
- Arranging simply-cut vegetables and fruit in rainbows of color can add a dazzling touch to a meal.
- Vegetables left whole add an interesting, wholesome flair to more complicated meals.
- Cut vegetables or fruit in unusual ways and arrange them on odd-shaped dishes with contrasting colors.
   Examples:
   —Arrange a handful of slivered carrots, sprinkled with nuts, on an oak leaf.
   —On a square white plate, arrange grated beets and garnish with one carrot flower and a mint leaf.
- Let the large leaves form the base of the salad. Split the center so they will lie flat.
- Arrange leaves so they form a circle or fan.
- Arrange smaller vegetables or fruit so they overlap each other until they reach the center of the ring.
- Cut vegetables slightly larger than the beans for a bean salad, so it will look more harmonious.
- Raw shredded zucchini or yellow squash make a beautiful bed for cooked vegetables.
- Use a melon baller or two spoons to form round and oval shapes.
   —Make a beautiful multi-colored melon salad.
   —Scoop out balls from cooked turnips, squash, zucchinis, potatoes, and yams.
   —Form elegant ovals from purées and add to salads.
- Use cookie cutters to cut out shapes from thinly sliced cucumbers, turnips, and bread.

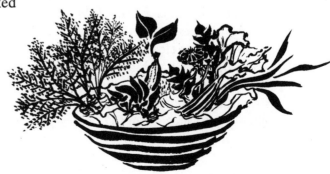

TOSSED GARDEN SALAD

- Use one or more leafy greens in season. Chop or leave whole.
- Add radish slices, grated onion, fresh corn kernels, cauliflower or broccoli flowers, slivered roots.
- First rub the inside of a wooden bowl with a clove of peeled crushed garlic.
- If you use oil, first toss the vegetables lightly with it. Next add lemon juice, vinegar, and herbs. They will cling well to the oiled vegetables.
- If you use a dressing, pour it on the bottom of the salad bowl and toss lightly from the bottom just before serving. This will prevent sogginess.

Notes on Parasites and Poisons

Salads often include raw vegetables and fruits which may contain hosts in the form of parasites and other undesirable microorganisms. To remove these, soak all greens, roots, fruits, and other produce to be eaten raw in a mild solution of apple cider vinegar for 15 minutes. Use one tablespoon vinegar per gallon of soak water or $\frac{1}{4}$ cup vinegar in a sinkfull.

Hydrogen peroxide also removes parasites, and denatures the poison sprays found on non-organic produce more effectively than vinegar. Though more costly than the bleach bath (below), it is ideal because of its effectiveness and purity. One may use regular hydrogen peroxide; convenient quart or gallon sizes can be ordered at drug stores. See page 84 for directions.

Another method of removing sprays and parasites is the bleach bath, a recommendation of the U.S. State Department for overseas military families. Like hydrogen peroxide, the bleach bath is extremely rich in oxygen and acts as a powerful oxidizer that destroys all fungi, viruses, bacteria and parasites. Vegetables soaked in it will often taste fresher and stay that way longer. Directions: add $\frac{1}{2}$ teaspoon Clorox™ bleach to each 1 gallon soak water. Soak produce 10 minutes, then place in clean rinse water for 10 minutes. *Note:* use only Clorox brand bleach—other bleaches may produce inadequate results.

*   *   *

Of all salad greens, cabbage is perhaps the only one that never harbors parasites that infest humans. In fact, cabbage is the only common raw salad green used in India and other parts of Southeast Asia. In most areas of the world, raw salad is a rarity. Nevertheless, salad clearly benefits the *excessive* and robust individual accustomed to a rich diet. Since the great majority of people become infected with parasites, it is important in a healing program to stop the influx of new parasites from all sources, including raw produce. Once a person reaches a high level of vitality, parasites generally do not proliferate but are destroyed by the concentrated digestive secretions.

SPRING SALADS

DANDELION SALAD

½ pound dandelion greens
Dressing:
    1 clove garlic (optional)
    2 teaspoons lemon juice
    ½ teaspoon umeboshi paste
    1 teaspoon oil (optional)

- Blend dressing ingredients in a mortar and pestle until creamy.
- Toss with greens.

HOT AND SOUR CHINESE SALAD

2 cups snow peas or early peas, cooked slightly
4 cups noodles, cooked and drained and cut into 2-inch lengths
Dressing:
    1 green onion, chopped (optional)
    1 tablespoon umeboshi paste
    2–3 teaspoons mustard
    Juice of 1–2 lemons

- Gently combine peas with noodles.
- Blend ingredients for dressing with a mortar and pestle or blender.
- Add dressing to noodle mixture.
- Mix lightly and serve before noodles become mushy.

MARINATED ASPARAGUS

1 bunch asparagus spears
1–1½ cups vinaigrette dressing with umeboshi (p. 577)

- Place 2 inches boiling water in a coffee pot.
- Stand asparagus up in the pot with tough ends on the bottom. Cover and simmer 10 minutes or until vivid green.
- Toss with dressing and marinate for several hours.
- Serves 4–6.

SIMPLE SPROUT SALAD

2 cups alfalfa sprouts
2 cups mung sprouts
1 cup sunflower sprouts

- Arrange an outside ring of alfalfa sprouts on a plate.
- Next make a ring of mung sprouts.
- Place sunflower sprouts in the center.
- Serve with your favorite salad dressing.

SUMMER SALADS

FRENCH GREEN BEAN SALAD

4 cups whole green beans, slightly cooked
1 cup seed yogurt (p. 613)
½ head lettuce, shredded
4 tablespoons fresh chervil or savory, minced
1 tablespoon almonds, slivered

- Arrange beans over lettuce and dress with seed yogurt.
- Sprinkle with chervil and almonds.

PRESSED CUCUMBER SALAD

Cucumbers, sliced paper-thin
½ teaspoon salt in 1 cup water
Pinch of dill

- Soak cucumbers in brine 30 minutes.
- Drain and dry slightly by pressing slices between paper towels.
- Sprinkle with dill and serve.

RICE SALAD

4 cups cooked brown rice
1 green onion, chopped (optional)
2 tablespoons parsley, finely chopped
1 cup peas, slightly cooked

Dressing:
2 tablespoons umeboshi vinegar
1 tablespoon soy sauce
1 teaspoon olive oil (optional)
1 tablespoon sesame seeds, toasted, or pine nuts

- Mix ingredients together.
- Toss gently with dressing.
- Let marinate several hours.
- Serves 4.

KOHLRABI SALAD WITH CILANTRO

2 medium kohlrabi, peeled and shredded
1 cup Chinese cabbage, shredded
1 carrot, cut into matchsticks
¼ cup fresh cilantro, chopped, or parsley
Ginger-Sesame Dressing (p. 579)

- Lightly toss each group of vegetables with dressing.
- Arrange vegetables in ribbons of color on a serving platter.

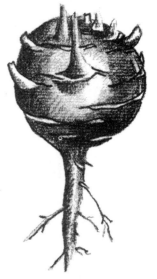

Variation Substitute zucchini rounds for kohlrabi.

FALL SALADS

RUTABAGA-PARSLEY SALAD

    1 cup salted boiling water
    ½ bunch parsley
  1–2 large rutabagas or turnips
    ½–1 teaspoon salt
    2 tablespoons tofu mayonnaise (p. 579)
    ¼ cup sauerkraut (pp. 586 and 609)

- Plunge parsley into salted boiling water for 2–3 minutes. Remove and chop finely.
- Cut rutabagas into rounds and cook until tender in a little of the parsley water.
- Spread each rutabaga round with tofu mayonnaise, and arrange them on a bed of parsley mixed with sauerkraut.

LEEK SALAD

    6 leeks, halved lengthwise
Dressing:
    ½ cup oatmeal yogurt
    2 tablespoons lemon juice
    1 teaspoon horseradish
    Soy sauce to taste

- Wash leeks well.
- Cook in a little water until just tender.
- Mix ingredients for dressing. If too thick, add leftover leek broth.
- Dress leeks and chill.

COLESLAW WITH CARAWAY

    1 head cabbage, shredded
    1 large carrot, grated
    2 tablespoons sunflower seeds, roasted
    2 tablespoons fresh chives, chopped
Dressing:
    2 tablespoons grated onion (optional)
    1 tablespoon umeboshi paste in 1 tablespoon water
    1 tablespoon oil (optional)
  1–2 teaspoons caraway seeds

- Prepare dressing using a mortar and pestle.
- Mix ingredients together.
- Toss lightly with dressing.

WINTER SALADS

Salting, then pressing raw vegetables or simply pressing cooked vegetables removes excess liquid and breaks down their cell structures, making the vegetables relatively more warming. Raw pressed salads are ideal in mild winters. Cooked, pressed vegetables are for more wintry climates. Use one or more leafy greens: kale, bok choy, chard, watercress, cabbage, or parsley. Root vegetables: rutabagas, turnips, carrots.

RAW PRESSED SALADS

- Cut roots into thin slices or slivers.
- Chop greens fine or into 1-inch pieces.
- Place vegetables into a large bowl. Sprinkle with salt and cover with a flat dish. Put a weight on top or use a pickle press.
- Press for 30 minutes to 3 days, pouring off water as it is expressed.
- The longer the vegetables are pressed, the more like pickles they become.
- Serve 1–2 tablespoons per person.

COOKED PRESSED SALAD

- Plunge whole leaves into scalding water and cook 2–3 minutes.
  Method 1: Roll leaves in a bamboo mat and press out excess water.
  Method 2: Place leaves on a plate. Cover with a flat dish. Put a weight on top. Let stand 30 minutes. Pour off water.
- Chop finely.
- Add miso, toasted nuts or seeds, or salad dressing.

RUSSIAN SALAD WITH SAUERKRAUT

1 cup beets, cooked and cut into rounds or diced
1 cup carrots, cooked and cut into rounds or diced
1 cup turnips, cooked and cut into rounds or diced
1 cup garbanzo beans, cooked and drained
1 cup sauerkraut
3 green onions, chopped fine
Dressing:
½ cup umeboshi vinegar
1–2 teaspoons sesame butter or sesame meal

- Mix ingredients together and toss lightly with dressing.

DRESSINGS

BASIC SALAD DRESSING (Vinaigrette)

- Mix 1–3 parts unrefined oil to 1 part vinegar or citrus juice.
- Add seasonings and choice of herbs or spices until the flavors blend well.
- Shake and let stand 10 minutes before serving.

Unrefined Oils	Vinegar	Juice	Seasonings
Sesame	Rice	Lemon	Sea Salt
Olive	Umeboshi Plum	Orange	Soy Sauce
Cold-pressed flax	Apple Cider	Grapefruit	Miso
Oleic Sunflower	Tangerine	Dry Mustard	
Oleic Safflower	Lime	Honey	
Almond		Umeboshi Plum	
Avocado			

Herbs: Basil, thyme, rosemary, tarragon, marjoram, oregano, dill, sage, mint, ginger, chives, onion, garlic.
Spices: Anise, curry, chili, cinnamon, coriander, cloves, nutmeg, cumin.

Note: The above oils must be unrefined in order to avoid unhealthful results. In addition, flax and all other polyunsaturated oils that you may choose should be "fresh"—recently cold-pressed, kept cool, and protected from light since pressing. Vinaigrette is not recommended for those with weak and *deficient* conditions, and it should be used sparingly by others.

CREAMY SALAD DRESSING

Add nut butters, raw or cooked vegetables, tofu, or cooked grain to Basic Salad Dressing and blend.

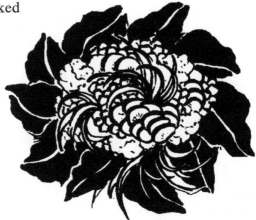

AVOCADO DRESSING

1 avocado
Juice of ½ lemon
½ cup water or broth
½ teaspoon dill
¼ teaspoon sea salt

- Combine ingredients and blend until smooth.
- Yield: 1½ cups.

To extend the dressing for groups or to make it less concentrated in avocado for people who tend toward *coldness,* the following variations will still have a rich and creamy taste

Variations   Dry-roast 2 tablespoons rice flour in a skillet until golden brown. Add 1½ cups water, stirring rapidly to prevent lumping. Simmer about ½ minute until a thick sauce develops. Place sauce and all dressing ingredients (except the ½ cup water) in blender, blend to creamy consistency. To extend the dressing even further, the rice flour and water of the sauce as well as the salt can be increased up to double. The avocado, lemon, and dill flavors continue to come through strongly.

BEET MAYONNAISE

4 beets, quartered
¼ cup beet cooking water
2 tablespoons vinegar
1 tablespoon onion, minced
5–6 tablespoons mayonnaise (p. 579)

- Combine ingredients and blend until smooth and cooked.
- Yield: 2 cups.

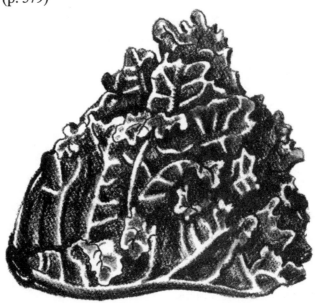

GINGER-SESAME DRESSING

1 tablespoon grated ginger juice
1 tablespoon umeboshi vinegar
1 teaspoon roasted sesame oil

- Blend ingredients until creamy.
- Toss with salad or vegetables.

TOFU MAYONNAISE

1 cake tofu
1 cup water
2 tablespoons umeboshi or
  brown rice vinegar
2 tablespoons lemon juice
½ teaspoon sea salt
¼ teaspoon ground coriander
1 tablespoon sesame oil (optional)

- Blend ingredients until creamy.
- Will keep refrigerated for several days.
- If the mixture separates, stir well before serving.

SOY SAUCE-LEMON DRESSING

1–2 tablespoons soy sauce
5–6 drops lemon juice

- Mix together.
- Toss with salad or use as marinade.
- Serves 4.

GREEN GRAIN DRESSING

2 teaspoons umeboshi paste
¼ onion (optional)
1 cup water
½ cup parsley, chopped
1 cup cooked brown rice
2 tablespoons sesame butter
  (optional)
1 teaspoon miso

- Combine ingredients and blend until creamy.

YOGURT DRESSING

1 cup oat or seed yogurt
  (pp. 613–614)
1 beet, cooked or raw, diced
1 clove garlic (optional)
Juice of 1 lemon
Miso or soy sauce to taste

- Combine ingredients and blend until creamy.

Seaweeds

The powers of sea vegetables (seaweeds) have been drawn upon for thousands of years for their ability to prolong life, prevent disease, and impart beauty and health for happier and longer lives.* In myth (as well as biology), the sea is the source that all things arise from and return to. The human body begins its development in a saline solution in the womb and is nourished and cleansed by blood that has almost the same composition as sea water.

Sea vegetables are classified by colors: reds, browns, greens, blue-greens, and yellow-greens. The particular color is related to the spectrum of light available to the plants for photosynthesis. The pigmentation, light exposure, depth, temperature, tides, and seashores all create different environments that correspond to the distribution of nutrients and variety among sea plants.

Sea plants contain ten to twenty times the minerals of land plants and an abundance of vitamins and other elements necessary for man's metabolism, making them an excellent source for food and medicine. Certain ones actually remove radioactive and toxic metal wastes from the body.

Properties of Seaweeds

Seaweeds (marine algae) share the ocean as a common bond. Thus, most seaweeds have a number of properties in common. In addition, each seaweed exhibits a distinct nutrient profile, although the scientific study of their nutritional attributes has only recently begun.

General Properties of Seaweeds: Cooling thermal nature; salty flavor; soften hardened areas and masses in the body; detoxify; moisten *dryness;* transform phlegm; diuretic; remove residues of radiation in the body; build the *yin* fluids and improve water metabolism; act as lymphatic cleansers; alkalize the blood; alleviate liver stagnancy (activate liver *qi*); beneficial to the thyroid. Seaweeds are useful in weight-loss programs and for lowering cholesterol and fat in the blood. Marine plants have a "sinking" quality and hence direct the energy of the body lower and more internally. They contain soothing, mucilaginous gels such as algin, carrageenan, and agar, which specifically rejuvenate the lungs and gastrointestinal tract.

---

*The book *Vegetables from the Sea* by Arasaki (Japan Publ., 1983) is a good source of further information on the healing potential of seaweeds.

Seaweeds in general are used to treat swellings, nodules, lumps, goiter, swollen lymph glands, edema, chronic cough with *heat* signs such as yellow or green phlegm, all skin diseases marked with redness, and tumors. They are also useful in the cure of cancer and fibroid tumors. According to ancient Chinese texts, "there is no swelling that is not relieved by seaweed."

Consider that our blood contains all one hundred or so minerals and trace elements in the ocean. Seaweeds contain these in the most assimilable form because their minerals and elements are integrated into living plant tissue. In fact, as a group they contain the greatest amount and broadest range of minerals of any organism, and hence make superb mineral-rich foods. On account of this unusual mineral content, they are effective even in relatively small, supplementary amounts such as a few kelp tablets. Normally, the ideal way to use seaweed is regularly as an ingredient in meals. Taken with other foods in this way, the dosage in the dried state (before soaking or cooking) is $\frac{1}{6}$–$\frac{1}{2}$ ounce (5–15 grams) daily.

As with land plants, it is important where seaweeds originate, because certain areas of the oceans are polluted, particularly with heavy metals. Since no body of water can now be considered pristine, it is helpful to know that wherever seaweeds grow, they do not simply absorb and concentrate toxins. Rather they detoxify and transform a certain amount of toxic metals, converting them to harmless salts, which the body excretes through the intestines.

In addition to a wealth of minerals, vitamins, and amino acids, seaweeds are especially excellent sources of iodine, calcium, and iron. A comparison of selected seaweeds in their customary dried state with other high sources of these nutrients looks like this: Hijiki, arame, and wakame each contain more than ten times the calcium of milk; sea lettuce contains twenty-five times the iron, hijiki eight times the iron, and wakame and kelp about four times the iron of beef; depending on when they are harvested, kelp, kombu, and arame contain one hundred to five hundred times more iodine than shellfish, and six hundred to three thousand times the iodine average of other marine fish. Seaweeds are also one of the few good sources of fluorine, a halogen that boosts the body's defenses and strengthens the teeth and bones. Since fluorine is lost with even minimal cooking, one must eat dried seaweeds raw (after soaking) to gain any fluorine benefit.

A bacteriological test indicates seaweeds are abundant in vitamin B_{12}. However, much of what tests as B_{12} is actually a B_{12} "analogue," which is not an effective form of the vitamin. Therefore, seaweeds are not a viable B_{12} source.

This chapter presents the most common seaweeds available commercially throughout the country, the majority being the popular Japanese varieties. However, this picture is rapidly changing and an expanding number of excellent-quality seaweeds are being wild-crafted on the shores of America and Europe. Examples not included in this section but becoming increasingly available are sea lettuce (*Ulva species*), sea palm (*Postelsia palmaeformis*), bladderwrack (*Fucus* species), and ocean ribbons (*Lessionopsis littoralis*). (To obtain, see Resources Index.) The properties of these sea plants generally follow those laid out above.

Bladderwrack is exceptional in that it is considered the most medically effective of the seaweeds for low thyroid gland function, obesity, high blood pressure, blood-clots, and edema. It also has the strongest anti-coagulant effect on the blood.

Cooking with Sea Vegetables

- If you are sensitive to salt, rinse the plants before using them.
- Introduce them gradually to your diet. It takes a week or so for the body to adapt its enzyme system to digest the sea vegetables. It also takes a while to adjust to their flavor and effect on the body.

Preparing Sea Vegetables

- Fresh sea vegetables need only be gathered, washed, and used as they are; or stored in a refrigerator.
- Keep dried ones in dark glass jars or hung in dark, dry rooms (keep for years).
- Prepare by freshening in water. The longer they soak, the easier they are to digest. Keep in refrigerator in soak-water or drained. Save the liquid for cooking grains, for soups, or feed to animals or plants.
- Sea vegetables are best cooked in ceramic pots, glassware, or stainless steel.
- Experiment with sea vegetables by adding them to your favorite recipes.

AGAR-AGAR

Agar-agar (also known as agar, and in Japan, as *kanten*) is a product of the mucilage of several species of seaweeds, collectively classified as "agarophytes." Three or so agarophytes are usually combined into one agar-agar formula. The majority of agar-agar is generally composed of *Gelidium* species seaweeds. Agarophytes grow at varying depths of 15–200 feet into fern-like fronds waving in browns, reds, and purples or into feather-like red blades up to three feet long. Hundreds of years ago, the Chinese and Japanese discovered how to freeze-dry and dehydrate the fronds until they became transparent and could be formed into kanten bars and readily used as gelatin. However, agar-agar is superior to gelatin in some respects— it doesn't easily melt and also has a firmer texture. Additionally, for those who value food low in caloric content, agar-agar contains no calories.

Healing Properties

Very cooling thermal nature; slightly sweet flavor; benefits lungs; influences the liver; reduces inflammations and other *heat* conditions affecting the heart and lungs; mildly laxative.

This seaweed product is used to promote digestion and weight loss, treat hemorrhoids, and to carry toxic and radioactive waste out of the body. A good source of dietary calcium and iron.

Cautions: Individuals with signs of *coldness* and/or weak digestion with loose or watery stools should use agar-agar carefully.

Preparation

Agar-agar comes in flakes, powder, or kanten bars.

- Soaking: Break kanten bar into pieces. Wash and wring out. Soak in liquid 30 minutes. Strain through a cheesecloth.
- Soften flakes or powder in liquid.
- Dissolving: Bring almost to a boil in water, juice or broth. Stir constantly until agar dissolves. Add ingredients.
- Molding: Turn mixture into a premoistened mold or glass bowl. Allow to set at room temperature or in refrigerator.
- Serving: Unmolded, in glass bowl or cut into cubes or slices. Arrange attractively.
- Uses: Pies, fruit desserts, jams, aspics, and vegetable molds.

Notes: Agar will not set in distilled and wine vinegars or foods with large amounts of oxalic acid (spinach, chocolate, rhubarb). Substitute with Irish moss.

1 kanten bar = $\frac{1}{4}$ teaspoon powder = 3 tablespoons light flakes = 5 tablespoons dark flakes. 1 kanten bar will gel 2 cups liquid.

AGAR-AGAR FRUIT GEL

3–4 tablespoons agar-agar flakes
4 cups apple juice
$\frac{1}{2}$ cup raisins
2 cups fresh fruit, chopped or puréed
1 teaspoon vanilla or almond extract or squeeze of lemon

- Soften agar in juice.
- Bring mixture to boil with raisins.
- Simmer 5 minutes.
- Stir in fruit and flavoring.
- Pour into mold and allow to set.
- Serves 6–8.

AGAR-AGAR FRUIT JAMS AND TOPPINGS

3 tablespoons agar-agar flakes
$\frac{1}{3}$ cup fruit juice
2 cups mashed or chopped fruit
$\frac{1}{2}$ cup sweetener (optional)
$\frac{1}{4}$ teaspoon each: allspice, cinnamon, cloves
1 teaspoon lemon juice

- Dissolve agar-agar in juice. Bring almost to a boil.
- Stir in fruit, sweetener, and other ingredients.
- Return to boil. Cook for 1 minute.
- Serves 4–6.

Jams: Pour into sterilized jars and seal.
Toppings: Cool slightly and pour over cakes and pies.

Variations Use apples, strawberries, blueberries, pineapple, pears, plums, apricots

AGAR-AGAR VEGETABLE MOLD WITH AVOCADO

2–3 tablespoons agar-agar flakes
  3 cups water
  1 teaspoon lemon juice
Pinch kelp powder
  2 carrots, grated
½ cup greens or sprouts
  1 avocado
  1 tablespoon grated onion
    (optional)
⅓ cup sunflower or pumpkin seeds
½ teaspoon cumin powder
  1 cup vinaigrette (p. 577)
Lettuce or chrysanthemum leaves

- Prepare agar-agar (p. 583). Remove from heat.
- Add lemon juice and kelp. Allow to cool slightly.
- Place carrots into pre-moistened mold or glass bowl. Cover with agar-agar liquid. Allow to partially set.
- Layer greens or sprouts over carrots and almost cover with liquid.
- Mash avocado and blend with onion and remaining liquid. Pour the mixture over the greens or sprouts.
- Allow to set.
- Before serving, dry-toast seeds and cumin. Stir into vinaigrette.
- Unmold onto a bed of chopped lettuce or arranged chrysanthemum leaves. Top with vinaigrette.
- Serves 4.

Variations Use combinations of cooked vegetables and your favorite homemade salad dressing

DULSE

Dulse *(Palmaria palmata)* has a red and blue pigmentation and grows with other seaweeds in flat, smooth fronds shaped like mittens that measure six to twelve inches long and up to six inches wide.

Healing Properties

Very cooling thermal nature; salty flavor; exceptionally concentrated in iodine; rich in manganese, which activates enzyme systems; prevents scurvy; induces sweating; remedy for seasickness and herpes virus; a good substitute for salt.

Has been traditionally used in soups and as a condiment in Europe.

Preparation

- Freshen in water and drain. Look for bits of shells.
- Use like spinach or any leafy vegetable.
- Toast in oven or pass over low flame (do not soak). Eat like chips.

- Sauté in oil and eat as a condiment.
- Use as a thickener in gravies and sauces.
- Layer in casseroles or in sandwiches.
- Blend with mashed potatoes, soups, croquettes, spreads, vegetable burgers, grains, salads, and desserts.

VEGETABLES WITH DULSE

1 cup dulse, soaked and sliced
1 carrot, cut into matchsticks
1 cup daikon, turnip, or parsnip, cut into matchsticks
1 teaspoon sesame oil (optional)
¼ teaspoon sea salt (optional)

- Sauté (in oil) vegetables 5–7 minutes on medium heat, or simmer until tender in ¼ inch of water.
- Add dulse and salt.
- Cover and cook on low heat 10 minutes.
- Remove cover and cook off excess liquid.
- Serves 4.

DULSE-SPROUT-TOFU SANDWICH

2 slices whole-wheat bread
½ cup sprouts
½ cup dulse, soaked or toasted
2 thin slices tofu
Lettuce or greens
Dressing:
1 teaspoon lemon juice
1 teaspoon sesame butter

- Mix dressing together. Spread on bread.
- Layer with ingredients.

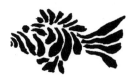

DULSE CHOWDER

¼ onion, diced
1 clove garlic, diced
1 teaspoon sesame oil
½ cup celery, diced
2 small potatoes, sliced
2 cups corn
2 carrots, cut into flowers
1 bay leaf
4 cups water
2 cups almond, cashew, or soy milk
½ cup dulse, soaked and chopped
¼ teaspoon each: thyme, parsley
½ teaspoon sea salt
Pinch of pepper

- Sauté onion and garlic in oil until transparent.
- Add celery and potatoes. Sauté 10 minutes.
- Add 1 cup corn, carrots, bay leaf, salt, and 2 cups water. Cover. Simmer 20 minutes.
- Blend 1 cup corn with 2 cups water. Add to chowder with nut or soy milk, dulse, thyme, and pepper. Simmer 10 minutes. Do not boil.
- Serve with sprig of parsley.
- Serves 6–8.

PICKLED VEGETABLES WITH DULSE

Marinade:

    ½ cup rice or umeboshi vinegar
    ½ teaspoon olive oil
    2 bay leaves
    1 teaspoon basil
    ½ teaspoon kelp powder

    1 pint vegetables, diced (celery, carrot, cabbage, red cabbage, beet, cucumber, daikon, pearl onions, zucchini, and/or yellow squash)
    ¾ cup dulse
  3–4 cups boiling water

- Prepare marinade and set aside.
- Drop vegetables in boiling water. Turn off heat.
- Cover. Let stand 3–4 minutes.
- Drain vegetables.
- Combine with dulse in sterilized jar.
- Pour in marinade. It should cover vegetables.
- Seal or refrigerate. Keeps for several weeks refrigerated.

SAUERKRAUT WITH DULSE

    1 cabbage, grated or chopped fine
    ½ cup dulse, soaked and sliced

- Save outer leaves of cabbage.
- Mix cabbage and dulse together. Pound with a wooden mallet to crush and release juices. Place in a ceramic pot or glass container.
- Cover with outer leaves, and then with a plate that rests directly on cabbage.
- Place a 3- to 5-pound weight on the plate; next cover the container with a piece of cheesecloth, and then a loose lid.
- Set in a cool place for 1–2 weeks.
- Discard leaves. Store kraut in refrigerator in glass jar. Lasts for weeks.

HIJIKI AND ARAME

Hijiki has brown branches that grow over the rocks and sea bottom like a carpet of stem-roots, or erect like a bush up to six feet high. The harvested plants are cut and dried in the sun, boiled until soft, and dried again until they are black.

Healing Properties of Hijiki

Very cooling thermal nature; salty flavor; diuretic; resolves *heat*-induced phlegm (yellow or green); detoxifies the body; softens hardened tissue areas and masses; benefits the thyroid; moistens *dryness*.

Excellent source of calcium, iron, and iodine; richly supplied in vitamins B_2 and niacin; helps normalize blood sugar level; aids in weight loss; builds bones and teeth; soothes nerves; supports hormone functions.

Arame has a dark yellow-brown pigmentation. It grows in bouquets of fronds with other seaweeds, especially with hijiki. It is so tough that it is chopped into string-like strips that resemble hijiki and is also boiled and dried to charcoal black.

Healing Properties of Arame

Very cooling thermal nature; salty flavor; moistens *dryness;* softens hardened areas and masses in the body; benefits the thyroid.

One of the richest sources of iodine; highly concentrated in iron and calcium; excellent for alleviating high blood pressure; builds bones and teeth; traditionally used to treat feminine disorders and mouth afflictions. Hijiki, arame, wakame, or any member of the kelp family, when consumed daily, can promote the growth of glossy hair and prevent its loss. They also help provide a clear complexion and soft, wrinkle-free skin.

Preparation

- Soak 5–15 minutes; expands to twice its original volume.
- Chop and cook with grains, soups, breads, stuffings, salads, baked potatoes, curries, tofu, and vegetable dishes.
- Sautéing in oil facilitates the digestion of oil-soluble vitamins and cuts the fishy taste.
- Arame does not have as strong a flavor as hijiki and is therefore more versatile.

All the following recipes can be prepared with either hijiki or arame.

SPICY CHINESE TOFU AND HIJIKI

1 teaspoon oil
1 clove garlic, minced
1 tablespoon ginger, chopped
¼ cup hijiki, soaked and chopped
1 block tofu, drained and cubed
1 scallion, chopped
Dash cayenne pepper
Sauce:
   1 cup water
   1 tablespoon kuzu or arrowroot
   2 tablespoons soy sauce
   ½ teaspoon anise seed or seven-spice powder

- Prepare sauce and set aside.
- Sauté garlic and ginger in oil 1 minute.
- Add hijiki and sauté 1 minute, until most of the oil is absorbed.
- Add tofu and sauce. Stir constantly until it thickens.
- Add scallion, season with pepper.
- Serve over rice.
- Serves 4.

CABBAGE IN MUSTARD SAUCE

1 tablespoon sesame oil
1 head cabbage, chopped
⅔ cup arame, soaked and cut

Sauce:

½ tablespoon mustard powder
2 tablespoons soy sauce
1 tablespoon sake or mirin

- Combine ingredients for sauce and set aside.
- Sauté cabbage in oil 1 minute.
- Add arame and sauté until tender.
- Add sauce. Simmer 2–3 minutes.
- Serve hot or let flavors marry and serve as a salad.
- Serves 4–6.

JAPANESE MUSHROOM STIR-FRY

6 shiitake mushrooms
1 tablespoon oil
⅓ cup arame, soaked and cut
1 cup carrots, sliced diagonally
1 cup bamboo shoots, slivered
¼ pound snow peas, slivered
¼ teaspoon kelp powder
2 tablespoons rice or umeboshi vinegar
¼ teaspoon sea salt

- Soak shiitakes in hot water 15 minutes, until soft. Slice (save stems for soup stock) and set aside.
- Stir-fry arame and carrots in oil until crispy.
- Add mushrooms, bamboo shoots, and snow peas, plus salt, and stir-fry 2 minutes.
- Add kelp powder and vinegar.
- Serves 4.

HIJIKI SALAD

1 cup hijiki, soaked and cut
1 teaspoon oil or ½ cup water
2 tablespoons umeboshi vinegar or rice vinegar, or lemon juice
1 carrot, grated
¼ onion, chopped (optional)
Sea salt to taste

- Sauté hijiki in oil 20–30 minutes or cook in water.
- Allow to cool.
- Mix all ingredients together and serve on chopped greens.
- Serves 4.

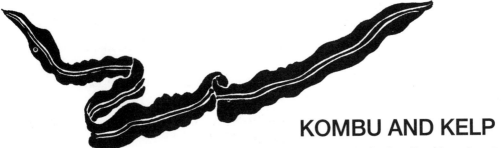

KOMBU AND KELP

Kombu is a member of the kelp family (*Laminaria* species).
The kelps have yellow-brown pigmentation and are the largest and longest
of all sea plants (up to 1,500 feet). They prefer to live in cool climates.

Healing Properties

Very cooling thermal nature; salty flavor; moistens *dryness;* increases *yin* fluids; softens hardened areas and masses in the body; helps transform *heat*-induced phlegm (yellow or green); benefits kidneys; diuretic; anti-coagulant effect on the blood; is a natural fungicide; relieves hormone imbalances and especially affects the thyroid.

Used to treat goiter, arthritis, rheumatism, high blood pressure, prostate and ovarian problems, lymphatic swellings, swollen and painful testes, edema, leukorrhea, diabetes, sterility in males, rheumatic fever damage, heart pain, blood clots, difficulty in swallowing, and anemia. Reduces tumors and other growths; cools and soothes the lungs and throat; relieves coughing and asthma; aids in weight loss; guards the heart at high altitudes; increases depth of breath and restores tired muscles; eradicates fungal and candida yeast overgrowths; used in ointments for wounds and cosmetics for facial beautification.

Greatly increases nutritional value of all food prepared with it, as it is considered the most completely mineralized food.

Kelp is often taken as a supplement, and is commonly available in powder, tablet, pill, or granular forms (dosage is 3 or more grams daily). It is now being gathered off the American shores and can be purchased like kombu, in dried fronds. Kelp substitutes well for salt because of its high mineral content and can be kept in a salt shaker for table use.

Both kombu and kelp are excellent added to beans, as the minerals help to balance the protein and oils in them and increase digestibility. They also soften and break down tough fibers in beans and other foods cooked with them.

Cautions: Use sparingly, if at all, during pregnancy; avoid if there is digestive fire deficiency (loose, watery stools and signs of *coldness*).

Preparation

- Break or cut with scissors.
- To soften, soak for 20–30 minutes in warm water. Cook 1–2 hours covered with water or until soft.
- Roast and grind into a powder to use as a condiment.
- Use in soups, salads, bean dishes, pickles.
- Wakame can be substituted for kombu

KOMBU SEASONING OR SOUP STOCK

3 inches kombu
5–6 cups water

- Wipe kombu with damp cloth.
- Add to water or dish (beans, stews, soups).
- Simmer 10–15 minutes.
- Remove kombu, allow to dry on bamboo mat or screen.
- Save to use in other dishes.

KOMBU BOUILLON ASPIC

2 bars kanten (agar-agar)
4–5 cups kombu soup stock
2 tablespoons soy sauce
1 scallion, chopped (optional)
1 tablespoon parsley, chopped

- Shred agar-agar and soak for 1 hour. Drain and squeeze out excess water.
- Add agar-agar to soup stock along with soy sauce.
- Bring to boil. Simmer 10–15 minutes, stirring.
- Add scallion and parsley. Remove from heat.
- Pour into pre-moistened mold. Allow to set.
- Serves 6

LAYERED KOMBU VEGETABLE BAKE

20 inches kombu, cooked and cut into squares
2 carrots, sliced diagonally
2 cups turnips, diced
2 cups cabbage, shredded
Sauce:
½ cup water
1 tablespoon ginger, minced
3 tablespoons soy sauce

- Preheat oven to 300°F.
- Prepare sauce and set aside.
- Layer vegetables in a baking dish in order given, beginning with kombu. Dash each layer with sauce.
- Cover and bake 45 minutes.
- Serves 6.

KOMBU KNOTS

1–2 inches kombu
Oil

- Wipe kombu with wet towel to soften it.
- Cut with scissors into strips ⅛-inch wide and 3 inches long.
- Tie into knots.
- Deep-fry in oil until crispy, about 1 minute.
- Serve like chips.

SWEET KOMBU

1 cup cooked kombu, cut in ½-inch pieces
5 tablespoons barley malt

- Mix together.
- Allow to cool. Refrigerate.

This is a "full sweet" food and will help to satisfy cravings for sweets when eaten in small amounts.

NORI

Nori (*Porphyra tenera* and related species) is dusky-jade colored. The fronds are hollow tubes that flutter in the water—some are like ruffled fans, while others are large and flat. The fibers of nori are more tender than other seaweeds. In Ireland, nori is called *sloke;* the Scottish call it *laver.*

Healing Properties

Very cooling thermal nature; sweet-and-salty flavor; increases *yin* fluids; diuretic; softens hardened body areas (such as nodules); transforms and resolves *heat*-induced phlegm (yellow or green).

Highest protein content (48% of dry weight) and most easily digested of the seaweeds; rich in vitamins A, B_1, and niacin; decreases cholesterol; treats painful and difficult urination, goiter, edema, high blood pressure, cough with yellow mucus, beriberi, fatty cysts under the skin, warts, and rickets; aids in digestion, especially with fried foods.

Preparation

- Comes in sheets and can be used as is.
- Can be crisped by passing over a low flame or in a 300°F oven, until color changes.
- Cut with scissors into strips or crumble over salads, stews, casseroles, dressings, spreads, or desserts.
- Also available in dried fronds gathered off the American coasts. In this form, nori is typically added to soups and stews, or is used as a condiment: oven- or pan-roast until crisp, then flake by rubbing between the palms of your hands. Sprinkle on grains, salads, soups, etc.

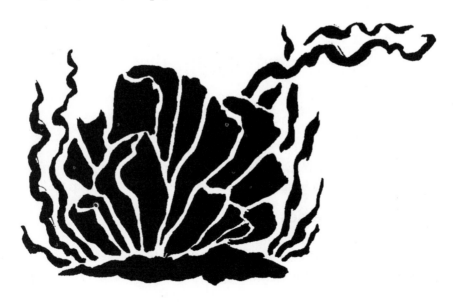

NORI ROLLS

2 cups cooked rice, hot
2 tablespoons rice or umeboshi
    vinegar
½ teaspoon kelp powder
4 sheets nori, toasted

Filling:
¼ cup grated cucumber
Dash soy sauce
1 teaspoon sesame seeds, toasted

- Mix up filling and set aside.
- Mix vinegar and kelp with rice.
- Place a sheet of nori on a small bamboo mat or heavy cloth napkin.
- Spread ½ cup of rice over the sheet, leaving a 2-inch edge uncovered at the end of the sheet.
- Arrange ¼ of filling in a line across the middle on the rice. Roll the nori in the mat.
- Place roll with seam down to seal.
- Slice 1 inch thick.

Variation   Use any grain or cooked vegetable combination. Mix umeboshi plum pulp or paste, miso, or natto miso with the grain.

Umeboshi plum and vinegar both help preserve the grain, making nori rolls containing either of these ingredients an excellent travel food. A simple and convenient variation for travelling is the rice ball—described on page 476. Use vinegar in these in the proportions given above for nori rolls.

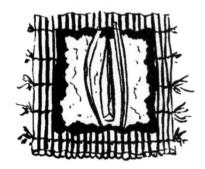 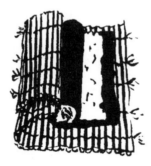 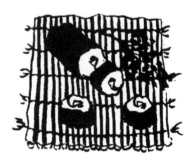

WAKAME

Wakame *(Undaria pinnatifida)* is olive-colored and grows in wing-like fronds up to twenty inches long in shallow water or twenty feet in deep water.

Inherent Properties

Very cooling thermal nature; salty flavor; diuretic; moistens *dryness;* softens hardened tissue and masses; tonifies the *yin* fluids; transforms and resolves phlegm (used for coughs with yellow or green mucus); counteracts growths and tumors.

One of the seaweeds highest in calcium content (hijiki is first); rich in niacin and thiamine; promotes healthy hair and skin. Used in Japanese tradition to purify the mother's blood after childbirth.

It softens beans and the hard fibers of foods cooked with it.

Alaria *(Alaria marginata)* is harvested in American coastal waters and exhibits properties and an appearance somewhat like those of wakame. Its preparation can be the same as wakame.

Preparation

- Soak for 3–4 minutes. Drain and save liquid for cooking.
- Cut into lengths and trim out the tough midrib to use in dishes that require longer cooking. Cook 45 minutes.
- Use like a leafy green vegetable; excellent in soups, salads, stews, sandwiches, baked vegetable and stir-fry dishes, spreads, and grains.

SNOW PEAS WITH CREAMY WAKAME DRESSING

2 cups snow peas
1 teaspoon oil (optional)
1 cake tofu
1 tablespoon sesame butter
1 tablespoon miso
½ cup cooked wakame, cut into small pieces
Dash of nutmeg and cayenne
Greens

- Parboil or sauté snow peas in oil until a deep green.
- Drop tofu into boiling water for 30 seconds. Drain and cool.
- Prepare tofu dressing by mashing tofu with sesame butter, miso, wakame, and spices.
- Arrange peas on a bed of chopped greens.
- Top with dressing.
- Serves 4

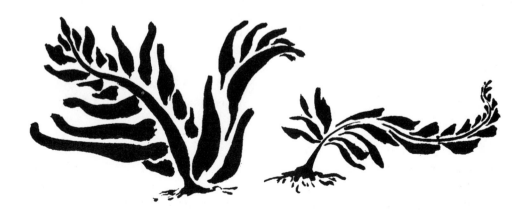

SUMMER WAKAME WITH GREENS

½ cup wakame, soaked and
    chopped
1 bunch greens, chopped
1 teaspoon oil (optional)
Dash of sea salt
½ teaspoon lemon juice

- Sauté wakame in oil 20 minutes (add a little water). Or cook wakame until tender in a small amount of water.
- Add greens, salt, and lemon. Reduce heat, cover and simmer 5 minutes or until bright green.
- Serves 4.

WAKAME VEGETABLE STEW

3 tablespoons whole-grain flour
½ teaspoon kelp powder
⅓ teaspoon each thyme and
    oregano
1 onion, cut into rings
½ cup soaked wakame, cut into
    pieces
1 tablespoon oil
2 burdock roots, sliced
4 small potatoes, chopped
1 cup broccoli, chopped
2 cups water
Sea salt to taste

- Mix flour, kelp, and herbs together. Coat onion and wakame by sprinkling with the mixture. Sauté in oil 2 minutes.
- Add burdock, sauté 2 minutes.
- Add potato, sauté 2 minutes.
- Add water and simmer 20 minutes.
- Meanwhile, boil broccoli in a bit of salted water until it turns bright green. Add broccoli plus water to stew last 5 minutes of cooking.
- Salt to taste. Simmer 2 minutes.
- Serves 4.

WAKAME CASSEROLE

2 cups wakame, chopped and
    cooked
½ onion, cut into crescent moons
    (optional)
2 cups bechamel sauce (p. 602)
¼ cup toasted sesame seeds
¼ teaspoon sea salt

- Preheat oven to 350°F.
- Simmer onion in a little water 5 minutes.
- Prepare bechamel sauce.
- Mix with wakame, onion, and salt.
- Pour into baking dish.
- Sprinkle with sesame seeds.
- Cover and bake 30 minutes.
- Remove cover and let brown 10 minutes.
- Serves 6.

IRISH MOSS AND CORSICAN

Irish moss *(Chondrus crispus)* fronds grow like broad forked fans in colors from reddish-purple to reddish-green.

Healing Properties

Cooling thermal nature; salty flavor; resolves phlegm (especially yellow or green phlegm); soothes and moistens the lungs; contains carrageenan, a gelatinous substance that treats peptic and duodenal ulcers, inhibits arteriosclerosis, guards against fat and cholesterol buildup, and has a mild anti-coagulant effect on the blood; contains calcium chloride, which acts as a heart tonic and glandular balance; treats chronic lung diseases, dysentery, diarrhea, and disorders of kidneys and bladder.

Traditional Irish used it as a food; they also extracted the carrageenan as a remedy for respiratory diseases. Irish moss is now being harvested along the eastern coast of North America.

Preparation

- Dissolving: Rinse twice, soak 10 minutes. Place in saucepan with liquid. Cook over medium heat until dissolved. Add ingredients. Place in mold. Allow to set at room temperature or in refrigerator.
- ½ cup will gel 4 cups thin liquid or 3 cups heavy liquid.
- Use as thickener in stews, gravies, salad dressings, aspics, pies, gels. A substitute for agar-agar.

Corsican *(Alsidium helminthocorton)* is sold as a tea. It discharges worms—especially pinworms and roundworms—from the body. Harvested in the Mediterranean waters off the island of Corsica, it has a laxative property and also has been a remedy for fibroid tumors.

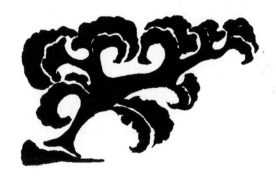

Soups

Soups are a part of every culture's diet. They can contain any food as an ingredient in their watery medium. The nature of water is *yin* and receptive—it takes the shape of its container. By eating foods that are water-saturated, we strengthen the fluids in our body. Very often the base for soups is something that needs or attracts water: salt, seaweeds, miso, and meats are examples of strong foods that require more water in their metabolism than most other foods.

Lighter soups (those that do not contain a strong base) are usually a balance for other concentrated ingredients in the meal; they also provide a relaxing, moistening quality to nurture those who are overheated from the climate or vigorous activity. The place of soup in a vegetarian diet varies depending on how much salt, bread, grain, seeds, nuts, and other concentrated food is consumed and also according to the metabolic rate of the person. Those with more concentrated diets and physiologies that run hotter will do well to include more fluid as well as soup in their diet.

In the meat-centered diet, soup will ideally be a main feature. In fact, for those who choose to eat meat, we suggest soup as the best way to modify its extreme nature. The water of soup in combination with included vegetables and herbs acts to dilute and predigest the proteins and fats in meat.

In many cases when there is a nutritional need for a meat soup or broth, miso or soy sauce will not only be more nutritionally balancing, but more flavorful. Next are listed examples of the options available in meatless soups.

Soups can be made from many ingredients including various seasonings, garnishes, and thickeners.

Examples:

Main ingredients: grains, beans, noodles, vegetables, tofu, seitan, tempeh

Seasonings: miso, sea salt, seaweeds, ginger, herbs, vinegar, mustard, garlic, onions, nut butters

Garnishes: scallions, parsley, toasted nuts, croutons, sprouts, toasted flaked nori or dulse

Thickeners: flours, kuzu (kudzu), arrowroot, puréed vegetables, couscous, oatmeal, amaranth, Irish moss

Soups can be adapted to the seasons by changing their texture and cooking method. Hearty winter soups are rich, creamy, and thick. They are cooked longer and help to generate heat for the colder months. Summer broths are light, clear, cooling, and are cooked quickly. Soups are a good way to combine various ingredients and qualities for certain illnesses and temperaments. They can be nourishing, soothing, refreshing, and revitalizing. Wild plants and medicinal herbs can be added to soups.

Salty, enzyme-rich miso soups eaten at the beginning of a meal help one to relax and prepare the digestive system for the rest of the meal. Soups with little or no salty flavor quench thirst and can be eaten as meals by themselves or in smaller amounts at the end of a meal so as not to overly dilute digestive juices.

Be creative and vary your soups to stimulate the senses daily.

- Use various soup stocks for full-bodied flavors.
    1. Cook vegetable scraps and ends slowly for an hour. Strain and squeeze out broth.
    2. Bean broth, seaweed broth, or herbal tea
    3. Leftover soak water from seaweeds or sprouts
- Roast grains before adding to soups.
- Simple soups can be more interesting. Use only one type of vegetable or simple combinations.
- Sauté or cook vegetables in small amount of broth. Then add heated broth or water and simmer. Vegetables will cook quicker and retain their color, flavor, and vitality.

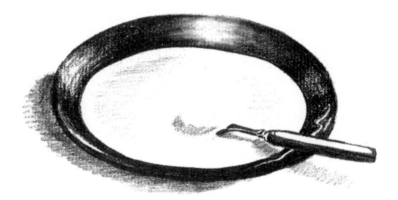

SPRING SOUPS

CHINESE NOODLE SOUP

2 cups noodles, cooked and drained
4 cups vegetable broth
1 carrot, cut into flowers
1 green onion, chopped (optional)
2 cups spring greens, finely cut
½ cup sprouts
Sea salt to taste

- Heat broth.
- Add carrots, onion, and salt.
- Simmer 10 minutes, until verging on tenderness.
- Add greens and cook until bright-colored.
- Serves 4–6.

Variations Hot and Sour Soup—
Add lemon juice or vinegar with hot sauce.

GREEN PEA SOUP

2 cups whole or split peas,
  presoaked
¼ onion diced (optional)
1 cup celery, diced
1 cup carrots, diced
1 bay leaf
5–6 cups water
½ cup dulse
¼ teaspoon dry mustard
1 teaspoon sea salt
2 tablespoons vinegar (optional)

- Layer vegetables in a pot in order given.
- Add peas, water, and bay leaf.
- Bring to boil. Reduce heat and simmer 1 hour. (Whole peas require longer cooking time.)
- Add dulse, mustard, and salt. Simmer 10 minutes more.
- Add vinegar before serving.
- Serves 6.

GREEN SPRING SOUP

6 cups water or broth
4 medium potatoes, chopped
¼ medium onion or leek, chopped
  (optional)
2–3 cups kale (or spring greens),
  chopped
2 cloves garlic
1 teaspoon sea salt
1 teaspoon olive oil (optional)

- Bring liquid to boil.
- Add potatoes, onion, and salt. Cover.
- Reduce heat. Simmer until tender.
- Add kale and garlic. Simmer until kale is tender and bright green.
- Purée all ingredients together.
- Add olive oil before serving.
- Serves 6.

SUMMER SOUPS

CORN SOUP

¼ onion, minced (optional)
½ teaspoon ginger, grated
1 teaspoon sesame oil (optional)
1 3-inch piece of kombu
Kernels from 6 ears of corn
6 cups water
1 teaspoon sea salt
½ cup oatmeal puréed in ½ cup
  water
2 tablespoons sesame butter
2 tablespoons croutons

- Sauté onion and ginger for 5 minutes.
- Add kombu, corn, water, and salt.
- Bring to scald. Reduce heat. Simmer 20 minutes.
- Add oat mixture and salt. Simmer 15 minutes more.
- Add sesame butter at end of cooking.
- Remove kombu.
- Garnish with croutons.
- Serves 6.

CHILLED CUCUMBER SOUP

4 cups cucumber, chopped
2 cups water or broth
1 cup oatmeal yogurt (p. 614)
1 clove garlic (optional)
Several fresh mint leaves
½ teaspoon sea salt
¼ teaspoon dill weed

- Purée everything in the blender.
- Serve chilled.
- Serves 4–6.

JADE GREEN SOUP

½ cup tofu, diced
2 cups leafy greens, chopped
¼ teaspoon sea salt
½ teaspoon oil (optional)
3 cups broth
½ tablespoon kuzu dissolved in 2 tablespoons water

- Sauté or steam tofu 5 minutes. Add salt.
- Add greens. Sauté 2 minutes.
- Add broth and simmer until greens are bright-colored.
- Add kuzu mixture and simmer until thickened.
- Serves 3–4.

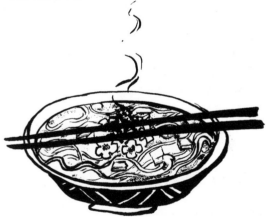

FALL SOUPS

SHEPHERD'S BARLEY SOUP

¼ onion, chopped (optional)
4 carrots, grated
2 parsnips, diced
1 tablespoon oil
2 quarts water
1 cup barley
⅓ teaspoon ginger, grated
1 teaspoon sea salt or 1 tablespoon natto miso
Parsley

- Sauté onion, carrots, and parsnips in oil (optional).
- Add water, barley, and ginger. Simmer 1½ hours.
- Add salt or miso and simmer 15 minutes more.
- Garnish with parsley.
- Serves 8.

LIMA BEAN-TURNIP SOUP

   5 inches wakame, broken into
      pieces, then soaked
   1 cup lima beans, soaked
   ¼ onion, diced (optional)
   2 carrots, cut into chunks
   4 small turnips, quartered
   1 cup cabbage, shredded
5–6 cups water
   1 tablespoon miso

- Place wakame, beans, and water in a pot. Bring to boil.
- Reduce heat and simmer 45–60 minutes.
- Add onion, carrots, turnips, and cabbage.
- Simmer about 20 minutes, until beans and vegetables are tender.
- Add miso and simmer 5–7 minutes.
- Serves 6.

CAULIFLOWER SOUP

   1 cauliflower
   ¼ onion, minced (optional)
   6 cups broth
Sea salt to taste
   ½ cup oat flakes or flour
   2 tablespoons sesame butter

- Separate flowerets from cauliflower. Cut off as much stem as possible and chop into small pieces. Set flowerets aside.
- Bring 4 cups of broth to boil.
- Add stems, onion, oats, and salt. Cover. Reduce heat and simmer 10 minutes until tender.
- While soup is cooking, bring the other 2 cups of broth to a boil. Drop in the flowerets and simmer 5 minutes. Remove with a slotted spoon and set aside.
- Add broth and sesame butter to soup.
- Remove soup from heat and purée all ingredients in blender.
- Garnish with flowerets.
- Serves 6.

WINTER SOUPS

WINTER ROOT SOUP

   ½ cup whole oat groats, cooked
5–6 cups water
   1 leek, sliced into rounds
   1 cup rutabaga, sliced
   1 carrot, cut into wedges
   ½–1 teaspoon sea salt

- Blend oats until creamy in water.
- Sauté leeks, rutabaga, and carrots for 8 minutes.
- Add oat mixture and salt. Simmer 15 minutes until vegetables are tender.
- Serves 6.

CREAM OF CARROT SOUP

1 tablespoon sesame oil
6 tablespoons flour
5–6 cups hot broth
2 medium carrots, cut into wedges
Sea salt to taste
Parsley

- Cook flour in oil 3–5 minutes.
- Remove pan from heat and slowly add broth, stirring constantly.
- Add carrots and salt. Simmer until tender. Stir occasionally to prevent scorching.
- Garnish with parsley.
- Serves 6.

GYPSY SOUP

1 leek, diced (optional)
2 carrots, sliced
1 cup cabbage, chopped
2 cups winter squash or pumpkin, diced
2 quarts hot water
½ teaspoon sea salt
1 teaspoon oil

- Sauté leeks, carrots, cabbage, and squash for 10 minutes.
- Add water and salt.
- Reduce heat. Simmer 35 minutes.
- Serves 8.

WINTER SUNSHINE SOUP—This is a good soup to brighten up a dark day.

1 cup yellow split peas, soaked
2 quarts water
1 5-inch piece kombu, soaked
½ onion, cut into crescent moons (optional)
2 carrots, cut into flowers
1 cup winter squash, diced
½ cup parsley, chopped
¼ teaspoon salt
Miso to taste

- Place kombu and peas in a pot with water.
- Bring to scald. Reduce heat and simmer 30 minutes.
- Add onion, carrots, squash, and salt. Simmer until peas and vegetables are tender.
- Add miso diluted in stock and simmer 5 minutes more.
- Serves 8.

Sauces

BASIC SAUCE (BECHAMEL)

1 tablespoon oil
2 tablespoons flour
1 cup water, broth, or almond or
    other nut milk (p. 612), heated
Seasonings: sea salt, miso, or soy
    sauce
Dash of nutmeg
Suggested flours:
    Whole wheat
    Rice
    Garbanzo
    Barley
    Corn
    Amaranth

- Heat oil in a heavy saucepan.
- Stir in flour. Whisk 1–2 minutes over low heat.
- Remove from heat. Add heated liquid and stir briskly until smooth.
- Return to heat. Add seasonings. Bring almost to a boil. Turn to low heat and simmer until thickened.
- Yields 1 cup.

Notes: Oil can be omitted: dry-toast flour and dilute in a small amount of liquid; add rest of liquid slowly. For a darker sauce, toast flour until brown.

GRAVY

- After sautéing vegetables, add flour to drippings in the pan.
- Finish as for Basic Sauce.

MUSHROOM SAUCE

- Add ¼ pound sliced mushrooms to 1 cup Basic Sauce.
- Simmer 10–15 minutes.

VEGETABLE SAUCE

- Add ½ cup diced, cooked vegetables to 1 cup Basic Sauce and simmer 5 minutes.

HERBAL SAUCE

- Add 1–2 teaspoons herbs to 1 cup Basic Sauce and simmer 5 minutes.
- Suggested combinations:
    Thyme, nutmeg, garlic
    Thyme, sage, parsley
    Coriander, cumin, ginger

NUT SAUCES

1 tablespoon nut butter: peanut, sesame, walnut, almond, sunflower, cashew
1 onion, minced
1 tablespoon lemon juice or vinegar or ¼ cup orange juice

- Thin nut butter with liquid.
- Combine all ingredients and add to 1 cup Basic Sauce, omitting oil.
- Simmer 5–8 minutes.

TOFU-ALMOND SAUCE

½ cake tofu, cubed
½–1 cup water
¼ cup almonds, chopped
2 tablespoons wheat germ
1 teaspoon miso
Chopped scallions (optional)

- Simmer tofu in water 20 minutes.
- Combine all ingredients and blend together, adding water slowly until desired thickness.
- Yields 1–1½ cups.

TOFU-SESAME BUTTER SAUCE

- Add 2 tablespoons sesame butter instead of almonds in the above recipe.

TOFU-AVOCADO SAUCE

- Add ½ avocado instead of almonds in the above recipe.

KUZU OR ARROWROOT SAUCE

1–1½ tablespoons kuzu or arrowroot
1 cup water or broth
Sea salt or soy sauce to taste

- Dilute kuzu or arrowroot in a little liquid.
- Add to remaining liquid and simmer until thickened.
- Add to soups or vegetable dishes.

SESAME BUTTER-LEMON SAUCE

¼–½ cup sesame butter
½ cup water or broth
1 clove garlic, crushed (optional)
½ cup lemon juice
1 scallion, minced (optional)
¼ cup parsley, minced
½ teaspoon cumin
Salt or soy sauce to taste

- Combine all ingredients.
- Beat well with a whisk, or in blender. It becomes thicker when whipped more.
- Yields 3–4 cups.

SALSA MEXICANA

1 medium tomato, diced
3 green chilies, minced
6 sprigs coriander leaves, chopped
  fine
Sea salt to taste
⅓–½ cup water
  ¼ onion, diced fine (optional)

- Mix together and serve.
- Yields 1½ cups.

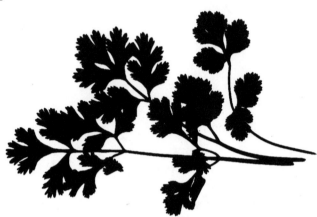

SALSA DE LA SIERRA (MOUNTAIN SAUCE)

1 tomato, whole
3 green chilies, whole
1 clove garlic (optional)
Dash sea salt

- Place tomato and chilies in a dry skillet. Let them heat through and roast until slightly charred, turning them over from time to time.
- With a mortar and pestle, grind salt and garlic together into a paste.
- Add tomato and chilies and grind together into a sauce.
- Yields 1 cup.

CHINESE GINGER SAUCE

1 clove garlic, mashed (optional)
3 slices ginger root
¼ teaspoon sesame oil (optional)
Stalk of celery, sliced diagonally
½ bell pepper, diced
¼ onion, diced (optional)
2 tablespoons soy sauce
1 teaspoon molasses
1 cup water or broth
1 tablespoon kuzu dissolved in ¼
  cup water

- Sauté garlic and ginger.
- Add rest of ingredients except kuzu and bring to just below boil.
- Cook 5 minutes.
- Add kuzu and simmer 5 minutes longer.
- Yields 1½ cups.

SWEET AND SOUR SAUCE

1 cup water or stock
¼ cup syrup or molasses
¼ cup cider or rice vinegar
1 tablespoon kuzu dissolved in ¼
  cup water
Sea salt or soy sauce to taste

- Heat liquid with sweetener and vinegar. Bring to boil.
- Stir in diluted kuzu and salt or soy sauce.
- Simmer 5–10 minutes.
- Yields 2 cups.

PASTA SAUCE

1 medium onion, minced
  (optional)
1 cup carrots, minced
1 stalk celery, minced
1 tablespoon olive oil (optional)
4 medium beets, cooked and
  puréed
2 tablespoons rice flour
1 tablespoon soy sauce
1 pinch oregano
1 clove garlic, minced (optional)
3 cups water
Chopped parsley

- Sauté onions (in oil) 2 minutes.
- Add carrots. Sauté 2 minutes.
- Add celery. Sauté 2 minutes.
- Add puréed beets. Simmer 5 minutes.
- Add 1 cup water. Bring to a scald. Simmer covered 20 minutes on low heat.
- Dilute rice flour in 2 cups water. Add with soy sauce to beet mixture. Simmer 10 minutes.
- Add garlic, oregano, and parsley. Simmer 5–10 minutes more.
- Serve over pasta, polenta, burgers, or pizza.
- Yields 1 quart.

TOMATO SAUCE

- Use red or green tomatoes, minced finely, rather than beets in the Pasta Sauce.

SQUASH SAUCE

- Use puréed squash instead of beets in the Pasta Sauce. Makes a sweet golden sauce.

KETCHUP

- Follow directions for Pasta Sauce, adding vinegar and puréeing all ingredients together.

Condiments

Condiments aid in digestion and add extra vitamins and minerals to meals. They can be used instead of salt for flavor. Sprinkle on grains and cereals. The methods used here for preparing gomasio and the seed mixtures result in very low salt content compared with commercial products. Also, the oxalic acid in sesame seeds is neutralized by the soaking and roasting procedures.

GOMASIO (sesame salt)—high in calcium, iron, and vitamins A and B

1 cup sesame seeds
½ tablespoon sea salt

- Wash and soak seeds with salt 6–8 hours. Drain.
- Dry-toast seeds in skillet over medium heat until they have a nutty aroma, are golden brown, and begin to pop.
- Grind sesame seeds with mortar and pestle or suribachi using even, gentle pressure in a circular motion until each seed is half-crushed.
- Store in a closed glass jar.

WAKAME-SESAME SEED MIXTURE—improves mineral balance; iron and iodine

1 ounce wakame
¼ cup sesame seeds, soaked and drained

- Roast wakame in oven at 350°F for 10–15 minutes until dark and crispy.
- Grind to a fine powder.
- Dry-toast sesame seeds until they have a nutty aroma and begin to pop.
- Add to wakame and grind until seeds are 90% crushed.

DULSE-SESAME SEED MIXTURE—high in iron

1 ounce dulse
½ cup sesame seeds, soaked and drained

- Dry-toast dulse in skillet until crispy.
- Prepare as in above recipe.

DAIKON RADISH—diminishes appetite; helps digest fried foods and beans

- Grate daikon radish and serve small portions (too much causes fatigue).
- Can add grated carrot and ginger.

CHUTNEYS AND RELISHES

These condiments freshen and enhance other flavors to give variety and color to simple grain and vegetable dishes. They can make each bite of the same food different and add to the digestibility and nutrition as well. The spicier combinations should be well balanced with something bland. Use in small amounts.

MIXED FRUIT CHUTNEY

4 apples
4 pears
6 dried apricots
Juice of 2 lemons
2 tablespoons grated lemon rind
1 cup raisins
2 tablespoons cinnamon
2 tablespoons ginger, grated
1 teaspoon cardamom
1 teaspoon caraway or cumin seeds
⅛ teaspoon cayenne
½ teaspoon salt

- Cut fruit into small pieces.
- Mix all ingredients together.
- Cook gently for 40 minutes.
- Cool and bottle. Store in refrigerator.
- Yields 2 quarts.

CARROT CHUTNEY

6–8 carrots, diced
1 teaspoon sea salt
2 tablespoons mustard seed
2 teaspoons cumin seed
2 teaspoons ginger, chopped fine
1 teaspoon black peppercorns
2–3 teaspoons honey (optional)
3 tablespoons rice vinegar
Juice of 1 lemon
A little water

- Mix ingredients together and simmer gently until carrots are tender.
- Cool and bottle. Store in refrigerator.
- Yields 1 quart.

PARSLEY AND MINT RELISH

1 cup parsley or Chinese parsley (coriander leaves)
½ cup mint leaves
1 green chili
1 clove garlic (optional)
2 dried apricot halves (soaked and minced) or juice of 1 lemon
½ teaspoon sea salt

- Wash greens.
- Chop and grind together with chili.
- Mix with rest of ingredients.
- Yields 1½ cups.

Spreads and Patés

VEGETABLE-WALNUT PATÉ

1½ cups cooked green beans
¼ cup toasted walnuts
½ onion, minced and sautéed
   (optional)
1–2 tablespoons mayonnaise
   (see p. 579)
¼ teaspoon sea salt
Pinch of nutmeg

- Combine all ingredients and blend together.
- Use as a sandwich spread or dip.
- Yields 2 cups.

BABAGANOUJ (Greek Eggplant Paté)

2 eggplants
Juice of 1 lemon
¼ cup sesame butter
½ cup fresh parsley, chopped
¼ teaspoon sea salt
1 teaspoon olive oil (optional)

- Preheat oven to 400°F.
- Prick eggplants with a fork.
- Roast until slightly charred and popped (45 minutes). Cool.
- Scoop the insides out and mash well or purée.
- Combine with all ingredients except olive oil.
- Drizzle oil over top before serving.
- Serve with vegetables or pita bread.

VEGETABLE OR BEAN SPREAD

1 cup cooked vegetables or beans
1 teaspoon miso
1 tablespoon sesame butter
¼ onion, chopped (optional)
1 tablespoon parsley, chopped
Pinch of coriander

- Mash vegetables or beans with a fork.
- Combine with remaining ingredients.
- Serve in sandwiches or as a dip; as fillings for crêpes or pastries.
- Yields 1 cup.

Pickles

A small serving of pickles after meals aids in digestion. All pickles can be made from carrots, daikon radish, broccoli, cucumbers, cabbage, cauliflower, greens, turnips, etc.

The pickles in these recipes can be beneficial for restoring the intestinal flora by promoting the growth of healthful *Lactobacillus acidophilus.* For those with candida overgrowth, cancer, and other degenerative conditions of impaired immunity, salt is restricted, and so the raw saltless sauerkraut is recommended in these cases. In addition, cabbage itself has important immune-enhancing properties (see "Vegetables"). Raw saltless sauerkraut is also recommended in the treatment of ulcers.

RAW SALTLESS SAUERKRAUT* (with Salt Option)

Minimum of 25 pounds of vegetables. Use mainly cabbage with beets and carrots. If desired: add celery, garlic, herbs, and soaked, chopped seaweeds such as dulse, wakame, and kelp. Any other vegetable can also be used. Option: add salt ($\frac{1}{2}$% to $1\frac{1}{4}$% of vegetable weight).

- Use stainless steel or ceramic crock (a 5-gallon container will hold approximately 35 pounds of vegetables).
- Grind up vegetables with a food processor, Champion Juicer (remove the screen), standard-size grater; or cut them up.
- If you don't use salt, the vegetables must be made juicier: put them in a stainless steel bowl or other unbreakable container and pound them with a baseball bat or board until some juice flows out—the more juice, the better.
- Place the vegetables in the crock. Don't fill to the brim (the fermenting vegetables will expand). If salt is used, mix it in now.
- Put many fresh cabbage leaves on top of the vegetables.
- Gently, yet firmly and evenly, compress the leaves using your hands and body weight.
- Put a plate as wide as possible on the crock.
- Put a rock or other weight on the plate. Do not put so much weight that the juice is forced up above the fermenting vegetables. Check that the weight is right and the plate is sitting even and flat a few times in the next 24–36 hours.
- Let the vegetables sit in a well-ventilated room at room temperature (between 60–72°F). After 5 to 7 days (6–7 days at 62°F and 5–6 days at 70°F), throw away the old cabbage leaves and moldy and discolored vegetables on the top.

---

*The technique for making *raw* sauerkraut is adapted from *Raw Cultured Vegetables* by Evan Richards. Note: Most commercial sauerkraut is pasteurized. For a source of raw sauerkraut, see Resources Index, p. 704.

- Put the remaining sauerkraut in glass jars and refrigerate. Will keep for 4 to 8 months when kept at 34°F and opened minimally. Do not freeze. If salt is used, then the kraut can be kept at temperatures as high as 40°F.

Note: The best fermentation takes place when at least 25 pounds of vegetables are used; however, smaller amounts of sauerkraut can be made with acceptable results. For instance, for a first attempt at kraut-making, try two large heads of cabbage in this recipe, or try "Sauerkraut with Dulse" on page 586, which uses one head of cabbage.

CABBAGE KIMCHEE (Korean Pickles)

1 head cabbage, cut into 2-inch pieces
1 pound white radish, cut into half-moons
5 cups water
2 tablespoons sea salt
2 tablespoons ginger, minced
1 clove garlic, minced (optional)
1 green onion, chopped
½ teaspoon cayenne
2 teaspoons sweetener (optional)

- In a large bowl combine water, 1½ tablespoons salt, cabbage, and radish. Set aside 12 hours.
- Remove cabbage and radish from soaking liquid and combine with ginger, garlic, scallions, cayenne, and ½ teaspoon salt.
- Put into a jar or crock. Stir sweetener into soaking liquid and pour over vegetables up to 1 inch from the top.
- Cover loosely with a clean cloth and set aside for 3–7 days.
- Yields 2 quarts.
- 1 cup serves 6–8.

SWEET AND SOUR LIME PICKLES (Indian)

6 limes (or lemons)
Cardamom from 4 pods
2 tablespoons whole cumin seeds
Cinnamon stick (2 inches)
12 whole cloves
1 tablespoon sea salt
6 tablespoons lime juice
1 teaspoon chili powder (optional)

- Cut limes into small pieces.
- Sprinkle with salt and spices. Put in a jar.
- Pour in juice.
- Cover tightly and keep in a warm place for a week until skins are tender.
- Shake jar daily.
- Yields 1 quart.

UMEBOSHI PICKLES

3–4 umeboshi plums
1 quart water
4 cups sliced vegetables

- Mash plums and put in a large jar with water and vegetables. Cover with cheesecloth. Put in a cool place.
- Ready to serve in 4–6 days.
- Yields 1½–2 quarts.

KOSHER DILL CUCUMBER PICKLES

1 quart cucumbers, scrubbed well
1 pint boiling water
1 tablespoon sea salt
1 clove garlic, whole (optional)
1 bay leaf
1/8 teaspoon cayenne
2 sprigs fresh dill or 1 tablespoon
dill seed

- Sterilize jar and new lid.
- Put spices in bottom of jar and pack with cucumbers.
- Boil water and salt and pour into jar up to 1 inch from top.
- Seal and store for 2 weeks or all winter.
- Yields 1 quart.

QUICK JAPANESE PICKLES

3–4 cups sliced root or round
vegetables
1/4 pint soy sauce
3/4 pint water
1 tablespoon ginger, grated

- Combine all ingredients.
- Set aside for 1–3 hours.

RICE-SALT PICKLES (*Nuka* Pickles)

5 pounds organic brown rice,
ground into coarse flour
10 cups water
1 cup sea salt
1 cup miso (optional)
Vegetables

- Boil water and salt. Cool.
- Dissolve miso completely in water.
- Dry-toast flour slightly in skillet to sterilize against microorganisms. Cool.
- Make a thick paste by mixing flour and salt water together.
- Stir thoroughly and place in crock or glass container.
- Bury vegetables in mash. They should not touch.
- Cover crock lightly. Store in cool place. (Refrigerate in warmer weather.)
- Allow vegetables to pickle 3 days to 1 week.
- Stir daily.
- To eat: Rinse pickles in water and cut into pieces. Use sparingly.

Notes: Firm vegetables work best (radish, carrot, turnip, cauliflower). Small pieces will pickle faster. Leave whole if small. If going on vacation, remove all vegetables from mash and refrigerate. This mash will last for years if cared for properly.

Add more flour and salt occasionally. Nuka pickles are usually made with rice bran, but most available bran is so heavily sprayed that the pickles do not ferment correctly. Thus, many nuka enthusiasts now use coarse ground organic brown rice.

Grain and Seed Milks

SEED MILK

½ cup seed (pumpkin, sesame,
  sunflower)
1 cup warm water
Dash kelp or sea salt

- Soak seeds overnight.
- Drain and throw away soak water.
- Blend with warm water and kelp or sea salt.
- Use as is, or strain and use pulp in breads, cookies, etc.

ALMOND MILK

¼ cup almonds (walnuts or other
  nuts may be substitutes)
2 cups warm water
Dash kelp or sea salt

- Follow recipe above.
- Option: remove skins after soaking almonds, especially for persons with sensitive digestion.

ALMOND MILK SHAKE

- Replace water with warm fruit juice in Almond Milk recipe.
- Or add fruit, 2 tablespoons grain coffee, or ½ cup carob powder.
- Blend all ingredients together.

SPROUTED GRAIN MILK

1 cup grain (oats, rice, millet,
  barley)
2 cups water

- Sprout grain for 3 days (p. 569).
- Blend with water and strain.
- Use pulp for bread, soups, etc.

COOKED GRAIN MILK

1 cup grain, soaked
7–10 cups water

Method 1:
- Bring water and grain to a boil.
- Lower heat. Cover and simmer 2 hours.

Method 2:
- Cover and cook on a low heat overnight.
- Strain through a cheesecloth. Use pulp in other grain dishes, burgers, sauces, breads, etc.

Variation Cook vanilla bean with whole oats.
Add a small amount of rice syrup or barley malt.

Rejuvelac and Yogurt

Rejuvelac is a fermented drink that provides an inexpensive source of friendly bacteria helpful for creating healthy intestinal flora.

REJUVELAC

2 cups wheat berries
1 quart water

- Soak 2 cups of wheat berries for one day. Discard soak water. Soft white wheat berries work best. Rinse berries and soak them again in a jar containing one quart water. Cover the mouth of the jar with a cloth or sprout screen and let stand for two days. Pour off rejuvelac. Add one quart of water to the wheat. After one day, pour off second batch of rejuvelac and compost wheat. Begin soaking more wheat berries to make a fresh batch of rejuvelac.

- Makes 4 cups.
- Rejuvelac tastes a little sour, somewhat like whey. If too sour, reduce the fermentation time. If it tastes foul, discard. This happens if it ferments for too long or the wheat is poor quality. Rejuvelac brews faster in hot weather. Once made, keep it refrigerated.
- For a stronger sour drink: after rejuvelac is first made, refrigerate it and keep wheat berries in the jar. Each time you pour off a drink, refill the container. Rejuvelac can be kept for several weeks.

Use rejuvelac as a drink, to make seed yogurts and dressings, in soups and sauces. Use as a natural leavener in breads. Follow the recipe for sourdough bread (p. 493) and replace the sourdough starter with rejuvelac.

SEED YOGURT

1 cup sesame or sunflower seeds or almonds, soaked (discard soak water)
1 cup rejuvelac or water
½ teaspoon unpasteurized soy sauce or miso (when not using rejuvelac)

- Blend seeds at high speed. Slowly pour in the rejuvelac or water and soy sauce or miso and blend until creamy.
- Add some previously made seed yogurt to speed fermentation.
- Set in warm place and cover. Do not seal.
- Let ferment 6–10 hours to desired sourness. Then refrigerate.

Seed yogurt is one of the finest predigested proteins and ferments. It is easily assimilated. The rancidity and oil of seed yogurt are reduced by the fermentation. Use in spreads, sauces, and dressings.

613

OAT YOGURT

1 cup rolled oats or whole oats,
   coarsely ground
1 cup water or rejuvelac
½ teaspoon unpasteurized soy
   sauce or miso (when not using
   rejuvelac)

• Follow recipe above for seed yogurt.

Fruit

The natural sugars and refreshing quality of fruit make it a wonderful substitute for food containing refined or chemical sweeteners. Even sour fruits such as the grapefruit and lemon balance the need for the sweet flavor according to the Five Element "Control Cycle." Fruit also contains valuable minerals, vitamins, enzymes, and fiber.

Whenever fruit is to be used extensively in the diet, it is of primary importance that it be tree- or vine-ripened. This is particularly true with citrus fruit. Citrus picked several weeks before ripening, which is most often the case, contains harmful amounts of acids and does not ripen with the same healthful benefits of the sun-ripened variety. Citric acid in citrus has a strong effect on the body. Its action is buffered when the fruit is eaten in its whole form rather than as juice alone. Eating a few seeds and some of the inner rind also creates balance. Other ripe-picked fruit is likewise more nutritious, although its use is not essential in short fasts or when fruit is a small percentage of the diet. When unripe fruit is purchased, it should be allowed to ripen at room temperature before eating. An exception is the intentional use of certain unripe fruit for its medicinal effect.

And when you crush an apple with your teeth, say to it in your heart,
"Your seeds shall live in my body,
And the buds of your tomorrow shall blossom in my heart,
And your fragrance shall be my breath,
And together we shall rejoice through all the seasons."

—Kahlil Gibran, *The Prophet*

The majority of the very popular fruits such as oranges, apples, and bananas are heavily sprayed to the point where their value is undermined. Even though sprays and chemical fertilizers are not put inside the fruit, they eventually work their way through the whole plant, influencing its growth and overall quality. With a little effort, fruit grown without chemicals can usually be obtained.

Fruit is easily digested and can offer a pleasant break from foods that take more effort to prepare and digest. In addition, most fruit is alkalizing, cleansing, and cooling, and thus balances the overuse of rich foods, particularly those containing concentrated proteins. Fruit is also a remedy for people who are stressed or over-heated from mental pressure, excessive physical activity, or a hot climate. The alkaline element in fruit combined with its acids stimulates the liver and pancreas, giving a natural laxative effect. In contrast, certain fruit including blackberries, sour plum, and pineapple can treat diarrhea.

If sweet fruit is used as a major part of the diet for a long time, its moistening quality, which can promote yeast overgrowth and other forms of *dampness,* is best offset by periodic non-fruit fasts, which have a drying effect. The sour fruits have a contractive astringent property, which also balances the sweet varieties.

Other helpful information on fruit:

- It is easier to adapt to fresh local fruit in season than to fruit from far away.
- Most summer and tropical fruits are cooling and refreshing. When eaten in winter, they may cause coldness and weakness, unless eaten by people with excess *heat* signs. Fall fruits that store, such as apples and dried fruit, are more suited to the winter.
- When fruits are juiced, their cooling and cleansing properties are concentrated. The juice is the cleansing/eliminating part of fruit; the relatively more building and warming parts are the rinds, skins, peels, pulpy sections, as well as seeds of fruit like papaya, watermelon, and other melons. Eat some of all parts for greater stamina. Heating juices or cooking fruit makes it less cooling. Drinking fruit juices all day long between meals is invariably weakening. Observe infants who drink apple juice most of the day—they often lose their appetite and become irritable and weak.
- Fruit can be canned in its own juices without additional sweeteners; to retain sweetness and flavor, can fruit in apple juice.
- Fruit does not mix well with other foods according to simple food-combining principles. Exceptions are the following combinations:
  a) fruit with lettuce or celery;

b) acid fruit with nuts, seeds, dairy, or other high-fat protein; and c) fruit, especially when cooked, with aduki beans. Adukis, lettuce, and celery all have the property of drying the *damp* yeast and fermented conditions in the digestive tract that easily arise from eating fruit.

- If the sweet and refreshing quality of fruit is strongly craved, it is usually best to satisfy the craving with an exclusively fruit meal or snack. Otherwise one may overeat heavier foods in a failed attempt to get the refreshing, cleansing quality offered by fruit. For best results, fruit juices should be drunk at least four hours after and one hour before a meal.

- *General dosage:* For chronic conditions that require the properties of fruit, the fruit meal is also superior. For example, as a remedy for rheumatic-induced numbness, a bowl of cherries for one daily meal can be eaten four or more times a week. If only very small amounts of fruit can be tolerated, the fruit snack is a better choice. For acute situations, fruit can be used more often and according to need. For example, to protect against *summer heat* (the effect of a very hot climate on the body), watermelon, apple, or lemon juice may be consumed as often as necessary. For relief of dysentery, figs may be eaten several times a day.

- Raw fruit must be used carefully, if at all, by individuals who are weakened with *cold* and/or *deficient* conditions, although moderate amounts of dried or cooked fruit are usually acceptable in these cases. There are a number of systems for categorizing warming and cooling properties of fruit. In previous sections in this text, fruit in general has been consistently identified as cooling because it most often generates a long-term cooling effect and also does not warm the deeper root *yang* associated with the kidney-adrenal function. Perhaps the nearest a fruit approaches deep warming action is the astringent property of the dried, unripe raspberry. Such astringency controls the urinary system, much like the warming *yang* energy of healthy kidneys. Another common fruit, the cherry, creates warmth but its effect is neither deep nor enduring.

None of the remaining fruits listed below exhibit warming properties. They are either neutral or cooling. In addition to the ability to alter personal temperature sensations, each fruit has certain specific healing actions as well as attributes which balance environmental influences of its native habitat and the time of year it ripens. The following list itemizes key properties of selected fruit drawn from traditions in the East, the West, and from modern nutrition.

Healing Properties of Fruit
Apple

Cooling thermal nature; sweet-and-sour flavor; reduces *heat,* especially *summer heat;* produces fluids for the body in general, but particularly to moisten *dryness* and cool *heat* in the lungs—protects the lungs from cigarette smoking; stimulates appetite; remedies indigestion—this ability is due in part to the presence of malic and tartaric acids in apples, which inhibit the growth of ferments and disease-producing bacteria in the digestive tract. Contains pectin, which removes cholesterol, toxic metals such as lead and mercury, and the residues of radiation. Benefits low blood sugar conditions and the emotional depression associated with it. A poultice of grated apple over the eyes for twenty minutes helps relieve swelling and irritations such as sunburn or "pink eye." Apples and their juice are also cleansing and beneficial for the liver and gallbladder, actually softening gallstones. (See "Gallbladder flush" in index.)

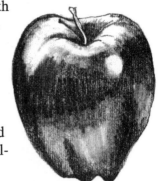

Apricot

Neutral thermal nature; sweet-and-sour flavor; moistens the lungs and increases the *yin* fluids: used for dry throat, thirst, asthma, and other lung conditions when there is fluid deficiency. Because of its high copper and cobalt content, it is commonly used to treat anemia. Apricots originated in China, where they are considered weakening if consumed abundantly. They must be used cautiously during pregnancy, and avoided in cases of diarrhea.

Avocado

Cooling thermal nature; sweet flavor; builds the blood and *yin,* harmonizes the liver, lubricates the lungs and intestines.

A natural source of lecithin, a brain food; more than 80% of its caloric content is easily digested fat, primarily in the form of monounsaturated oils. Individuals with cravings for oils but who do poorly with most fatty foods can usually tolerate avocado. Rich in copper, which aids in red blood cell formation. A nutritious protein source often recommended for nursing mothers. Used as a remedy for ulcers; also known to beautify the skin.

Banana

Very cooling thermal nature; sweet flavor; lubricates the intestines and lungs; treats constipation and ulcers. Strengthens the *yin* and benefits conditions of thirst and *dryness.* For *dry* lung conditions and *dry* cough, eat bananas that have been sliced and cooked into a thick soup. Before their completely ripe stage, bananas have an astringent property: use partially ripened steamed bananas for diarrhea, colitis, and hemorrhoids. For hemorrhoids, steam the whole banana until very soft and eat one organic banana with skin twice a day on an empty stomach.

Bananas detoxify the body. In addition, their cold nature and high sugar content are useful in the treatment of drug addiction (especially alcoholism) marked by *heat* signs and sugar cravings during withdrawal.

Rich in potassium, bananas are used universally for hypertension. Because they can reduce blood pressure, are easy to digest, and also moisten dryness, bananas are a good food for many elderly people (blood pressure, dryness, and digestive weakness tend to increase with age). Bananas are commonly given to children and infants, although they should be used cautiously with children who are *cold,* inactive, or frail.

Cherry

Warming thermal nature; sweet flavor; increases *qi* ener-gy, tonifies the spleen-pancreas, and prevents involun-tary seminal emission. Cherries are a well-known remedy for gout, arthritis, and rheumatism. They also help overcome numbness in the limbs and paralysis as a result of rheumatism. Part of their action in rheumatic disorders occurs from their ability to eliminate excess body acids. Cherries are most beneficial for treating disorders accompanied by *coldness,* such as when the person feels perennially cold. Richly supplied in iron, cherries are often used to improve the blood and treat anemia.

Fig

Neutral thermal nature; sweet flavor; influences the stomach and spleen-pancreas and moistens the lungs and large intestine. Has detoxifying action and is used for skin discharges and boils. One of the most alkalizing foods; balances acidic con-ditions that result from a diet rich in meat and refined food.

For dry cough, signs of lung *heat,* asthma, or sore throat, drink ½ cup of the water and eat 1–2 figs from a lightly cooked fig soup several times a day. The high mucin content of figs makes them a soothing laxative for treating constipation, especially the "fluid deficiency" type. Figs also clean the intestines and treat dysen-tery and hemorrhoids.

Milk from the unripe fruit applied twice daily directly to warts helps to remove them. For toothaches, rub fresh fig into the gums.

Grape

Neutral thermal nature; sweet-and-sour flavor; increases *qi* energy; used in the East and West as a blood tonic—contains valuable cell salts known to build and purify the blood and improve the cleansing function of the glands; benefits the kidneys and liver and thus strengthens their corresponding tissues—the bones and sinews. Used to treat rheumatism and arthritis, especially when these conditions are marked with signs of *coldness.* Diuretic: reduces edema and treats urinary difficulty including painful urination. Grape juice is also a valuable remedy for liver malfunctions such as hepatitis and jaundice.

A poultice of mashed grapes purifies infected areas and reduces growths. For this purpose, a fresh poultice is applied daily and kept in place for at least 8 hours. Continue using poultices until the condition improves.

Grapes make a good energy snack for children. The dark varieties of grapes are better for blood-building needs such as anemia; they are also more strengthening.

Caution: Excessive use of grapes may diminish visual acuity.

Dosage: Approximately 8 ounces once daily for chronic conditions, twice daily for acute conditions.

Grapefruit

Cooling thermal nature; sweet-and-sour flavor; treats poor digestion, belching, and increases appetite during pregnancy. Helps overcome alcohol intoxication. The juice, when combined with a tea of the pulp, will reduce fevers (simmer the pulp for 10 minutes in 6 ounces of water, then sip slowly the juice/tea combination and abstain from solid foods).

Grapefruit peel has warming energy, a pungent, sweet, and bitter flavor. Like most citrus peel, it moves and regulates the spleen-pancreas digestive energy, and can be used to alleviate intestinal gas, pain, swelling, and promote peristalsis. It also helps resolve mucus conditions of the lungs and can treat lung congestion and coughs that have *cold* signs. The bioflavonoid activity of the peel in conjunction with its vitamin C is useful for strengthening the gums, the arteries, and circulation in general. To extract the properties of the peel, make a tea by simmering the fresh or dried peel for about 20 minutes. For frostbite, apply a compress of the room-temperature tea to help restore circulation to the damaged tissue.

Citrus seed extract, an extremely potent natural antibiotic derived primarily from the seeds of grapefruit, was developed after observing that citrus seeds do not readily decompose in nature from microbial action. Slightly warming in thermal nature and exceptionally bitter, citrus seed extract works in the body like most bitters, but more effectively for purposes of drying *damp* conditions in the body. (Pathogenic microbes can cause as well as feed off *damp* excesses in the body.) This extract has been found to inhibit members of several classes of microbes and parasites, among them: protozoa, amoebas, bacteria, viruses, and at least thirty different types of fungi, including the candida yeast-like fungi. It is available as a major ingredient in liquid extracts, capsules, sprays, ointments, and a variety of other forms for treating a host of maladies. Among its more common internal uses are diarrhea (take daily while traveling to prevent "traveler's diarrhea"), allergies including hay fever, candida overgrowth, giardia and most other parasites, flu, strep throat, and staph infections. Externally it is applied in various dilutions for warts, athlete's foot, nail fungi, dandruff and other scalp problems, and poison oak; specific liquid formulations containing the extract treat vaginal yeast infection, nasal and sinus problems, and ear infections. Uses in the home involve adding a few drops of the extract to water for soaking produce to remove parasites and pesticides, sterilizing laundry (used this way in hospitals), cleaning contaminated surfaces, kitchen utensils and cutting boards, and ridding drinking, bathing, and swimming water of microbes. Dosages for internal use depend on the strength of the extract; information on other uses is available from the manufacturer.

Cautions: Individuals with signs of *dryness* and/or *deficiency,* including the *deficient yin* syndrome, should use citrus seed extract sparingly.

Lemon (and Lime)

Cooling thermal nature; very sour, astringent flavor; and antiseptic. Perhaps the most valuable fruit therapeutically for people who have eaten a high-fat/protein diet. Destroys putrefactive bacteria in both the intestines and mouth; used to purify the breath. Its antiseptic, anti-microbial, and mucus-resolving action make it useful during dysentery, colds, flus, hacking coughs, and parasite infestation. Benefits the liver, encouraging the formation of bile; improves absorption of minerals; promotes weight loss; cleanses the blood; treats high blood pressure, thick, poorly circulating blood, and weak blood vessels. Alleviates flatulence and indigestion in general.

Lemon increases the production of fluids in the body. Its juice, diluted with water, is often used for reducing the effects of *summer heat,* calming the nerves, treating sore throat, cramps, and diabetes, which are often marked by fluid deficiency.

Lemon is used externally to heal sores (apply juice), to relieve itching from insect bites (rub in juice), and to soften and reduce corns (poultice). One drop of fresh juice combined with warm water makes a cleansing eye wash.

In general, limes can be substituted and are grown with fewer chemicals. The citric acid content of lemons and limes is 4–6 times higher than oranges and at least three times that of grapefruit. Thus these fruits should not be used by those with too much stomach acid or ulcers. In addition, citric acid thins the blood, and so citrus should be used cautiously by those with weak blood signs such as pale complexion and tongue, insomnia, irritability, and thinness.

Dosage: Start with 1–3 lemons daily for one week and increase according to need and desire (9–12 lemons daily can be tolerated by the robust person in need of their properties).

Lemon peel is used similarly to grapefruit peel, although it has stronger ability to move stagnant liver *qi;* lime peel has even more specific action on the liver.

Mulberry

Cooling thermal nature; sweet flavor; builds the *yin* fluids and blood; moistens the lungs and gastrointestinal tract; strengthens the liver and kidneys; treats *wind* conditions, including vertigo and paralysis. Beneficial for blood deficiency signs such as anemia, prematurely gray hair, irritability, insomnia, and constipation from fluid dryness; also is used in treating stomach ulcers, diabetes, dry cough, ringing in the ears, and poor joint mobility. At one time in the West, mulberries were highly regarded as a general tonic for the whole system, which corresponds to some degree with the Chinese view of their tonic action on the kidneys, liver, and blood.

Orange

Cooling thermal nature; sweet-and-sour flavor; general tonic for weak digestion and poor appetite; regenerates body fluids; helps cool and moisten those who are *dry* and over*heated* from disease processes, physical activity, or hot weather. Oranges have been valuable for inflammatory, highly acidic diseases such as arthritis; they also help lower high fever; their vitamin C/bioflavonoid content benefits those with weak gums and teeth. The peel has *qi*-stimulating, digestive, and mucus-resolving properties similar to grapefruit peel above. The inner white lining, placed directly on the eyelids, helps to dissolve eye cysts.

Tangerines make a good substitute for commercial oranges since they have many of the same properties but are sprayed less with chemicals.

Papaya

Neutral thermal nature; sweet-and-bitter flavor; tonifies the stomach; acts as a digestive aid; moistens the lungs and alleviates coughing. Used for treating dysentery, indigestion, mucus excesses, and the pain of rheumatism. Underripe papaya and its seeds are rich in the digestive enzyme papain, which helps digest protein, break down deposits on the teeth, resolve mucus, and has strong vermicidal action capable of destroying most intestinal worms including tapeworm. Its worm-destroying capacity is bolstered by removing the skin and soaking in cider vinegar for one day. Then eat eight ounces of this pickled papaya and drink two ounces of the vinegar solution daily for four days. Another vermicidal remedy: eat one tablespoon of the seeds, or drink one cup of tea made by steeping them, each day for seven days. Papaya also contains carpaine, a compound providing anti-tumor activity.

Peach

Cooling thermal nature; sweet-and-sour flavor; builds body fluids; moistens the lungs and intestines; used for dry cough and other *dry* conditions of the lungs; relieves high blood pressure. The slightly sour quality of the peach is astringent and tends to limit perspiration while tightening tissues. For a "peaches and cream" complexion apply a poultice of blended fresh peach on the face, let dry, rinse, and pat dry.

The kernel inside the peach pit strengthens *qi* and blood circulation and is used to clear congealed blood; it appears in tumor formulas including those for uterine fibroids.

Peach leaf taken as a tea destroys worms.

The very soft nature of peach flesh makes it ideal for those with acute gastrointestinal inflammations, in which case it should be cooked and puréed.

Pear

Cooling thermal nature; sweet and slightly sour flavor; specifically affects the lungs, eliminating *heat* and excess mucus; stops coughing associated with *hot* lungs; moistens the lungs, throat, and *dryness* in general; quenches thirst resulting from *heat* conditions. Used for diabetes, injuries to the skin, constipation, loss of voice, and gallbladder inflammation and obstruction.

Caution: Not for those with deficient digestive fire. Symptoms include loose or watery stools, signs of *coldness,* and a swollen, pale tongue. Excessive use of pears during pregnancy may cause poor fetal development and miscarriage.

Persimmon

Very cooling thermal nature; sweet flavor; cools *heat,* especially lung *heat;* builds body fluids, moistens the lungs and resolves phlegm; tonifies the spleen-pancreas; soothes mucous membranes in the digestive tract to relieve gastrointestinal inflammations; treats common *hot* and/or *dry* conditions such as often occur in thirst, canker sores, and chronic bronchitis.

The unripe persimmon has an "astringent" taste that makes the lips pucker from its tannic acid content; as persimmon ripens, the tannic acid is converted until none is left in the fully ripe state. The astringent property of partially ripe persimmon is desirable in treating these conditions: diarrhea, dysentery, hypertension, and spitting up, coughing up, or vomiting blood.

Pineapple

Neutral thermal nature; sweet-and-sour flavor; removes *summer heat;* contains the enzyme bromelin which increases digestive ability and destroys worms. Is thirst-quenching; diuretic; treats sunstroke, indigestion, anorexia, diarrhea, and edema. Pineapples should be ripe, very sweet, juicy, and not acidic. Underripe pineapple is very acidic and can damage teeth.

Caution: Not to be used by those with peptic ulcers or skin discharges.

Plum

The purple variety is slightly cooling while the yellow varieties tend to be neutral; sweet-and-sour flavor; builds body fluids. Used for liver diseases and diabetes; stewed prunes are a traditional remedy for constipation and are especially beneficial when *excess* liver and *heat* signs are present. Plums also treat cirrhosis of the liver, hardened or expanded liver conditions in general, and dehydration. The purple plums are best in liver conditions that express themselves as emotional repression, pain, and nervous disorders.

Cautions: The plum is not good for people with delicate digestion or gastrointestinal ulcers or inflammations. Rich in oxalic acid, plums can deplete calcium in the body.

Umeboshi salt plums (very sour and salty) treat indigestion, diarrhea, dysentery, remove worms, and act on the liver. Highly alkalizing, umeboshi are sometimes called "Japanese Alka-Seltzer" because of their use in treating digestive upset. Habitual consumption can add too much salt to the diet. Unfortunately, the Japanese salt plum and most other varieties are customarily made with refined salt. Umeboshi plums are available whole, and they are also made into a variety of extracts including liquids, tablets, vinegars, and pastes.

Pomegranate

Sweet-and-sour flavor; used as a remedy for bladder disturbances; destroys worms in the intestinal tract; strengthens gums; soothes ulcers of the mouth and throat.

Raspberry

Neutral thermal nature; sweet-and-sour flavor; benefits liver and kidneys; enriches and cleanses the blood of toxins; regulates the menstrual cycle; controls urinary functions; treats anemia, as well as excessive and frequent urination, especially at night. Can be used to induce and promote labor at childbirth.

Raspberry leaf, a widely available herb, strengthens the uterus, checks excessive menstrual flow, and restrains bleeding in general; it is of exceptional benefit for tonifying the uterus and supporting optimum hormonal patterns during pregnancy.

The dried unripe raspberry fruit, a prominent, slightly warming Chinese herb (*Rubus chingii;* Mandarin: *fu pen zi),* is considered beneficial to the kidneys through its astringent action. It controls excessive and frequent urination like ripe raspberry, but more effectively; it also astringes the *jing* essence and thereby treats impotence, involuntary seminal emission, spermatorrhea, and premature ejaculation. It improves visual acuity and thus is used for blurred vision. Ripe raspberry also seems to benefit vision. In animal experiments, the unripe raspberry has estrogen-like effects on the female sex organs; quite possibly the ripe raspberry and its leaf have these same effects.

The blackberry is closely related to the raspberry and has similar astringent and blood-building properties. It is used for treating diarrhea, anemia, and for astringing the urinary system.

Strawberry

Cooling thermal nature; sweet-and-sour flavor; benefits the spleen-pancreas and improves appetite; moistens the lungs and generates body fluids. Used for thirst, sore throat, and hoarseness. Eat before meals to treat poor digestion accompanied by abdominal pain and swelling. Relieves urinary difficulties including painful urination and inability to urinate.

Very rich in silicon and vitamin C: useful for arterial and all connective tissue repair. To strengthen the teeth and gums and help remove tartar, cut a strawberry in half and rub onto the teeth and gums; leave on 45 minutes and rinse with warm water.

One of the first fruits to appear in the spring, strawberries are good for spring cleansing. Allergic reactions to strawberries are often caused by berries that are not vine-ripened.

Watermelon

Very cooling thermal nature; sweet flavor; removes *heat* including *summer heat* problems; influences the heart, bladder, and stomach; builds body fluids; diuretic; moistens the intestines. Used to treat thirst, urinary difficulty, edema, canker sores, depression, and kidney and urinary tract inflammations such as nephritis and urethritis.

Caution: Not to be used by those with weak digestion, anemia, or excessive or uncontrolled urination.

The seeds of watermelon benefit the kidneys and act as a general diuretic. They contain cucurbocitrin, a compound which dilates capillaries, lowering high blood pressure. They also are a remedy for constipation. Dried seeds are decocted into a tea. Fresh seeds can be consumed if chewed well.

The rind is rich in silicon and its outer green skin is concentrated in chlorophyll. Rind can be used in all the ways listed above for the inner fruit. It additionally treats diabetes and high blood pressure. Watermelon rind can be juiced and drunk; or small amounts (1 ounce 2–3 times daily) can be eaten; or a tea may be made from the dried rind (dry ¼-inch strips in the sun or in a food dryer). Rind can also be pickled in salt, following the same procedure for vegetable pickles (not for high blood pressure though, because of salt content).

Desserts

Traditionally, desserts are the sweetest, lightest, and last part of the meal. In earlier times, they often contained spices, herbs, and fruit as digestive aids. Our desserts also emphasize these ingredients as well as sweeteners that are very mild, similar in strength to the semi-refined sugars of centuries ago.

One purpose of desserts is to end a meal of heavy meats and greasy food with a lighter quality. Also, high-protein food calls for greater amounts of carbohydrates, which are abundantly available as simple sugars in fruit and most desserts.

Unfortunately, the sensually stimulating combination of meat with sweets causes fermentation and gastric difficulty, since sugars and proteins at the same meal typically combine poorly, especially in those with sensitive digestion. One partial solution is to use food that limits the production of putrefactive bacteria. The first choice is bitter green vegetables, particularly celery and lettuce, as explained in *Food Combinations,* Chapter 19. Thus, our suggestion for those who include sweet food at the meal's end is to precede it with an abundance of green salad comprised primarily of celery and lettuce.

An even better practice is to use quality desserts as small meals by themselves or perhaps as the dessert following a "meal" of celery- and lettuce-based salad. The desserts listed in this section all have wholesome ingredients—unrefined grains, vegetables, legumes, nuts, seeds, fruit, herb seasoning, and quality sweeteners.

Because they contain hearty ingredients with concentrated sweeteners, all of which are usually well cooked, these desserts can be considered energizing and strengthening. This follows the principle that cooked, sweet food tonifies the body. Of course, such principles quickly reverse (extreme *yang* changes to *yin*) if taken to the limit. For example, conditions that can occur from too much sweet food—diabetes, hypoglycemia, obesity, and various pathologic yeasts, growths, and inflammations—suggest that the major segment of the current generation with such imbalances has been weakened from overconsumption of extremely sweet food. The fact that most treats people eat contain denatured ingredients only adds to the problem.

However, we should consider the therapeutic use of quality desserts. The *deficient, cold,* thin, or *dry* person may benefit from *moderate* amounts of cooked dessert containing ingredients like those in the following recipes. Individuals with serious disorders and sensitive digestion should use even simpler sweet food. Recall that well-cooked grain ("congees," for instance) and starchy vegetables such as parsnip, carrot, potato, and winter squash are tonifying and sweet. In addition, simple fruit meals can be cooked for these persons.

The robust, strong, *excessive,* or *overheated* person does best with raw fruit desserts. This is because most fruit, though sweet, generally reduces *excess.* Eating it raw preserves its cooling, reducing attributes. When this person uses sweeteners, the best choices are stevia and raw honey. An example of a sweet, cooling, and detoxifying dessert is the "Agar-Agar Fruit Gel" on page 583. Another is slices of ripe, green apple, which is a customary ending to a traditional French meal.

The *damp,* sluggish individual (those with edema, candida overgrowth, tumors, or growths) should use desserts with caution since highly sweetened food is moistening and growth-promoting. This person, however, can normally tolerate "desserts" made of these kind of ingredients: fresh flax oil, stevia powder, ground cinnamon, and/or dulse powder sprinkled over rice, millet, rice cakes, or winter squash.

The use of sweeteners varies according to individual tastes. Try out quality sweeteners to find the right one and amount, keeping in mind the value of fruits and spices (see *Sweeteners*, chapter 11). Below is a conversion chart to help you substitute wholesome sweeteners in recipes containing refined sugar and adjust the proportion of liquid ingredients.

Substitutions for Recipes Containing Refined "White" Sugar		
Sweetener	**Substitution for each cup refined sugar**	**Reduction of total liquid per cup sugar**
Barley Malt and Rice Syrup	1½ cups	slightly
Honey	¾ cup	⅛ cup
Fruit Juice Concentrate	¾ cup	⅛ cup
Maple Syrup	¾ cup	⅛ cup
Maple Granules	1 cup	—
Molasses	½ cup	—
Unrefined Cane Juice Powder	¾ cup	—
Stevia	1 teaspoon	add ⅛ cup

Of the growing number of people who eat primarily wholesome foods, a surprising percentage continue eating commercial treats of poor quality. Even when "natural," such treats frequently contain rancid oils and flours, chemical ingredients such as baking soda, huge amounts of fruit sweeteners that concentrate toxins from pesticide-drenched fruit, and soybeans that have been through a dozen devitalizing processes. The following sizeable collection of desserts is offered with encouragement for the many who struggle indefinitely with this area of dietary transition, and to stimulate awareness and creativity in dessert-making with foods that have healing potential.

PUMPKIN PIE

1 medium pumpkin
½ cup rice syrup
½ cake tofu
1 cup sprouted wheat flour (p. 491)
½ teaspoon each cinnamon, ginger, cloves
¼ teaspoon nutmeg
¼ teaspoon sea salt
2 pie crusts (p. 499)

• Prepare crusts.
• Peel and cut pumpkin into small pieces.
• Add rice syrup. Cover and cook until tender. Add a little water if needed.
• Add tofu last 10 minutes of cooking.
• Mix and purée all ingredients together.
• Pour into pie crusts and bake 1 hour at 300°F.
• Yields 2 pies.

SQUASH CAKE

1 cup whole-wheat pastry flour
1 cup brown rice flour
½ teaspoon sea salt
1 teaspoon each coriander,
 cinnamon, grated ginger
1 cup apple juice or grain coffee
¼ cup chopped nuts
3 cups cooked, puréed squash or
 sweet potatoes
⅓ cup maple syrup or unrefined
 cane juice powder

- Preheat oven to 350°F.
- Mix dry ingredients.
- Add remaining ingredients and beat well by hand.
- Pour into oiled cake pan.
- Bake 1 hour.
- Serves 8.

CARROT CAKE

- Use 2 cups grated carrots in place of squash in Squash Cake.
- Add ½ cup soaked raisins and increase maple syrup or dried cane juice to ⅔ cup.

APPLE CAKE

- Use 2 cups chopped apples and 1 cup apple sauce in place of squash in Squash Cake.

PERSIMMON CAKE

- Use 2 cups raw, chopped persimmon in place of squash in Squash Cake.

APPLE PIE

6–8 apples, sliced
1 tablespoon lemon juice
1 cup apple juice
½ cup raisins, soaked
1 teaspoon vanilla
1 tablespoon cinnamon
1½ tablespoons arrowroot, dissolved
 in ½ cup apple juice
1 flaky pie crust for top and
 bottom crust (p. 499)

- Prepare the crusts.
- Preheat oven to 375°F.
- Sprinkle apples with lemon juice.
- Combine raisins, apple juice, vanilla, and cinnamon in a saucepan and simmer 5 minutes.
- Add arrowroot mixture and stir constantly until thickened.
- Fill pie crust with apples. Pour in raisin sauce.
- Cover with top crust and flute edges with a fork. Poke small holes in top with fork.
- Bake 35–40 minutes.
- Yields 1 pie.

SWEET POTATO PIE

4–6 sweet potatoes, cooked
¼ teaspoon cardamom
¼ teaspoon cinnamon
Dash of nutmeg
¼ cup raisins
2 tablespoons sesame butter
½ teaspoon sea salt
1 pie crust (p. 499)

- Prepare pie crust.
- Preheat oven to 350°F.
- Mash potatoes and mix all ingredients together.
- Fill pie crust with potato mixture.
- Bake 35–40 minutes.
- Yields 1 pie.

APPLE CRISP

4–6 apples, sliced
Juice of 1 lemon
¼ cup apple juice with ½ teaspoon cinnamon
½ cup oatmeal
½ cup whole-wheat pastry flour
¼ cup sesame seeds, toasted and ground
¼ cup ground nuts
2 tablespoons apple juice
2 tablespoons water
⅓ teaspoon sea salt

- Preheat oven to 350°F.
- Combine oatmeal, flour, sesame seeds, nuts, water, lemon juice, 2 tablespoons apple juice, and salt to make a crumbly crust.
- Arrange half the apples in an oiled casserole dish and pour apple juice over them.
- Sprinkle half the crust over the apples.
- Make a second layer of apples and cover with remaining crust.
- Bake 40 minutes.
- Serves 6.

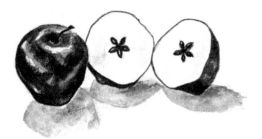

TOFU PIE

1 cake tofu
2 tablespoons sesame butter
½ cup rice syrup
½ cup apple juice
2 tablespoons lemon juice
¼ teaspoon sea salt
1½ teaspoons vanilla
Buckwheat pie crust (p. 500)

- Prepare pie crust.
- Preheat oven to 350°F.
- Purée all ingredients together.
- Pour into pie crust.
- Bake 30–35 minutes, until top is lightly golden.
- Cool and top with Fruit Topping (see p. 631).
- Yields 1 pie.

TAPIOCA PUDDING

¼ cup almonds, soaked
1 quart water
4 ounces tapioca pearls
⅓ cup maple syrup
1 teaspoon vanilla

- Blend almonds in water to make almond milk.
- Pour into saucepan.
- Add tapioca pearls. Soak 15 minutes.
- Add maple syrup and bring to boil. Reduce heat. Simmer 10 minutes.
- Add vanilla. Allow to cool.
- Serve plain with a fruit topping or as a cake topping.
- Serves 4–6.

FESTIVE RICE PUDDING

2 cups sweet brown rice
6 cups apple juice
1 stick cinnamon
1 vanilla bean, split
½ teaspoon sea salt
¾ cup raisins
¼ cup almonds or chestnuts, toasted
1 tablespoon sesame butter
2 tablespoons grated orange peel
2 tablespoons kuzu or arrowroot, diluted
1 tablespoon anise seed

- Cook rice in 5 cups apple juice with salt, cinnamon stick, and vanilla bean (remove after cooking).
- Purée rice.
- Simmer raisins in 1 cup apple juice for 10 minutes.
- Mix puréed rice, raisin mixture, almonds, sesame butter, kuzu, and orange rind together.
- Place in an oiled casserole dish and bake 30 minutes.
- Sprinkle anise seeds on top and bake 10 minutes more.
- Serves 6–8.

BREAD PUDDING

3 cups stale bread, cubed
1 cup dried fruit
2 cups apple juice or grain coffee
1 teaspoon cinnamon
½ teaspoon cardamom
1 tablespoon grated lemon or orange rind
Sea salt to taste
¼ cup chopped nuts
½ cup wheat germ

- Soak bread cubes, dried fruit, cinnamon, cardamom, rind, and salt in liquid for several hours.
- Preheat oven to 300°F.
- Spoon mixture into a casserole and sprinkle with nuts and wheat germ.
- Cover and bake for 30 minutes.
- Remove cover and bake until browned on top.
- Serves 6.

Variation Add vanilla extract or rose water.

APRICOT MOUSSE

2 pints fresh apricots, halved, or
   1 pint dried apricots, soaked
1 teaspoon agar-agar powder
2 cups apple juice
¼ teaspoon sea salt
1 vanilla bean, split lengthwise
⅓ teaspoon stevia powder
   (optional)
1 cup rice cream or cooked
   oatmeal
Fresh strawberries

- Simmer apricots, agar-agar, salt, stevia, and vanilla bean in juice for 15 minutes.
- Remove vanilla bean.
- Purée cereal and agar mixture together.
- Pour into a mold and let set until firm.
- Unmold and garnish with strawberries.
- Serves 4–6.

BLUEBERRY COUSCOUS PUDDING

1 pint blueberries
3 cups apple juice
1 cup couscous
1 teaspoon grated lemon or orange
   rind
¼ teaspoon sea salt

- Mix all ingredients together.
- Cover and simmer 10 minutes.
- Turn off heat and let sit undisturbed 15 minutes.
- Spoon onto a platter and arrange into a mound.
- Garnish with fresh blueberries and strawberry leaves.
- Serves 6.

OATMEAL ALMOND CUSTARD

3–4 cups cooked oatmeal
1–2 apples, grated
1 teaspoon cinnamon
Sea salt to taste
¼ cup barley malt or ⅓ teaspoon
   stevia powder (optional)
½ cup toasted oat flakes
¼ cup ground almonds

- Preheat oven to 350°F.
- Brush pie pan with oil or liquid lecithin.
- Sprinkle bottom and sides with oat flakes.
- Combine oatmeal, apples, cinnamon, sweetener, and salt.
- Fill pie pan and sprinkle almonds on top.
- Bake 30 minutes.
- Cool and cut into slices.
- Yields 1 pie.

BAKED FRUIT

- Core apples and pears.
- Place in a casserole and cover.
  Slow method: Bake at 250°F for 1½–2 hours.
  Fast method: Bake at 400°F for 30 minutes.

STUFFED BAKED FRUIT WITH TOPPING

- Stuff cored apples and pears with raisins, chopped nuts, and cinnamon.
- Pour enough apple juice over apples and pears to cover ½ inch of the bottom of pan.
- Bake until soft.

FRUIT TOPPING

1 cup fresh fruit, chopped
½ cup apple juice
⅛ teaspoon sea salt
1½ tablespoons arrowroot diluted in 2 tablespoons apple juice

- Combine fruit, apple juice, and salt in a saucepan. Bring to a simmer.
- Add arrowroot mixture and stir gently until thick.
- Pour topping over pie, fruit, or cake.

SNOWY FRUIT TOPPING

½ cup sweet rice flour or sprouted wheat flour (p. 491)
1 tablespoon sesame butter (optional)
1 vanilla bean, split lengthwise
3 cups apple juice
2–3 tablespoons maple syrup or ⅛ teaspoon stevia powder (optional)
¼ teaspoon sea salt

Toasted sesame seeds
- Mix flour and sesame butter together.
- Add juice, vanilla bean, sweetener, and salt.
- Simmer 15–20 minutes until thick.
- Remove vanilla bean.
- Serve over baked fruit.
- Sprinkle with sesame seeds.

STRAWBERRY AND PEAR DELIGHT

1 pint fresh strawberries
1 pint pears, halved and cooked
2 cups mint tea or apple juice
¼ teaspoon sea salt
1 bar agar-agar

- Rinse agar-agar in cold water. Squeeze out excess water and tear into small pieces.
- Simmer in tea or juice 15 minutes. Skim off foam.
- Arrange pear halves on the bottom of a glass dish or mold. Cover with strawberries.
- Pour agar-agar over fruit and let set until firm.
- Serves 6.

Amasake: This fermented sweet rice is made from koji, a starter treated with a special yeast culture—*Aspergillus oryzae*—which converts the starch in rice into a simpler sugar. This sugar is not refined and is not as concentrated as honey, molasses, etc. Use as a sweetener in desserts, breads, pancakes, muffins, drinks. Most whole-food stores either carry or have access to koji.

Note: Certain commercial types of amasake, usually from Japan, are very concentrated syrups and should be diluted or used in smaller amounts.

AMASAKE

2 cups sweet brown rice, brown rice, or brown basmati rice soaked in
3½ cups water
¼ cup koji soaked in ½ cup water

- Soak rice and koji separately overnight.
- Simmer rice in water 1 hour.
- Transfer rice to a ceramic or glass container and let cool until warm (80°F).
- Add koji and mix gently.
- Cover and let sit in a warm place 12 hours. Stir occasionally for uniform fermentation.
- To store: Add ¼ teaspoon sea salt and simmer over low heat to stop fermentation. Refrigerate up to 2 weeks.

SAKE—sweet rice wine

- Let amasake stand for 2–3 days until it releases a yeasty odor.
- Add 2 cups water to 1 cup amasake and bring to just below boil.
- Add 1 teaspoon grated ginger. Serve warm or use in cooking.

AMASAKE PUDDING

- Add cinnamon, vanilla, and raisins to regular amasake.
- Sprinkle with toasted almonds or sunflower seeds.

AMASAKE CORN CAKE

4 cups cornmeal
2 cups amasake
1 cup apple juice or fennel tea
Juice and grated rind of ½ lemon
1 teaspoon sea salt
4 tablespoons unrefined cane juice powder (optional)

- Combine all ingredients together.
- Spoon into a preheated and oiled cake pan.
- Bake in a 350°F oven for 45 minutes to 1 hour, or steam 3 hours on stove top (p. 497).
- Serves 8–12.

Variation Use grain coffee, cinnamon, and orange peel in place of juice and lemon. Add vanilla extract or rose water.

AMASAKE FRESH FRUIT SHAKE

- Purée amasake with seasonal fruit (blueberry, peach, strawberry, cherry).

AMASAKE OAT BALLS

2 cups oat flakes
½ cup rice flour
¾ cup amasake
½ cup raisins, washed and soaked
(or any other dried fruit, e.g.,
apricots, apples, currants. Dice
large fruit.)
½ cup coarse-ground almonds,
lightly roasted
½ teaspoon sea salt

- Mix all ingredients together, form into 1-inch-high balls, and place on cookie sheet (no need to oil sheet).
- Bake in preheated oven at 350°F for 15–20 minutes.
- Yields 12 balls.

LEMON COOKIES

1½ cups brown rice flour
1½ cups oat flour
1½ cups amasake
½ teaspoon sea salt
1 tablespoon sesame oil
¼ cup roasted sesame seeds
Juice and grated rind of 1 lemon

- Preheat oven to 350°F.
- Mix all ingredients together.
- Roll dough into small balls and press onto preheated and oiled cookie sheet with the tines of a wet fork.
- Bake 10 minutes on one side. Turn cookies over and bake 5 minutes more.
- Yields 3 dozen.

RAINBOW DREAM COOKIES

2 cups whole-wheat pastry flour
1 cup chestnut or rice flour
1 teaspoon sea salt
¼ cup oil or sesame meal
2 teaspoons vanilla
¼ cup beet purée
¼ cup squash purée
¼ cup amasake
¼ cup raisin purée

- Mix dry ingredients together.
- Mix vanilla and oil and rub into flour.
- Divide mixture into 4 equal portions. Place in separate bowls.
- Add one purée to each bowl and mix until a ball of dough begins to form. (Add apple juice if dough is too dry.)
- Chill 2 hours.
- Preheat oven to 350°F.
- Roll out each piece of dough ¼-inch thick.
- Stack to make 4 layers. Press lightly together.
- Cut stacks into various shapes.
- Bake 10–15 minutes.

CRUNCHY OATMEAL COOKIES

3 cups oat flakes
2 cups boiling fruit juice
½ cup rice flour
½ cup whole-wheat pastry flour
½ cup chopped almonds
1 tablespoon oil (optional)
½ teaspoon sea salt
1 teaspoon cinnamon
1 teaspoon vanilla or almond
 extract
½ cup raisins

- Dry-toast flakes until golden.
- Pour into a mixing bowl and scald with hot juice. Let sit 5–10 minutes.
- Mix with remaining ingredients.
- Drop tablespoons of dough onto a preheated oiled cookie sheet.
- Bake at 350°F for 12–20 minutes.
- Yields 3 dozen.

FIG BARS

1 cup chopped figs, dried
½ cup puréed chestnuts
1 cup grain coffee or soy milk
Juice and rind of 1 orange
2 tablespoons rice flour
¼ teaspoon sea salt
Light pressed pie crust (p. 500)

- Preheat oven to 350°F.
- Simmer all ingredients together 5 minutes until thick.
- Spoon into pie crust and sprinkle with extra dough.
- Bake 30–40 minutes.
- Cool and cut into bars.
- Yields 24 bars.

ADUKI-CAROB BROWNIES

1 cup aduki beans, soaked and
 drained
3 cups apple juice
1 vanilla bean, split lengthwise
½ cup carob powder
¾ cup applesauce
½ cup rice flour
1 cup whole-wheat pastry flour
½ teaspoon sea salt
1 teaspoon cinnamon
1 tablespoon sesame oil or sesame
 butter (optional)
½ cup chopped nuts
½ cup raisins

- Cook beans with apple juice and vanilla bean until soft.
- Remove vanilla bean and mash beans until creamy.
- Preheat oven to 350°F.
- Mix with other ingredients and pour batter into a preheated oiled cake pan.
- Bake 1 hour and 15 minutes until top is dark and firm.
- Cut into 20 squares.

GOLDEN SQUASH PUFFS

1 butternut squash, cooked
¼ cup whole-wheat pastry flour
¼ cup rice flour
¼ teaspoon cardamom
Pinch of nutmeg
Juice and grated rind of 1 lemon or orange
4 tablespoons unrefined cane juice powder, or ¼ teaspoon stevia powder (optional)
¼ teaspoon sea salt
Almonds, blanched

- Preheat oven to 350°F.
- Mash squash and mix with rest of ingredients.
- Drop tablespoons of dough onto a preheated and oiled cookie sheet and top with an almond.
- Bake 30 minutes until brown on bottom.
- Yields 2 dozen.

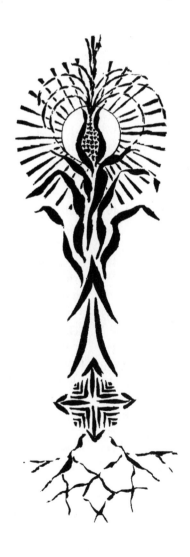

Recipe Locator

Note: Foods marked with an asterisk (*) have their healing properties listed on the pages shown.

SUMMARY

Sattva: Food as Medicine for the Mind and Body

A major unifying theme throughout this book is the relationship of diet to the vitality of the mind and body. This theme is summarized here in the context of the guiding principles of Ayurveda regarding food, its preparation and selection, and healing in general. Ayurveda of India, an ancient therapeutic system still widely in use, has identified the positive and negative attributes of diets that today, over 3,000 years later, are finally recognized in the West by modern nutritional science. This traditional approach interprets dietary categories and their healing attributes. We have chosen Ayurveda to summarize the basic intention of this volume because it uniquely realizes how greatly food and other life habits influence one's thinking and feelings.

A Foundation for Immunity and Renewal: The Traditional Sattva Plan of Equilibrium and Essence[1,2,3,4,5]

Many people seek a dietary and lifestyle plan that supports high-level wellness and mental/spiritual evolution. The ancient Ayurvedic Sattva plan is a model of life-affirming principles, which are highly adaptable to individual needs. This plan provides a goal toward which individuals can aspire, while balancing specific health and constitutional requirements. The Sattva plan presents comprehensive moral and spiritual practices, lifestyle guidelines and nutrition developed over the millennia. Sattva ideals, although ascribed mainly to the teachings of India, can generally be found among the ultimate truths at the core of every spiritual tradition. The identifying features of such traditions have been a sense of heightened awareness, peace and tranquillity among its followers.

*   *   *

Transliterated from Sanskrit, Sattva means *the path of equilibrium and essence.* Sattvic practices, which bring one to a state of balance, are an ultimate therapeutic approach; they are the foundation that can unify all other therapies. Building immunity and improving the healing response in general hinge on the strength of one's spirit. This view from traditional Chinese healing was explored in the Fire Element chapter in discussions on the heart/mind concept: the spirit provides direction, intelligence and awareness in healing. More specifically, spirit leads the *qi* energetic functions in their healing activities. Because a primary effect of Sattva practice is to strengthen the mind and spirit, one can say the path of equilibrium and essence resides at the foundation of healing.

In this summary we present a discussion of the three prime attributes or *gunas*—Sattva, Tamas, and Rajas—and their relationship to contemporary civilization.

How does one live a Sattvic lifestyle? Following are a few of the most basic principles:

Activity should be appropriate, relaxed, and not excessive. Work is balanced with rest; study of an uplifting nature is borne out through spiritual practices. By strengthening the spirit, the heart flourishes, and mental conflict can be transformed in the heart's flame of awareness. Activities such as yoga and t'ai chi (Chinese yoga) are beneficial because they help us see the body as a facet of mind. Carefully moderating sexual activity substantially improves the vitality of the body and mind. (*Ojas,* a concept discussed later, represents the vital essence of the entire human organism, and it depends largely on ample reproductive reserves.)

Diet is lacto-vegetarian, of absolute quality, freshness and life-force. Food categories include grains (e.g., rice, bread, pasta), vegetables, fruits, nuts, seeds, dairy products, and legumes (especially tofu, lentils, peas, mung beans, and aduki beans—most other beans lack the soothing quality of Sattva). All food is recently prepared, cooked to perfection—not over- or undercooked, not oily or greasy; spices are used in moderation, and the mind of the cook should be in the Sattvic state. Likewise, the food should be eaten in this state.

Sattvic food is simple. But the practice of simplicity is a challenge for most of us in developed countries. In this present "age of excess," over 50,000 different types of foods and food products from around the world are now available in America. Sampling dozens of ingredients in each meal, people experience tremendous mental and digestive stimulation that is impossible to assimilate harmoniously. This is difficult to prove in lab experiments, but you may try this experiment for yourself: Eat simply for a day or two—according to food combining plan B, for example, on page 265. Then notice how your mind and body feel. Most people feel much clearer, brighter, and stronger. After a few weeks, many report feeling the best they have felt in their lives.

The Sattvic individual avoids overeating. This practice, like eating simple food, often presents difficulty in wealthy countries. As we learned earlier in Chapter 18, however, overeating directly reduces life span.

Updating Sattva dietary principles for the Twenty-first Century. Originally Sattvic foods, like all foods at the time, were "organic"—grown and prepared without pesticides, herbicides, chemical fertilizers, hormones, genetic modification, irradiation to prevent spoilage, microwave cooking (toxic effects described on page 60), and so on. They were also unrefined, whole foods, or with at most minor refinements such as occur in *ghee* and other naturally extracted, unrefined oils. The modern denaturing of foods through massive refining and chemical treatment deranges their pranic-qi life force, making them unable to foster Sattva equilibrium and essence.

The Sattvic emphasis on complex carbohydrates and dairy products promotes brain chemistry rich in tryptophan, serotonin, and melatonin. (These, along with specific foods that support their generation in the body, are discussed a little later in the "Chemical and Drug Sattva" section.) Modern researchers now find that when these substances are abundant in the body, they promote deep sleep, calmness, strong immunity, and a relaxed, focused mind—all of which are Sattvic qualities.

The **sweet flavor** is one of the least well-understood areas of the Sattva plan. The reference to sweet foods in the *Bhagavad-Gita* (Section 17) suggests that moist, pleasant-tasting, naturally sweet foods promote longevity, strength, purity, and happiness. Sweet foods in general are said to promote "Shakti" (awareness).[6] This corresponds with Chinese traditional healing and its designation of "sweet" as the central flavor that counteracts deficiency and strengthens and nourishes the body and mind; however, white refined sugar and highly refined sweeteners are a perversion of the sugar cane, sugar beets and other foods they are derived from, much as German social philosopher Rudolf Steiner considered grain alcohol a perversion of grain. (Note: alcohol is also a sugar.) We now focus on white sugar as an example of extreme food processing in this present age.

White refined sugar did not exist at the time ancient teachings and disciplines originated. However, it is amply clear that products refined to such an extent are in the realm of medicines, and that regular use violates human health and integrity (see pages 189–190), making the Sattvic goal of a clear, focused mind difficult indeed. This is due to the way white sugar is unbalanced, i.e., lacking virtually all metabolism-controlling minerals that were part of its original structure, which tends to cause the mind to reel out of control. The effect is not far different from alcohol although, in our personal observation, a little wine or beer sometimes de-stabilizes the metabolism less. A number of Ayurvedic doctors as well as yogis have realized that regular use of white sugar, like many extremely refined substances, can ultimately contribute to spiritual demise. They experience refined sugar as a degenerate, "Tamasic" substance[7] that distorts and depletes their *"ojas,"* which is the essence required for spiritual development.

People who are addicted to white sugar often claim that food doesn't matter; this represents a separation of mind from substance. Once there is an addiction to alcohol, white sugar, or any other strong substance, addictive denial blinds one to the simplicity of reality.

Equally as unbalancing to the body as highly processed sugar, chemical- or pesticide-laden foods are not Sattvic in quality;[8] neither are prepackaged, canned or stale foods.[9] All intoxicants, including alcohol, marijuana, psychoactive mushrooms and synthetic drugs such as LSD destroy the purity and subtlety of the Sattvic experience.[10] All meats, including chicken, fish and eggs—because their consumption destroys sentient life—reside outside the domain of Sattva. If milk is included, it must be *freshly* drawn from healthy animals, not pasteurized or homogenized.[11,12] (For a perspective on pasteurized/homogenized processes, see the dairy section, pages 286–287.)

The primary non-Sattvic vegetables are those of the onion family; these, according to various ancient teachings, are said to bring excessive desires and mental dullness to the person, making mental/spiritual equilibrium difficult. One such teaching from Gautama Buddha regarding the onion family is: "Those who eat the five pungent plants [garlic, onions, leeks, scallions and chives] ... will not be protected by the Good Spirits of the Ten Directions; immensely powerful demons will disguise themselves as Buddhas and speak false dharma to them, resulting in lust, rage and delusion."[13] Thus, some Sattvic individuals will use the onion family only as medicine; others totally abstain.

This family of vegetables has remarkable healing potential and, because of its ability to resolve the deposits in the body from meat-eating, suits those who partake of meat and often those who are still in early transition from meat-based diets. The anti-Sattvic aspect of onions and their relatives presents some difficulty in the West because of their pervasiveness in both vegetarian and general diets. Garlic has been promoted as a near cure-all for an extensive list of ailments (page 546), as it should be, but it is helpful to remember that powerful herbs and strongly medicinal foods ought to be used cautiously in the normal daily diet. A Chinese folk saying warns that "Healthy people who regularly use medicines become ill."

What about other pungent foods? The basic rule is to use spices with caution, and in small amounts. The common Sattvic spices are turmeric, ginger, cinnamon, cardamom, coriander, fennel, and anise. Black pepper and other very hot peppers promote a fiery "Rajas" temperament.

Raw foods are not considered purely Sattvic, in part because of the parasites and microbes they often harbor. Some teachings also suggest that raw foods bring on anger.[14] In addition, as noted in the Earth Element chapter, raw foods can weaken one's "center," making digestion and assimilation weak. This in turn reduces the body's ability to build life-essence or *"ojas."* Ojas, essentially synonymous with the *jing* (pages 360–365) of Chinese healing, represents the vital essence of the body, without which life ceases. *Ojas* is derived from reproductive essences in the body, and is necessary for growth, development, and immunity. Proper functioning of the mind also depends on this vital essence; spirit is a transformation of *ojas.*

Without abundant *ojas,* mental and spiritual enlightenment are an impossibility. Nevertheless, individuals on a generally Sattvic program will often eat some raw foods for a limited time for cleansing and renewal; this is especially recommended in the West for most of those embarking on Sattva, until their excess is purged. Raw foods should be purified of parasites before eating (see page 572 for an effective method).

Oils and fatty foods are taken sparingly in the Sattvic plan,[15] but they are important for the development of the mind and should not be absent from the diet except for specific short-term therapeutic plans to reduce dangerous buildup of fats in the body's tissues. As a young child, the legendary East Indian saint known as Krishna was notoriously fond of *ghee* (clarified butter), quite possibly to fuel his tremendous intellectual and spiritual development. *Ghee* enhances *ojas* in the body, and other quality dairy products also provide suitable foundation materials.

Finding sources of quality dairy is a challenge for many vegetarians and, since

Western peoples have an extremely high fat intake to begin with, most should partake of fatty foods—including *ghee*—with restraint in any case. If consumed excessively, dietary fat causes liver upset, which easily provokes responses such as anger, impatience, mental depression, resentment, and other deep and obstructed emotions (pages 159 and 318). Thus some Sattvic individuals seldom eat fried foods and, when needing oil to feel more earthy and grounded, will obtain it naturally in their diet of whole, unrefined foods, and also will follow the Sattvic practice of rubbing natural oils on their bodies after bathing. Three traditional oils for external use are coconut butter, unrefined sesame oil, and virgin olive oil.

When using commercial soaps, shampoos, body lotions, perfumes, deodorants, various kinds of makeup, and other such items, it is best to avoid those made with chemical solvents and synthetic additives—these are directly absorbed into the body through the skin[16] and interfere with immunity. Even so-called "natural" toiletries frequently contain health-damaging chemicals. A general rule: avoid rubbing substances into your skin that you wouldn't eat. There are alternatives; for example, whole, unrefined oils including those mentioned above make excellent body lotions. If aroma is desired in these oils, simply add pure essential oils such as lavender or rosemary, which contribute their own aromatherapeutic effects. Body-care products for external use can be made at home using a variety of wholesome foods. (See note 17 on page 700.) Bathing and cleanliness in general is important to health. A daily bath is recommended, and keeping the body and clothing clean is considered a helpful support for pursuits of a sublime nature.

Finally we consider **salt** (see "Salt" chapter), an extremely yin substance manifesting a cooling, strongly descending nature. Salt is so yin that it brings forth an opposite, yang, warming nature in the deep, internal and lower parts of the body. The extremely descending nature of salt counteracts the natural upward surges of nutritional essences that fuel the higher centers of the body: the integrated "heart/mind" center and its spirit, and the brow and crown (head top) chakra areas and their supporting pineal and pituitary glands. Therefore salt is used sparingly or even omitted by those intent on Sattva.

How does Sattva manifest in the human personality? From Ayurvedic writers, we know that the Sattvic person has a clear and focused mind. They find joy in simple everyday activities. They refrain from dishonesty, the destruction of life, thievery, sexual misconduct and intoxicant usage because Sattvic training has enabled them to innately know how these activities stress the body and disrupt mental and emotional equilibrium. One has little need for extreme emotional or mental releases (catharsis)—the emotions are harmonized, as are the body and intellect. The equilibrium of Sattva is energized through guidance by spiritual essence, in contrast to the experiences of most of us, who are driven by base desires and emotions.

If you regularly find yourself with great excesses of emotional baggage, consider which elements of your life are least Sattvic. The balance of Sattva has been empirically proven over the centuries to quell emotional turbulence.

How long before improvements result from Sattvic life patterns? Many begin to notice improvements right away; with others, it may take weeks or months. It depends in part on one's karmic remainder—the physical, emotional and psychic residues from previous poor life habits. In most cases, however, one must adhere to a consistent Sattvic pattern for several years to reach benefits that work comfortably into the entire personality.

TAMAS. To truly appreciate the harmonious state of Sattva, it helps to know about an imbalance known as "Tamas." This state describes a sizable percentage of peoples in the "advanced" civilizations of the world. The key words describing Tamas are *stagnation and degeneration*. Tamasic personalities exhibit dark obsessions and dull, warped personality traits; they are filled with stagnant desires and cravings, and are unusually self-serving, with little regard for the welfare of others. They may be obstructed in relationships and personal finances. Their nervous systems, hearts, and minds degenerate first. Other organs go next and thus in the United States there exist epidemics of cancer, tumors, heart and emotional/mental diseases, arthritis, chronic fatigue syndromes, sexually transmitted diseases, moral and spiritual degeneration, and so on. (Modern people with serious degenerations sometimes have significant Sattvic mentality, which unfortunately, is often insufficient to overcome the greatly Tamasic and toxic state of common foods and the planet in general.)

The lifestyle of Tamasic individuals sharply contrasts with that of Sattva: they are often slothful as well as unaware of uplifting pursuits; rather than being helpful, they prefer to be entertained and sedentary; they may be blindly addicted to prepackaged, processed and very rich-tasting foods, excessive and/or poor-quality meats, intoxicants of one kind or another, overly sweet, spicy, salty, fatty and/or stale foods, and actually may have little sense of diet other than mindless desires. Overeating, even of Sattvic foods, brings one into Tamas.

RAJAS. In contrast with the stagnancy of Tamas and the balance-point of Sattva is the activity of Rajas. The key words here are *action and aggression*. Their quest in diet and other dimensions of life is for sensual stimulation. They are interested in prosperity, power, prestige and position, but not obsessed with these as is Tamas. A Rajas lifestyle may benefit the warrior, politician, competitive athlete, or aggressive business person.

The Rajasic diet contains all the ingredients of the Sattvic diet, and therefore must be fresh and of high quality.[18] In addition, compared with Sattva, cooking time can vary more; it may contain a bit more spice and oil, and greater amounts of protein foods, which can include legumes (beans, peas, lentils and their products) and any wild game such as fish, deer, pheasant, etc. (Feedlot animals promote Tamas.) Many early American colonists as well as Native Americans ate diets with a substantial Sattvic/Rajasic element; this undoubtedly contributed to their strength and clear, simple values. The trend among modern Americans to embrace fundamental values characteristic of the founding colonists would be greatly supported by returning to a simpler, fresher diet.

Nutritional science now seems in agreement with a key facet of Rajas theory: The amino acid tyrosine, which is abundantly supplied in protein-rich diets, produces in the brain the chemical dopamine; a behavioral marker of dopamine is enhanced activity and aggression.

Those who unwittingly propel their Rajas temperament with stimulants such as cocaine, coffee, cigarettes, excesses of spices, refined-sugar treats, meats and poor-quality fats reap only near-term benefits; ultimately nervousness, agitation and depletion result.

From the perspective of the aggressive action of Rajas and the stagnancy of Tamas, **the power of Sattva** is the power inherent in equilibrium. The simplicity of balance affords a sufficient sense of security to let go of attachments, which in turn allows a "universal" power to come through, and the person becomes a conduit for Guidance. According to the ancient teachings, Sattva ultimately bestows limitless access to knowledge, strength, and awareness.

More specifically, with long-term Sattvic practices, one has fewer feelings of ownership and separation, while gaining a greater sense of belonging and unity. Stress melts and one feels light, clear, easy, content, and as if continually immersed in an ocean of peace. The Chinese sages claim that few people have these kinds of experiences, which they describe as "middle path." Many individuals strive for one or more of these or similar attributes, so that, in a sense, these individuals strive for Sattvic qualities; most, however, do not know how to achieve it. Numerous ills of modern culture simply represent an unskillful attempt to reach the natural benefits of Sattva. For example, some try mind-altering drugs in pursuit of a permanently elevated state of awareness; others try thrill-seeking or gathering fabulous amounts of data in this current information age; while many believe that an abundance of sex or money is the answer. Most of us seek out exceptional highs and rushes of personal power, not realizing that just around the corner are depressions and other psychic pits. There is a shift, however, as aware people, who in only rare instances actually know the term "Sattva," in growing numbers accept its principles—patience, moderation, appropriate use of the Earth's resources, and guidance by spirit rather than by greed. The high of the middle (Sattvic) path is better described as a "centered" experience; similarly, the sense of power is more evolved, more sublime—beyond the personality, it is the universal essence expressing itself through one's center.

People who use strong substances and extreme measures that take advantage of others, in hopes of gaining for themselves wisdom, enlightenment, power, financial security and so on, are misguided; these gifts are available on a long-term basis with Sattvic practices. Such practices take discipline and commitment, and they not only succeed but continue to function over time—they are the quality approach. The Rajasic route, and especially the tamasic one, promise "everything now" but fail to deliver enduring benefits.

Sattva—a major (unconscious) direction of nutritional science. Sattva dietary practices have gradually eroded, especially in the last hundred years, as a result of the deterioration of fresh, high-quality food and the onset of truck and chemical farming, refrigeration, food processing, and so on. As sound dietary practices are undermined on every front by the agricultural and food industries, a wave of irrefutable information based on landmark studies[19] by nutritional science is beginning to look like Sattvic dietary advice: many nutritionists are now encouraging us toward diets centered on whole grains, beans and other legumes, fresh fruits and vegetables, and caution with regard to salt and fats. (Recommended supplementary items typically include a variety of animal products.)

The intense anxiety and mentality many modern people experience arise from our deep involvement in **the information age;** rooted, balanced mental faculties are needed to handle abundant information without stress. The mental/spiritual dimension is all too often deranged in modern people, who are often unable to sleep well or concentrate; and increasing numbers of children are diagnosed each year with signs of attention deficit disorder (ADD). The centered, balancing attributes of Sattva practices can remedy the fragmentation we experience from information overload.

Where is Sattva available? Even though many elements of society are gradually moving in a Sattvic direction to counteract widespread physical and moral degeneration, the actual high standards of Sattva are seldom found. For example, food-conscious persons who eat pure Sattvic diets may lack evolved mental/spiritual attitudes or practices; on the other hand, good numbers of spiritually evolved individuals eat denatured diets. Finding both the dietary and mental elements of Sattva integrated in one person is uncommon.

When ancient yogis followed Sattva, the choices were simpler: the default diet available to everyone was not processed or, at most, minimally so; it contained no synthetic chemicals, and was primarily composed of local ingredients. The main focus was freshly prepared vegetarian foods. The situation today is far different. As we shall soon see, the contemporary person needs to be ever-mindful of several variables regarding food and how it is prepared, to ensure even a vague semblance of Sattva.

The West brought the technology for highly refined white sugar, white rice, processed and hydrogenated oils and finally petro-chemical agriculture to India, China, Japan and most other Asian nations. Now, not only have these foods and farming practices replaced the original relatively pure diets of these countries, but Asian teachers and immigrants in their move to the West have brought with them their habit of eating these denatured foods. In Chinese and other Asian restaurants, the menu often includes dishes containing white "polished" rice, refined sugar and oils, older, stale ingredients from Western-style cans and packages, and other poor-quality items. Asian-inspired monasteries, ashrams, and meditation centers around the world frequently serve up similar food, heavily processed and cooked in aluminum pots. These foods often contain immunity-destroying synthetic ingredients (the wonderful traditional *ghee* of India is quickly being replaced among the Indian masses by hydrogenated margarines).

Highly refined foods lack most of the minerals, essential fatty acids, vitamins, and much of the protein required for proper immunity and other body functions. For example, magnesium is all but lost in such refined items as white sugar, white rice, and white flour products, including white-flour pastries, white bread, white noodles and other white pastas. Magnesium provides, among other functions, a flowing quality so that bodily functions can occur smoothly. In magnesium-depleted "white" diets, the bones atrophy (see pages 9–12, 218) while the bowels, menses, heart and arteries, kidneys and other organs and their processes tend to malfunction and become obstructed.

The dairy products served in these awareness centers are commonly pasteurized, homogenized, and derived from cows fed pesticide-sprayed feeds, hormones, antibiotics, and so on. The cows are virtually always part of the meat industry and are slaughtered after they stop milk production. The use of dairy products so closely associated with the meat industry, which violates the Sattvic principle that forbids taking sentient life, is one reason such diets are not truly Sattvic.

Similarly, the millings from the refined rice, refined sugar, refined wheat bread and other refined foods are used primarily in feed for pigs, cattle, chicken, and other animals destined for slaughter.* In short, a good number of awareness centers in the Far East and West based on teachings with Sattvic traditions serve the ultra-refined, chemically contaminated, lifeless, degeneration-promoting *(Tamasic)* diets characteristic of meat-centered diets in the West—without the meat.

A more difficult situation arises in Western churches that require priests, monks and nuns to take vows of chastity and poverty while eating meat-based Tamasic/Rajasic diets that drive emotions and passionate desire. Such emotional heat may have influenced thousands in religious orders worldwide to drop out in recent years. Of course, the social disarray in our current society fuels the situation, and is a reflection of the life-depleting food intake that becomes the brain chemistry influencing thinking and emotions. It should be noted that, with enough faith and strength of purpose, the unfavorable influences of poor diet can undoubtedly be overcome; but it seems that the great expenditure of effort in doing so could be better spent.

A change is underway as a number of these groups move to the country,[21] learning the simpler ways of other religious groups that never left. There they have taken to growing their own foods and milking their own contented cows and goats; most have begun to eat less meat. A growing number of city-based Western as well as Eastern religious communities are also using freshly prepared foods and such traditional unrefined staples as brown rice and whole-grain noodles and breads.

---

* In Asian countries, food millings are often used in human nutrition, e.g., Japanese "nuka" or rice-bran pickles contain rice bran in the pickling medium.

Chemical and Drug Sattva. Synthesized melatonin is the chemical shadow of what people strive naturally for in Sattva. Melatonin, a hormone produced by the pineal gland, which is located near the center of the brain, is said to reduce stress, boost immunity, deepen sleep, and promote longevity. An Eastern medical perspective can help us better understand melatonin.

The raw material from which all brain hormones are made, according to traditional Chinese medical theory, originally comes from the kidney-adrenal hormones and fluids, known as "kidney yin." Processing of these hormones and fluids may occur in the liver and various other glands. When kidney yin—including its *ojas* transformation—is deficient, the heart, mind, and brain yin (hormones and chemicals) also become deficient, and result in insomnia, stress, poor immunity, and so on. So the real problem of melatonin deficiency appears traceable to an underlying kidney depletion, which in turn can be brought on by any number of stressors, among them sexual excess, infection, overwork, alcohol, tobacco and drug use (see note 22 on page 701 for modern and traditional viewpoints on marijuana and psychoactive drugs), excessive intake of salt and spices, worry, ELF and VLF radiation from various electromagnetic sources including computer monitors, and weak kidney yin inherited from stressed parents who also lacked ample yin essence.

Soon after its introduction to the nutrition market, melatonin became a much sought-after product, while a media blitz touted its benefits. Since that time great numbers of Americans have used this hormone, and for good reason: Millions are severely stressed, and their suffering can at least be temporarily reduced with melatonin. Instead of addressing stress-related depletion with rest, renewal practices, and a sensible diet, however, many in the melatonin-ingesting population have chosen, partly out of lack of knowledge of alternatives, to simply eat these pills synthesized in the chemist's laboratory (although some individuals who take melatonin clearly have metabolic deficiencies not easily overcome without it).

A major problem with hormone supplements is the tendency to become dependent on them. This dependency arises as the body slows the natural production of hormones being supplied from an outside source. For instance, one person who took melatonin for approximately twenty years finds that he must continue to take it; otherwise he experiences an immediate bodily weakness as well as decreased resistance to common infectious diseases.[30]

A more holistic approach to counteracting stress is to increase the body's own melatonin through the intake of foods that nurture the *yin*. Some of these foods were listed earlier as complex carbohydrates (page 65), which also form the foundation of a Sattvic diet. Interestingly, the complex carbohydrates are shown to increase melatonin because when amply supplied in the diet, they maximize tryptophan, one of its precursors. (The body uses tryptophan to produce serotonin; serotonin is then used to produce melatonin.)

Eating foods rich in tryptophan is also effective. Good sources include spirulina, soy products (e.g., tofu, tempeh, soy milk, soy sauce), pumpkin seeds, brewer's yeast, and almonds; rich animal-product sources include dairy products and most fowl, including chicken and turkey. Certain foods even supply actual melatonin. Among the best sources are oats, sweet corn, daikon radish, rice, tomato, and banana.[31] Other nutrients, including B vitamins that help the body manufacture tryptophan and serotonin (and thus melatonin), are abundantly supplied in a varied diet of whole, unrefined vegetal foods. All the above food options seem a wise choice to try before experimenting with synthetic hormones. According to some health professionals melatonin, especially in its synthetic form, has not been adequately tested for human safety.[33]

As the hormones melatonin, DHEA (dehydroepiandrosterone), human growth hormone, the brain chemical phosphatidylserine and a host of other synthetic mood- and thought-altering substances make their way to the marketplace, we repeat a tired theme of modern medicine—we continue to invest in pills and palliatives rather than addressing the origin of our problems. At the same time, a more responsible approach is gaining momentum as a sensible alternative to synthetic pill therapy—more people are choosing to live beyond the chaos of this era with Sattva-like life patterns, including an emphasis on mindfulness, prayer and meditative practices, and a calming vegetarian diet.

Nevertheless, an enlightened Sattvic experience is not guaranteed within any given timeframe by a dietary regime or any other practice; for instance, one cannot say: "Now that I have eaten pure foods, kept moral precepts, and done awareness practices, I have therefore arrived at such-and-such a level of enlightenment." There are simply too many factors in our lives, and mental and spiritual evolution occur in various unchartable ways—sometimes in quantum leaps that defy understanding. Sattva can never be precisely or objectively measured, but the things we do and the foods we eat either *support* or *detract* from Sattva.

Are Sattva-type plans the **inevitable survival models** for the human species? The Earth's peoples, over thousands of years, have experimented with extremes—economically, politically, morally and with regard to nutrition. In industry, continual expansion has been the rule and, as business leaders tell us, without growth there is failure. If there is truth to the idea that humans need to participate in an endless frontier of growth, we can embrace the Sattvic paradigm as a solution, as it can help us focus our growth on the internal regions of persona. Understanding our emotional nature, our spiritual journey and the infinite complexity of the soul provides endless opportunities for growth.

We are ready finally for what will make life not only possible in the coming years on Earth, but to create a harmonious Sattva equilibrium. This is not the balancing of one pathogenic extreme with another, such as "balancing" a rabid, fascist devotion with anger and prejudice; these approaches too have been tried. The Sattva approach is most successful when balancing life patterns and processes that are both virtuous and "middle path"—near the balance point already. This implies moderation in diet as well as all other areas in which we utilize the Earth's resources.

With such an approach, we will naturally, as our inspired way of living, preserve the environment. Simply reducing meat consumption would greatly reduce planetary pollution (meat production creates massive pollution from chemical fertilizers and pesticides—more than fifty percent of all United States water pollution results from growing feed for livestock.[34]) As Sattva requires freshly prepared foods—not prepackaged,* not chemically adulterated or transported across continents there is less reliance on chemical agriculture and long-range transportation.

> For perfect health, food should always be eaten as fresh as possible both after plucking as well as after cooking. The more it is kept, the more it will lose it vital quality and the less likely it is to produce vitality in us.
>
> —Vanamali, from her book
> *Nitya Yoga: Essays on the Sreemad Bhagavad Gita*

The skeptic will ask, "How can this bold plan occur?" The person with common sense will reply: "How can it not occur? We will fail to survive if we continue as we are." Sattva provides the ultimate tool for transformation of a difficult nature—a strong spirit and the wisdom that grows from it.

In preserving the Earth's resources, we also preserve our own personal resources. As exterior pollution diminishes, our immune systems can begin to function correctly; they will no longer be depleted by the fight against environmental poisons. With a life low in stress, we preserve our *ojas*, the foundation of our immune response to stress.

From biomedical statistics, it seems that we may be on the verge of extinction for another reason. Over the last half-century since World War II, human sperm counts in industrialized countries have dropped 50% on average, and are predicted to be near zero within the next few generations.[36,38,39,40,42] [See note 44 on page 702 for discussion of the sperm-count controversy.] Likely causes are various toxic pesticides, herbicides and industrial chemicals (DDT, PCBs, and others), estrogen compounds (including chemicals that mimic estrogens), hormones in animal products, and stress from modern urban lifestyles.[37,41,42] Preserving our *ojas* through reduced environmental stress, we directly improve the strength and richness of our reproductive capacities, including sperm (recall that *ojas* arises through the transformation of reproductive substances).

Clearly a Sattvic approach purifies the current earthly environment, and our personal bodily environment as well—but what about the future? Sattva establishes the middle path, the center where yin and yang, past and future, merge. At this merger point all things are known, because it is the source of our thinking and

---

*Foods in aseptic packages are among the best examples of hyper-processed products that last, without refrigeration, for months, even years, before deteriorating. Common aseptically packaged foods are juices, tofu, soy milk and rice milk. We have seen poor results from the use of these lifeless products; when eaten regularly, they seem to produce mucoid deposits that all too frequently lead to *damp* excesses in the body and especially to lung infections with excess phlegm.

our existence. The enlightened individual, therefore, sees into the beginningless past and distant future, and thereby navigates upcoming challenges skillfully. Thus Sattva is not only a cure for our current system of toxicity and greed, but can help lay the foundation for a golden age.

Since it is the rare, fully enlightened individual who has the above Sattvic abilities in their most evolved form, one may question whether the novice stages of these abilities are of any practical use. Consider that relative wisdom, though less than absolute, is far better than none. As an example of one who developed wisdom throughout life, Thomas Jefferson, the author of the Declaration of Independence, had profound insight at a young age into how he could help others in the future, and from that point forward changed his life from one focused on comfort and social status to one of service. It is our belief that most people, by developing their wisdom, can have an insight of this level of magnitude when obstructed mental conditioning is at least partially transformed and clarified through Sattvic practices.

Ancient wisdom teaches a *soma-psyche* unity: **We all eat perfect diets** insofar as our diets and all else that we do are perfect reflections of who we are. In this perfect relationship between *what we do* and *who we are,* it behooves us to be mindful of all that we do. More specifically, this theory suggests that how we live—our particular desires, how we think, how we treat others and ourselves, and the foods we choose to eat corresponds perfectly with all that we receive in our lives, including health and awareness. If we find the results we receive through our choices in life, including disease and pain, to be intolerable, we need only make better choices. Conversely, when we live in balance, a Sattvic diet and lifestyle become the way that is most agreeable to us.

This karmic equation is not always immediately enforced; some individuals eat moderately and live uplifting lives for a year or longer before beneficial results manifest. Apparently this out-of-phase experience between how one lives and what one receives occurs because the brightness of right living erases and is therefore spent overcoming—both physical and psychic toxins from previous poor diets and other stressful behavior. With perseverance, however, the toxic residues diminish, and one nears the other shore of transcending difficulties, pain, and suffering.

Recalling the healing priority discussed earlier; opening and purifying the mind and strengthening the spirit through consistent awareness practices is considered the most efficient way to begin. Thus with Sattva comes the knowledge that food alone is insufficient for our healing and evolution.

Sattva/Rajas/Tamas and their attributes are much more than a philosophy; they are a pathway that inspires living beyond the darkness of emotional obstruction, by drawing near to the peace of Sattva equilibrium and essence.

Epilogue

The major intention of this text has been to assist the reader in making skillful and enduring changes on the pathways of awareness and healing. In order to gain skill, we fully embrace our experiences. The following verse by the venerable Chinese Zen patriarch Hsuan Hua speaks to us about the nature of "everything":

Everything's a test,
to see what you will do;
Mistaking what's before your eyes,
you have to start anew!

This message counsels us to see everything clearly as it is—right before our eyes—and to apply this experience of truth to "everything," all of life's challenges. Otherwise we must face the same test again and "start anew." This passage also teaches us about the root of disease: our stale, repetitive, addictive behavior patterns, whether in the dietary/intoxicant realm or any other. So often, when we simply stop for a moment and clearly see the nature of our destructive patterns, the brightness of our awareness causes them to dissolve—without a struggle.

APPENDIX A

Parasite Purge Program
by Suzanne Shaw and Paul Pitchford

An understanding of parasite infestation and its treatment is essential for true vitality and strong immunity. Our observations indicate that more people are infected with worms and harmful micro-organisms than previously suspected. If parasites are identified as a source of imbalance, a parasite cleanse is in order before attempting to heal other aspects of the body. This comprehensive program extends beyond the Prevention Program described on pages 114–115, as it includes broad dietary strategies, further preventive measures, and additional natural remedies. It is also customized for several constitutional types, ranging from frail to robust individuals. Powerful herbs and substances that are appropriate for the healthy or robust may debilitate the weaker person.

This Purge Program is ideal for those with pronounced signs of parasite infection, whether determined from observed symptoms or laboratory analysis. In our experience, however, this program should also be followed by virtually everyone with lingering illnesses or degenerative conditions (e.g., cancer, arthritis, AIDS, chronic fatigue syndromes, alcoholism, etc.); parasitic pathogens nearly always play a role in the etiology of degeneration.

The Nature Of Parasites

The general usage of "parasite" refers to any organism that invades and lives at the expense of another organism, known as the host. For the purposes of this book we will refer to "parasite" not only as those organisms scientifically categorized as parasites, such as protozoa and tapeworms, but also yeasts, fungi, viruses, and bacteria. It is rare that a person is affected only by yeasts, or by one type of germ. People often harbor many species of pathogenic organisms, which contribute to a wide spectrum of health problems ranging from arthritis and diabetes to depression and irritable bowel syndrome. In the bodily milieu, such organisms disrupt normal functioning of the organs and continually excrete toxic waste products, which stress the body and wear down immunity.

This Purge Program also provides a response to the many new varieties of microbes that resist conventional treatment. Considering the weakening immunity of many contemporary individuals, the potential for future widespread epidemics is not small; in Africa and some areas of Asia, long-standing epidemics of AIDS and other sexually transmitted diseases have already begun.

About a decade before the onset of these epidemics, the late Dr. John Christopher, a revered herbalist, predicted that the near future would be characterized by uncontrollable plagues. He believed that herbal and nutritional remedies would protect those wise enough to choose such gifts from nature's healing bounty. We have endeavored to provide a program that offers not only some of the most potent biologic remedies but the nutritional and hygienic plans needed to rid the bodily terrain of pathogenic organisms—and protect the terrain from future invasions. Without the burden of parasitic stress, the immune system can naturally regenerate.

The broad range of parasite-induced health problems is evident once the nature and extent of parasitic infection is understood. A general misconception about parasites is that they inhabit only the intestines of the host. However, there are parasites that live in the host's blood, lymph system, vital organs, and/or other body tissues. Some parasites may infect the entire body. Yeasts often proliferate first in the intestines, then spread throughout the body, becoming "systemic." Other parasites attack specific organs; for example, hookworms enter the body through the skin, travel in the blood, and eventually inhabit the lungs and small intestine; if left untreated they can remain in these organs for years, causing such symptoms as nausea, pneumonia and anemia. Not counting the thousands of parasitic germs, fungi, viruses and other such microbes, scientific sources list 3200 varieties of parasites which fall into four major categories:

Protozoa: *Giardia lamblia, cryptosporidium, trichomonas, and Endolimax nana;* these are microscopic organisms that travel through the blood stream and infect all body parts.

Trematoda: blood, liver, lung, intestinal, kidney and bladder flukes. Flukes are approximately 1–2.5 centimeters in length.

Cestoda: beef, pork, dog and fish tapeworms that infect the intestines. Tapeworms are large by parasitic standards and can measure up to twelve meters in length.

Nematoda: pinworms, hookworms, roundworms; these enter the intestines, lymphatic system, pancreas, heart, lungs and liver. Nematodes vary in size from .2 to 35 centimeters. This group is easily transmitted, especially by children.

Considering the extensive terrain of parasites, the vast number of adverse health effects they cause is not surprising.

Symptoms of Parasitic Infection

Abdominal pain and diarrhea are the most frequently observed symptoms of acute parasitic infection; however, if left untreated, the condition becomes chronic, causing more complicated patterns that may mimic other syndromes. Following is a list of symptoms of parasite infection:

Digestive: gas, bloating, belching, diarrhea, constipation, intestinal tract burning and cramping, changeable bowel movements, irritable bowel syndrome, mucus in the stools, malabsorption of nutrients, inability to digest fats, lactose or gluten intolerance, low blood sugar, high blood sugar, insatiable appetite, weak appetite, anorexia, over-weight, under-weight, cravings for sweet, burnt, and/or crunchy foods.

Immune system dysfunction: chronic fatigue, weakness, frequent colds and flus.

Nervous and muscular system dysfunction: mental fog, memory problems, sleep disturbances, insomnia, teeth grinding (especially during the full moon), hearing loss, eyesight impairment, joint and muscle aches and pains.

Excess mucus: a sign of *dampness.* This may manifest as mucus in the stools, chronic post nasal drip, or frequent sinus infections.

Exterior signs: allergies, skin rashes, hives, swellings, eczema, acne, white spots around the mouth, swelling of the lips, blue coloring in the whites of the eyes, and itching in the anus and the ears.

Emotional signs: apathy, depression, nervousness, anxiety, restlessness, irritability, hyperactivity in children.

Laboratory testing is an option. Accurate testing for parasites is a difficult procedure. Many laboratories only test for intestinal parasites. The most reliable and thorough tests are available in dedicated parasitology laboratories, which are frequently located in academic or research settings. (See "Publications and Organizations" in Resources index for parasite test labs.)

How Parasites Spread

According to an article by the New England Medical Center, Tufts University School of Medicine, parasites are easily spread through normal daily activities.[1] Parasites "often find their way into water supplies, where they resist chlorination and are incompletely filtered from processed drinking water supplies, even when filtration is working optimally." Transmission can occur through fecally contaminated swimming-pool water, municipal water supplies, food, sexual activity, dogs, cats and other animals. Those at greatest risk are immunocompromised persons and children in day-care centers.[2] The following is a list of sources of contamination:

* Water sources: Rivers, lakes, wells, and tap water are potentially contaminated with harmful organisms. Drinking or swimming in water containing parasites is a primary way to become infected.
* Animals: Pets and farm animals are carriers of parasites. All animals contact parasites (particularly worms) outdoors, and if allowed indoors, expose their owners.
* Worldwide travel: The climate and conditions of various countries may support organisms that are easily communicated to foreigners. Travelers, who may not develop symptoms until returning, frequently bring parasites back to their native country where the organisms may be passed on to others.
* Raw and undercooked foods: Parasites are found in many raw and

undercooked foods, especially meat, fish and nuts. (Microwave cooking is often inadequate to destroy parasites.) Improperly treated raw fish in sushi is a frequent source of parasites. An infected food handler working in a restaurant kitchen can transmit parasites.

- Physical contact: Parasites are often spread through the close contact, especially by children during play and lack of proper hand-washing habits. Parasites are easily transmitted during sexual contact.
- Overuse of antibiotics: Antibiotics greatly interfere with the balance of the intestinal bio-culture, allowing the proliferation of harmful microorganisms.

Healing Strategy

Parasites affect the whole body chemistry; therefore other healing methods will not be fully effective until they are eradicated. A view from traditional Chinese medicine: Taking tonic herbs to strengthen a deficient, weakened digestive system of the person infected with parasites may further debilitate the person—the herbs may nourish primarily the parasites, causing them to proliferate. Making beneficial dietary changes is difficult when you are feeding both yourself and your parasites. Once the parasites are eliminated, the remaining health issues can be successfully addressed. Three key factors are collectively responsible for the effectiveness of this program. The first is to change the external environment to remove both the source of parasites and the factors that contribute to their spread. The second factor is to eliminate the internal environment that supports parasites. Conditions that promote parasites include a *damp* internal climate with excess mucus, imbalance in the intestinal flora, and/or chronic constipation. The program includes strategies for correcting these situations. Finally, we eliminate the unwanted organisms. Herbs and substances that destroy parasites accomplish this goal. The combination of these strategies produces a unique and highly effective anti-parasite plan.

Natural Therapies in the Parasite Purge Program

A. Prevention

During and after the program it is essential to prevent new parasitic infections:

- Checking your water source and buying a filter if necessary is a positive step toward avoiding re-infection. Avoid swallowing water when swimming.
- Parasites can be eliminated by treating all foods to be eaten raw with a parasiticide (treatment methods are listed on page 572). All meat, chicken, and fish need to be thoroughly cooked. Avoid microwave cooking for two reasons: Microwave ovens do not heat foods, particularly animal products, sufficiently to destroy parasites; and secondly, reliable research demonstrates that they denature and toxify foods (see page 60). Use a

separate cutting board for animal products, and wash it thoroughly after each use.
- Have pets routinely checked for worms. Putting a little garlic in their food regularly helps eliminate their parasites. Especially vulnerable are people who sleep with their animals or allow animals to lick their faces. The safest practice is to not have dogs, cats, birds or other animals live inside your house.
- Wash your hands thoroughly with soap and warm water after touching pets, using the bathroom, working in garden soil and before eating or preparing food.
- When traveling in foreign countries drink only bottled, purified, or boiled water. Eat only thoroughly cooked food. Avoid raw foods, dairy products, and iced drinks. Many travelers, who are careful with food and drink still become infected; often the culprit is ice in tea, water or other beverages, as ice is usually not made with purified water. Take citrus-seed extract or anti-parasitic herbal remedies between meals when traveling.

B. Intestinal Cleansing During Parasite Purge

A clogged, sluggish colon may be impacted with waste from years of poor dietary habits. This type of internal environment supports parasites, which can lie dormant in the gastrointestinal tract and resurface when the immune system is weakened. Keeping the intestines functioning effectively is an important part of any parasite purge.
- If constipation is a problem laxative herbs may be needed to assist the body in eliminating parasites. To determine which remedy is best for your constitutional type refer to information on pages 383–386.
- For breakfast eat ¼ to ⅓ cup of rinsed, raw brown rice. Chew until liquid, eat nothing else for three hours (hypoglycemic individuals may need to eat again sooner). Those with weak teeth may grind the raw rice coarsely (e.g., in a grain, coffee, or nut/seed mill), then soak it in water overnight, before eating. A daily raw-rice breakfast benefits all constitutional types during the program and is a key therapy. Eating raw rice deeply cleanses the intestines, removing impacted residues that shelter parasites. A parasite plan may be unsuccessful without this level of intestinal cleansing, regardless of the strength of the remedies.
- Options for those with gas and bloating: 1) "Papain" enzymes found in papaya are helpful in digesting accumulated mucus in the colon. Papain is available in capsule form. Follow directions on the product container. Avoid products containing ox bile, as it encourages the growth of giardia. 2) To relieve indigestion and balance the acid/alkaline level in the intestines, take a teaspoon of apple cider vinegar at the beginning of each meal. This increases beneficial gastric secretions and stimulates digestion. Try to obtain high quality vinegar (see page 205).

C. Re-establish Healthy Intestinal Microorganisms

1. Raw, saltless sauerkraut is an excellent food for regenerating the intestines. It harmonizes the digestion by balancing the secretions of the stomach, helps in the formation of enzymes and vitamins, strengthens the function of the pancreas, and improves the digestion of fats. Raw, saltless sauerkraut also helps maintain the acid-alkaline balance of the body, strengthens the nerves and the immune system, and stimulates blood formation. Its numerous benefits help to rejuvenate the whole body.

For maximum benefits sauerkraut is best eaten on a daily basis. Gradually introduce the new bacteria into the body by adding small amounts of sauerkraut at each meal. Eating large amounts of sauerkraut in the beginning can cause gas and bloating. One tablespoon per meal is good for the first week and the amount can be gradually increased to ¼–cup per meal. For a raw saltless sauerkraut recipe refer to page 609.

2. Nearly everyone needs to take a good-quality, viable pro-biotic supplement during the plan to re-establish healthy intestinal flora (examples are given at chart bottom on page 386). This recommendation is crucial for those who do not take the suggested fermented foods in this section. It is also helpful to take pro-biotic supplements daily when traveling.

3. Rejuvelac, and oat yogurt made with rejuvelac supply a source of friendly bacteria helpful in creating a balanced intestinal environment (recipes listed on pages 613–614).

D. Food Therapy Program

- It is essential to avoid overeating, and to chew all food thoroughly. This allows the food that is eaten to be digested properly, and facilitates the absorption of nutrients. Parasites thrive in *damp* conditions often created by inadequately digested foods. The most available and low-cost remedy is proper chewing.
- The dietary plan for the duration of this Purge Program is the candida diet on pages 73–75. Complying with the candida suggestions, or at least adapting them as much as possible to your current dietary needs, will improve the program's effectiveness. This is particularly the case if your previous diet has been poor, or if there is an acute or dangerous infection with a parasite or other pathogen. Eating the simple diet of the candida plan eliminates foods that encourage pathogenic organisms to spread quickly. This diet can also be used as a safeguard during an epidemic of infectious disease of any kind.
- If you are following a Regeneration DIET A, B or C (beginning on page 407), you can easily adapt to the candida plan during the Parasite Purge by simply avoiding certain items in some regeneration diets: fruit, wheat, corn, sweet potatoes, yams and concentrated sweeteners (except for stevia). Also avoid cooked rice although the previously recommended raw rice

breakfast is essential. If you have pronounced candida overgrowth signs (listed on page 72), it is best to continue with the candida diet after completing the Parasite Purge, until symptoms subside. The herbs recommended (later) in this program should be combined with those of the regeneration diets.

- Avoid eating foods that may carry parasites: In addition to undercooked meats mentioned earlier, avoid raw walnuts, which may harbor parasites; roast walnuts or cook them into food before eating. All produce, particularly watercress, lettuce, parsley, celery and water chestnuts, should not be eaten raw unless treated (see page 572).
- Choose foods that repel parasites. Add foods to the diet that contain the bitter, hot, and sour flavors; these assist the body in eliminating parasites.

The following foods and herbs have anti-parasitic properties:

Beneficial vegetables are beet, cabbage, carrot, garlic, leek, onion, radish, and sorrel. These vegetables have stronger anti-parasitic actions when eaten raw.

Helpful spices to use with foods are fennel, clove, cayenne, garden sage, ginger, horseradish and thyme.

Additional helpful foods are almond (use sparingly), kelp and umeboshi plum.

Roasted pumpkin seeds are especially helpful as they destroy parasites. (Lightly pan or oven roast to destroy *E. coli* on their surface.) They can be eaten with meals or as snacks although avoid them if you have difficulty digesting fats.

E. Herbs and Remedies

Prescription drugs may eliminate only one type of parasite, but herbs have a broad-spectrum effect. When using herbs or oxygen products, knowing the type of parasite infecting you is not usually necessary for your remedy to be effective. Herbs in the suggested formulas treat a wide variety of parasites, help dry the *damp* environment that parasites favor, and increase digestive function.

Herbs and other traditional remedies for parasites fall into several major groups, according to their flavor, thermal properties and other attributes.

Bitter and cold herbs such as *Chaparro armagosa,* black walnut *(Juglans nigra),* rhubarb root *(Rheum palmatum)* and wormwood *(Artemisia absinthium)* have been used effectively to treat parasite-induced chronic digestive disturbances because they are formidable parasiticides.

Chaparro armagosa is a specific remedy for giardia and amoebic dysentery, while black walnut is helpful for all types of parasites and could be included in most plans to eradicate harmful microorganisms of any type. It has traditionally been used for eczema, acne, boils, tumors, cancers and ulcers as well as parasites. Wormwood has been used by many natural healers for parasites; it stimulates liver and gall-bladder secretions and is a nervine (helps relax nerves). However, wormwood is potentially toxic and should be used with caution. Rhubarb also called Turkey rhubarb root, is a valuable laxative herb; it tonifies the digestive system and gently cleanses the intestines. It is safe to use for children.

In the formula section, these cold, bitter herbs will be used in combination with other herbs that modify their strong and somewhat noxious properties.

Garlic *(Allium sativum)*, prickly ash bark *(Xanthozylum americanum)*, and thyme *(Thymus vulgaris)* have warming and stimulating properties, destroy parasites and fungi, treat abdominal pain caused by *cold,* and have a tonic effect on the digestion. They are best taken before meals, to help stimulate gastric secretions.

Oil of Oregano, an exceptional antiseptic, has warming, drying, aromatic and acrid properties. It is frequently used as a broad-spectrum "antibiotic," but has potent antiviral and antifungal properties not found in standard antibiotics. It is taken against colds and flus, candidiasis, fungi, muscular pain including arthritis and fibromyalgia, virtually all dangerous microbes including anthrax, and parasites of all kinds, including the spirochete of Lyme disease. For lung conditions such as asthma, whooping cough, pneumonia, and tuberculosis, one may take the oil both internally and via vapor steaming (see below). For external diseases, e.g., acne, warts, psoriasis, ringworm, dandruff, bee stings and venomous bites, teeth and gum infections (rub in with finger), and athlete's foot, one may apply the oil topically as well as take it internally.

Researchers in Mexico have used oregano oil successfully against the tenacious giardia parasite. And according to research at Georgetown University completed in November, 2001, the oil may be may be more effective than antibiotics for some "staph" (staphylococcus) infections. A study in *Phytotherapy Research* demonstrates Oregano oil as a potent painkiller, particularly where inflammation is present.

Oregano oil is available in capsules, as a pure essential oil, or diluted in olive oil. *Dosages:* for the pure essential oil, take exactly one drop daily, diluted in a glass of water or in $\frac{1}{2}$ teaspoon of cold pressed flax oil or organic olive oil. The dilution in oil is better for sensitive individuals. If one drop makes the dilutions too acrid to ingest, take just $\frac{1}{2}$ of the water or oil each time. For commercially diluted products and capsules, follow product recommendations. As vapor-steaming therapy, place three to six drops of pure oil in a container of two quarts water that has set for 1 minute after boiling, and breathe the vapors. Repeat twice or three times daily. As an option, enclose a towel over your head down to the container so that the vapors are contained.

Note that many of the medicinal properties of oregano oil parallel those of raw garlic. (The healing properties of garlic are listed on pages 545–547.)

The extract of citrus seeds is bitter, sour, and slightly warming; it is an effective remedy for most constitutional types and is widely active against protozoa, viruses, pathogenic bacteria, and most other forms of parasites. Non-toxic, it can be used long-term. Taking citrus-seed extract is especially good for prevention when traveling.

Aloe vera gel and colloidal silver (a colloidal suspension of silver in water) are anti-parasitic and support the *yin* (the tissues and fluids) of the body.

When using the aloe vera plant, most people benefit from the gel unless there is a need for the cathartic effect of aloe powder. Aloe powder is a strong, bitter, cold cathartic-laxative, and should be used with caution. In contrast, the juice or gel of the aloe vera plant is a *yin* tonic, rejuvenative for the liver, spleen, intestines and the female reproductive system. (A further discussion of the properties of unrefined aloe vera gel appears on page 437.)

Silver-protein solutions, prior to the introduction of antibiotics, were used in the West as broad spectrum anti-microbial agents; nevertheless, such solutions could accumulate in the body, causing argyria, a permanent grayish discoloration of the skin. With the recent failure of antibiotics to cure a number of infectious diseases, silver is re-emerging as a natural antibiotic without the side effects of conventional antibiotics.

According to traditions of the Far East, metals such as gold, iron and silver are tonifying, with each metal doing so in unique ways. Deficient people cannot tolerate intensely bitter, hot, or aromatic herbs or substances for long periods of time. If they can withstand a small amount for short intervals, these strong substances can be balanced with silver colloid because of its *yin*-building effects, which cool and moisten the body, nurture the immune system and support tissue-building. Severely *deficient,* frail people with lengthy infections may exhibit deficient yin signs of heat and inflammation. This is where silver colloid truly shines.

True colloidal silver is electro-colloidally manufactured from just two ingredients—silver and water—at concentrations of 5 to 150 parts per million with a particle size of 4 to 25 nanometers. (See Resources index.) Any excess of silver is easily eliminated from the body. In contrast, many silver products are chemical solutions, not true colloids (even though they may be advertised as such) and contain stabilizers and nitrates—not listed on product labels. With silver concentrations of 50 to more than 500 parts per million, they, like the early compounds mentioned above, can cause argyria.

Formulas: The following herbal formulas are tailored to specific body constitutions; they destroy and expel parasites, and tonify the digestive system. The addition of concentrated green foods such as micro-algae and cereal grasses amplifies the cleansing effect of the herbs. (More information on green foods is given in Chapter 16.) Choose the plan that most closely fits your body type and signs.

Schedule: Due to the life-cycle of the parasites, the herbal remedies should be taken according to a schedule of ten days on, five days off, for a minimum of three, and as many as nine, times. The five days off gives parasite eggs an opportunity to hatch. If this cycle is not followed, the symptoms could become much worse when you stop the program. Most individuals who have marked degeneration and are following the Regeneration Diets (beginning on page 407) benefit from nine cycles. To decide on an appropriate number of cycles, you can add more cycles according to the number and strength of these signs: thick tongue coating, history of parasites, many signs of parasites, and deep or long-term illness. When following a program for several months, you may need to change which of the five options below you use, as your symptoms change.

1. Remedies for the **person with *deficient yin* signs** such as fresh-red cheeks and tongue, frequent thirst, tidal or afternoon fevers, night sweats, restlessness:
- Aloe vera juice—1–3 oz., 1–2 times daily
- Use colloidal silver at manufacturer's recommended dosage
- Green black walnut tincture—10 drops one time daily
- Wormwood leaf, Spearmint leaf, Fennel seed—25 drops or one capsule, two times daily.
- Chlorella or spirulina may be the most beneficial concentrated green food for *deficient yin* signs

2. Remedies for the ***deficient* person with normal thermal nature or with *cold* signs** such as cold hands and feet, pale face and pale, puffy tongue, weak, soft voice, low life-spark, fatigue:
- One small clove of raw garlic chopped finely into food with meals
- Oregano oil—see dosage on page 661
- Prickly ash bark, Sagebrush leaf, Ginger root, Thyme, Orange peel—25 drops or two capsules, 30 minutes before each meal
- Chlorella may be the most beneficial concentrated green food for *deficiency* or *deficiency* with *cold* signs

3. Remedies for the **very *deficient* person**—thin, frail, weak, introverted, pale, weak voice:
- Use colloidal silver at manufacturer's recommended dosage
- Oregano oil—see dosage on page 661
- Chlorella or spirulina may be the most beneficial concentrated green food for extreme *deficiency*

4. Remedies for the **person with *heat* signs** such as red face and tongue, aversion to heat, desire for large amounts of cold water or other drinks, frequent constipation, dark yellow urine, foul-smelling breath and stools:
- Green black walnut tincture—25 drops one time daily
- Wormwood leaf, Spearmint leaf, Fennel seed—25 drops or two capsules, 30 minutes before each meal
- Citrus seed extract—5–10 drops two times daily
- Blue Green Algae, wheat- or barley-grass, or alfalfa tablets may be the most beneficial concentrated green food for the over*heated* person
- For the robust individual with constipation, laxative herbs with specific parasite-expelling properties include: *Cascara sagrada,* and Turkey rhubarb root *(Rheum palmatum);* the formula on page 384 may be included with parasite herbs

5. Remedies for **robust person with normal signs or with *cold* thermal nature** such as pale face and tongue, aversion to cold, dislike of cold drinks, lack of thirst, clear water-like urine:

- One clove of raw garlic before meals
- Oregano oil—see dosage on page 661
- Prickly ash bark, Wormwood leaf, Sagebrush leaf, Ginger root, Thyme, Orange peel—20 drops or two capsules, 30 minutes before each meal
- Citrus seed extract—3 drops two times daily
- Alfalfa tablets or wheat- or barley-grass may be the most beneficial concentrated green food for the robust person with possible *cold* signs

How to make formulas: The preparation of all herbs in this section follows the guidelines in the *Dietary Transition* chapter on pages 110–111 except for (green) black walnut husk tincture: Black walnuts with husks should be harvested in the fall when they are green and beginning to ripen, but before they turn dark. Pack the whole walnuts with husks tightly into a glass jar and cover with 60–80 proof alcohol, place a lid on the jar, let set for two days only, and then pour off the alcohol tincture.

- Use equal proportions of herbs listed when making the herbal formulas in plans 1, 2, 4, & 5.
- All formulas listed are best used as tinctures but may be used in capsule form. Recommended capsule size—00. Herbs in capsules may cause digestive problems for those with weak digestion.
- Formulas are most effective taken on an empty stomach 1 hour to 30 minutes before a meal.

Notes: Green black walnut extract and herbal formulas similar to those above are frequently available at herbal outlets, and may be used as substitutes for the formulas in the above plans 1, 2, 4, & 5. (See also: Resources index.)

Though less than optimal, the herbal formulas will still be effective if one or more of the major ingredients is missing; the requirement for formula effectiveness is that at least one of the following ingredients is present: green black walnut, oregano oil, wormwood leaf, sagebrush leaf.

Additional Remedies:

Chaparro armagosa is an effective remedy for acute stage of amoebic dysentery and giardia. For acute symptoms (burning diarrhea and vomiting) take 25 drops 4–5 times daily until symptoms subside. *Chaparro* may be added (25 drops 1–2 times daily for two ten-day cycles) to any plan where chronic giardia is suspected.

Oxygen therapy is an especially powerful addition to any parasite program, as it destroys many types of parasites, viruses, amoebas, fungi and yeasts. A variety of oxygen products is now available and they need to be used with care. Two of the safest oxygen products are various compounds of stabilized oxygen and magnesium oxide. These products are often available at health food stores or by mail-order. Each manufacturer markets a different potency. Use the recommended dosage on the product. Hydrogen peroxide and ozone are other options (see pages 78–84). The green foods in the parasite program help protect the body from over-oxidation.

Artemisia Annua has been used for over two thousand years as a remedy for parasites and is being researched by the army as a therapy for drug-resistant malaria. At the present time there is a world-wide resurgence of malaria. Malaria is a parasite-borne disease spread by mosquitoes. The drug chloroquine which has been used successfully in the past, is often ineffective in killing the pathogen.[3] Many travelers to tropical countries return with difficult to treat malarial infection.

Artemisia annua is also used in the treatment of giardia; in addition, in the latter part of 2001, substantial evidence from research at the University of Washington was reported in *Life Sciences* journal suggesting that an extract of this plant can completely destroy breast cancer cells as well as leukemia cells.

It should be noted that we have discussed other plants in the artemisia family in this text, all of which have parasiticidal value: mugwort, wormwood, and sagebrush. *Artemisia annua* and citrus seed extract formulas are available through herb outlets and mail-order (see Resources index).

Important considerations:

- These plans are not recommended for pregnant and nursing mothers or children under age six. Young children respond well to treatment if they are on a good diet. A remedy for children is given on page 297. Children can also benefit from adding lightly roasted pumpkin seeds to their diet and following the hygienic and prevention ideals of this plan.
- The herbs and dosages included in this article are relatively non-toxic. If symptoms persist, see a health care professional.
- *Maintenance Plan:* Take anti-parasite remedies for two short cycles each year, and as a preventative measure when traveling. Suggested maintenance schedule: Every six months, take the indicated herbal remedies for two cycles: one week on and five days off. The best times to purge parasites are springtime and late summer.

The Purge Program is intended to provide an enduring solution to the very significant problem of parasites. Rejuvenating the digestive and immune systems from a debilitating parasitic infection may take years. A serious commitment is necessary to completely restore the body to health. The traditional American herbal remedies and modern nutritional strategies presented here have proven effective in a majority of cases.

Scabies

Scabies is a skin disease caused by an almost invisible organism *(Sarcoptes scabiei),* the "itch mite." It appears as a red, itchy rash found in mite burrows between fingers and toes, on elbows, wrists or in any sensitive areas, creases or folds in the skin. The itching intensifies at night.

The "itch" is highly contagious. There have been numerous epidemics in the past, especially during World War I and World War II. It spreads easily among schoolchildren due to their close contact, and is then transmitted to their family members by direct skin-to-skin contact or by sharing infected towels and clothing.

A major resurgence in the frequency of scabies infections is underway in the United States.[4] If you think you are infected you can obtain positive identification with a simple test at a medical clinic. The common treatment for scabies is Lindane™, a toxic drug.[5,6] With overuse Lindane has been thought to cause nerve and brain damage.

A less toxic, but highly effective folk remedy used in China and America is Sulfur Sublimed (or Flowers of Sulfur) available at drugstores. Nevertheless, some individuals are allergic to sulfur; if in doubt, test the following formula on a small patch of skin for one day, and monitor the patch for any adverse reaction.

Scabies Treatment Formula: Mix thoroughly 1 part Sulfur Sublimed and 5 parts quality oil such as coconut, virgin olive, or unrefined sesame, over low heat. After an evening shower, apply over entire body from the neck down before bed; pay careful attention and apply to all creases and folds of the skin, and under finger-and toenails. Shower in the morning. Do this for four consecutive nights.

This sulfur formula is also used in the treatment of psoriasis, eczema and impetigo.

APPENDIX B

The Effect of Root Canals on Health*

The dental procedure known as "root canal" is one whereby the nerve of a tooth is removed and the tooth is then filled with any of various materials. It is often performed on seriously infected teeth that cannot be saved in any other way, thus making it possible to retain teeth that would otherwise be extracted.

This well-intended procedure, however, can unfortunately seriously weaken health, according to well-documented research performed by the person some dentists believe to be the foremost dental researcher in history—Dr. Weston Price. It seems that root canals may cause dangerous weakening of the internal organs; people with seriously imbalanced health who have had root canals performed or recommended should consider how to treat this dental problem as a priority in their healing process.

Dr. Weston Price, former Director of Research of the American Dental Association for fourteen years, spent thirty-five years of his career researching the relationship between certain systemic diseases of the body, such as kidney and heart disease, and toxins that seep out from root-canal-filled teeth. His findings challenged the safety of the accepted dental practice of performing root canals and, as a result, caused quite a controversy in the dental community.

Price's research indicated that many people cannot tolerate root canals.[1,2] He found that if he removed root-filled teeth from people suffering from kidney and heart disease, in most cases their condition would improve. To establish a relationship between the tooth and the disease, he inserted the root-filled teeth under the skin of rabbits, whose immune systems are similar to that of humans. When he did this, the rabbits died within two days, and sometimes within twelve hours. If only a very small fragment were implanted, within two weeks the rabbit would lose over 20% of its body weight and die of either kidney or heart disease, correlated to the condition that the human donor had.

To further demonstrate the relationship, Price successively implanted the same tooth fragment in one hundred rabbits, and each died from the same disease the human had had. In contrast, a normal, non-infected tooth can be inserted under the

---

*Much of the dental information in this article is adapted from a paper by Dr. Hal A. Huggins, D.D.S., M.S., entitled "How Root Canals Generate Toxins." The options for oxygen, essential oil, and herbal treatment are suggestions of the present author.

skin of a rabbit for a year with no adverse reactions. Dr. Price's experiments clearly showed a relationship between root-filled teeth and degenerative diseases.

Price's further investigation into the root canal procedure revealed that inadequate sterilization of the teeth is the source of the problem. Streptococcal bacteria normally inhabit the mouth, and when a tooth begins to decay, they invade the tooth and start destroying tooth tissues. Once inside the tooth, they invade not only the pulp tissue, but also the "dentin" of the tooth. Dentin is composed of thousands of tiny tubules, which can house billions of Streptococcus bacteria. The problem is that the chemicals the dentist uses to sterilize the tooth for the root canal do not reach these dentin tubules. After the dentist seals the tooth, the remaining bacteria are left in the tooth chamber to proliferate.

There is no oxygen within the sealed tooth. In this anaerobic environment, the streptococci mutate to adapt to the new conditions. The normal bacteria produce only slightly offensive waste products in aerobic conditions. The anaerobic mutants, however, produce poisonous substances that seep out through tiny holes in the tooth. Unfortunately, our immune system cells are too large to fit through the holes and destroy the bacteria inside the tooth; but nutrient-rich fluids can seep into the tooth to feed the bacteria, allowing them to flourish. The bacteria are protected inside the tooth, releasing toxins into the body.

The body can have various responses to these toxins released from the tooth. Price's insights on these reactions challenged conventional thinking of the day. For instance, the body may form pus around the tooth in response to toxins. Price discovered that this pus is nearly sterile, and that it successfully quarantines toxins inside the tooth. His peers, on the other hand, saw the pus as a sign to administer antibiotics—which allows the poisons to continue to seep out. In other cases, there may be no pus formation or pain around the tooth, but enzymes may stimulate the formation of "condensing osteitis," a heavier substance than bone, around the tooth, fusing the tooth to the bone. In conventional medicine, this is considered to reflect excellent healing. However, Price knew that toxins can still seep out, and that if a person's immune system is weak, these toxins will attack internal organs.

Several risk factors predispose a person to developing problems from root canals. From 140,000 determinations in 1200 patients, Price found that hereditary factors make a person more susceptible to having adverse reactions to root canals. Specifically, a high frequency of degenerative disease in patients' families for two generations back puts them at higher risk. But certain stressors can make someone of healthy genetic stock more likely to develop disease from root canals. Dr. Price learned that the two greatest stressors were pregnancy and influenza. Under the influence of either of these conditions, the toxins from root-filled teeth are more apt to produce disease. Other risk factors are grief, anxiety, chilling, severe hunger, and acute or chronic infections.

To remove an offending root canal, more than just the tooth must be pulled. Studies show that the lymphocytes of auto-immune disease become embedded at least a millimeter into the bone. Therefore, this bone surface in addition to the tooth must be removed for best results.

Price's research, published in many peer reviewed journals, has never been refuted. Commercial expediency has, no doubt, discouraged dentists from changing their thinking on the root canal procedure, much to the misfortune of root canal recipients. Fortunately, however, a growing number of people are being educated about the dangers of root canals.

Alternatives and Recommendations: According to some holistically oriented dentists, when a root canal is indicated, there are alternatives, though all are less than ideal. Some feel that simply pulling the tooth is a less toxic procedure, and therefore preferable to a root canal. However, a missing tooth may weaken surrounding teeth, resulting in the possible loss of more teeth. Two other alternatives are: 1) an implanted tooth that is secured with a relatively non-reactive metal such as titanium, and 2) a "bridge."

Following are a few simple remedies to help keep toxicity low in a root canaled tooth: Ingest an oxygen supplement or an essential oil such as oregano oil or lavender oil three times a week, for example, on Monday, Wednesday, and Friday. One of the safest oxygen supplements for prolonged use is any of various stabilized oxygen compounds available in many health food stores or through mail-order (see Resources index). For using either essential oil, follow dosage guidelines on page 661 for ingestion of oregano oil. Because the body tends to adjust to the effects of these detoxifying substances, it may be ideal to cycle between them on a weekly basis, for example, one week take oregano oil, the next week, stabilized oxygen, and the final week, lavender oil. Then repeat.

If you have an imbalance that you believe is caused by root canals, you should experience better health before week seven on this protocol of essential oils and oxygen. If not, then you may increase the frequency of taking the remedies—to 4, 5, or 6 times a week—until there is improvement. If improvement is not evident at a dosage of once daily, 6 times per week, then these remedies may not be appropriate in your case or, your imbalance may stem from a cause other than root canals.

Another useful supplement is the herb "horsetail" *(Equisetum arvense)*, which has a strong affinity for teeth, strengthening and purifying their entire structure. The supplement form of this herb, either in tablets or capsules, must be specially prepared to be non-toxic (see Resources index); decocted horsetail tea is also non-toxic (see page 110 for "decoction" and dosage). We recommend taking horsetail as a foundation remedy to support the action of the stabilized oxygen and essential oils.

Resources: see "Publications and Organizations" in Resources Index for information on dental referral services that provide access to holistically oriented dentists.

Bibliography

with Selected Annotations

East-Asian Philosophy

Chan, Wing-Tsit. *A Source Book in Chinese Philosophy.* Princeton, NJ: Princeton Univ. Press, 1973

Deng, Ming-Dao. *The Wandering Taoist.* San Francisco, CA: Harper and Row, 1983. Records of practices of one of the last traditional Taoist communities in China.

Feng, Gia-Fu and English, Jane [translators]. *Chuang Tsu.* New York: Vintage Books, 1974

Mitchell, Stephen. *Tao Te Ching: A New English Version, with Foreword and Notes.* New York, NY: HarperPerennial, 1992. A superb translation that captures the inner intention of this ancient text. The foreword and notes provide important insights.

Liu, Wu-Chi and Lo, Irving Y. [editors]. *Sunflower Splendor—3000 Years of Chinese Poetry.* New York: Anchor Books, 1975

Vanamali. *Nitya Yoga: Essays on the Sreemad Bhagavad Gita.* Vanamali Publications, Vanamali Gita Yogashram, PO Tapovan 249-192, Via Shivananda Nagar, Rishikesh. U.P. (Himalayas) India. Provides lucid, easily understood, and practical insights into the East Indian classic—*Bhagavad Gita.*

Wilhelm, Richard and Baynes, Cary [translators]. *I Ching* or *The Book of Changes.* New York: Pantheon Books, 1966

Chinese Medicine: Theory and Foundations

Beinfield, Harriet and Korngold, Efrem. *Between Heaven and Earth: A Guide to Chinese Medicine.* New York: Ballantine Books, 1992. A skillful Five Element presentation integrated into other theories of Chinese medicine.

Connelly, Dianne M. *Traditional Acupuncture: The Law of the Five Elements* [2nd Edition]. Columbia, MD: Centre for Traditional Acupuncture Inc., 1994. An easily understood and creative treatment of Five Element theory.

Kaptchuk, Ted J. *The Web that has no Weaver: Understanding Chinese Medicine* [Revised Edition]. Chicago, Ill: Contemporary Books, 2000. A modern classic of Chinese medicine fundamentals with superb references.

Jarrett, Lonny S. *Nourishing Destiny: The Inner Tradition of Chinese Medicine.* Stockbridge, MA: Spirit Path Press, 1998. Chinese medicine and the evolution of consciousness. Encourages the reader to connect with the roots of Chinese healing arts.

Maciocia, Giovanni. *The Foundations of Chinese Medicine: A Comprehensive Text for Acupuncturists and Herbalists.* London: Churchill Livingstone, 1989. A clearly written, complete volume which sets the standard for foundation texts in Chinese medicine.

Ming, Zhu [translator]. *The Medical Classic of the Yellow Emperor.* Beijing: Beijing Foreign Language Press: 2001. Includes extremely informative annotations and commentaries. One of the most authoritative translations.

Ni, Maoshing. *The Yellow Emperor's Classic of medicine: a new translation of the Neijing Suwen with commentary.* 1st ed. Boston: Shambhala, 1995. An important translation with helpful interpretations.

O'Connor, John, and Bensky, Dan [translators]. *Acupuncture: A Comprehensive Text/Shanghai College of Traditional Medicine.* Seattle, WA: Eastland Press, 1981. In addition to acupuncture, contains a concise discussion of Chinese medical theory.

Omura, Yoshiaki. *Acupuncture Medicine.* New York: Japan Pub., 1982

Porkert, Manfred and Ullmann, Christian. *Chinese Medicine;* translated and adapted by Mark Howson. 1st Owl book ed. New York: H. Holt, 1990.

Veith, Ilza [translator]. *The Yellow Emperor's Classic of Internal Medicine.* Berkeley, CA: Univ. of California Press, 1972. The first commonly available translation of this text into English. An academic work that lacks detail needed for use in Chinese medicine.

Wiseman, Nigel [translator]. *Fundamentals of Chinese medicine.* [Rev. ed.] Brookline, MA: Paradigm Publications, 1995. Describes major disease patterns and presents basic herbal and acupoint remedies.

Chinese Dietary Therapy

Flaws, Bob. *The Tao of Healthy Eating: Dietary Wisdom According to Traditional Chinese Medicine.* Boulder, CO: Blue Poppy Press, 1998. Explains vegetarianism, cooked and raw food, candida, obesity and other topics in terms of Chinese medicine.

Lu, Henry C. *Chinese System of Foods for Health & Healing.* [edited by Laurel Ornitz]. New York: Sterling Publ., 2000. Offers a wealth of remedies and a valuable discussion of the principles of using food for healing.

Lu, Henry C. *Doctors' Manual of Chinese Medical Diet.* Vancouver, B.C., Canada: Academy of Oriental Heritage, 1981

Ni, Maoshing with Cathy McNease. *The Tao of Nutrition.* Santa Monica, CA: SevenStar Communications, 1993. A welcome text on Chinese dietary therapy, which recognizes the plight of American health as a problem resulting from excess animal products and refined foods.

Ayurvedic and Tibetan Medicine

Badjajew, Peter; Badjajew, Vladimir; and Park, Lynn. *Healing Herbs: The Heart of Tibetan Medicine.* Berkeley, CA: Red Lotus Press, 1982

Chopra, Deepak *et al. Perfect Health.* New York: Harmony Books, 1990. Uses principles of Ayurveda to provide creative insights into mental and physical health.

Donden, Yeshi. *Healing from the source: The Science and Lore of Tibetan Medicine.* Ithaca, NY: Snow Lion Publications, 2000. Imparts the basics of holistic Tibetan medicine and includes spiritual perspective.

Frawley, David. *Ayurvedic Healing: A Comprehensive Guide.* Sandy, UT: Passage Press, 1990. One of the most complete books on Ayurveda, with information suitable to both the layman and professional.

Lad, Vasant. *Ayurveda: The Science of Self-Healing.* Santa Fe, NM: Lotus Press, P.O. Box 6265, Santa Fe, NM 87502, 1984. A clear and simple explanation of the fundamentals of Ayurveda.

Rapgay, Lopsang. *The Tibetan Book of Healing.* Salt Lake City, UT: Passage Press, 1997. Applications of Tibetan medicine and Buddhist psychological guidelines. The Tibetan approach has points in common with Ayurveda from India and Chinese medicine.

Svoboda, Robert. *Prakruti: Your Ayurvedic Constitution.* Albuquerque, NM: Geocom, 1988. Contains invaluable insights into Ayurvedic diagnosis.

Thakkur, C.G. *Ayurveda: The Indian Art & Science of Medicine;* New York: ASI Publ., 1974

Tiwari, Maya. *Ayurveda Secrets of Healing: The Complete Ayurvedic Guide to Healing through Pancha Karma Seasonal Therapies, Diet, Herbal Remedies, and Memory.* Twin Lakes, WI: Lotus Press, 1995.

Tiwari, Maya. *A Life of Balance.* Rochester, VT: Healing Arts Press, 1995. Presents traditional Ayurveda with numerous excellent recipes.

Western Approach to Nutrition

Appleton, Nancy. *Lick the Sugar Habit.* Garden City Park, NY: Avery Pub., 1988. Demonstrates how sugar devastates immunity, leading to many disorders. Includes a self-help plan for overcoming sugar addiction and leading a healthy life. This plan cured the author of her sugar habit and chronic illnesses.

Ballentine, Rudolph. *Diet and Nutrition: A Holistic Approach.* Honesdale, PA: Himalayan International Institute, 1978. A seminal text for understanding nutrition from a blend of traditional and scientific perspectives.

Ballentine, Rudolph. *Transition to Vegetarianism: An Evolutionary Step.* Honesdale, PA: The Himalayan International Institute, 1987. Provides a readily workable method for becoming vegetarian.

Chaitow, Leon. *Amino Acids in Therapy.* Rochester, VT: Thorsons, 1985

Colbin, Annemarie. *Food and our Bones: The Natural Way to Prevent Osteoporosis.* New York: Plume, 1998

Cousens, Gabriel. *Conscious Eating.* Berkeley, CA: North Atlantic Books, 2000. A look at intuitive wisdom in helping make appropriate food choices. Dispels "one size fits all" diets through research and common sense.

Dean, Carolyn, MD. *The Miracle of Magnesium.* New York: Ballantine Books, 2003. Clearly written—latest research on the many health effects of the mineral magnesium.

Erasmus, Udo. *Fats that Heal, Fats that Kill: The Complete Guide to Fats, Oils, Cholesterol, and Human Health.* [Rev., updated and expanded ed.] Burnaby, BC, Canada: Alive Books, 1993

Fuchs, Nan Kathryn. *Overcoming the Legacy of Overeating: How to Change Your Negative Eating Patterns.* Los Angeles, CA: Lowell House, 1999

Gates, Donna. *The Body Ecology Diet: Recovering Your Health & Rebuilding Your Immunity.* [7th Edition] B.E.D. Publications. Helpful protocols for treating candidiasis.

Gittleman, Ann Louise. *Guess What Came To Dinner.* Garden City Park, NY: Avery Publishing Group Inc., 1993. All about parasites.

Guyton, Arthur C. *Textbook of Medical Physiology.* Philadelphia, PA: W.B. Saunders, 1990. A useful text for the nutritionist, especially for new understandings of the metabolic processes of protein and amino acids in the body.

Hendler, Sheldon Saul. *The Doctor's Vitamin and Mineral Encyclopedia.* New York: Simon and Schuster, 1990. Based on scientific experimentation, contains insights on the effectiveness of supplementation with vitamins, minerals, amino acids, lipids, herbs, and many other therapeutic substances.

Jarvis, D.C. *Folk Medicine.* Greenwich, CT: Fawcett Crest, 1958. A popular Vermont folk medicine classic, with numerous remedies based on apple cider vinegar, honey, kelp, and other foods. Precaution: the vinegar and honey remedies may not be appropriate for many long-term vegetarians.

Jenson, Bernard and Anderson, Mark. *Empty Harvest: Understanding the Link Between Our Food, Our Immunity, and Our Planet.* Garden City Park, NY: Avery Pub. Group, 1990

Jensen, Bernard. *The Chemistry of Man.* Escondido, CA: Bernard Jensen Pub., 1983

Meinig, George E. *Root Canal Cover-up.* Ojai, CA: Bion Pub., 1994. Exposes the suppression of information regarding the "root canal" dental procedure.

Murray, Michael and Pizzorno, Joseph. *Encyclopedia of Natural Medicine.* Rocklin, CA: Prima Publ., 1998. [Revised 2nd Edition.] A well-researched naturopathic guide to healing common diseases.

Price, Weston A. *Volume I: Dental infections, oral and systemic; Volume II: Dental infections and the degenerative diseases.* Cleveland, OH: The Penton publishing company, 1923. [Volume I presents researches on fundamentals of oral and systemic expressions of dental infections; volume II presents researches on clinical expressions of dental infections.

Price, Weston A. *Nutrition and Physical Degeneration.* La Mesa, CA: The Price-Pottenger Nutrition Foundation, 1945

Rudin, Donald O. and Felix, Clara. *The Omega-3 Phenomenon.* New York: Avon Books, 1988

Schaeffer, Severen L. *Instinctive Nutrition.* Berkeley, CA: Celestial Arts, 1987

Seely, Stephen *et al. Diet-Related Diseases.* New York: AVI Pub., 1985

Stanway, Penny. *Healing Foods: For Common Ailments.* London: Gaia Books Limited, 1998

Wilhelmi-Buchinger, Maria. *Fasting: The Buchinger Method.* Essex, England: Saffron Walden, the C.W. Daniel Co., 1986

Wood, Rebecca. *The New Whole Foods Encyclopedia: A Comprehensive Resource for Healthy Eating.* New York, NY: Penguin/Arkana, 1999. A catalog of healthful foods with inspired tips and valuable information.

Healing the Mind and Spirit

Cheung, C.S. *et al. Mental Dysfunction As Treated by Traditional Chinese Medicine.* San Francisco, CA: Traditional Chinese Medical Pub., 1986

Hammer, Leon. *Dragon Rises, Red Bird Flies.* Barrytown, NY: Station Hill Press, 1990. Explores connections between psychology and Chinese medicine.

Hanh, Thich Nhat. *Peace is Every Step: The Path of Mindfulness in Everyday Life.* New York, NY: Bantam Books, 1991. A world spiritual leader teaches how to adapt simple Zen principles for daily living and the way to peace.

Millenson, J.R. *Mind Matters: Psychological Medicine in Holistic Practice.* Seattle, WA: Eastland Press, 1995. Includes practical "mind-body" techniques for use in phsychological healing.

Nutrition and Mental Health. Sponsored by the U.S. Senate Select Committee on Nutrition and Human Needs, 1980. Documents the effects of nutrient deficiencies on learning disorders and behavioral problems.

Pfeiffer, Carl C. *Nutrition and Mental Illness: An Orthomolecular Approach to Balancing Body Chemistry.* Rochester, VT: Inner Traditions, 1988

Raheem, Aminah. *Soul Return: Integrating Body, Psyche, and Spirit.* Boulder Creek, CA: Aslan Publ., 1991. Uses psychotherapeutic models as well as Chinese Five Element theory in emotional therapy and to reveal dimensions of the soul in healing the whole person.

Werbach, Melvyn R. *Nutritional Influences on Mental Illness: Sourcebook of Clinical Research.* Tarzana, CA: Third Line Press, 1991. Integrates important literature concerning food therapies for many types of mental and behavior problems.

Wurtman, Judith. *Managing Your Mind and Mood Through Food.* New York: Rawson Associates, 1986

Chinese Herbology

Bensky, Dan, and Gamble, Andrew, with Kaptchuk, Ted. *Chinese Herbal Medicine: Materia Medica* [Revised] Seattle, WA: Eastland Press, 1993. An in-depth work covering more than 400 herbs and substances—for the serious student of Chinese herbalism.

Bensky, Dan and Barolet, Randall. [Translators] *Chinese Herbal Medicine: Formulas and Strategies* [Revised Edition]. Seattle, WA: Eastland Press, 1990. An invaluable contemporary classic that includes explanations of the inner workings of Chinese medical theory and herbology.

Fratkin, Jake. *Chinese Herbal Patent Medicines, A Clinical Desk Reference.* Boulder,

CO: Shya Publications, 2001. Greatly expanded edition. Covers over 1300 formulas with notes regarding endangered species, heavy metals, pharmaceuticals and research.

Hsu, Hong-Yen. *Oriental Materia Medica.* Long Beach, CA: Oriental Healing Arts Institute, 1986

Smith, F. Porter, and Stuart, G.A. *Chinese Medicinal Herbs.* San Francisco, CA: Georgetown Press, 1973

Western Herbology

Blumenthal, Mark [editor], *et al. The complete German Commission E monographs, Therapeutic guide to herbal medicines / developed by a special expert committee of the German Federal Institute for Drugs and Medical Devices.* Austin, Texas: American Botanical Council; Boston: Integrative Medicine Communications, 1998

Christopher, John R. *School of Natural Healing.* Provo, UT: Bi World Pub., 1978. One of the best collections of remedies in the American herbal tradition.

Felter, Harvey and Lloyd, John. *King's American Dispensatory.* Portland, OR: Eclectic Medical Publications, 1983. This is a modern printing of an 1898 classic that lists the medicinal uses and dosages of important herbs and pharmaceutical drugs. Much of its information on herbs is unavailable elsewhere.

Kloss, Jethro. *Back to Eden: A Human Interest Story of Health and Restoration to be Found in Herb, Root, and Bark.* Loma Linda, CA: Back to Eden Books Pub., 1988. In the early 20th century, Jethro Kloss developed timeless herbal and food therapies still in use today.

Santillo, Humbart. *Natural Healing with Herbs.* Prescott Valley, AZ: Holm Press, 1985

Tierra, Michael. *Planetary Herbology.* Santa Fe, NM: Lotus Press, 1988. A combination of Eastern (Ayurvedic and Chinese) and Western herbal traditions.

Worwood, Valerie. *The Complete Book of Essential Oils and Aromatherapy.* San Raphael, CA: New World Library, 1991. Covers a wide range of essential oil use, including cooking.

Green Foods

Henrikson, Robert. *Earth Food: Spirulina.* Laguna Beach, CA: Romore Enterprises, 1989

Hills, Christopher. *Secrets of Spirulina: Medical Discoveries of Japanese Doctors.* Boulder Creek, CA: INM Books, University of the Trees Press, 1980

Meyerowitz, Steve. *Wheatgrass, Nature's Finest Medicine: The Complete Guide to using Grass, Foods & Juices to help your Health.* [6th ed.] Great Barrington, MA: Sproutman Publications, 1999

Scientific Research Digest on Chlorella. Hokkaido, Japan: Medicinal Plant Institute of Hokkaido, 1987 [on Medline Data Base computer network, information retrieval: 1737191]

Vonshak, Avigad. [editor] *Spirulina platensis (Arthrospira): physiology, cell-biology, and biotechnology.* London; Bristol, PA: Taylor & Francis, 1997.

Seaweeds

Arasaki, Seibin and Teruko. *Vegetables from the Sea.* Tokyo, Japan: Japan Pub. Inc., 1983

Bradford, Peter and Montse. *Cooking With Sea Vegetables: A Collection of Naturally Delicious Dishes Using to the Full the Bountiful Harvest of the Oceans.* Rochester, VT: Healing Arts Press, New York: 1985

Ellis, Lesley. *Seaweed: A Cook's Guide: Tempting Recipes for Seaweed and Sea Vegetables.* Tucson, AZ: Fisher Books, 1999

Erhart, Shep and Cerier, Leslie. *Sea Vegetable Celebration.* Summertown, TN: Book Pub. Co., 2001

Lewallen, Eleanor and John. *The Sea Vegetable Gourmet Cookbook and Forager's Guide.* Order from Mendocino Sea Vegetable Co., Box 372, Navarro, CA 95463.

Children

Conners, C. Keith. *Feeding the Brain: How Foods Affect Children.* New York: Plenum Press, 1989

Cournoyer, Cynthia. *What About Immunizations? Exposing the Vaccine Philosophy.* Santa Cruz, CA: Nelson's Books, 1995

Crook, William G. *Help for the Hyperactive Child.* Jackson, TN: Professional Books, 1991. Includes nutritional methods for helping the hyperactive child without drugs.

Green, Nancy S. *The Nontoxic Baby.* (204 N. El Camino Real, Suite E214,) Encinitas, CA: Natural Choices, 1991. Identifies common toxins in the baby's room, care products and foods.

Johnson, Roberta Bishop. *Whole Foods for the Whole Family: Cookbook.* Franklin Park, IL: La Leche League International,1993

Neustaedter, Randall. *The Immunization Decision: A Guide for Parents.* Berkeley, CA: North Atlantic Books, 1990

O'Mara, Peggy. *The Way Back Home: Essays on Life and Family.* Santa Fe, NM: Mothering, 1991. Mothering also publishes books on vaccinations, circumcision, schooling at home, teens, being a father, midwifery and the law; for a catalog, write Mothering, P.O. Box 1690, Santa Fe, NM 87504.

Samuels, Mike and Nancy. *The New Well Pregnancy Book.* New York: Simon & Schuster, 1996

Schauss, Alexander; Meyer, Barbara; and Meyer, Arnold. *Eating for A's.* New York: Pocket Books, 1991. A program for replacing refined and poor-quality foods with nutritious whole foods rich in the "learning nutrients" used by the brain.

Scott, Julian. *Natural Medicine for Children.* New York: Avon Books, 1990. An excellent guide to treating and preventing childhood illness (from birth through age twelve) with diet, herbs, homeopathy, massage, and awareness methods. The reader may make choices for many of the remedies by following simple evaluation tests of the child, which are often based on Chinese healing principles.

The Womanly Art of Breastfeeding. Schaumburg, IL: La Leche League International, 1997

Whole Foods for Kids to Cook. Schaumburg, IL: La Leche League Inter national, 1995

Ecology, Politics, and Ethics of Food

Adams, Carol, J. *The Inner Art of Vegetarianism: Spiritual Practices for Body and Soul.* New York: Lantern Books, 2000. Well-written; deepens the experience of vegetarianism.

Anderson, Luke. *Genetically Engineered Food and our Environment.* White River Junction, VT: Chelsea Green Publishing, 1999

Berthold-Bond, Annie. *Better Basics for the home: Simple Solutions for Less Toxic Living.* New York, Three Rivers Press, 1999. A handbook of over 800 recipes for alternatives to common household toxins.

Lappé, Frances M. *Diet for a Small Planet—20th Anniversary Edition.* New York: Ballantine Books, 1991. An appropriate dietary plan for the present condition of the planet. This edition is an improvement over the original, recognizing that protein requirements are easily met in vegetarians without complementing amino acid profiles among plant foods.

Lappe, Frances M. and Baily, B. *Against the grain: Biotechnology and the Corporate Takeover of your food.* Cambridge, MA: Common Courage Press, 1998. The serious risks to health and ecosphere from genetic engineering. Exposes biotechnology's propaganda.

Lappé, Frances M. *Rediscovering America's Values.* New York: Ballantine Books, 1991

Nestle, Marion. *Food and Politics: How the Food Industry Influences Nutrition and Health.* Berkeley, CA: U-CAL Press. 2002. A nutritionist writes about the big corporations pushing junk food and soft drinks; the food pyramid and food policies.

Phelphs, Norm. *The Dominion of Love: Animal Rights According to the Bible.* New York: Lantern Books, 2002. Encourages all who revere Biblical scripture to find ways to halt the suffering inflicted on animals.

Robbins, John. *The Food Revolution: How Your Diet Can Help Save Your Life and the World.* Berkeley, CA: Conari Press, 2001. An inspiring document indicating the devastating effect of poor food choices on the fate of the earth. A political and ecologic foundation for plant-based diets.

Teite, Martin and Wilson, Kimberly A. *Genetically Engineered Food: Changing the Nature of Nature.* Rochester, VT: Park Street Press, 1999. Excellent explanation of genetic engineering and explores the health risks.

Towns, Sharon and Daniel. *Voices from the garden: Stories of Becoming a Vegetarian.* New York, NY: Lantern Books, 2002

Degenerative Diseases and Immunity

Addanki, Sam. *Diabetes Breakthrough.* New York: Pinnacle Books, 1982

Borell, G.L. *The Peroxide Story.* Box 487, Stanton, CA 90680

Gerson, Max. *A Cancer Therapy: Results of Fifty Cases.* Bonita, CA: Gerson Inst., 1986

Jochems, Ruth. *Dr. Moerman's Cancer Diet.* Garden City Park, NY: Avery Pub., 1990. First tried in Holland in the 1930s, these dietary plans have been gradually accepted as useful therapy, and now are approved by the government of Holland. This text includes the Moerman diets in detail, with an explanation of how they work.

LeBeau, Conrad. *Hydrogen Peroxide Therapy.* Hales Corners, WI: Vital Health Publ., 1989

Levine, Stephen A. and Kidd, Parris M. *Antioxidant Adaptation: Its Role in Free Radical Biochemistry.* San Francisco: Biocurrents Press, 1985

Viebahn, Renate. *The use of ozone in medicine.* Heidelberg, Germany: K.F. Haug Publisher, 1994. A fine treatise on the many uses of ozone; this book was also published in 1987 by Medicina Biologica, Portland, Oregon.

Whitaker, Julian. *Reversing Heart Disease.* New York: Warner Books, 1985. Based on results of Dr. Whitaker's experience with 2,000 heart patients, this text shows why modern research is finding heart disease generally easy to prevent and cure. Contains a complete natural care program for avoiding and repairing heart disease without drugs or surgery.

Toxins and Radiation

Dadd, Debra Lynn. *The Non-Toxic Home: Protecting Yourself and Your Family from Everyday Toxics and Health Hazards.* Los Angeles, CA: Jeremy P. Tarcher, Inc., New York: Distributed by St. Martin's Press, 1986

Dadd, Debra Lynn. *Nontoxic, Natural, and Earthwise.* New York: St. Martins, 1990. Lists sources for healthful, nontoxic products; over 2,000 products—from building materials to clothing to foods—are rated based on personal and planetary environmental impact.

Farlow, Christine. *Dying to Look Good: The Disturbing Truth About What's Really in Your Cosmetics, Toiletries and Personal Care Products.* Escondido, CA: KISS for Health Publishing, 2001

Farlow, Christine. *Food Additives: A Shopper's Guide to What's Safe and What's Not.* Escondido, CA: KISS for Health Publishing, 1999

Mott, Lawrie and Snyder, Karen. *Pesticide Alert: A Guide to Pesticides in Fruits and Vegetables.* San Francisco, CA: Sierra Club Books, 1988

Schechter, Steven R. *Fighting Radiation with Foods, Herbs and Vitamins.* Brookline, MA: East-West Health Books, 1988

Schwartz, George R. *In Bad Taste: The MSG Syndrome.* Santa Fe, NM: Health Press, 1988. Documentation of mild-to-severe reactions caused by monosodium glutamate, a flavor enhancer found (and often disguised) as an additive in many common foods.

Webb, Tony and Lang, Tim. *Food Irradiation—Who Wants It?* Rochester, VT: Thorson's Pub., 1987

Cookbooks

Beeby, Max and Rosie. *Cafe Max and Rosies: Vegetarian Cooking with Health and Spirit.* Berkeley, CA: Ten Speed Press, 2000

Brown, Edward Espe and Madison, Deborah. *The Greens Cookbook: Extraordinary Vegetarian Cuisine from the Celebrated Restaurant.* New York: Bantam, 1987

Fallon, Sally. *Nourishing Traditions: The Cookbook That Challenges Politically Correct Nutrition and the Diet Dictocrats.* Washington DC: New Trends Publishing,1999. Unites traditional dietary patterns, often based on the research of Weston Price, with scientific research.

Kaufmann, Klaus and Schoneck, Annelies. *The Cultured cabbage: Rediscovering the Art of Making Sauerkraut.* Alive Books. 1998. How to make sauerkraut, in a crock, jar, or a barrel. Has a score of tasty recipes.

Lair, Cynthia. *Feeding the Whole Family.* Seattle, WA; Moon Smile Press, 1997. Sound advice on simple, nutritionally healthful cooking for parents with children of all ages.

McCarthy, Meredith. *Sweet and Natural: More Than 120 Naturally Sweet and Dairy-Free desserts.* New York: St. Martin's Press, 1999

Meyerowitz, Steve. *Sproutman's Kitchen Garden Cookbook.* Great Barrington, MA: Sproutman Publications, 1999. Recipes using sprouts in everything from bread to ice cream.

Mollison, Bill. *The Permaculture Book of Ferment and Human Nutrition.* Australia: Tagari Publications, 1998. An extensive study and explanation of cultured food and how to store and make it—a basic survival handbook.

Morningstar, Amita, and Desai. *The Ayurvedic Cookbook: A Personalized Guide to Good Nutrition and Health.* Sante Fe, NM: Lotus Press, 1990

Pickarski, Brother Ron, O.F.M. *Friendly Foods: Gourmet Vegetarian Cuisine.* Berkeley, CA: Ten Speed Press, 1991

Shurtleff, William and Akiko Aoyagi. *The Book of Tofu and Miso.* Berkeley, CA: Ten Speed Press, 2001

Sources of Data for Tables, Charts, and Nutritional Statistics

Pennington, Jean [revised by]. Bowes and Church's *Food Values of Portions Commonly Used: 15th Edition.* Philadelphia, PA: J.B. Lippincott, 1989

National Research Council. *Recommended Dietary Allowances: 10th Edition.* Washington, D.C.: National Academy Press, 1989

Agriculture Handbook No. 8, Revised. *Composition of Foods, Raw, Processed,*

Prepared. Washington, D.C.: U.S. Dept. of Agriculture:

8-1 Dairy and Egg Products, Nov 1976

8-4 Fats and Oils, June 1979

8-5 Poultry Products, Aug 1979

8-9 Fruits and Fruit Juices, Aug 1982

8-11 Vegetables and Vegetable Products, Aug 1984

8-12 Nut and Seed Products, Sep 1984

8-16 Legumes and Legume Products, Dec 1986

Agriculture Handbook No. 456, *Nutritive Value of American Foods in Common Units.* U.S. Dept. of Agriculture, 1975

U.S. Dept. of Agriculture Provisional Tables, Washington, D.C.: Fatty Acid and Cholesterol Content of Selected Foods, March 1984

Data supplied by various food manufacturers and companies

References and Notes

Chapter 1: Origins & Access to Healing with Whole Foods

1. Combs, G.F. Jr., Selenium in global food systems. *British Journal of Nutrition* 85(5): pp 517–547, May 2001

2. Rayman, M.P. The importance of selenium to human health. *Lancet* 356(9225): pp 233–241, July 15 2000

3. *Ibid.*

4. Pizzulli, A.and Ranjbar, A. Selenium deficiency and hypothyroidism: A new etiology in the differential diagnosis of hypothyroidism in children. *Biological Trace Element Research* 77(3): pp 199–208, Dec 2000

5. Whanger, P.D. Selenium and the brain: A review. *Nutrition Neuroscience* 4(2): pp 81–97, 2001

6. *Op cit.* reference 1

7. Sandstrom, P.A., Murray, J., *et al.* Antioxidant defenses influence HIV-1 replication and associated cytopathic effects. *Free Radical Biology and Medicine* 24(9): pp 1485–1491, June 1998

8. Deidda, D.and Lampis, G., Antifungal, antibacterial, antiviral and cytotoxic activity of novel thio- and seleno-azoles. *Pharmacological Research* 36(3): pp 193–197, Sep 1997

9. Sinatra, S.T. and DeMarco, J. Free radicals, oxidative stress, oxidized low density lipoprotein (LDL), and the heart: Antioxidants and other strategies to limit cardiovascular damage. *Connecticut Medicine* 59(10): pp 579–588, Oct 1995

10. Vijaya, J., Subramanyam, G., *et al.* Selenium levels in dilated cardiomyopathy. *Journal of the Indian Medical Association* 98(4): pp 166–169, Apr 2000

11. Darlington, L.G.and Stone, T.W. Antioxidants and fatty acids in the amelioration of rheumatoid arthritis and related disorders. *British Journal of Nutrition* 85(3): pp 251–69, Mar 2001

12. Mai, J., Sorensen, P.S., Hansen, J.C. High dose antioxidant supplementation to MS patients. Effects on glutathione peroxidase, clinical safety, and absorption of selenium. *Biological Trace Element Research* 24(2): pp 109–17, Feb 1990

13. Standing Committee on the Scientific Evaluation of Dietary Reference Intakes. *Dietary Reference Intakes for Calcium, Phosphorus, Magnesium, Vitamin D, and Fluoride.* Washington, DC: National Academy of Sciences; 1997.

14. Iannello, S. and Belfiore, F. Hypomagnesemia.

A review of pathophysiological, clinical and therapeutical aspects. *Panminerva Medica* 43(3): pp 177–209, Sep 2001

15. Saris, Nils-Erik L., Mervaala, E. *et al.* Magnesium: An update on physiological, clinical and analytical aspects. *Clinica Chimica Acta; International Journal of Clinical Chemistry* Volume 294 (1–2), pp 1–26, April 2000

16. Durlach, J., Pages, N., *et al.* Biorhythms and possible central regulation of magnesium status, phototherapy, darkness therapy and chronopathological forms of magnesium depletion. *Magnesium Research* 15(1–2): pp 49–66, Mar 2002

17. Dean, Carolyn, MD. *The Miracle of Magnesium.* New York: Ballentine Books, 2003

18. *Op cit.* reference 16

19. Russell, I.J., Michalek, J.E., Flechas, J.D., Abraham, G.E. Treatment of fibromyalgia syndrome with Super Malic: A randomized, double blind, placebo controlled, crossover pilot study. *Journal of Rheumatology* 22(5): pp 953–958, May 1995

20. Magaldi, M., Moltoni, L., *et al.* Changes in intracellular calcium and magnesium ions in the physiopathology of the fybromyalgia syndrome [Article in Italian]. *Minerva Medica* 91(7–8): pp 137–140, Jul-Aug 2000

21. Ng, S.Y. Hair calcium and magnesium levels in patients with fibromyalgia: a case center study. *Journal of Manipulative Physiological Therapeutics* 22(9): pp 586–93, Nov-Dec, 1999

22. Chilton, S.A. Cognitive behaviour therapy for the chronic fatigue syndrome. Evening primrose oil and magnesium have been shown to be effective. *BMJ* 312(7038): pp 1096; discussion 1098, Apr 26, 1996

23. Shilis, M.E. Magnesium in health and disease. *Annual Review of Nutrition* 8: pp 429–460, 1988

24. *Op cit.* reference 17, pp 139, 155

25. *Op cit.* reference 23

26. Haas, Elson M., MD. *Staying Healthy with Nutrition* Berkeley, CA: Celestial Arts Publ, p 167, 1992

27. Squier, T.C. Oxidative stress and protein aggregation during biological aging. *Experimental Gerontology* 36(9): pp 1539–1550, Sep 2001

28. Seelig, Mildred S.. *Magnesium Deficiency in the Pathogenesis of Disease: Early Roots of Car-*

diovascular, Skeletal, and Renal Abnormalities. New York: Plenum Medical Book Co., 1980

29. Kawahara, M. and Kuroda, Y. Intracellular calcium changes in neuronal cells induced by Alzheimer's beta-amyloid protein are blocked by estradiol and cholesterol. *Cellular and Molecular Neurobiology* 21(1): pp 1–13, Feb 2001

30. O'Neill, C., Cowburn, R.F., *et al.* Dysfunctional intracellular calcium homoeostasis: a central cause of neurodegeneration in Alzheimer's disease. *Biochemical Society Symposia* (67): pp 177–194, 2001

31. Johnson, S. The multifaceted and widespread pathology of magnesium deficiency. *Medical Hypotheses* 56(2): pp 163–170, Feb 2001

32. *Op cit.* reference 15

33. Dean, Carolyn, MD. *The Miracle of Magnesium.* New York: Ballentine Books, 2003, p 23

34. Mattson, M.P.and Chan, S.L., *et al.* Presenilin mutations and calcium signaling defects in the nervous and immune systems. *Bioessays* 23(8): pp 733–44, Aug 2001

35. Anderson, I., Adinolfi, C., *et al.* Oxidative signalling and inflammatory pathways in Alzheimer's disease. *Biochemical Society Symposia* (67): pp 141–149, 2001

36. Morris, M.C., Evans, D.A., *et al.* Dietary intake of antioxidant nutrients and the risk of incident Alzheimer disease in a biracial community study. *Journal of the American Medical Association* 287(24): pp 3230–3237, Jun 26 2002

37. Rock, E., Astier, C., *et al.* Magnesium deficiency in rats induces a rise in plasma nitric oxide. *Magnesium Research* 8(3): pp 237–242, Sep 1995

38. Ornish D., Scherwitz, L.W., *et al.* Effects of stress management training and dietary changes in treating ischemic heart disease. *Journal of the American Medical Association* 249(1): pp 54–59, Jan 7 1983

39. *Op cit.* reference 14

40. Davis, M.M. and Jones, D.W. The role of lifestyle management in the overall treatment plan for prevention and management of hypertension. *Seminars in Nephrology* 22(1): pp 35–43, Jan 2002

41. Milan, A., Mulatero, P., *et al.* Salt intake and hypertension therapy. *Journal of Nephrology* 15(1): pp 1–6, Jan-Feb 2002

42. Ornish D., Scherwitz L.W., *et al.* Intensive lifestyle changes for reversal of coronary heart disease. *Journal of the American Medical Association* 280(23): pp 2001–2007, Dec 16 1998

43. Contact: Dean Ornish, MD, Founder and President, Preventive Medicine Research Institute, Clinical Professor of Medicine, University of California, San Francisco, 900 Bridgeway, Suite 1, Sausalito, California 94965, USA; email: DeanOrnish@aol.com

44. The National Institute of Arthritis and Musculoskeletal and Skin Diseases.

45. Atkins, Robert C.. *Dr. Atkins' New Diet Revolution.* New York : Quill, 2002.

46. Qureshi, A.A., Sami, S.A., *et al.* Effects of stabilized rice bran, its soluble and fiber fractions on blood glucose levels and serum lipid parameters in humans with diabetes mellitus Types I and II. *Journal of Nutritional Biochemistry* 13(3): pp 175–187, Mar 2002

47. Qureshi, A.A., Mo, H., *et al.* Isolation and identification of novel tocotrienols from rice bran with hypocholesterolemic, antioxidant, and antitumor properties. *Journal of Agricultural and Food Chemistry* 48(8): pp 3130–3140, Aug 2000

48. Kim, K.M., Yu, K.W. et al. Anti-stress and anti-fatigue effects of fermented rice bran. *Bioscience, Biotechnology, and Biochemistry* 65(10): pp 2294–2296, Oct 2001

49. Macdonald, I.A. Carbohydrate as a nutrient in adults: Range of acceptable intakes. *European Journal of Clinical Nutrition* 53 Suppl 1: pp S101–S106, Apr 1999

50. Cicero, A.F. and Gaddi, A. Rice bran oil and gamma-oryzanol in the treatment of hyperlipoproteinaemias and other conditions. *Phytotherapy Research* 15(4): pp 277–289, Jun 2001

51. Wei, Y.H., Lu, C.Y., *et al.* Oxidative stress in human aging and mitochondrial disease-consequences of defective mitochondrial respiration and impaired antioxidant enzyme system. *Chinese Journal of Physiology* 44(1): pp 1–11, Mar 31, 2001

52. Mai, J., Sorensen, P.S., Hansen, J.C. High dose antioxidant supplementation to MS patients. Effects on glutathione peroxidase, clinical safety, and absorption of selenium. *Biological Trace Element Research* 24(2): pp 109–17, Feb 1990

53. Darlington, L.G. and Stone, T.W. Antioxidants and fatty acids in the amelioration of rheumatoid arthritis and related disorders. *British Journal of Nutrition* 85(3): pp 251–69, Mar 2001

54. Linnane, A.W., Zhang, C., *et al.* Human aging and global function of coenzyme Q10. *Annals of the New York Academy of Sciences* 959: pp 396–411; discussion 463–465, Apr 2002

55. Lamson, D.W. and Plaza, S.M. Mitochondrial factors in the pathogenesis of diabetes: A hypothesis for treatment. *Alternative Medical Review* 7(2): pp 94–111, Apr 2002

56. Beal, M.F. Coenzyme Q10 as a possible treatment for neurodegenerative diseases. *Free Radical Research* 36(4): pp 455–460, Apr 2002

57. Lister, R.E. An open, pilot study to evaluate

the potential benefits of coenzyme Q10 combined with Ginkgo biloba extract in fibromyalgia syndrome. *Journal of International Medical Research* 30(2): pp 195–199, Mar-Apr 2002

58. Sen, C.K., Khanna, S., *et al.* Oxygen, Oxidants, and Antioxidants in Wound Healing: An Emerging Paradigm. *Annals of the New York Academy of Sciences* 957: pp 239–249, May 2002

59. Bagchi, D., Bagchi, M., *et al.* Cellular Protection with Proanthocyanidins Derived from Grape Seeds. *Annals of the New York Academy of Sciences* 957: pp 260–270, May 2002

60. Levinson, Harold N.. *Total Concentration : How to Understand Attention Deficit Disorders, with Treatment Guidelines for You and Your Doctor.* New York : M. Evans, 1990.

61. Ladd, S.L., Sommer, S.A., *et al.* Effect of phosphatidylcholine on explicit memory. *Clinical Neuropharmacology* 16(6): pp 540–54, Dec 1999

62. Sahakian, B., Joyce, E., Lishman, W.A. Cholinergic effects on constructional abilities and on mnemonic processes: A case report. *Psychological Medicine* 17(2): pp 329–333, May 1987

63. Rosenberg, G.S. and Davis, K.L. The use of cholinergic precursors in neuropsychiatric diseases. *American Journal of Clinical Nutrition* 36(4): pp 709–720, Oct 1982

64. Filla, A. and Campanella, G. A six-month phosphatidylcholine trial in Friedreich's ataxia. *Canadian Journal of Neurological Sciences* 9(2): pp 147–150, May 1982

65. Hsu, H.H., Grove, W.E., *et al.* Gastric bezoar caused by lecithin: An unusual complication of health faddism. *American Journal of Gastroenterology* 87(6): pp 794–796, Jun 1992

66. Ghoneum, M. and Jewett, A. Production of tumor necrosis factor-alpha and interferon-gamma from human peripheral blood lymphocytes by MGN-3, a modified arabinoxylan from rice bran, and its synergy with interleukin-2 in vitro. *Cancer Detection and Prevention* 24(4): pp 314–324, 2000

67. Herberman, R.B. Cancer immunotherapy with natural killer cells. *Seminars in Oncology* 29 (3 Suppl 7): pp 27–30, 2002 Jun

68. Ghoneum, M. Anti-HIV activity in vitro of MGN-3, an activated Arabinoxylane from rice bran. *Biochemical Research Communications.* 243: pp 25–29, 1998

69. Basse, P.H., Whiteside, T.L., Herberman, R.B. Cancer immunotherapy with interleukin-2-activated natural killer cells. *Molecular Biotechnology* 21(2): pp 161–170, Jun 2002

70. Ghoneum, M. and Manatalla, G. NK immunomodulatory function in 27 patients by MGN-3, a modified arabinoxylane from rice bran. Abstract. 87th Annual Meeting of the American Association of Cancer Research, Washington, DC, Apr. 1996

71. Ghoneum, M. Immunomodulatory and Anticancer properties of MGN-3, a modified xylose from rice bran, in 5 patients with breast cancer. Abstract. American Association for Cancer Research Special Conference: The Interface between basic and applied research, Baltimore, MD., Nov. 1995

72. Ghoneum, M. NK Immunorestoration of Cancer Patients by MGN-3, a modified arabinoxylane rice bran (study of 32 patients up to 4 years). Abstract, 6th International Congress on Anti-Aging and Bio-medical Technologies (American Academy of Anti-Aging Medicine), Las Vegas, Nevada, December 1998

73. A report in progress, regarding over 100 patients, by Mamdooh Ghoneum, PhD, Chief of Research, Dept of Otolaryngology, Charles D. Drew University of Medicine and Science, 1621 East 120th Street, Los Angeles, CA 90059 USA

74. *Op cit.* reference 66

75. Jariwalla, R.J. Inositol hexaphosphate (IP6) as an anti-neoplastic and lipid-lowering agent. *Anticancer Research* 19(5A): pp 3699–3702, Sep-Oct 1999

76. Grases, F. and Costa-Bauza, A. Phytate (IP6) is a powerful agent for preventing calcifications in biological fluids: Usefulness in renal lithiasis treatment. *Anticancer Research* 19(5A): pp 3717–3722, Sep-Oct 1999

77. El-Sherbiny, Y.M., Cox, M.C., *et al.* G0/G1 arrest and S phase inhibition of human cancer cell lines by inositol hexaphosphate (IP6). *Anticancer Research* 21(4A): pp 2393–2403, Jul-Aug 2001

78. Deliliers, G.L., Servida, F., *et al.* Effect of inositol hexaphosphate (IP6) on human normal and leukaemic haematopoietic cells. *British Journal of Haematology* 117(3): pp 577–587, Jun 2002.

79. Shamsuddin, A.M. Metabolism and cellular functions of IP6: A review. *Anticancer Research* 19(5A): pp 3733–3736, Sep-Oct 1999

80. Valencia, S., Svanberg, U. *et al.* Processing of quinoa (Chenopodium quinoa, Willd): effects on in vitro iron availability and phytate hydrolysis *International Journal of Food Science and Nutrition* 50(3): pp 203–211, May 1999

81. Centeno, C. and Viveros, A. Effect of several germination conditions on total P, phytate P, phytase, and acid phosphatase activities and inositol phosphate esters in rye and barley. *Journal of Agricultural and Food Chemistry* 49(7): pp 3208–3215, Jul 2001

82. Rowland, R.. American Heart Association weighs in on fat substitutes; *AHA Scientific Statement* June 10, 2002

83. Shide, D.J. and Rolls, B.J. Information about the fat content of preloads influences energy intake in healthy women. *Journal of the American Dietetic Association.* 95: pp 993–998, 1995

84. Young, L.R. and Nestle, M. The contribution of expanding portion sizes to the US obesity epidemic. *American Journal of Public Health* 92(2): pp 246–249, Feb 2002

85. Smith, B.L. Organic foods vs supermarket foods: element levels. *Journal of Applied Nutrition* 45(1), 1993

86. Worthington, V. Nutritional quality of organic versus conventional fruits, vegetables, and grains. *The Journal of Alternative and Complementary Medicine* 7(2): pp 161–173, April, 2001

87. Troubled times amid commercial success for roundup ready soybeans: Glyphosate efficacy is slipping and unstable transgene expression erodes plant defenses and yields: by Dr. Charles M. Benbrook, Northwest Science and Environmental Policy Center, Sandpoint Idaho, www.biotech-info.net, May 3, 2001

88. *The Calgary Herald,* Wed, June 2, 1999 page B8; by Charles Clover and George Jones, Reprinted from *The Daily Telegraph* (London, UK)

89. *The Daily Telegraph* (London, UK), "GM crop firms should be liable for any damage done, says Prince" by Caroline Davies in Lubeck. Edited, June 12, 2002

90. Sierra Legal Defence Fund organization website: www.sierralegal.org June 17, 2002.

91. "Genetically modified organisms 25 years on." The Institute of Science in Society Feature Articles. [Presented at the First National Conference on Life Sciences, Selangor, Malaysia, May 21–22, 2002]. www.i-sis.org.uk

92. Pollock, K.M. Exercise in treating depression: broadening the psychotherapist's role. *Journal of Clinical Psychology* 57(11): pp 1289–1300, Nov 2001

93. Lane, A.M. and Lovejoy, DJ. The effects of exercise on mood changes: the moderating effect of depressed mood. *Journal of Sports Medicine and Physical Fitness* 41(4): pp 539–545, Dec 2001

94. Somer, Elizabeth.. *Food & Mood : The Complete Guide to Eating Well and Feeling Your Best.* New York: Henry Holt, 1999.

95. Atkins, Robert C.. *Dr. Atkins' new diet revolution.* New York: Quill, 2002.

96. The Stillman Diet in the 1960's; Dr. Atkins Diet in the 1970's; The Scarsdale diet in the late 1970's and 1980's; More recently, in the 1990's and continuing into the early 21th Cenury: Dr. Atkins New Diet Revolution; Sugar Buster's Diet; The Carbohydrate Addict's Diet by Rachael and Richard Heller; Suzanne Somer's Diet; Protein Power by Mary and Michael Eades, and others.

97. Alford, B.B., Blankenship, A.C., Hagen, R.D. The effects of variations in carbohydrate, protein, and fat content of the diet upon weight loss, blood values and nutrient intake of adult obese women. *Journal of the American Dietetic Association* 90: pp 534–540, 1990

98. Sarwer, D.B. and Wadden, T.A. The treatment of obesity: what's new, what's recommended. *Journal of Womens Health and Gender Based Medicine* 8(4): pp 483–493, May 1999

99. Swaminathan R. Nutritional factors in osteoporosis. *International Journal of Clinical Practice* 53(7): pp 540–548, Oct-Nov 1999

100. Taal, M.W. and Brenner, B.M. Evolving strategies for renoprotection: non-diabetic chronic renal disease. *Current Opinion in Nephrology and Hypertension* 10(4): pp 523–31, Jul 2001

101. Brand-Miller, J.C., Holt, S.H. *et al.* Glycemic index and obesity. *American Journal of Clinical Nutrition* 76(1): pp 281S-285S, 2002 Jul

102. *Ibid.*

103. Lichtenstein, A.H. and Schwab, U.S. Relationship of dietary fat to glucose metabolism. *Atherosclerosis* 150(2): pp 227–243, Jun 2000

104. Chen, H., Ward, M.H., *et al.* Dietary patterns and adenocarcinoma of the esophagus and distal stomach. *American Journal of Clinical Nutrition* 75(1): pp 137–144, Jan, 2002

105. Brown, W.V. and Karmally, W. Coronary heart disease and the consumption of diets high in wheat and other grains. *American Journal of Clinical Nutrition* 41(5 Suppl): pp 1163–1171, May 1985

106. Fleming, R.M. The effect of high-, moderate-, and low-fat diets on weight loss and cardiovascular disease risk factors. *Preventive Cardiology* 2002 Summer; 5(3): pp 110–118

107. Cordain L, Miller JB, Eaton SB, Mann N. Macronutrient estimations in hunter-gatherer diets. *American Journal of Clinical Nutrition* 72(6): pp 1589–92, Dec 2000

108. Cordain, L., Miller, J.B., Eaton, S.B., *et al.* Plant-animal subsistence ratios and macronutrient energy estimations in worldwide hunter-gatherer diets. *American Journal of Clinical Nutrition* 71(3): pp 682–92, Mar 2000

109. Dickson, J.H. Scientists analyze Stone Age

man's last meal. *Archaeology Today* 10/24/2001

110. Nestle, M. Animal v. plant foods in human diets and health: Is the historical record unequivocal? *Proceedings of the Nutrition Society* 58(2): pp 211–218, May 1999

111. USDA/NASS Monthly Reports from the year 2001

112. Frank Waters, Oswald White Bear Fredericks. *The Book of The Hopi;* Reprint edition, Viking Press, 1985

113. Székely, Edmond Bordeaux.. *The Essene Gospel of Peace* San Diego, CA: Academy of Creative Living, 1971–74.

114. A number of biblical scholars, modern-day Essenes, vegetarians, Christians and nutritionists are interested in whether Jesus was vegetarian. Some arguments in favor of the idea include: 1) Jesus was never described in the Bible as eating meat. The biblical story that Jesus created fish to feed the multitude is similar to the scripture that describes Gautama Buddha creating meat for his disciples. Orthodox Buddhists sometimes claim that such meat created by a Christ or Buddha carries no karma for those who ingest it. 2) There is some evidence that Jesus was connected with the Essenes, a vegetarian desert community in the region where Jesus lived most of his life. The forty-day fast by Jesus in the desert, described in the New Testament of the Bible, was a standard purification protocol for Essene masters. 3) The Dead Sea Scrolls, discovered in the mid-Twentieth Century, are thought by some scholars to be older and have greater validity than other scriptural sources. Some of these documents have been interpreted to suggest that Jesus was an Essene. In fact, one document—*The Humane Gospel of Christ*"—liberated from Jesuit priests by John Allegro of the scroll team, is a record of the teachings of Jesus as an Essene master. (This document is not considered valid by some established churches today.)

A similar finding predating the Dead Sea Scrolls occurred in 1891. A clergyman from Great Britain, Reverend G. J. Ouseley, received and translated a document that had reportedly been hidden by ancient Essenes in a Buddhist monastery in Tibet. The document, which he translated as *The Gospel Of The Holy Twelve* contains much of what the standard four gospels contain but also includes the teachings of Jesus against the killing of animals and eating of flesh meat. From the book's introduction: "... the Roman Churchmen at Nicea opposed these doctrines and eliminated them from the Gospels, which they radically changed so as to be acceptable to Constantine, who loved the red meats and flowing wine of his midnight feasts too much to accept a religion that prohibited these pleasures, which was a main reason why he so bitterly persecuted the early Christians who advocated these doctrines. For this reason the Church Fathers changed the Gospel in such a way that Love and Compassion were limited only to human beings but the animal expressions of life were excluded from receiving these benefits."

The Hungarian physician, Professor Edmond Bordeaux Székely, discovered an evangelical text in the royal library in Wien [Vienna], written in ancient Slavonian language. Later he found the original, written in Aramaic, in the Vatican library. From this document, Székely extracted the areas attributed to the teachings of Jesus that dealt with bodily health including recommendations for vegetarian diet. He published this in German under the name *Heliand* in 1937. Later it was published in English as *The Essene Gospel of Peace.*

Various other texts and fragments have also been discovered in recent years. Like the above documents, many carry similar messages, sometimes in identical wording.

This information is important in that Christian thought permeates the laws, morals, social attitudes and customs, and the development of our way of life in the West perhaps more than any other force. If we come to accept that the original Christian teachings recommend compassion toward animal life, this would, in my opinion, dramatically and positively influence how we live on the planet.

None of the above information is presented as proof that original Christians were vegetarians. I hope, however, it will stimulate creative thought and encourage further investigation.

115. Yamori, Y., Miura, A., Taira, K. Implications from and for food cultures for cardiovascular diseases: Japanese food, particularly Okinawan diets. *Asia-Pacific Journal of Clinical Nutrition* 10(2): pp 144–145, 2001

116. *Op cit.* reference 110

117. Pitskhelauri, G.Z. trans/edited by Gari Lesnoff-Caravaglia. *The Longliving of Soviet Georgia.* New York: Human Sciences Press, 1982

118. Atkins, Robert C.. *Dr. Atkins' New Diet Revolution.* New York : Quill, 2002.

119. Shintani, T.T., Beckham S., *et al.* The Hawaii Diet: ad libitum high carbohydrate, low fat multi-cultural diet for the reduction of chronic disease risk factors: obesity, hypertension, hypercholesterolemia, and hyperglycemia. *Hawaii Medical Journal* 60(3): pp 69–73, Mar 2001

120. Campbell, T. Colin & Cox, Christine. *The China Project: Revealing the Relationiship Between Diet and Disease.* Ithaca, NY: Paracelsian, Inc, p 10. Tel order # for book: 607-257-4224. www.paracelsian.com, 1996

121. *Op cit.* reference 119

122. *Op cit.* reference 120, all pages.

123. Grogan, Bryanna Clark. *Authentic Chinese Cuisine: For the Contemporary Kitchen.* Summertown, Tenn.: Book Pub. Co., 2000.

124. "Universally regarded as the most outstanding Buddhist of the Chinese order in the modern era." (Richard Hunn) "Dharma successor of all five Chan schools; main reformer in the Chinese Buddhist Revival (1900–50). Born Chuan Chou (Quan Zhou), Fukien (Fujian) province. Left home at 19. At 20 took precepts with master Miao Lien and received Dharma name Ku Yen [Hsu Yun]. In 56th year achieved final awakening at Kao Min Ssu in Yang Chou (Yang Zhou). Thereafter began revival and teaching work. Eventually invited to take charge of the Sixth Patriach's temple (Tsao-Chi/Chao Xi), then very rundown; restored it along with temples and monasteries; also founded many schools and hospitals. Died in his 120th year. Had also traveled in Malaysia and Thailand, and taught the King of Thailand. Autobiography: *Empty Cloud* (translated by Charles Luk)." –From *The Seeker's Glossary of Buddhism*

125. Sturm R, Wells KB. Does obesity contribute as much to morbidity as poverty or smoking? *Public Health* 115(3): pp 229–35, May 2001

126. Gillman, M.W., Rifas-Shiman, S.L., *et al.* Risk of overweight among adolescents who were breastfed as infants. *Journal of the American Medical Association* 285(19): pp 2461–7, May 16, 2001

127. Kruzel, M.L. and Janusz, M. Towards an understanding of biological role of colostrinin peptides. *Journal of Molecular Neuroscience* 17(3): pp 379–389, Dec 2001

128. Ogra, P.L. and Dayton, D.H. (editors) Immunology of breast milk: A monograph of the National Institute of Child Health and Human Development. New York: Raven Press, 1979

129. Janusz, M. and Lisowski, J. Proline-rich polypeptide (PRP)—an immunomodulatory peptide from ovine colostrum. *Archivum Immunoogiae et Theapiae Experimentalis* (Warsz) 41(5–6): pp 275–279, 1993

130. Ley, B.M. *Immune system control: colostrum & lactoferrin.* Detroit Lakes, MN : BL Publications, 2000

131. Ballard, F.J., Nield, M.K. *et al.* The relationship between the insulin content and inhibitory effects of bovine colostrum on protein breakdown in cultured cells. *Journal of Cellular Physiology* 110(3): pp 249–254, March 1982

132. Mero, A., Miikkulainen, H., *et al.* Effects of bovine colostrum supplementation on serum IGF-I, IgG, hormone, and saliva IgA during training. *Journal of Applied Physiology* 83(4): pp 1144–1151, Oct 1997

133. Sporn, M.B., *et al.* … Bovine colostrum used for wound healing. *Science,* 219: pp 1329–1331, 1983

134. Rump, J.A. and Arndt, R. Treatment of diarrhoea in human immunodeficiency virus-infected patients with immunoglobulins from bovine colostrum. *Clinical Investigations* 70(7): pp 588–594, July 1992

135. Greenberg, P.D. and Cello, J.P. Treatment of severe diarrhea caused by Cryptosporidium parvum with oral bovine immunoglobulin concentrate in patients with AIDS. *Journal of Acquired Immune Deficiency Syndromes and Human Retrovirology* 13(4): pp 348–354: Dec 1996

136. Mortensen, E.L., Michaelsen, K.F., *et al.* The association between duration of breastfeeding and adult intelligence. *Journal of the American Medical Association* 287(18): pp 2365–71, May 8, 2002

137. Hanson, L.Å., Strömbäck, L., *et al.* The immunological role of breast feeding. Pediatric Allergy and Immunology. 12(s14) p 15, May 2001

138. Hanson, L.Å. Human milk and host defence: Immediate and long-term effects. *Acta Paediatrica* Supplement 88(430): pp 42–46, Aug 1999

139. *Dr. Schulze's Bi-Monthly Newletter* [Natural Healing Publications; Tel: 877-832-2463] p 5, May, 2002

140. McCullough, M.L., Feskanich, D., *et al.* Adherence to the Dietary Guidelines for Americans and risk of major chronic disease in men. American Journal of Clinical Nutrition 72(5): pp 1223–1231, November 2000

141. According to the National Association of Specialty Food Trade (NASFT), 2002

Chapter 4: Heat/Cold, Chapter 5: Interior/Exterior: Building Immunity and Chapter 6: Excess/Deficiency

1. O'Connor, J., Bensky, D. *Acupuncture: A Comprehensive Text.* Seattle, WA: Eastland Press, 1981, p 39

2. Russell-Manning, B. *Self-Treatment for AIDS.* San Francisco: Greensward Press, 1989, p 58

3. Clifford, D.P. and Repine, J.E. Hydrogen peroxide mediated killing of bacteria. *Molecular and Cellular Biochemistry* 49: pp 143–149, 1982

4. For information on hydrogen peroxide from Fr. Wilhelm, contact him in writing at 6600 Trail Blvd., Naples, FL 33940

5. Freibott, G. *et al.* Oxidation—the key to cancer and degenerative diseases. *Cancer News Journal* 18(4): Winter 83–84.

6. Pang, T.Y. *Chinese Herbal.* Rt 1, Box 117, East Sound, WA: Tai Chi School of Philosophy and Art (Publisher), 1982, p 38

7. Teff is tiny, native Ethiopian grain-like seed that is now being grown in the United States; it is becoming more widely available at stores carrying unrefined foods. Teff excels at regulating blood sugar levels and has a rich nutritional profile, being especially concentrated in protein and iron. It can enrich other grain dishes such as millet, oats or rice. It imparts a uniquely substantial and nourishing quality not found in other foods, and Ethiopians prefer it above all other grains. We find that teff, especially the common dark varieties, strengthens the kidneys, particulary their *yin* aspect, which in turn helps reduce stress and support renewal, fluid metabolism, and growth and development of the body.

Chapter 7: Dietary Transition

1. Chen, J., Campbell, T.C. *et al. Diet, Lifestyle and Mortality in China: a Study of the Characteristics of 65 Counties.* Ithaca, NY: Cornell Univ. Press [co-publishers: Oxford Univ. Press and The China People's Medical Publishing House], 1990, p 97

2. King, R.G. Do raised brain aluminum levels in Alzheimer's dementia contribute to cholinergic neuronal deficits? *Medical Hypotheses* 14: pp 301–306, Jul, 1984

3. Roberts, E. A systems approach to aging, Alzheimer's disease, and spinal cord regeneration. *Progress in Brain Research* 86: pp 347–348, 1990

4. Candy, J.M. *et al.* Aluminosilicates and senile plaque formation in Alzheimer's disease. *The Lancet* 1(8477): pp 354–357, Feb 15, 1986

5. Jones, H.B. and Jones, H. *Sensual Drugs.* Cambridge, England: Cambridge University Press, 1977, pp 255, 306. In this same well-researched volume, additional effects of marijuana use are documented: RNA/DNA damage, brain atrophy as well as irreversible brain damage, cell metabolism upset, and others. A sequel, *The Marijuana Question* (New York: Dodd, Mead & Co., 1985), by Helen Jones and Paul Lovinger, discusses further studies on marijuana use.

6. Jacob, S.W. and Francone, C.A. *Structure and Function in Man.* Philadelphia, PA: W.B. Saunders and Co., 1974, p 42

Chapter 8: Water

1. Adapted from Federal water studies by cancer researcher Dr. Wm. D. Kelley, author of *One answer to cancer: an ecological approach to the successful treatment of malignancy.* Kelley Foundation, 1974

2. Bridges, M.A. *Bridges' Dietetics for the Clinician.* 5th Ed. Revision [See Dr. H.J. Johnson's study on vitamin E] Philadelphia, PA: Lea & Febiger, 1949

3. Price, J.M. *Coronaries, Cholesterol & Chlorine.* New York: Jove Publications, 1984

4. Bensky, D. and Gamble, A. *Chinese Herbal Medicine—Materia Medica.* Seattle: Eastland Press, 1986, p 576

5. Yiamouyiannis, J. *Fluoride: The Aging Factor.* Delaware, OH: Health Action Press, 1986

6. Von Mundy, V.G. Influence of fluorine and iodine on the metabolism, particularly on the thyroid gland. *Muenchener Medicishe Wochenschrift* 105: pp 182–186, 1963

7. Stolc, V. *et al.* Effect of fluoride on the biogenesis of thyroid hormones. *Nature* 188(4758): p 855, 1960

8. Yiamouyiannis, J. *op. cit.,* pp 43–69

9. Robbins, J. *Diet for a New America.* Walpole, NH: Stillpoint Pub., 1987, p 367

10. *Ibid.* p 373

11. Lappé, F., Collins, J. *et al. Food First.* Boston, MA: Houghton-Mifflin, 1977. Recommended for information on how the world food shortage is a result of types of food consumed as well as global political and financial manipulation.

Chapter 9: Protein and Vitamin B$_{12}$

1. One of the first books to emphasize "complete" protein for vegetarians was *Diet for a Small Planet* by Frances Moore Lappé. Since the time of its first printing in 1972, however, she has had different thinking on the subject: "As I said in my first editions, it is true that we do get more protein if we combine grains and beans, for example, rice and lentils. . . . But over the years I've come to the conclusion that if we eat a very balanced diet (not junk food and not one solely of certain root crops), there is absolutely no danger of not getting enough protein. I've showed that even with no accounting for complementarity [of foods for maximum protein] and having no animal food in your diet—meat, fish, eggs, dairy, etc.—you can still get all the protein if you eat a healthy grain and vegetable diet."—*East West Journal*, Feb, 1982

2. Rose, W. The amino acid requirements of adult man. *Nutritional Abstracts and Reviews* 27: p 631, 1957

3. Guyton, A.C. *Textbook of Medical Physiology.* Philadelphia, PA: W.B. Saunders Co., 1986, p 831

4. Hua, H. *Buddha Root Farm.* San Francisco, CA: Buddhist Text Translation Society, 1731 15th St. San Francisco, CA 94103, 1976, p 64. In a transcription of this 1975 lecture at a Pure Land retreat in Oregon, Chinese Zen Partriach Hsuan Hua suggested that taking the life of a higher animal, because of its concentration of sentience, may be the karmic equivalent of destroying an entire species of plants. If this is true, the taking of plant life in quantities necessary for an entire human lifetime is certainly preferable to the effect (karma) accumulated from the killing of even one animal.

5. Deng Ming-Dao. *The Wandering Taoist.* San Francisco: Harper and Row, 1983

6. Gerras, C. *The Complete Book of Vitamins.* Emmaus, PA: Rodale Press, p 222

7. Bensky, D. and Gamble, A. *Chinese Herbal Medicine—Materia Medica.* Seattle: Eastland Press, 1986, p 475

8. Briggs, D.R. *et al.* Vitamin B_{12} activity in comfrey (Symphytum sp.) and comfrey products. *Journal of Plant Foods.* (London) 5: pp 143–147, 1983

9. Dagnelie, P.C. *et al.* Vitamin B_{12} from algae appears not to be bioavailable. *American Journal of Clinical Nutrition.* 53: p 695, Mar 1991

10. Areeku, S. *et al.* The source and content of vitamin B_{12} in the tempehs. *Journal of the Medical Association of Thailand.* 73: pp 152–156, Mar 1990

11. Albert, M.J., Mathan V.I. and Baker S.J. Vitamin B_{12} synthesis by human small intestinal bacteria. *Nature.* 283: pp 781–782, Feb 21, 1980

12. Lindenbaum, J. *et al.* Neuropsychiatric disorders caused by cobalamin deficiency in the absence of anemia or macrocytosis. *New England Journal of Medicine.* 318: pp 1720–1728, 1988

13. Craig, G.M. *et al.* Masked vitamin B_{12} and folate deficiency in the elderly. *British Journal of Nutrition* 54(3): pp 613–619, Nov 1985

14. Giugliana, E.R.J. *et al.* Serum vitamin B_{12} levels in parturients, in the intervillous space of the placenta and in full-term newborns and their interrelationships with folate levels. *American Journal of Clinical Nutrition* 41: pp 330–335, Feb 1985

15. Van Den Berg, H., Dagnelie, P.C., and Van Staveren, W.A. Vitamin B_{12} and seaweed. *The Lancet* pp 242–243, Jan 30, 1988

16. Herbert, V. and Drivas, G. Spirulina and vitamin B_{12}. *Journal of the American Medical Association* 248(23): pp 3096–3097, 1982

17. Stabler, S.P. *et al.* Inhibition of cobalamin-dependent enzymes by cobalamin analogues in rats. *Journal of Clinical Investigation* 87: pp 1422–1430, Apr 1991

18. Dostalova, L. Vitamin status during puerperium and lactation. *Annals of Nutrition and Metabolism* (Basel, Switzerland) 28: pp 385–408, Nov/Dec 1984

19. [Editorial.] Pregnant vegetarian. *Nutrition and the M.D.* (Van Nuys, CA) 10: pp 4–5, May 1984

20. Specker, B. *et al.* Increased urinary methylmalonic acid excretion in breast-fed infants of vegetarian mothers and identification of an acceptable dietary source of vitamin B_{12}. *American Journal of Clinical Nutrition* 47(1): p 89, Jan 1988

21. Craig, G. *et al.* Masked vitamin B_{12} and folate deficiency in the elderly. *British Journal of Nutrition* (Cambridge, U.K.) 54: pp 613–619, Nov 1985

22. Abramsky, O. Common and uncommon neurological manifestations as presenting symptoms of vitamin B_{12} deficiency. *Journal of the American Geriatrics Society* 20: pp 95–96, Feb, 1972

23. McLaren, D.S. A fresh look at protein-calorie malnutrition. *The Lancet* 2: pp 485–488, 1966

24. Winick, M. *Nutrition and Drugs.* New York: Wiley, 1983

25. Shinwell, E.D. and Gorodischer, R. Totally vegetarian diets and infant nutrition. *Pediatrics* 70: pp 582–586, Oct 1982

26. Hendler, S. *The Doctor's Vitamin and Mineral Encyclopedia.* New York: Simon and Schuster, 1990, pp 377–379; also see index references to "mental functioning," p 489

27. Steenblock, D. *Chlorella: Natural Medicinal Algae.* El Toro, CA: Aging Research Inst., 1987, p 4

28. Hills, C. [Editor] *The Secrets of Spirulina: Medical Discoveries of Japanese Doctors.* Boulder Creek, CA: University of the Trees Press, 1980, pp 11, 206

29. Allen, L.H. *et al.* Protein-induced hypercalcuria: a longer-term study. *American Journal of Clinical Nutrition* 32: pp 741–749, Apr 1979

30. Lu, H. *Doctor's Manual of Chinese Medical Diet.* Vancouver, B.C., Canada: Academy of Oriental Heritage, 1981

31. Flaws, B. and Wolfe, L. *Prince Wen Hui's Cook* Brookline, MA: Paradigm Pub., 1983

32. Ni, M. *The Tao of Nutrition.* Los Angeles, CA: The Shrine of Eternal Breath of Tao, 1987

Chapter 10: Oils and Fats

1. Carroll, K.K. Dietary fats and cancer. *American Journal of Clinical Nutrition* 53(4 Suppl): pp 1064S-1067S, Apr 1991

2. Statland, B.E. Nutrition and cancer. *Clinical Chemistry* 38(8B Pt 2): pp 1587–1594, Aug 1992

3. Chen, J., Campbell, T.C. *et al. Diet, Lifestyle and Mortality in China: a Study of the Characteristics of 65 Counties.* Ithaca, NY: Cornell Univ. Press [co-publishers: Oxford Univ. Press and The China People's Medical Publishing House], 1990, p 97

4. Dannenberg, A.L. and Kannel, W.B. Remission of hypertension: the "natural" history of blood pressure treatment in the Framingham Study. *Journal of the American Medical Association* 257: pp 1477–1483, 1987

5. O'Brien, J.S. *et al.* Quantification of fatty acid and fatty aldehyde composition of ethanolamine, choline and serine glycerophosphatides in human cerebral grey and white matter. *Journal of Lipid Research* 5: pp 329–338, 1964

6. Walker, B.L. Maternal diet and brain fatty acids in young rats. *Lipids* 2: pp 497–500, 1967

7. Lamptey, M.S. and Walker, B.L. A possible essential role for dietary linolenic acid in the development of the young rat. *Journal of Nutrition* 106: pp 86–93, Oct 1976

8. Simopoulos, A.P. Omega-3 fatty acids in health and disease and in growth and development. *American Journal of Clinical Nutrition* 54: pp 438–463, Sep 1991

9. Harris, W.S. *et al.* Will dietary omega-3 fatty acids change the composition of human milk? *American Journal of Clinical Nutrition*, 40: pp 780–785, 1984

10. Sinclair, A.J. Incorporation of radioactive polyunsaturated fatty acids into liver and brain of the developing rat. *Lipids* 2: pp 175–184, 1975

11. Mohrhauer, H. and Holman, R.T. The effect of dietary essential fatty acids upon composition of polyunsaturated fatty acids in depot fat and erythrocytes of the rat. *Journal of Lipid Research* 4: pp 346–350, 1963

12. "Earthrise Newsletter" Number 10: Earthrise Company (P.O. Box 1196, San Rafael, CA 94915), 1988; references for research in China and Mexico are cited on page 4.

13. Putnam, J.C. *et al.* The effect of variations in dietary fatty acids on the fatty acid composition of erythrocyte phosphaticylcholine and phosphatidylethanolamine in human infants. *American Journal of Clinical Nutrition* 36: pp 106–114, 1982

14. Rudin, D.O. "Omega-3 Fatty Acids in Medicine." *1984–85 Yearbook of Nutritional Medicine.* J. Bland, Editor. New Canaan, CT: Keats Pub., 1985, p 41

15. Begin M.E., Ells G., Das U.N., and Horrobin D.F. Differential killing of human carcinoma cells supplemented with n-3 and n-6 polyunsaturated fatty acids. *Journal of the National Cancer Institute* 77(5): pp 1053–1062, Nov 1986

16. Keane, W.R. *et al.* Hyperlipidemia and the progression of renal disease. *American Journal of Clinical Nutrition* 47: pp 157–160, 1988

17. Rudin, D.O. and Felix, C. *The Omega-3 Phenomenon.* New York: Rawson Associates, 1987, pp 46, 47, 87

18. Lee, T.H. *et al.* Effects of dietary fish oil lipids on allergic and inflammatory diseases. *Allergy Proceedings* 12: pp 299–303, Sep-Oct, 1991

19. Ornish, D., Schorwitz, L., and Doody, R. Effects of stress management training and dietary changes in treating ischemic heart disease. *Journal of the American Medical Association* 249(1): p 54, Jan 7, 1983

20. Blaufox, M.D. *et al.* The dietary intervention study of hypertension (DISH). *Cardiovascular Reviews and Reports* 6: p 1036, Sep 1985

21. Bland, J.S. *Review of Molecular Medicine* Vol I. 3215 56th St. NW, Gig Harbor, WA: JSB and Associates, 1985, p 198

22. Horrobin, D.F. *et al.* The reversibility of cancer: the relevance of cyclic AMP, calcium, essential fatty acids and prostaglandin E1. *Medical Hypotheses* 6(5): pp 469–486, May 1980

23. Vaddadi K.S. Use of gamma-linolenic acid in the treatment of schizophrenia and tardive dyskinesia. *Prostaglandins Leukotrienes and Essential Fatty Acids* 46: pp 67–70, May 1992

24. Campbell, A. and MacEwen, C. Systemic treatment of Sjogren's syndrome and the Sicca syndrome with Efamol (evening primrose oil), vitamin C, and pyridoxine. *Clinical Uses of Essential Fatty Acids,* D.F. Horrobin, Editor. Montreal, Quebec, Canada: Eden Press, 1982, pp 129–137

25. Horrobin, D.F. and Manku, M.S. Possible role of prostaglandin E1 in the affective disorders and in alcoholism. *British Medical Journal* 280(6228): pp 1363–1366, Jun 7, 1980

26. Horrobin, D.F. A biochemical basis for alcoholism and alcohol-induced damage including the fetal alcohol syndrome and cirrhosis interference with essential fatty acid and prostaglandin metabolism. *Medical Hypotheses* 6(9): pp 929–942, Sep 1980

27. Horrobin, D.F. "Gamma-linolenic Acid in Medicine," *1984–85 Yearbook of Nutritional Medicine,* J. Bland, Editor. New Canaan, CT: Keats Pub., 1985, p 31

28. Cunnane, S.C., Manku, M.S., *et al.* Abnormal essential fatty acid composition of tissue lipids in genetically diabetic mice is partially corrected by dietary linoleic and gamma-linolenic acids. *British Journal of Nutrition* 53(3): pp 449–458, May 1985

29. Horrobin, D.F. The use of gamma-linolenic acid in diabetic neuropathy. *Agents and Actions, Supplements* 37: pp 120–144, 1992

30. Houtsmuller, A.J. *et al.* Favourable influences of linoleic acid on the progression of diabetic micro- and macroangiopathy. *Nutritional Metabolism* 24: pp 105–118, 1980

31. *Ibid,* pp 253, 258–259

32. Horrobin, D.F. [Editor]. *Clinical Uses of Essential Fatty Acids.* Montreal, Quebec, Canada: Eden Press, 1982

33. Fredericks, C. *Nutrition Guide for the Prevention and Cure of Common Ailments and Diseases.* New York: Simon and Schuster, 1982

34. Horrobin, D.F. "Gamma-linolenic Acid in Medicine," *1984–85 Yearbook of Nutritional Medicine*, J. Bland, Editor. New Canaan, CT: Keats Pub., 1985, p 25

35. Erasmus, U. *op. cit.,* p 252

36. Horrobin, D.F. *Journal of Holistic Medicine* 3(2): p 118, 1981

37. Regtop, H. "Nutrition, Leukotrienes and Inflammatory Disorders," *1984–85 Yearbook of Nutritional Medicine*, J. Bland, Editor. New Canaan, CT: Keats Pub., 1985, p 63

38. Bland, J.S. *op. cit.,* p 37

39. Bland, J.S. *Review of Molecular Medicine, Vol II.* Gig Harbor, WA: HealthComm, Inc., 1987, p 65

40. *The Shurangama Sutra*, commentary by Tripitaka Master Hsuan Hua, Vol VII. Box 217, Talmage, CA: Buddhist Text Translation Society, 1981, p 14

41. Mensink, R.P., Katan, M.B. Effect of dietary trans fatty acids on high-density and low-density lipoprotein cholesterol levels in healthy subjects. *New England Journal of Medicine* 323(7): pp 439–445, Aug 16, 1990

42. Grundy, S.M. Trans monounsaturated fatty acids and serum cholesterol levels. *New England Journal of Medicine* 323(7): pp 480–481, Aug 16, 1990

43. Erasmus, U. *Fats and Oils.* Vancouver, B.C., Canada: Alive Pub., 1986, p 100

44. Ballentine, R. *Diet and Nutrition.* Honesdale, PA: The Himalayan International Institute, 1978, pp 96–98

45. Erasmus, U. *op. cit.,* p 304

46. Carroll, K.K. Dietary fats and cancer. *American Journal of Clinical Nutrition* 53(4 Suppl): pp 1064S-1067S, Apr 1991

47. Ballentine, R. *Transition to Vegetarianism.* Honesdale, PA: The Himalayan International Institute, 1987

48. For information and products regarding peanut oil and other remedies, contact Edgar Cayce Heritage Products, Virginia Beach, N.C. 23458

49. Erasmus, U. *op. cit.,* p 110

50. Atkins, R.C. *Dr. Atkin's Nutrition Breakthrough.* New York: William Morrow and Co., 1981

51. Smith, R.S. The macrophage theory of depression. *Medical Hypotheses* 35: pp 298–306, Aug, 1991

52. Kromhout, D. The importance of N-6 and N-3 fatty acids in carcinogenesis. *Medical Oncology and Tumor Pharmacotherapy* 7(2-3): pp 173–176, 1990

53. Trichopoulou, A. *et al.* Consumption of olive oil [and margarine] and specific food groups in relation to breast cancer risk in Greece. *Journal of the National Cancer Institute.* 87(2): pp 110–116; Jan. 18, 1995

Chapter 11: Sweeteners

1. Ballentine, R. *Diet and Nutrition.* Honesdale, PA: The Himalayan International Inst., 1978, pp 53–61; 483–491

2. Rohe, F. *The Complete Book of Natural Foods.* Boulder, CO: Shambhala Pub., 1983, pp 43–51

3. Yudkin, J. *Pure, White and Deadly: Problem of Sugar.* New York: Penguin Pub., 1988

4. Dufty, W. *Sugar Blues.* New York: Warner Books, 1975

5. McDougall, John and Mary *The McDougall Plan.* Piscataway, New Jersey: New Century Pub., 1983, pp 110–116

6. Beguin, M.H. *Natural Foods, Healthy Teeth.* La Chaux-de-Fonds, Switzerland: Edition de l'Etoile, 1979

7. Price, Weston, *Nutrition and Physical Degeneration.* La Mesa, CA: The Price-Pottenger Nutrition Foundation, 1945

8. *International Congress Series* International Federation of Diabetes, Buenos Aires, no. 209, Aug 1970

9. Miguel, O. A new oral hypoglycemate. *Medical Review of Paraguay* 8: no. 5 and 6, p 200, July-Dec 1966

10. Kinghorn, A.D. and Soejarto, D.D. Current status of stevioside as a sweetening agent for human use. *Economic and Medicinal Plant Research* 1: Academia Press Inc., 1983

Chapter 13: Condiments, Caffeine, and Spices

1. Jarvis D.C. *Folk Medicine.* Greenwich, CT: Fawcett Crest, 1956

2. Kirschmann, J.D. *Nutrition Almanac.* New York: McGraw-Hill, 1984, p 44

3. Hunter, B.T. *Fact/Book on Food Additives and Your Health.* New Canaan, CT: Keats Pub., 1972, pp 70–74

4. Zeegers, M.P.A. *et al.* Are coffee and tea consumption associated with urinary tract cancer risk? A systematic review and meta-analysis. *International Journal of Epidemiology* 30: pp 353–362, 2001

5. Rohe, F. *The Complete Book of Natural Foods.* Boulder, CO: Shambhala Pub., 1983, pp 258–259

6. Williams, P. Coffee intake of elevated cholesterol and apolepoprotein B levels in women. *Journal of the American Chemical Society* 253: p 1407, 1985

7. Li Shih-Chen (compiler), Smith, F.P. and Stuart, G.A.(translators) *Chinese Medicinal herbs.* San Francisco: Georgetown Press, 1973, p 82

8. Stoner, G.D. *et al.* Polyphenols as cancer chemopreventive agents. *Journal of Cellular Biochemistry.* 22: pp 169–180; Suppl 1995

9. Mazumder, A. *et al.* Effects of tyrphostins, protein kinase inhibitors, on human immunodeficiency virus type 1 integrase. *Biochemistry.* 34(46): pp 15111–15122; Nov 21, 1995

10. Burke, T.R. Jr. *et al.* Hydroxylated aromatic inhibitors of HIV-1 integrase. *Journal of Medicinal Chemistry.* 38(21): pp 4171–4178; Oct 13, 1995

11. Carper, Jean. *Food—Your Miracle Medicine.* New York: Harper-Row/Collins, 1993

12. Porta, Porta, *et al.* Association between coffee drinking and K-ras mutations in exocrine pancreatic cancer. *Journal of Epidemiology and Community Health* 53: pp 702–709, 2001.

Chapter 14: Vitamins and Supplements

1. Livesley, B. Vitamin C and plasma cholesterol. *The Lancet* 2(8414): p 1275, Dec 1, 1984

2. Cameron, E. and Pauling, L. *Cancer and Vitamin C.* New York: W.W. Norton and Co.[Distributors], 1979, p 208

3. Stone, I. *The Healing Factor.* New York: Grosser and Dunlap, 1972

4. Kirschmann, J.D. *Nutrition Almanac.* New York: McGraw-Hill, 1984, p 44

5. Teraguchi, S., Ono, J. *et al.* Vitamin production by *Bifidobacteria* originated from human intestine [Thiamine, riboflavin, pyridoxine, niacin, folacin, vitamin B_{12}, vitamin C]. *Nippon Eiyo Shokuryo Gakkaishi [Journal of the Japanese Society of Nutrition and Food Science]* 37(2): pp 157–164, 1984 (language: Japanese with summary in English)

6. Cameron, E. and Pauling, L. *op. cit.,* p 210

7. Lane, B.C. *1984–85 Yearbook of Nutritional Medicine.* New Canaan, CT: Keats Publ. 1985, p 244

8. *Ibid,* p 245

9. Finley, E.B. and Cerklewski, F.L. Influence of ascorbic acid supplementation on copper status in young adult men. *American Journal of Clinical Nutrition* 37(4): pp 553–556, 1983

10. Staff of Prevention Magazine. *The Complete Book of Vitamins.* Emmaus, Pa: Rodale Press, 1977, p 292

11. Pauling, L. *Vitamin C and The Common Cold.* San Francisco: W.H. Freeman and Co., 1977

12. Eaton, S.B. Konner, M. Paleolithic nutrition. A consideration of its nature and current implications. *New England Journal of Medicine* 312(5): pp 283–289, Jan 31, 1985

13. Roberts, H.J. Perspective on vitamin E as therapy. *Journal of the American Medical Association* 246(2): pp 129–31, 1981

14. Bland, J.S. *Review Of Molecular Medicine, Vol I.* JSB & Assoc, 1985, p 220

15. Chandra, R.K. Excessive intake of zinc impairs immune responses. *Journal of the American Medical Association* 252(11): pp 1443–1446, Sep 21, 1984

16. The study of the healing value of phytochemicals (plant chemicals) is being applied more rigorously to foods in recent years. Phytochemicals frequently exhibit properties that differ from those found in standard nutrients such as vitamins, minerals and amino acids. In total, millions of phytochemicals are found in common foods, making this a fertile area of study. However, one should first consider the basic properties of a food before eating it for its chemical value. For instance, the basic properties of soybeans include moistening and cooling attributes, making them especially useful for the *dry, overheated* person. They also contain the phytochemical genistein that is thought to help prevent breast cancer; nonetheless, a person with a *cold* constitution (feels cold often) and with *damp* signs (mucus excess and water retention) may become *colder* and *damper* with soybean consumption. In addition, cancer becomes more likely with *damp* food intake (see page 410). Using the extracted, isolated phytochemical may solve this problem, but, as discussed earlier, taking isolated nutrients can also imbalance the body.

One of the best uses of phytochemicals is as a

marker for choosing from among those foods with the appropriate basic properties. For example, one ideally first eats according to one's constitution and condition—warming foods for *coldness,* bitter foods for *excessive* conditions, tonic foods for weakness and frailty, detoxifying foods for toxicity, and so on. After doing this, it then seems in order to choose which of these foods to emphasize according to any of their known nutrient parameters—their phytochemicals, nutraceuticals, vitamins, minerals, fatty acids, enzymes, and so on. Even their color, shape, aroma, and texture can be taken into account. Intuition should play role too, and is enhanced with objective information on foods. The more that is known, the more confidence one has in making choices for food as medicine.

Note: A "nutraceutical" is a phytochemical with pharmaceutically recognized healing properties.

17. Omenn, G.S. *et al.* Effects of a combination of beta carotene and vitamin A on lung cancer and cardiovascular disease. *New England Journal of Medicine.* 334(18): pp 1150–1155; May 2, 1996

18. Hennekens, C.H. Lack of effect of long-term supplementation with beta carotene on the incidence of malignant neoplasms and cardiovascular disease. *New England Journal of Medicine.* 334(18): pp 1145–1149; May 2, 1996

19. Greenberg, E.R. and Sporn, M.B. Antioxidant vitamins, cancer, and cardiovascular disease [editorial; comment] *New England Journal of Medicine* (334(18): pp 1189–1190; May 2, 1996

20. The Alpha-Tocopherol, Beta Carotene Cancer Prevention Study Group. The effect of vitamin E and beta carotene on the incidence of lung cancer and other cancers in male smokers. *New England Journal of Medicine* 330(15) pp 1029–1035; Apr. 14, 1994

21. Greenberg, E.R. *et al.* A clinical trial of antioxidant vitamins to prevent colorectal adenoma. Polyp Prevention Study Group. *New England Journal of Medicine.* 331(3): pp 141–147; July 21, 1994

Chapter 15: Calcium

1. Abraham, G. Role of nutrition in managing the premenstrual tension syndromes. *Journal of Reproductive Medicine* 32(6): pp 405–422, June 1987

2. Regtop, H. Is magnesium the grossly neglected mineral? *International Clinical Nutrition Review* 3: pp 18–19, July 1983

3. Levine, B. and Coburn, J. Magnesium: the mimic/antagonist of calcium. *New England Journal of Medicine* 310: pp 1253–1255, May 10, 1984

4. Miller, R. Osteoporosis, calcium and estrogens. *FDA Consumer* 18(9): p 17, Nov 1984

5. Writing Group for the Women's Health Initiative Investigators. Risks and benefits of estrogen plus progestin in healthy postmenopausal women: principal results From the Women's Health Initiative randomized controlled trial. *Journal of The American Medical Association* 288(3): pages 321–333, Jul 17, 2002

6. Paty, J. Bone mineral content of female athletes. *New England Journal of Medicine* 311: p 1320, 1984

7. Ellis, F. *et al.* Incidence of osteoporosis in vegetarians and omnivores. *American Journal of Clinical Nutrition* 25: pp 555–558, 1972

8. Faelton, S. *et al. Complete Book of Minerals for Health.* Emmaus, PA: Rodale Books, 1981, p 22

9. Kervran, C.L. *Biological Transmutations, and their Application in Chemistry, Physics, Biology, Ecology, Medicine, Nutrition, Agriculture, Geology.* Binghampton, NY: Swan House Publ., 1972

Chapter 16: Green Food Products

1. Rudolph, T. *Chlorophyll.* San Jacinto, CA: Nutritional Research, 1957

2. Wiznitzer, T. *et al.* Acute necrotizing pancreatitis in the Guinea pig; effect of chlorophyll-alpha on survival times. *American Journal of Digestive Diseases* 21(6): pp 459–464, Jun 1976

3. Negishi, T. *et al.* Inhibitory effect of chlorophyll on the genotoxicity of 3-amino-1-methyl-5H-pyrido (4,3-b) indole (Trp-p-2). *Carcinogenesis* 10(1): pp 145–149, 1989

4. Yoshida, A. *et al.* Therapeutic effect of chlorophyll-a in the treatment of patients with chronic pancreatitis. *Gastroenterologia Japonica* 15(1): pp 49–61 1980

5. Ong, T. *et al.* Chlorophyllin: a potent antimutagen against environmental and dietary complex mixtures. *Mutation Research* 173: pp 111–115, Feb 1986

6. di Raimondo, F. Chlorophyll effects on development of bacteria and on streptomycin antibiosis. *Rivista dell Istituto di Sieroterapia Italiano* (sezione I) 24: pp 190–196, Jul-Sep 1949

7. Ammon, R. and Wolff, L. Hat Chlorophyll eine baktericide bzw. bakteriostatische Wirkung? *Arzneimittel-Forschung* 5: pp 312–314, Jun 1955

8. Kutscher, A., Chilton, N. Observations on clinical use of chlorophyll dentifrice. *Journal of the American Dental Association* 46: pp 420–422, April 1953

9. Lam, F. and Brush, B. Chlorophyll and wound healing; experimental and clinical study. *American Journal of Surgery* 80(1): pp 204–210, Aug 1950

10. Offenkrantz, F. Water-soluble chlorophyll in treatment of peptic ulcers of long duration. *Review of Gastroenterology* 17: pp 359–367, May 1950

11. Patek, A. Chlorophyll and regeneration of blood; effect of administration of chlorophyll derivatives to patients with chronic hypochromic anemia. *Archives of Internal Medicine* 57: pp 73–84, Jan 1936

12. Russell-Manning, B. *Wheatgrass Juice, Gift of Nature*. Los Angeles, CA: Greensward Press, 1974

13. Licata, V. *Comfrey and Chlorophyll*. Santa Ana, CA: Continental Health Research, 1971

14. Hills, C. [editor] *The Secrets of Spirulina/ Medical Discoveries of Japanese Doctors*. Boulder Creek, CA: University of the Trees Press, 1980

15. Private written communication with researcher Gregory M.L. Patterson, Dec 6, 1989

16. *Ibid,* pp 11, 206

17. Switzer, L. *Spirulina/The Whole Food Revolution*. Berkeley, CA: Proteus Corp., 1980, p 56

18. Yamane, Y. The effect of spirulina on nephrotoxicity in rats. Presented at The Annual Symposium of the Pharmaceutical Society of Japan, Pharmacy Dept., Chiba University, Japan, April 15, 1988

19. Troxler, R. and Saffer, B. (Harvard School of Dental Med. researchers) Algae derived phycocyanin is both cytostatic and cytotoxic (dose-response) to oral squamous cell carcinoma (human or hamster). Paper delivered at International Association for Dental Research General Session, 1987

20. Hills, C. *Rejuvenating the Body*. Box 644, Boulder Creek, CA: University of the Trees Press, 1980, p 58

21. Prudden, J. and Balassa, L. The biological activity of bovine cartilage preparations. *Seminars on Arthritis and Rheumatism* 3(4): pp 287–321, 1974

22. Day, C.E. Control of the interaction of cholesterol ester-rich lipoproteins with arterial receptors. *Atherosclerosis* 25: pp 199–204, Nov-Dec 1976

23. Kojima, M. *et al.* A *Chlorella* polysaccharide as a factor stimulating RES activity. Dept. of Pathology, Fukushima Medical College, Fukushima City, Japan. *Journal of the Reticuloendothelial Society* 14: pp 192–208, 1973

24. Kojima, M. *et al.* A new *Chlorella* polysaccharide and its accelerating effect on the phagocytic activity of the reticuloendothelial system. Paper delivered at: Symposium II: Phagocytic Activity of RES, Dept. of Pathology, Fukushi-

ma Medical College, Fukushima City, Japan

25. White, R. and Barber, G. An acidic polysaccharide from the cell wall of *Chlorella pyrenoidosa*. Research at: Dept. of Biochemistry, Ohio State Univ. 484 W. 12 Ave., Columbia, OH 43210

26. Komiyama, K. *et al.* An acidic polysaccharide Chlon A from *Chlorella pyrenoidosa*. (Antitumor activity and immunological response.) Research at: The Kitasato Institute, Japan

27. Vermeil, C. and Morin, O. Role experimental des algues unicellulaires prototheca et *Chlorella (Chlorellaceae)* dans l'immunogenese anticancereuse (sarcome muin BP 8). Societe de Biologie de Rennes. Seance du April 21, 1976

28. Hamada, M. *et al.* Immune responsiveness of tumor-bearing host and trial of modulation. Combined research at: 1) Dept. of Serology, Kanazawa Medical Univ., Uchinada, Ishikawa, 920-02, Japan. 2) Dept. of Biochemistry, Taipei Medical College, Taipei, R.O.C.

29. Konishi, F. *et al.* Antitumor effect induced by a hot water extract of *Chlorella vulgaris* (CE): Resistance to meth-a tumor growth mediated by CE-induced polymorphonuclear leukocytes. Dept. of Immunology, Medical Inst. of Bioregulation, Kyushu Univ., Fukuoka 812, Japan. In: *Cancer Immunology Immunotherapy*. Publisher: Springer-Verlag, 1985

30. Vermeil, O. *et al.* Anti-tumoral vaccination by peritoneal injection of micro-vegetable (yeasts and unicellular algae). Conceptual error or reality? *Archives Medicales de L'Oest-Tome* 14(10): pp 423–426

31. Tanaka, K. *et al.* Augmentation of antitumor resistance by a strain of unicellular green algae, *Chlorella vulgaris*. Dept. of Immunology, Medical Inst. of Bioregulation, Kyushu Univ., 69, 3-1-1 Maidashi Higashi-Ku, Fukuoka 812, Japan. In: *Cancer Immunology Immunotherapy* Publisher: Springer-Verlag, 1984

32. Hashimoto, S. *et al.* Effects of soybean phospholipid, chlorella phospholipid, and clofibrate on collagen and elastin synthesis in the aorta and on the serum and liver lipid contents in rats. In: *Scientific Research Digest on Chlorella* Hokkaido, Japan: Medicinal Plant Institute of Hokkaido, Hokkaido, 089-37, Japan, 1987, pp 481–487

33. Sano, T. and Tanaka, Y. Effect of dried, powdered *Chlorella vulgaris* on experimental atherosclerosis and alimentary hypercholesterolemia in cholesterol-fed rabbits. *Artery* 14(2): pp 76–84, 1987

34. Sawyer, P. *et al.* Demonstration of a toxin from *Aphanizomenon flos-aquae. Canadian Journal of Microbiology* 14: p 1199, 1968

35. Alam, M. *et al.* Purification of aphanizomenon flos-aquae toxin and its chemical and physiolog-

ical properties. *Toxicon* [Pergamon Press, Great Britain] II: pp 65–72, Jan 1973

36. Personal communication with Wm. Barry, Ph.D, in 1988

37. Barton, L.L. Studies on [Mice with] Dietary Supplements of Super Blue Green at Ultra High Levels. Research at: Dept. of Biology, Univ. of New Mexico, Albuquerque, N.M. 87131, April 20, 1984

38. Sawyer, P. *op. cit.,* p 1201

39. Kulvinskas, V. "Algae in your Salad" *Serenity Magazine* Fall, 1987

40. Hagiwara, Y. *Green Barley Essence.* New Canaan, CT: Keats Pub, 1986, pp 74, 135

41. Kubota, K. *et al.* Isolation of potent anti-inflammatory protein from barley leaves. Research at: Dept. of Pharmaceutical Sciences, Science University of Tokyo [Ichigaya-funa-gawara-machi, Shinjuku-ku], Tokyo, 162, Japan. Part of this paper is in: *Japanese Journal of Inflammation* v 3(4): 1983. A P4D1/steroid comparison is discussed in the paper: "A preliminary report on how the juice of young green barley plants can normalize and rejuvenate cells...," signed by Dr. Yasuo Hotta, Biology Dept., Univ. of California, San Diego, CA.

42. Christopher, J. *School of Natural Healing.* Provo, UT: BiWorld Pub., 1976, p 543

43. Hagiwara, Y. *op. cit.,* pp 83–132

44. Erasmus, U. *Fats and Oils.* Vancouver, B.C.: Alive Books, 1986, p 251

45. Hills, C. [editor] *The Secrets of Spirulina/Medical Discoveries of Japanese Doctors.* Boulder Creek, CA: University of the Trees Press, 1980 pp 55–66, 103

46. *Harvard Medical Area Focus* May 14, 1987

47. National Research Council. *Diet, Nutrition and Cancer:* the report of a blue-ribbon committee of experts published by the NRC. (Among its conclusions: "A growing accumulation of epidemiological evidence indicates that there is an inverse relationship between the risk of cancer and the consumption of foods that contain vitamin A ... The epidemiological evidence is sufficient to suggest that foods rich in carotenes or vitamin A are associated with reduced risk of cancer.")

48. Shekelle, R.B. *et al.* Dietary vitamin A and risk of cancer in the Western Electric study. *The Lancet* 2(8257): pp 1186–1190, Nov 28, 1981(This article reports on a nineteen-year study of 1,954 middle-aged men and concludes that incidence of lung cancer is inversely related to the intake of beta carotene; in other words, the more beta carotene in the diet, the fewer cancer cases.)

49. Omenn, G.S. *et al.* Effects of a combination of beta carotene and vitamin A on lung cancer and cardiovascular disease. *New England Journal of Medicine.* 334(18): pp 1150–1155; May 2, 1996

50. Hennekens, C.H. Lack of effect of long-term supplementation with beta carotene on the incidence of malignant neoplasms and cardiovascular disease. *New England Journal of Medicine.* 334(18): pp 1145–1149; May 2, 1996

Chapter 17: Survival Simplified

1. Strom, A. and Jensen, R. Mortality from circulatory diseases in Norway 1940–1945. *The Lancet* 1: pp 126–129, Jan 20, 1951

2. Rudin, D.O. and Felix, C. *The Omega-3 Phenomenon.* New York: Rawson Associates, 1987, pp 33–34

Chapter 18: Enjoyment of Food

1. Walford, R.L. *The 120 Year Diet—How to Double Your Vital Years.* New York: Simon and Schuster, 1986

2. Ross, M.H. Dietary behavior and longevity. *Nutr Reviews* 35(10): pp 257–265, Oct 1977

3. Szekely, E.B. *The Essene Gospel of Peace, Book One.* 3085 Reynard Way, San Diego, CA: International Biogenic Society, 1981

Chapter 20: Fasting and Purification

1. Cousens, G. *Spiritual Nutrition and The Rainbow Diet.* P.O. Box 2044, Boulder, CO: Cassandra Press, 1986, pp 147–148

2. Albright, J. *Our Lady of Medjugorje.* P.O. Box 7, Milford, Ohio 45150: The Riehle Foundation

3. Cousens, G. *op. cit.,* p 155

4. *Ibid,* p 147

5. The Bible. Moses fasting (twice): Exodus 34:28; Deuteronomy 9:9, 18; Jesus fasting: Matthew 4:2

Chapter 21: Food for Children

1. Ballentine, R. *Diet and Nutrition.* Honesdale, PA: Himalayan Inst., 1978, p 129

2. Leonard, J. Hofer, J. and Pritikin, N. *Live Longer Now.* New York: Grosset and Dunlap, 1974, p 10

3. Sampsidis, N. *Homogenized!* P.O. Box 25, Glenwood Landing, N.Y.: Sunflower Pub.

4. Svoboda, R. *Prakruti.* Albuquerque, NM: Geocom, 1989, p 72

5. Hergenrather, J. *et al.* Pollutants in breast milk of vegetarians. *New England Journal of Medicine* 304(13): p 792, Mar 26, 1981

6. Cunningham, A. Morbidity in breast-fed and artificially fed infants. *Journal of Pediatrics* 90: pp 726–729, 1977

7. Addy, D.P. Infant Feeding: a current view. *British Medical Journal* 1: pp 1268–1271, May 22, 1976

8. Newton, N. The uniqueness of human milk. Psychologic differences between breast and bottle feeding. *American Journal of Clinical Nutrition* 24: pp 993–1004, Aug 1971

9. Lippmann, M. *Chemical Contamination of the Human Environment.* Oxford, England: Oxford Univ. Press, 1979, p 146

10. Ballentine, R. *Diet & Nutrition.* Honesdale, PA: Himalayan International Inst., 1978, p 119

11. Wetzel, W.E., *et al.* Carotene jaundice in infants with "sugar nursing bottle syndrome." *Monatsschrift Kinderheilkunde* 137: pp 659–661, Oct 1989

12. Baker, J.P. *et al. Conscious Conception.* Monroe, UT: Freestone Pub., 1986

13. Chang, S. *The Great Tao.* San Francisco, CA: Harper and Row, 1985, p 325

14. Attention Deficit Disorder (ADD) is frequently associated with hyperactivity, or ADHD (Attention Deficit Hyperactivity Disorder). Excessive activity and inability to pay attention often have a common root in Oriental medicine: insufficient *yin,* where *yin* represents the calm and receptive dimension of human personality. In such childhood disorders, *yin* deficit frequently affects the kidneys and liver. (In Western terms, this could translate into a deficiency of liver and kidney metabolites and hormones, which are produced from a rich and balanced supply of vitamins, minerals, amino acids, fatty acids, enzymes, and so on.) The task of *yin*-building in children is not far different from that in adults.

One reason children may exhibit *yin* deficit is heredity, if not enough was available from the parents. Studies have shown that parents who are themselves subject to depression, attention deficit, hyperactivity, and other developmental imbalances have a greater likelihood of bearing children with ADHD [see notes 15,16,17 below]. Since children are in a *yang* growth phase of their life, which needs the support of their *yin* resources, they easily become at least somewhat deficient in *yin.* Because the *yin* and its supporting nutrients are depleted by refined foods, synthetic chemicals, pesticides, radiation from computers and TVs, highly spiced foods, fluorescent lights, smog and numerous other toxic elements of modern life, it is advisable for children with *yin* deficit to have as natural a diet and lifestyle as possible. Chaos in the home, along with other stresses discussed in the section "Food and Behavior," seems to contribute to this syndrome in children.

Specific nutritional remedies that frequently help, especially if given regularly over the years, include: sea vegetables, which supply the wealth of minerals needed to calm the mind and body,

and can be cooked into bean dishes and stews; also, many children with ADHD are benefited by taking a few kelp tablets daily. Foods such as spirulina, tempeh, butter and ghee, almonds, and various animal products in the deficiency section (pages 293–297) also may prove helpful in building *yin* essence. The omega-3 and GLA oils, e.g., in the form of flax and borage oils, greatly help the *yin* of the liver, and are indicated when the child is unruly or especially angry and disruptive. Studies suggest these fatty acids tend to be lacking in children with ADHD [see note 18 below]. ADHD is also frequently made worse by parasitic infections. As suggested in the "Food for Children" chapter, garlic can help with childhood parasites; but because of its intensely hot nature, which burns up *yin* hormones and fluids, these children are better balanced with aloe vera gel and colloidal silver, per the Parasite Purge Program, Appendix A. Both are generally safe for children, and help nurture their *yin,* receptive aspects while ridding the body of many forms of parasites and pathogens. Thus, aside from the parasite issue, some parents give one or both remedies to their children long-term simply to aid in *yin* nourishment.

Hyperactivity and attention deficit represent a mind and body that move, often chaotically, from one action, object, or idea to another. Chaotic and disruptive change, whether mental or physical, is described in Chinese medicine as *wind* syndrome. *Wind* conditions are made worse by heat-producing foods and stressful activity, by diets that cause liver stagnation (page 324), and by consuming eggs, crab meat, and buckwheat. Whether ADHD syndrome is brought about by injuries, parasites, heredity, dietary or environmental factors or any combination of these, it can be improved at least to some extent by consistently following basic guidelines such as those suggested in this note. Because children are growing, they frequently out-grow their imbalances when given the nutritional and emotional support to do so.

15. Roizen, N.J., *et al.* Psychiatric and developmental disorders in families of children with attention-deficit hyperactivity disorder. *Archives of Pediatric and Adolescent Medicine.* 150(2): pp 203–208; Feb, 1996

16. McCormick, L.H. Depression in mothers of children with attention deficit hyperactivity disorder. *Family Medicine.* 27(3): pp 176–179; Mar, 1995

17. Comings, D.E. Role of genetic factors in depression based on studies of Tourette syndrome and ADHD probands and their relatives. *American Journal of Medical Genetics.* 60(2): pp 111–121; Apr 24, 1995

18. Stevens, L. J. Essential fatty acid metabolism in boys with attention-deficit hyperactivity disorder. *American Journal of Clinical Nutrition.* 62(4): pp 761–768; Oct, 1995

Chapters 22 through 28: The Five Element and Organ Systems

1. Lane, B.C. "Nutrition and Vision." In *1984–85 Yearbook of Nutritional Medicine.* J. Bland, Editor. New Canaan, CT: Keats Pub., l985, p 244

2. Goldman, A.S. "Immunologic Aspects of Human Milk." Symposium on Human Lactation, U.S. Dept. of Health, Education, and Welfare, DHEW Publication (HSA) 79-5107, L. Waletsky, Editor. Arlington, VA. Oct 7–8, 1976

3. Mellander, O. and Valquist, B. Breast feeding and artificial feeding. Norrbotten Study, *Acta Paediatrica* suppl. 116, 48: p 1, 1959

4. Matthews, T., Nair, C. *et al.* Antiviral activity in milk of possible clinical significance. *The Lancet* 2(8000): pp 1387–89, Dec 25, 1976

5. Williams, R. "The Trusting Heart," *Psychology Today*, p 35, Jan/Feb 1989

6. Marx, J. Anxiety peptide found in brain. *Science* 227: p 934, 1985.

7. Belongia, E. *et al.* An investigation of the cause of the eosinophilia-myalgia syndrome associated with tryptophan use. *New England Journal of Medicine* 323(6): pp 357–65, Aug 9, 1990

8. The theory of pleomorphic microorganisms—particularly as proposed by Antoine Bechamp, a 19th century contemporary and critic of Pasteur—asserts that disease-producing microbes take on specific forms that correspond to the bodily milieu. Thus, the theory posits that the milieu, or total internal environment, "is everything," and the type and number of harmful viruses, bacteria, amoebas, or other microbes that develop from primitive, non-dangerous forms found in all bodies, merely reflect the degree of bodily toxicity, including *damp*-mucous conditions. Attempting to cure disease by simply destroying the so-called "causative" microbes makes a long-term healing unlikely: such microbes, according to the theory, are never truly eliminated but instead transform into more dangerous forms that proliferate later—sometimes years later—and contribute to deeper disorders. On the other hand, if the body is purified while microbes are "destroyed," then no toxic milieu will exist to support a pathogenic microbial transformation. Appropriate foods, herbs, exercises, and other wholesome treatments tend to both purify the body and eliminate pathogens, while most drugs appear to eliminate pathogens only. The theory of pleomorphic organisms is supported by numerous studies in bacteriology, and is a principle used in various holistic healing arts, but is not well-accepted by most practitioners of standard medicine. A number of 20th century writers as well as Bechamp have applied and/or described the theory, including the six listed in the following references (numbers 9–14):

9. West, J. *Important Facts You Should Know About AIDS: Diseases and Diets the Authorities Fail To Tell You: Pasteur, Bechamp & AIDS.* Bundaber, Queensland, Australia: AIDS biological Research Centre, 1988

10. Mattman, L. *Cell Wall Deficient Forms.* Cleveland, OH: CRC Press, 1974

11. Pearson, R.B. *Pasteur Plagiarist, Impostor. The Germ Theory Exploded.* Denver, CO: Health, Inc., 1942

12. Enby, E. *et al. Hidden Killers.* Sheehan Communications, 1990

13. Domingue, G.J. Naked bacteria in human blood. *Microbia* Tome 2, No. 2, 1976

14. Bechamp, A. *Sang et son troisieme element anatomique [The Blood and its Third Anatomical Element].* Australia: Veritas Press, 1988 [Reprint and translation; originally published: London: J. Ouseley, 1912]

15. O'Neill, M. "Eating to Heal: The New Frontiers." *The New York Times* p B5, Feb 7, 1990

16. West, D.W. *et al.* Dietary intake and colon cancer: sex- and anatomic site-specific associations. *American Journal of Epidemiology* 130: pp 883–94, Nov 1989

17. Harris, R.W. *et al.* A case-control study of dietary carotene in men with lung cancer and in men with other epithelial cancers. *Nutrition and Cancer* 15(1): pp 63–68, 1991

18. Singh, V.N. and Gaby, S.K. Premalignant lesions: role of antioxidant vitamins and beta carotene in risk reduction and prevention of malignant transformation. *American Journal of Clinical Nutrition* 53(1 Suppl): pp 386S-390S, Jan 1991

19. Fontham, E.T. Protective dietary factors and lung cancer. *International Journal of Epidemiology* 19 Suppl 1: pp S32–42, 1990

20. Statland, B.E. Nutrition and cancer. *Clinical Chemistry* 38(8B Pt 2): pp 1587–1594, Aug 1992

21. Dard, D. *et al.* [Hemorrhoids: dietary factors.] *Revue Medicale de la Suisse Romande* 110: pp 381–384, Apr 1990

22. Friedman, G.D. and Fireman, B.H. Appendectomy, appendicitis, and large bowel cancer. *Cancer Research* 50: pp 7549–7551, Dec 1990

23. Klurfeld, D.M. Dietary fiber-mediated mechanisms in carcinogenesis. *Cancer Research* 52(7 suppl): pp 2055s-2059s, Apr 1, 1992

24. Shankar, S. and Lanza, E. Dietary fiber and cancer prevention. *Hematology/Oncology Clinics of North America* 5: pp 25–42, Feb 1991

25. Melange, M. and Vanheuverzwyn, R. [Etiopathogenesis of colonic diverticular disease; role of dietary fiber and therapeutic perspectives] *Acta Gastroenterologica Belgica* 53: pp 346–350, May-Jun 1990

26. Yang, P. and Banwell, J.G. Dietary fiber: its role in the pathogenesis and treatment of constipation. *Practical Gastroenterology* 6: pp 28–32, 1986

27. Frank, B. *Nucleic Acid Therapy in Aging and Degenerative Disease.* New York: Psychological Library Publishers, 1968

28. Kirschmann, J.D. *Nutrition Almanac* New York: McGraw-Hill, 1984, p 31

29. *Ibid,* p 15

30. Kohler, G. *et al.* Growth-stimulating properties of grass juice. *Science* 83: p 445, 1936

31. Kohler, G. *et al.* The relation of the "grass juice factor" to guinea pig nutrition. *Journal of Nutrition* 15: p 445, 1938

32. Colio and Babb. Study of a new stimulatory growth factor. *Journal of Biological Chemistry* 174: p 405, 1948

33. Kohler, G. *et al.* The grass juice factor. *Journal of Biological Chemistry* 128: p 1w, 1939

34. Bensky, D. and Gamble, A. [translators] *Chinese Herbal Medicine: Materia Medica* Seattle, WA: Eastland Press, 1986, p 508

35. Allen, R. and Lust, J. *The Royal Jelly Miracle.* Simi Valley, CA: Benedict Lust Publ., 1958, pp 20, 21

36. Murray, M. *Sea Energy Agriculture.* Winston-Salem, NC: Valentine Books, 1976, p 12

37. Vorberg, G. Ginkgo Biloba Extract: A long-term study of chronic cerebral insufficiency in geriatric patients. *Clinical Trials Journal* 22: pp 149–157, 1985

38. Bauer, U. Six-month double-blind randomized clinical trial of Ginkgo Biloba Extract versus placebo in two parallel groups in patients suffering from peripheral arterial insufficiency. *Arzneim-Forsch* 34: pp 716–721, 1984

39. Hindmarch, I. and Subban, Z. The psycho-pharmacological effects of Ginkgo Biloba Extract in normal health volunteers. *International Journal of Clinical Pharmacological Research* 4: pp 89–93, 1984

40. Gebner, B. *et al.* Study of the long-term action of a Ginkgo Biloba Extract on vigilance and mental performance as determined by means of quantitative pharmaco-EEG and psychometric measurements. *Arzneim-Forsch* 35: pp 1459–1465, 1985

41. On June 7, 1995, the Venerable Master Hsuan Hua, Chinese Buddhist Patriarch, peacefully passed away. Upon cremation, his ashes yielded over 10,000 *sharira*. His teachings inspired many aspects of this book regarding awareness, including certain philosophical elements of Sattva (the middle path) discussed in the Summary, Chapter 52. To obtain information on his life and teachings, contact: City of Ten Thousand Buddhas, 2001 Talmage Road, P.O. Box 217, Talmage, CA 95481-0217, USA.

42. Mathe, G.. *et al.* A Pygeum africanum extract with so-called phyto-estrogenic action markedly reduces the volume of true and large prostatic hypertrophy. *Biomedicine and Pharmacotherapy.* 49(7–8): pp 341–343; 1995

Chapters 29 through 33: Diseases and Their Dietary Treatment

1. Van Eck, W.R. The effect of a low fat diet on the serum lipids in diabetes and its significance in diabetic retinopathy. *American Journal of Medicine* 27: pp 196–211, Aug, 1959

2. Sartor, G. *et al.* Dietary supplementation of fibre as a means to reduce postprandial glucose in diabetics. *Acta Medica Scandinavica* (suppl) 656: pp 51–53, 1981

3. Jenkins, D. *et al.* Decrease in postprandial insulin and glucose concentrations by guar and pectin. *Annals of Internal Medicine* 86: p 20, 1977

4. Holman, R. *et al.* Prevention of deterioration of renal and sensory-nerve function by more intensive management of insulin-dependent diabetic patients. *The Lancet* 1(8318): pp 204–208, Jan 29, 1983

5. Olefsky, J. *et al.* Reappraisal of the role of insulin in hypertriglyceridemia. *American Journal of Medicine* 57: pp 551–560, Oct 1974

6. Himsworth, H.P. Dietetic factor determining glucose tolerance and sensitivity to insulin of healthy men. *Clinical Science* 2: pp 67–94, Sep 1935

7. Wolf, H.J. and Priess, H Experiences with fat free diet in diabetes mellitus. *Deutsche Medizinische Wochenschrift* 81: pp 514–515, Apr 6, 1956

8. Barnard, R.J. *et al.* Response of non-insulin-dependent diabetic patients to an intensive program of diet and exercise. *Diabetes Care* 5: pp 370–374, Jul-Aug 1982

9. Singh, I. Low-fat diet and therapeutic doses of insulin in diabetes mellitus. *The Lancet* 1: pp 422–425, Feb 26, 1955

10. Lu, H.C. *Chinese System of Food Cures.* New York: Sterling Pub., 1986, p 139

11. Kloss, J. *Back To Eden.* Santa Barbara, CA: Lifeline Books, 1939, p 407

12. Jensen, B. *Nature Has a Remedy.* Santa Cruz, CA: Unity Press, 1978, p 167

13. Rudolph, T.M. *Chlorophyll*. San Jacinto, CA: Nutritional Research, 1957, p 31

14. Hills, C. *The Secrets of Spirulina*. Boulder Creek, CA: Univ. Of the Trees Press, 1980, pp 59–66

15. Jensen, B. *Health Magic Through Chlorophyll*. Provo, UT: BiWorld Pub., 1973, p 113

16. Addanki, S. *Diabetes Breakthrough*. New York: Pinnacle Books, 1982, p 6

17. Jensen, B. *Health Magic Through Chlorophyll*. Provo, UT: BiWorld Pub., 1973, p 113

18. *Ibid*, p 29

19. Erasmus, U. *op. cit.*, p 305

20. Addanki, S. *op. cit.*, p 110

21. *Ibid*, p 110

22. Kirschmann, J.D. *Nutrition Almanac*. New York: McGraw Hill, 1984, p 168

23. Jensen, B. *Nature Has a Remedy*. Santa Cruz, CA: Unity Press, 1978, p 224

24. Jacob, S.W. *Structure and Function in Man*. Philadelphia, PA: W.B. Saunders and Co., 1974, p 442

25. "Keep Taking Your Bran"[Editorial.] *The Lancet* 1: p 1175, June 2, 1979

26. Piepmeyer, J.L. Use of unprocessed bran in treatment of irritable bowel syndrome. *American Journal of Clinical Nutrition* 27(2): pp 106–107, Feb 1974

27. Painter, N.S. *et al*. Unprocessed bran in treatment of diverticular disease of the colon. *British Medical Journal* 2: pp 137–140, Apr 15, 1972

28. Hodgson, J. *et al*. Effect of methylcellulose on rectal and colonic pressures in treatment of diverticular disease. *British Medical Journal* 3: p 729, Sep 23, 1972

29. Dissanayake, A. *et al*. Lack of harmful effect of oats on small-intestinal mucosa in coeliac disease. *British Medical Journal* 4(5938): pp 189–191, 1974

30. Kirschmann, J.D. *op. cit.*, p 134

31. Singh, M.M. and Kay, S.R. Wheat gluten as a pathogenic factor in schizophrenia. *Science* 191(4225): pp 401–402, Jan 30, 1976

32. Ross-Smith, P. and Jenner, F. Diet and schizophrenia. *Journal of Human Nutrition* 34(2): pp 107–112, 1980

33. Frisch, R.E. Amenorrhoea, vegetarianism, and/or low fat? *The Lancet* 1(8384): p 1024, May 5, 1984

34. Frisch, R.E. *et al*. Magnetic resonance imaging of body fat of athletes compared with controls and the oxidative metabolism of estradiol. *Metabolism: Clinical and Experimental* 41: pp 191–193, Feb 1992

35. Kemmann, E. *et al*. Amenorrhea associated with carotenemia. *Journal of the American Medical Association* 249(7): pp 926–929, 1983

36. Baker, C.E. [publisher] *Physicians' Desk Reference*. Oradell, NJ: Medical Economics Co., 1982, pp 1899, 1900

37. Airola, P. *How to Get Well*. Phoenix, AR: Health Plus Pub., 1982, p 128

38. Report prepared by the National Cancer Institute: *Cancer Control Objectives for the Nation: 1985–2000*. Available for sale from Superintendent of Documents, U.S. Government Printing Office, Washington, DC 20402, Tel: (202) 783-3238; document order number 017-042-00191-9

39. Gerson, M. *A Cancer Therapy*. Bonita, CA: Gerson Institute, 1986

40. Pauling, L. and Cameron, E. *Cancer and Vitamin C*. Menlo Park, CA: Linus Pauling Inst. of Science and Medicine, 1979, p 190

41. *Ibid*, pp 99–210

42. Pauling, L. "Good Nutrition for the Good Life." Article reprinted in *The Complete Book of Vitamins*. Emmaus, PA: Rodale Press, 1977, p 80

43. Bendich, A. and Olson, J.A. Biological actions of carotenoids. *FASEB Journal* 3: pp 1927–1932, Jun 1989

44. Ziegler, R.G. A review of epidemiologic evidence that carotenoids reduce the risk of cancer. *Journal of Nutrition* 119: pp 116–122, Jan 1989

45. Suda, D. *et al*. Inhibition of experimental oral carcinogenesis by topical beta carotene. *Carcinogenesis* 7: p 711, 1986

46. Donden, Y. *Health Through Balance*. Ithaca, NY: Snow Lion Publ., 1986, pp 186, 198

47. Zhu, Y. *et al*. Growth-inhibition effects of oleic acid, linoleic acid, and their methyl esters on transplanted tumors in mice. *Journal of the National Cancer Institute* 81(17): pp 1302–1306, Sep 6, 1989

48. Adlercreutz, H. Does fiber-rich food containing animal lignan precursors protect against both colon and breast cancer? *Gastroenterology* 86: p 761, April 1984

49. Setchell, K.D.R. *et al*. Lignan formation in man—microbial involvement and possible roles in relation to cancer. *The Lancet* 2: p 4, July 4, 1981

50. Lederoq, G. and Henson, J.L. *Biochimica et Biophysica Acta* 560: p 427, 1979

51. Brown, G. and Mortimer, J. Remission of canine squamous cell carcinoma after nitriloside therapy. *Veterinary Medicine: Small Animal Clinic* 71: pp 1561–1562, Nov 1976

52. Yamamoto, I. and Maruyama, H. Effect of dietary seaweed preparations on 1,2-dimethylhydrazine-induced intestinal carcinogenesis in rats. *Cancer Letters* 26: pp 241–251, Apr 1985

53. Christopher, J.R. *School of Natural Healing.* Provo, UT: BiWorld Pub., 1978, pp 266–267

54. Chihara, G. *et al.* Fractionation and purification of the polysaccharides with marked anti-tumor activity, especially letinan, from *Lentinus edodes. Cancer Research* 30: pp 2776–2781, 1980

55. Sone, Y. *et al.* Structures and anti-tumor activities of the polysaccharides isolated from fruiting body and the growing *Ganaderma lucidum. Agricultural and Biological Chemistry* 49: pp 2641–2653, 1985

56. Leighton, Terrance, Chairman of Microbiology and Immunology at the University of California, Berkeley: press release on "quercetin" in *San Francisco Examiner*, p D-19, Nov 12, 1989

57. Block, E. "The Chemistry of Garlic and Onions." *Scientific American* 252: p 119, 1985

58. Barone, F. and Tansey, M. Isolation, purification, identification, synthesis and kinetic activity of the anti-candidal component of *Allium sativum*, and a hypothesis for its mode of action. *Mycologia* 79: pp 341–348, 1977

59. Caldes, G. A potential antileukemic substance present in *Allium ascalonicum. Planta Medica* 23: pp 90–100, 1973

60. Cummings, J.H. Short-chain fatty acids in the human colon. *Gut—The Journal of the British Society of Gastroenterology* 22: pp 763–779, Sep 1981

61. Whitehead, R.H. *et al.* A colon cancer cell line (LIM 1215) derived from a patient with inherited nonpolyposis colorectal cancer. *Journal of the National Cancer Inst.* 74: pp 759–765, April 1985

62. Leavitt, J. *et al.* Butyric acid suppression of the in vitro neoplastic state of Syrian hamster cells. *Nature* 271: pp 262–265, Jan 1978

63. Bensky, D. and Gamble, A. [translators], *Chinese Herbal Medicine: Materia Medica.* Seattle, WA: Eastland Press, 1986, p 194

64. Christopher, J.R. *op. cit.,* p 62

65. Erasmus, U. "The Value of Fresh Flax Oil" *Lipid Letter* issue no. 3, distributed by Spectrum Naturals, 133 Copeland St., Petaluma, CA 94952

66. Kremmer, J.M. Clinical studies of omega-3 fatty acid supplementation in patients who have rheumatoid arthritis. *Rheumatic Diseases Clinics of North America* 17: pp 391–402, May 1991

67. Robinson, D.R. and Kremer, J.M. Rheumatoid arthritis and inflammatory mediators. *World Review of Nutrition and Dietetics* 66: pp 44–47, 1991

68. Jantti, J. *et al.* Evening primrose oil in rheumatoid arthritis: changes in serum lipids and fatty acids. *Annals of the Rheumatic Diseases* 48: pp 124–127, 1989

69. McCarthy, G.M. and Kenny, D. Dietary fish oil and rheumatic diseases. *Seminars in Arthritis and Rheumatism* 21: pp 368–375, Jun 1992

70. Bjarnason, I. *et al.* Intestinal permeability and inflammation in rheumatoid arthritis: Effects of nonsteroidal and anti-inflammatory drugs. *The Lancet* 2: pp 1171–1174, Nov 24, 1984

71. Lee, T.P. *et al.* Effect of quercetin on human polymorphonuclear leukocyte lysosomal enzyme release and phospholipid metabolism *Life Sciences* 31: pp 2765–2774, Dec 13, 1982 [This research indicates that arachidonic acid release is inhibited by quercetin, which implies its metabolites—PGE-2 and leukotrienes—are also inhibited]

72. Middleton, E. The flavonoids. *Trends in Pharmacological Sciences* p 336, Aug 1984

73. di Fabio, A. *Rheumatoid Diseases Cured at Last.* Franklin, TN: Rheumatoid Disease Foundation, 1985. Among other things, this book discusses an early amoeba theory of rheumatoid arthritis, which to some extent has given way to a broader theory (see note 8 for Chapter 26 on page 696); the treatment developed from the amoeba theory is nevertheless beneficial in many cases. The book is available from the address in note 74, below.

74. Contact The Rheumatoid Disease Foundation, 5106 Old Harding Rd., Franklin, TN 37064, for information which includes a list of physicians, some of whom administer certain broad-spectrum antimicrobial drugs and treat rheumatoid arthritis with a variety of complementary as well as standard therapies.

75. Brinckerhoff, C.E. *et al.* Effect of retinoids on rheumatoid arthritis, a proliferative and invasive non-malignant disease. Ciba Foundation Symposium, 113: pp 191–211, 1985

76. Skoldstam, L. Fasting and vegan diet in rheumatoid arthritis. *Scandinavian Journal of Rheumatology* 15(2): pp 219–221, 1986

77. Roberts, J. and Hayashi, J. Exacerbation of SLE associated with alfalfa ingestion [letter]. *New England Journal of Medicine* 308(22): p 1361, June 2, 1983

78. These disorders (diagnostic patterns) are based on those supplied by the National Acupuncture Detoxification Association, 3115 Broadway #51, New York, NY 10027.

79. Anand, C. Effect of *Avena sativa* on cigarette smoking. *Nature* 233: p 496, 1971

80. Badgley, L. *Healing AIDS Naturally.* 370 W.

San Bruno Ave, San Bruno, CA: Human Energy Press, 1987

81. Hendler, S. *The Doctors' Vitamin and Mineral Encyclopedia.* New York: Simon and Schuster, 1990, p 425

82. Badgley, L. *op. cit.,* pp 41–43; 47–49; 52–53; 169–173

83. Block, E. *op. cit.,* pp 114–119

84. Badgley, L. *op. cit.,* p 170

85. Womble, D. and Helderman, J. Enhancement of allo-responsiveness of human lymphocytes by acemannan (Carrisyn). *International Journal of Immunopharmacology* 10(8): pp 967–974, 1988

86. Grindlay, D. and Reynolds, T. The aloe phenomenon: A review of the properties and modern uses of the leaf parenchyma gel. *Journal of Ethnopharmacology* 16: pp 117–151, Jun 1986

87. Meruelo, D. *et al.* Therapeutic agents with dramatic antiretroviral activity and little toxicity at effective doses: aromatic polycyclic diones hypericin and pseudohypericin. *Proceedings of The National Academy of Sciences* 85: pp 5230–5234, July 1988

88. Ito, M., Sato, A. *et al.* Mechanism of inhibitory effect of glycyrrhizin on replication of human immunodeficiency virus (HIV). *Antiviral Research* 10: pp 289–298, Dec 11, 1988

89. Nakashima, H., Kido, Y. *et al.* Purification and characterization of an avian myeloblastosis and human immunodeficiency virus reverse transcriptase inhibitor, sulfated polysaccharides extracted from sea algae. *Antimicrobial Agents and Chemotherapy* 31(10): pp 1524–1528, Oct 1987

90. Myers, D.E. *et al.* Production of a pokeweed antiviral protein (PAP)-containing immunotoxin, B43-PAP, directed against the CD19 human B lineage lymphoid differentiation antigen in highly purified form for human clinical trials. *Journal of Immunological Methods* 136: pp 221–237, Feb 15, 1991

91. Dworkin, R. Linoleic acid and multiple sclerosis. *Neurology* 34: p 1219, 1984

92. Barbul, A. *et al.* Arginine stimulates lymphocyte immune response in healthy human beings. *Surgery* 90: pp 244–251, 1981

93. Horrobin D.F. The relationship between schizophrenia and essential fatty acid and eicosanoid metabolism. *Prostaglandins Leukotrienes and Essential Fatty Acids* 46: pp 71–77, May 1992

94. Erasmus, U. *Fats and Oils.* Vancouver, B.C., Canada: Alive Pub., 1986, pp 251, 254

95. Vaddadi K.S. Use of gamma-linolenic acid in the treatment of schizophrenia and tardive dyskinesia. *Prostaglandins Leukotrienes and Essential Fatty Acids* 46: pp 67–70, May 1992

96. Lad, V. *Ayurveda: The Science of Self-Healing.* Santa Fe, NM: Lotus Press, 1985, p 131

97. Tierra, M. *Planetary Herbology.* Santa Fe, NM: Lotus Press, 1988, p 363

98. Omenn, G.S. *et al.* Effects of a combination of beta carotene and vitamin A on lung cancer and cardiovascular disease. *New England Journal of Medicine.* 334(18): pp 1150–1155; May 2, 1996

99. Greenberg, E.R. and Sporn, M.B. Antioxidant vitamins, cancer, and cardiovascular disease [editorial; comment] *New England Journal of Medicine* 334(18): pp 1189–1190; May 2, 1996

100. The Alpha-Tocopherol, Beta Carotene Cancer Prevention Study Group. The effect of vitamin E and beta carotene on the incidence of lung cancer and other cancers in male smokers. *New England Journal of Medicine.* 330(15) pp 1029–1035; Apr. 14, 1994

Chapter 52: Summary

1. Thakkur, C.G. *Ayurveda: The Indian Art & Science of Medicine;* New York: ASI Publ., 1974

2. Vanamali. *Nitya Yoga: Essays on the Sreemad Bhagavad Gita.* Vanamali Publications, Vanamali Gita Yogashram, PO Tapovan 249–192, Via Shivananda Nagar, Rishikesh. U.P. (Himalayas) India

3. Svoboda, Robert E. *Prakruti: Your Ayurvedic Constitution.* Albuquerque, NM: Geocom, 1989

4. Frawley, David. *Ayurvedic Healing: A Comprehensive Guide.* Salt Lake City, UT: Passage Press, 1989

5. Lad, Vasant. *Ayurveda: The Science of Self-Healing.* Santa Fe, NM: Lotus Press, 1985

6. Frawley, David. *op. cit.,* p 82

7. *Ibid,* p 82, 84

8. Thakkur, C.G. *op. cit.,* p 198 (appendix)

9. Vanamali. *op. cit.,* p 217

10. Lad, Vasant. *op. cit.,* p 131

11. Frawley, David *op. cit.,* p 82

12. Svoboda, Robert E. *op. cit.,* p 72

13. Gautama Buddha. *Shurangama Sutra, Volume 7;* available through: City of 10,000 Buddhas, Box 217, Talmage, CA 95481

14. *Ibid*

15. Frawley, David. *op. cit.,* p 84

16. Brain, K.R. *et al.* Percutaneous penetration of dimethylnitrosamine through human skin in vitro: application from cosmetic vehicles. *Food and Chemical Toxicology* 33(4): pp 315–322; Apr, 1995

17. One may obtain manuals with formulas for toiletry products that use herbs, lemon, avocado, oats, honey, clay, aloe vera gel, and so on.

Resources: *Kitchen Cosmetics* by Jeanne Rose, (North Atlantic Books); *Herbal Healing for Women,* by Rosemary Gladstar (Fireside Books (Simon & Schuster), 1993); *The Herbal Body Book* by Stephanie Touries (Storey Pub. Co, 1995); and *Jeanne Rose's Herbal Body Book* by Jeanne Rose (Perigee Books, 1982)

18. Ballentine, R. *Diet and Nutrition.* Honesdale, PA: The Himalayan International Institute, 1978, pp 549

19. Chen, J., Campbell, T.C. *et al. Diet, Lifestyle and Mortality in China: a Study of the Characteristics of 65 Counties.* Ithaca, NY: Cornell Univ. Press [co-publishers: Oxford Univ. Press and The China People's Medical Publishing House], 1990

21. One example is a group of scholarly contemplative nuns in the Cistercian order at Redwoods Monastery near Whitethorn, California; they are vegetarian, and make and distribute communion hosts made from whole-grain flour. They have incorporated into their practices some Oriental traditions such as quasi-zazen-style sitting meditation.

22. Marijuana has been shown to dramatically increase melatonin levels [Note 32 below]. (Presumably many other strongly psychoactive drugs will be shown to have similar effects.) The traditional Chinese medical view of such psychoactive substances is that their "high" results from large amounts of transformed *ojas/jing* essence being sent to the brain through the action of the substance, in which process the *ojas/jing essence* of the kidneys becomes depleted. It seems that science is confirming part of this traditional belief, as melatonin may be considered an element of the transformed *ojas/jing* essence. In our practice we have witnessed dozens of marijuana users who, in their terms, have "hit bottom." This appears to confirm the second part of the Chinese observation—that "hitting bottom" represents the depletion of the user's foundation *ojas/jing* essence from their kidneys, to the extent that they can no longer experience a "high." These individuals invariably look dried-out and aged far beyond their years. Such degeneration is yet another sign of *ojas/jing* depletion (see page 360 for a more complete discussion of *"jing"*). The point at which depletion via marijuana is clearly noticed ("hitting bottom") depends entirely on the individual; for some it's a matter of days or weeks; for others it's years. Nevertheless, from our observation, depletion occurs throughout the entire period of marijuana use.

Ayurvedic tradition also holds that marijuana damages the liver and brain [note 10 above]. The late Professor Hardin B. Jones of the University of California at Berkeley, lists in his book *Sensual Drugs* (Cambridge University Press, 1977, p 255) a comparison between brain damage from marijuana versus that from alcohol: "Irreversible brain changes are apparent after only three years of daily marijuana use; it takes decades for irreversible brain changes to appear in the heavy drinker." Evidence of cerebral atrophy, widening of synaptic clefts in the brain, disintegration of brain nerve cells, and deposits called "inclusion bodies" in the nuclei of brain nerve cells from regular marijuana use has been demonstrated in primates with electron microscopy and CAT scans [notes 23–27 below].

Structural damage of this type, which is similar to poisoning in the brain from toxic chemicals such as carbon tetrachloride, is generally considered permanent [note 28 below]. Our perception is that drug-induced brain damage can be partially overcome through long-term use of a regeneration diet (e.g., at least 6 months of DIET A, B, or C, beginning on p. 407; for application of diet and addictive therapy, see pp. 429–433) and certain herbs, especially calamus root (see "Drugs," pp. 113–114). A new awareness of marijuana is needed in response to misguided public thinking regarding its safety. This is due in part to early, somewhat superficial research [note 29 below] suggesting that marijuana was a "mild intoxicant." This opinion was widely broadcast in all news media at the time, misleading millions of Americans, many of whom today continue to underrate the potency of this powerful intoxicant. On the other hand, in a fashion similar to many natural and synthetic prescription drugs, virtually all intoxicants, including marijuana as well as alcoholic beverages, cocaine, psychoactive mushrooms, heroin, and amphetamines, have certain dramatic medicinal applications—that with prolonged use—one may pay for dearly with loss of health and vitality.

23. McGahan, J.P. *et al.* Computed tomography of the brains of rhesus monkeys after long-term delta-9tetrahydrocannabinol treatment. (Presented at: 67th Annual Meeting of Radiological Society of North America, Chicago, Nov, 1981.)

24. Kristensen F.W. Cannabis and psychoses [Danish language]. *Ugeskrift For Laeger.* 156(19): pp 2875–8, 2881; May 9, 1994

25. Harper, J.W. *et al.* Effects of *Cannabis sativa* on ultrastructure of the synapse in monkey brain. *Journal of Neuroscience Research.* 3: pp 83–93, 1977

26. Myers, W.A. and Heath, R.G. *Cannabis sativa:* ultrastructural changes in organelles of neurons in brain septal region of monkeys. *Journal of Neuroscience Research.* 4: pp 9–17, 1979

27. Heath, R.G. *et al. Cannabis sativa:* effects on brain function and ultrastructure in rhesus monkeys. *Biological Psychiatry.* 15(5): pp 688, 1980

28. Pollin, William. Health consequences of marijuana use. (hearing before U.S. Senate) pp 243–258, Jan 16, 1980

29. Weil, Andrew T. *et al.* Clinical and psychological effects of marihuana in man. *Science.* 162: pp 1234–1242, Dec 13, 1968

30. Reiter, R.J. and Robinson, J. *Melatonin.* Bantam Books, 1995, p 213

31. Ibid., p 193

32. Ibid., p 198

33. Turek, Fred W. Melatonin—hype hard to swallow. *Nature.* 379(6563): pp 295–6; Jan 25, 1995

34. Myers, Norman [editor] *Gaia, An Atlas of Planet Management.* Doubleday, 1984, p 64

35. Carlsen E. *et al.* Declining sperm counts and increasing incidence of testicular cancer and other gonadal disorders: is there a connection? *Irish Medical Journal.* 86(3): pp 85–86, May, 1992

36. Carlsen, E., Giwercman, A.J., Keiding, N., Skakkebaek, N.E. Decline in semen quality from 1930 to 1991.[Danish] *Ugeskrift For Laeger.* 155(33): pp 2530–2535; Aug 16, 1993

37. Sharpe, R.M. and Skakkebaek, N.E. Are oestrogens involved in falling sperm counts and disorders of the male reproductive tract? *Lancet.* 341(8857): pp 1392–1395; May 29, 1993

38. Auger J. Kunstmann JM Czyglik F., Jouannet P. Decline in semen quality among fertile men in Paris during the past 20 years. *New England Journal of Medicine.* 2;332(5): pp 281–285; Feb, 1995

39. Sharpe, R.M. On the importance of being earnest. Decline in semen quality among fertile men in Paris during the past 20 years. *Human and Experimental Toxicology.* 14(5): pp 463–464; May, 1995

40. Decline of the quality of male semen [German] *Deutsche Medizinische Wochenschrift.* 120(31-32): p 1107; Aug 4, 1995

41. Jensen, T.K., Toppari, J., *et al.* Do environmental estrogens contribute to the decline in male reproductive health? *Clinical Chemistry.* 41(12 Pt 2): pp 1896–1901; Dec, 1995

42. Wright, L. Silent Sperm. *The New Yorker.* Jan 15, 1996, pp 42–55

43. Olsen, G.W., Bodner, K.M., Ramlow, J.M., Ross, C.E., Lipshultz, L.I. Have sperm counts been reduced 50 percent in 50 years? A statistical model revisited. *Fertility and Sterility.*63(4): pp 887–93; Apr, 1995

44. Whether or not sperm counts are decreasing has been debated on the basis of the testing procedures used. In the United States there have been statistical studies derived from various tests involving different test parameters. Thus, some studies (funded by The Dow Chemical Company and others) suggest that certain previous statistical analyses used inappropriate statistical models in identifying declining sperm counts, and are therefore unreliable [see note 43 above]. However, there are a number of carefully controlled European studies that leave little doubt in any statistician's mind that sperm counts indeed are in rapid decline in many areas of the world [notes 36, 38, 39, and 40 above].

Some areas have declined faster than others; in Finland, where sperm counts are generally high, the counts in certain rural, isolated areas are considerably higher than in cities. This suggestion, coupled with research indicating that chemical, toxic, and stressful situations contribute to declining sperm counts, brings us a clear perspective: Sperm, the progenitor of life, is in decline because the vitality of the planet and her inhabitants is in decline. Excessive population is often cited as a cause. Certainly too many people are on the planet for the kinds of technology we are using. Waking up to this awareness intellectually is only part of the solution. Biologic forces are strong, and if many continue to eat the foods of degeneration (Tamas), then many will continue to participate in degenerative activities, regardless of how they conceptualize the problem and its solution. Providing statistical proof of the dire planetary situation (which has been amply done over the last generation) falls flat when faced with mindless desire and greed. When more people choose vital, uplifting foods, and find security in spiritual strength rather than material accumulation, we will experience a mental and biologic foundation that encourages living not only appropriately, but with wisdom and joy.

Appendix A: Parasite Purge Program

1. Keusch, G.T., Hamer, D., Joe, A., *et al.* Cryptosporidia—who is at risk? *Schweizerische Medizinische Wochenschrift.* 125(18): pp 899–908; May 6, 1995

2. Thorne, G.M. Diagnosis of infectious diarrheal diseases. *Infectious Disease Clinics of North America.* 2(3): pp 747–774; Sep, 1988

3. Verdrager, J. Localized permanent epidemics: the genesis of chloroquine resistance in Plasmodium falciparum. *Southeast Asian Journal of Tropical Medicine and Public Health.* 26(1): pp 23–28; Mar, 1995

4. Barrett, N.J. and Morse, D.L. The resurgence of scabies. *Communicable Diseases Report/CDR Review.* 3(2): pp R32–34; Jan 29, 1993

5. Boffa, M.J., Brough, P.A., Ead, R.D. Lindane

neurotoxicity. *British Journal of Dermatology.* 133(6): p 1013; Dec, 1995

6. Sarkar, M., Sarkar, A.K., Biswas, S.K. Gamma benzene hexachloride neurotoxicity. *Indian Pediatrics.* 30(11): pp 1358–1359; Nov, 1993

Appendix B: The Effect of Root Canals on Health.

1. Price, Weston A. *Volume I: Dental infections, oral and systemic; Volume II: Dental infections and the degenerative diseases.* Cleveland, OH: The Penton Publishing Company, 1923. [Volume I presents researches on fundamentals of oral and systemic expressions of dental infections; Volume II presents researches on clinical expressions of dental infections.]

2. Meinig, George E. *Root Canal Cover-up.* Ojai, CA: Bion Pub., 1994

Resources

UNREFINED FOODS

Diamond Organics. P.O. Box 2159, Freedom, CA 95019. (888) 674-2642. diamondorganics.com. Fresh organic fruits, vegetables, flowers, herbs and other food products.

Gold Mine Natural Food Co. Retail and wholesale. 7805 Arjons Dr., San Diego, CA 92126. (800) 475-3663. goldminenaturalfood.com. A wide variety of organic and traditional Oriental foods (grains, cereals, noodles, beans, seaweeds, soy sauces, etc.); also books, cookware, grain mills, water filters, and other household items.

The Grain and Salt Society. 273 Fairway Drive, Asheville, NC 28805 (800) 867-7258. www.celtic-seasalt.com. Unrefined sea salts, organic bulk whole foods, traditional cookware, hygienic products, and books.

Green Earth Farm. www.greenearthfarm.com. A variety of medicinal and culinary herbs; also vegetables, quinoa and rye.

Jaffe Bros. 760-749-1133. Organicfruitsandnuts.com. Organic fruits, nuts, vegetables, legumes, grains, oils and more.

Rapunzel Pure Organics. Wholesale and retail. 122 Smith Road Extension, Kinderhook, NY 12106. 800-207-2814 or 518-758-6398. www.rapunzel.com Producers of completely unrefined, dried organic cane juice, one of the only commercially available whole sugars in the West. Note: "cane juice" in most products is partially or completely refined sugar. Other products include organic: dried fruits and nuts, cocoa powder, chocolate, soup bases and others.

Rejuvenative Foods. Wholesale (for retail, contact them to locate sources of their products in your area). P.O. Box 8464, Santa Cruz, CA 95061. 800-805-7957. Organic raw cultured vegetables including raw saltless and salted sauerkraut (using unrefined salt), raw nut and seed butters.

South River Miso Company, Inc. Retail and wholesale. South River Farm, Conway, MA 01341. 413-369-4057. Southrivermiso.com. Unpasteurized, organic, handmade misos.

Seaweeds

Maine Coast Sea Vegetables. Shore Road, Franklin, ME 04634. (207) 565-2907.
Mendocino Sea Vegetable Co. Box 372, Navarro, CA 95463. (707) 937-2050.

HERBS

Alta Health Products. PO Box 990, Idaho City, ID 83631. (800) 423-4155. Altahealthproducts.com. Nontoxic Horsetail Silica tablets and other nutritional products.

Amazon Herb Co. 1002 Jupiter Park Lane, Jupiter, FL 33458. (800) 835-0850. Amazonherb.com. Herbs from the South American rainforest, including

Suma™ and pau d'arco. Providing this work for rainforest natives helps halt the destruction of the area by cattle raisers.

BioDelta. 220 Harmony Lane, Garberville, CA 95542. Herbal extracts, parasite remedies, organic oregano and lavender oils, citrus seed extract, nontoxic horsetail silica supplement, fulvic acid concentrate, chlorella and wild blue-green micro-algae. Also L. sporogenes, B. laterosporus intestinal biocultures, and stabilized oxygen compounds.

Blessed Herbs. Rt. 5, Box 1042, Ava, MO 65608. (800) 489-4372. Wildcrafted or organic herbs and tinctures.

East Earth Trade Winds. P.O. Box 493151, Redding, CA 96049. (800) 258-6878. Chinese herbal preparations and major tonic herbs.

Health Center for Better Living. 1414 Rosemary Ln., Naples, FL 34103. (800) 544-4225. www.hcbl.com. Individual and combinations of Western herbs in bulk and various preparations.

Health Concerns. Professional/wholesale only. 8001 Capwell Drive, Oakland, CA 94621. (800) 233-9355. Chinese herbal formulas adapted to Western needs, including parasite remedies.

Herbalist & Alchemist Inc. Retail and wholesale. P.O. Box 458, Bloomsbury, NJ 08823. www.herbalist-alchemist.com. Chinese and Western organic and wild-crafted herbs.

Kroeger Herb Products Co., Inc. 805 Walnut Street, Boulder, CO 80302. (800) 225-8787. Herbal formulas, including parasite remedies.

Mayway Trading Corp. 1338 Mandela Parkway, Oakland, CA 94607. 510-208-3113. Large selection of individual Chinese herbs, formulas, and products.

Mountain Rose Herbs. 85472 Dilley Lane, Eugene, OR 97405. (800) 879-3337. Mountainroseherbs.com. Herbs, teas, seasonings; many organic and wildcrafted varieties; herb seeds, quality body products, books, and supplies for herbalists.

San Francisco Herb & Natural Food Co. Wholesale/retail. 47444 Kato Rd., Fremont, CA 94538. (800) 227-2830. www.herbspicetea.com. Large selection of herbs, teas, and seasonings.

Simplers Botanical Co. Retail and Wholesale. PO Box 2534, Sebastopol, CA 95473. 800-652-7646. www.simplers.com. A variety of high quality herbal extracts and organic pure essential oils including oregano and lavender oils.

FOOD AND HERB SEEDS

Abundant Life Seed Foundation. P.O. Box 772, Port Townsend, WA 98368. Grains, beans, perennial woody plants, wildflowers; all untreated non-hybrid heirloom varieties; also books.

Bountiful Gardens. 18001 Shafer Ranch Rd., Willits, CA 95490. (707) 459-6410. Open-pollinated heirloom seeds of vegetables, herbs, flowers, and grains; also beneficial insects, fertilizers, and books.

Deep Diversity. P.O. Box 15189, Santa Fe, NM 87506-5189. Planetary gene pool service and resource center; organic non-hybrid herb, vegetable, and flower seeds; and trees.

Horizon Herbs. P.O. Box 69, Williams, OR 97544 (541) 846-6233, www.horizon-herbs.com. Medicinal seeds and live roots and plants.

Japonica Seeds. P.O. Box 729, Oakland Gardens, NY 11364. Seeds of Oriental herbs and vegetables.

Johnny's Selected Seeds. 310 Foss Hill Road, Albion, ME 04910. Wide variety of mainly untreated, organic, high-quality seeds.

Native Seeds/SEARCH. (Southwestern Endangered Aridland Resource Clearing House), 526 N. 4th Ave, Tucson, AZ 85705 (520) 622-5561 www.nativeseeds.org. Southwest desert traditional and wild seeds—preserving gardening heritage of Southwest drought-resistant varieties.

Nichols Garden Nursery. 1190 N. Pacific Highway, Albany, OR 97321. Good variety of herb seeds.

Seeds of Change. P.O. Box 15700, Santa Fe, NM 87506-5700. (800) 957-3337. Wide variety of organic seeds.

Southern Exposure Seed Exchange. P.O. Box 170, Earlysville, VA 22936

NUTRITIONAL PRODUCTS

Green Foods

Desert Lake Technologies/Rossha. Wholesale and retail. PO Box 489, Klamath Falls, OR 97601. (800) 736-2379. www.rossha.com. Wild blue-green micro-algae *(Aphanizomenon)*. Harvested while in peak nutrient/bloom stage.

The Earth Rise Company. P.O. Box 60, Petaluma, CA 94953. (707) 778-9078 or (800) 949-7473. Spirulina and other nutritional products.

Klamath Blue-Green. Wholesale and retail. 301 S. Old Stage Road, Mt. Shasta, CA 96067. (800) 327-1956. Wild blue-green micro-algae *(Aphanizomenon)*.

Microlight Nutritional Products. 124 Rhodesia Beach, Bay Center, WA 98527. (800) 338-2821. Spirulina, dunaliella, and other nutritional products.

Pines International. Wholesale and retail. P.O. Box 1107, Lawrence, KS 66044. (800) 642-7463. Wheat- and barley-grass products.

Sunshine Chlorella Co. Wholesale and retail. 234-5149 Country Hills Blvd. NW, Suite 227, Calgary, Alberta T3A 5K8, Canada. 888-277-7330 or 403-547-3459. www.pure-chlorella.com. High quality chlorella.

Oils

Flora, Inc. Wholesale and retail. P.O. Box 73, 805 E. Badger Rd., Lynden, WA 98264. (360) 354-2110 or (800) 498-3610. Fresh, unrefined, cold-pressed flax and other oils, nontoxic horsetail silica supplement, herbal formulas, and other products.

Home Health Products, Inc. P.O. Box 2219, Virginia Beach, VA 23450-2219. (800) 284-9123. Cold-pressed, cold-processed castor oil.

Omega Nutrition. Wholesale and retail. 6505 Aldrich Road, Bellingham, WA 98226; and 165-810 West Broadway, Vancouver, B.C. V5Z 4C9, Canada. (800) 661-3529 in U.S. and Canada. Omeganutrition.com. Fresh, unrefined, cold-pressed flax, hemp seed oil, borage, and other oils, unrefined vinegar, and other products.

Spectrum Naturals. Wholesale only. 133 Copeland St., Petaluma, CA 94952. Fresh, unrefined, cold-pressed flax and wheat-germ oils, extra virgin olive oil, unfiltered vinegar, and a variety of other refined and unrefined oils (refined canola and other refined oils are not recommended).

Ferment Cultures and Bee Products

Gem Cultures. 30301 Sherwood Road., Fort Bragg, CA 95437, (707) 964-2922. www.gemcultures.com. A wide variety of ferment kits from around the world including organisms for making bread, yogurt, kefir, tempeh, miso, amasake, and others.

Honey Gardens Apiaries. Hinesburg, VT 05461 (802) 985-5852. www.honeygardens.com. Quality honey and medicinal products with honey and herbs.

Hyper-Oxygenation Therapies and Products

Aerobic Life Industries, Inc., 3045 S. 46th St., Phoenix, AZ 85040. (800) 798- 0707. Stabilized oxygen compounds: sodium chlorite and magnesium oxide; also aloe vera gel/hydrogen peroxide combination and bovine colostrum.

Family News, 9845 NE 2nd Ave., Miami Shores, FL 33138. (800) 284-6263. Information on and sales of food-grade hydrogen peroxide, ozone, B. laterosporus, and a variety of other remedies.

Matrix Health Products, 8400 Magnolia Ave., Suite N, Santee, CA 92071. (800) 736-5609. Stabilized oxygen and other oxygen compounds.

Dutch Pride Products, P.O. Box 1651, Cottonwood, AZ 86326. (520) 634-7066. Chlorine dioxide.

International Credible Medicine Assn., P.O. Box 610767, Dallas/Fort Worth, Texas 75261. Contact for locating a physician trained in complementary medicine and the intravenous/intra-arterial use of hydrogen peroxide.

International Oxidation Institute, P.O. Box 1360, Priest River, ID 83856. Glyoxlide.

International Ozone Assn., 83 Oakwood Terrace, Norwalk, CT 06850. Information on ozone.

The Secretariat of the Medical Society for Ozone Therapy, Nordring 8-10, D-7557 Iffezheim, Germany. Information on ozone.

Colloidal Silver

Electro-Pure. 2715 Walkers Creek Road, Middlebrook, VA 24459 (877) 355-9407. pure-silver-colloid.com. Electro-colloidal silver of high concentration and purity. A safe and very effective silver preparation.

KITCHEN WARE, SPROUTING SUPPLIES, HOUSEHOLD GOODS

Miracle Exclusives. Retail and wholesale. P.O. Box 349, Locust Valley, New York 11550. (800) 645-6360. Juicers, grain mills, wheat-grass juicers, sprouters, food mills, cookware.

Real Goods. 555 Leslie St., Ukiah, CA 95482. (800) 762-7325. (707) 468-9214 for foreign orders. Products for energy independence—home solar-powered electrical systems and devices, many environment-preserving household items including water purifiers, and books.

The Sprout House. P.O. Box 754131, Parkside Station, Forest Hills, NY 11375 800-777-6887. www.sprouthouse.com. Sprout bags and other items for making sprouts, seeds for sprouting, juicers, books.

PUBLICATIONS AND ORGANIZATIONS

Center For Food Safety. 660 Pennsylvania Ave. SE, Ste. 302 Washington, DC 2003 (202) 547-9359 www.centerforfoodsafety.org A non-profit organization fighting for strong organic standards, promoting sustainable agriculture, and protecting consumers from hazards of genetically engineered food and pesticides.

Chefs Collaborative. 282 Moody St., Ste. 21, Waltham, MA 02453. (781) 730-0635 www.chefnet.com. Restauranteurs and chefs, using locally grown, sustainably produced foods and boycotting swordfish and other destructive harvests.

Conservation Beef. 304 Main St., Ste. 11, Lander, NY 82520 (877) 749-7177 www.conservationbeef.org A coalition of ranchers using alternative, conservation-oriented techniques.

Council for Responsible Genetics. 5 Upland Road, Ste. 3, Cambridge, MA O2410 (617) 868-0870, www.gene-watch.org. A public forum that sponsors debates on implications of new gene technologies.

Dental Amalgam Syndrome (DAMS). Support Network, 725-9 Tramway Lane NE, Albuquerque, NM 87122-1601. (800) 311-6265. Dentist referral, books, and dental information.

EarthSave. 706 Frederick St., Santa Cruz, CA 95062. Information including newsletter based in part on John Robbins' book, *Diet for a New America,* which promotes vegetarianism and exposes the meat industry as a major contributor to pollution and disease.

Enviromental Dentistry Association (EDA). 10160 Aviary Drive, San Diego, CA 92131. (619) 586-7626 or (800) 388-8124. List of alternative dentists, and information on toxins in dentistry, root canals, and amalgam removal.

Great Smokies Diagnostic Laboratory. 18A Regent Park Blvd., Ashville, NC 28806. (800) 522-4762 or Fax (704) 253-1127. Parasite testing.

Food First/Institute for Food and Development Policy. 398 60th St., Oakland, CA 94618. (510) 654-4400. www.foodfirst.org. Information on business practices and politics which cause inequalities in food distribution, especially among Third World peoples.

Herb Research Foundation. 1007 Pearl St., Suite 200, Boulder, CO 80302. (303) 449-2265. Information on well-researched therapeutic herbs, an herb magazine *(HerbalGram),* and a large list of herb seed sources.

Oldways Preservation and Exchange Trust. 266 Beacon St., Boston, MA 02116 (617) 621-3000. A food history group promoting healthy eating, encouraging sustainable food choices and preserving traditional foodways.

Price-Pottenger Foundation. P.O. Box 2614, La Mesa, CA 92041. Books on the subject of physical degeneration in various cultures from refined foods.

People for the Ethical Treatment of Animals (PETA). P.O. Box 42516, Washington, D.C. 20077.

Rural Advancement Fund International. P.O. Box 640 and 655, Pittsboro, NC 27312 (919) 542-1396, www.rafiusa.org. An international non-government organization dedicated to conservation and maintenance of sustainable traditions of agricultural biodiversity.

The Soyfoods Center. P.O. Box 234, Lafayette, CA 94549. (925) 283-2991. Most extensive database in the world on soy foods and vegetarianism. Many bibliographies as well as 55 books in print, most for commercial purposes and research. For basic soy information and recipes contact The Soy Fan Club: www.thesoyfanclub.com or www.thesoydailyclub.com.

Unikey Health Systems. P.O. Box 7168, Bozeman, MT 59771. (800) 888-4353. Parasite testing and parasite remedies.

World Research Foundation. 15300 Ventura Blvd., Suite 405, Sherman Oaks, CA 91403. Both computerized and manual library searches on current health information and treatments available around the world. Often used by health care practitioners as well as individuals, for finding wider options than standard medical sources provide.

Marine and Fish Environmental/Sustainability Organizations

Audubon Living Oceans. 550 S. Bay Ave., Islip, NY 11751. 888-397-6649. www.audubon.org. email: livingoceans@Audubon.org. The marine conservation program of the Audubon Society. Seafood guides are available to help one choose fish which support sustainable marine fisheries.

Marine Stewardship Council. 2110 N. Pacific St., Suite 102, Seattle, WA 98103. 206-691-0188. www.msc.org. Email: info@msc.org. An international nonprofit organization that promotes environmentally responsible stewardship of ocean fish, dedicated to rewarding sustainable fishing practices. Their seal of approval on fish products indicates sustainable marine practices.

Monterey Bay Aquarium. 886 Cannery Row, Monterey, CA 93940 831-648-4800. www.mbayaq.org. A organization that inspires conservation of the oceans. "Seafood Watch Cards" are available to inform one when fish is caught or farmed in environmentally friendly ways.

Index

Note: Main page references are printed in **boldface** type; references to items in charts and tables are followed by a "t."

About the Author

Paul Pitchford is a teacher and nutrition researcher. In his healing work with individuals, he develops rejuvenative plans based on awareness and dietary practices. His early training, following ancient traditional practice, was primarily through apprenticeships and private instructions with masters of meditation and East Asian medicine. For more than three decades, he has applied the unifying wisdom of Far Eastern thought to the major dietary therapies available in the West to create a new vision of health and nutrition.

He has taught at various learning centers, including universities and schools of traditional Chinese medicine, and at numerous healing events. When possible, he takes an integrative approach that touches many facets of the human personality, and enjoys teaching diverse programs composed of any of his long-term practices: meditation, food and herbal therapy, zen shiatsu healing touch, and tai ji movement.

He finds spiritual awareness and the resulting guidance to be the essence of life in all its aspects, including diet. Out of preference and to learn more about the nutritive value of plant foods, he has followed a vegan diet devoid of animal products for the last thirty years. From this and his extensive healing practice, he has gained insights into the therapeutic nature of virtually every type of diet.

He currently lives in the Northern California coastal mountains at Heartwood Institute, where he directs the Asian Healing Arts and Integrative Nutrition Program and leads healing retreats.

If you have benefited from information in this book, the author would appreciate knowing this. Correspondence with him regarding retreats, telephone or in-person consultations, and upcoming training programs should also be addressed to him c/o Heartwood Institute, 220 Harmony Lane, Garberville, CA 95542.

www.healingwithwholefoods.com

North Atlantic Books Series: Food as Medicine, Food as Consciousness

North Atlantic Books has developed a series of unique books on food as medicine and the relationship between diet and consciousness. These books transcend traditional categories of nutrition, alternative medicine, and spiritual practice to discuss health, diet, and consumption in terms of our actual human situation. The three titles presently comprising the series are *Healing with Whole Foods: Oriental Traditions and Modern Nutrition* by Paul Pitchford (published originally in 1993; revised and updated in 2002); *Conscious Eating* by Gabriel Cousens, M.D. (published originally by Essene Vision Books in 1992; enlarged, revised, and republished by North Atlantic Books in 2000); and *How We Heal: Nutritional, Emotional, and Psychospiritual Fundamentals* by Douglas Morrison (published originally by Health Hope Publishing House as *Body Electronics Fundamentals* in 1993; enlarged, revised, and republished by North Atlantic Books in 2001). A fourth title, *Everyday Vegan* by Jeani-Rose Atchison, is a cookbook written in the spirit of conscious diet.

These books propose that every food is a medicine (and has long-term secondary effects on both our organs and our psyche) and that each medicine is likewise a food (and directly affects metabolic balance and energetic capacity).

In all three "food as medicine, food as consciousness" books, consumption is viewed not just as a mechanical event of nutrition and bodily maintenance nor as sensual recreation but also as a total psychospiritual process. Dietary sources and preparation, cooking procedures and utensils, levels of taste and consumption awareness, and diverse facets of digestion and fasting are explored. The authors are concerned with the assimilation and transmutation of what enters the body-mind (including enzymes, minerals, oils, type of water, type of air, etc.) rather than what is either enjoyable and pleasing to consume or rumored to be healthy. Each of these books explores the deeper cellular satisfaction and resonance that come from eating, drinking, and combining foods as part of a serious daily practice. Each ask: what makes food alive?; how does eating teach you who you are?; how can whole foods and conscious eating help you find your destiny?

Each of the books also deals with the impact human beings have on the Earth and its sentient beings (the role of compassion and responsibility in diet), plus the reciprocal effects of the planet's environment on health and food. They presume that eating must be attuned to communities and ecosystems.

Note: These books were written independently of one another. The individual authors' advice, while overlapping in some areas, disagrees in others, sometimes even offering contradictory solutions to the same issues (for instance, the advantages and drawbacks of cooking and consuming food raw). None of the authors specifically recommends the other two books or has any connection to them.

North Atlantic Books as a publisher is presenting these separate visions for readers to consider in creating their own diets and addressing their own self-healing. Individuals will find ideas in one or another book better suited to their own constitutions and temperaments, so every reader should use sound personal judgment and intuition in choosing a path of food.

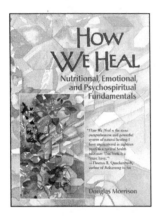

How We Heal:
Nutritional, Emotional, and Psychospiritual Fundamentals
By Douglas Morrison
ISBN: 1-55643-362-X
$27.50 trade paper, 488 pp.
illustrations

"… for healing to be possible, we must desire this healing and yet have no attachment to it: we must remain willing to not heal. We must be willing to put our full effort into the process and yet have no attachment to the outcome of that effort."

—from the book

This book addresses healing in the broadest conceivable context. Though *How We Heal* is a comprehensive resource on the physical basis of health, it goes far beyond the physical to examine the emotional and spiritual elements that cause illness and can block even the most powerful healing methods from success. Morrison's genius lies in explaining the full nature of the healing crisis and the role of resistance in preventing us from getting well. This book serves as an excellent introduction to the frontiers of healing, where the most advanced realms of molecular science meet the most esoteric aspects of spirit.

How We Heal explores some of the more cutting-edge methods of diagnosis and healing, including iridology, sclerology, and Body Electronics. An extensive section on nutrition includes cooking methods, the research of Dr. Weston A. Price, diet versus supplements, digestion, elimination, the role of friendly microbes within our digestive system, and the use of probiotics. Topics such as sleep, air and breathing, quantity and quality of water, exercise methods, bodywork techniques, and the dangers of amalgam dental fillings, root canals, fluoride, electromagnetic fields, vaccinations, drugs, and tobacco are considered in a clear, informative way. Yet, as thoroughly as Morrison presents all these physical factors, the author never loses sight of the much larger picture, and it is his ability to integrate the physical, emotional, mental, and spiritual aspects of health that is truly at the heart of this book.

Douglas Morrison studied Body Electronics with its founder, Dr. John Whitman Ray, and has been teaching seminars since 1988. He is a graduate of Harvard University and holds doctorate degrees in naturopathy, nutritional counseling, and alternative medicine.

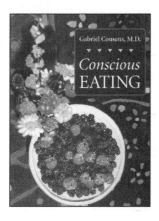

Conscious Eating

By Gabriel Cousens, M.D.
ISBN: 1-55643-285-2
$35.00 trade paper, 874 pp.
illustrations, charts, recipes

Long viewed as the bible of vegetarianism, *Conscious Eating* is a comprehensive effort to bring clarity and light to the most essential questions regarding our food choices and the process of living healthfully, happily, and in increased harmony with all beings on the planet.
Conscious Eating not only serves as an encyclopedia of vegetarian, vegan, live-food, and organic nutrition, but is really four books in one: Principles of Individualizing the Diet; The Choice of Vegetarianism; Transition to Vegetarianism and Live-Foods; and The Art of Live-Food Preparation. The mystery and mastery of *Conscious Eating* is that it integrates all four books into one. Read one book at a time, the entire text, or use it as a reference.

Conscious Eating, in a revolutionary approach, addresses the uniqueness of each human and empowers readers to deal with this scientific reality as opposed to the "one diet serves all" approach of fad books. Readers will learn how to individualize their diets for their particular psycho-physiological types—including four main perspectives: fast/slow oxidizer; parasympathetic/sympathetic autonomic; ayurvedic; and blood type—to optimize their health on all levels.

Explore chapter after chapter of new information including:

- How to heal the "biologically-altered brain"—the result of genetic weakness compounded by generations of poor diet and present poor diet combined with environmental and emotional toxicities.
- A mind-body-spirit approach to the vegetarian way of life.
- The importance of vegetarianism in healing self and ecology of the planet.
- The most complete scientific explanation of vegetarianism and vitamin B_{12}.
- How a vegan diet protects you from the dangers of radiation.
- Live-food and nutrition: from biophysics to metaphysics.
- An extensive chapter on enzymes—the secret of health and longevity.
- New theory of nutrition: why the material/mechanistic theory of nutrition (nutrition focusing on calories) is inadequate, misleading, and an inaccurate way of understanding nutrition.
- The art of live-food preparation: two hundred recipes included.
- In-depth discussion on the transition to vegetarianism, veganism, and live-foods.

Gabriel Cousens, M.D. and Diplomat of Ayurveda, is one of the foremost medical proponents of a vegetarian/vegan, live-food, one-hundred-percent organic diet as a key component to maximum health and spiritual awareness. He is the founder/director of the Tree of Life Rejuvenation Center located in Patagonia, Arizona.